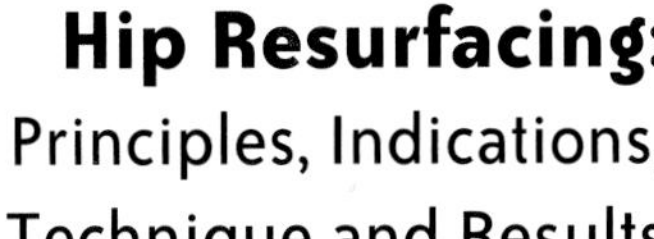

Hip Resurfacing:
Principles, Indications, Technique and Results

Hip Resurfacing:
Principles, Indications, Technique and Results

Harlan C. Amstutz, MD
Emeritus Professor
Orthopaedic Surgery
UCLA School of Medicine
Medical Director
Joint Replacement Institute
St. Vincent Medical Center
Los Angeles, California

SAUNDERS

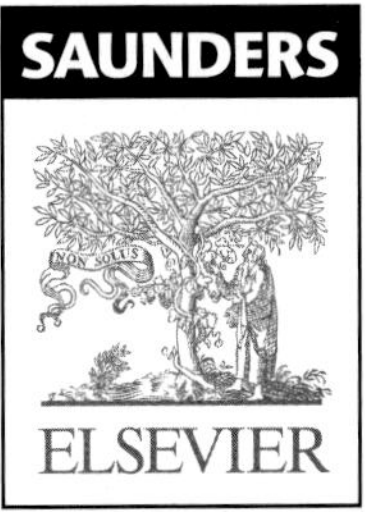

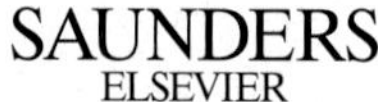

SAUNDERS
ELSEVIER

1600 John F. Kennedy Blvd.
Ste 1800
Philadelphia, PA 19103-2899

HIP RESURFACING: PRINCIPLES, INDICATIONS, TECHNIQUE AND RESULTS
ISBN: 978-1-4160-4724-7

Notice

Knowledge and best practice in this field are constantly changing. As new research and experience broaden our knowledge, changes in practice, treatment and drug therapy may become necessary or appropriate. Readers are advised to check the most current information provided (i) on procedures featured or (ii) by the manufacturer of each product to be administered, to verify the recommended dose or formula, the method and duration of administration, and contraindications. It is the responsibility of the practitioner, relying on their own experience and knowledge of the patient, to make diagnoses, to determine dosages and the best treatment for each individual patient, and to take all appropriate safety precautions. To the fullest extent of the law, neither the Publisher nor the Editor assumes any liability for any injury and/or damage to persons or property arising out or related to any use of the material contained in this book.

The Publisher

Library of Congress Cataloging-in-Publication Data

Amstutz, Harlan C., 1931-
Hip resurfacing : principles, indications, technique, and results / Harlan C. Amstutz.—1st ed.
p. ; cm.
Includes bibliographical references.
ISBN 978-1-4160-4724-7
1. Total hip replacement. 2. Hip joint–Surgery. I. Title.
[DNLM: 1. Arthroplasty, Replacement, Hip—methods. WE 860 A528h 2008]

RD549.A47 2008
617.5′80592—dc22 2007045162

Publishing Director: Kim Murphy
Developmental Editor: Julia Bartz
Project Manager: Bryan Hayward
Design Direction: Karen O'Keefe Owens
Illustrator: Bob Williams

Printed in China

Last digit is the print number: 9 8 7 6 5 4 3 2 1

Contributors

Harlan C. Amstutz, MD
Emeritus Professor, Orthopaedic Surgery, UCLA School of Medicine; Medical Director, Joint Replacement Institute, St. Vincent Medical Center, Los Angeles, California
Evolution of Hip Resurfacing; Surgical Technique; Indications for Metal-on-Metal Hybrid Hip Resurfacing; Results of Conserve®Plus Hip Resurfacing; Primary Osteoarthritis; Osteonecrosis of the Hip; Childhood Disorders; Post-Traumatic Arthritis; Rheumatoid Arthritis and Related Disorders; Hip Resurfacing for Other Conditions and Etiologies; Assessment of the Failed or Poorly Performing Hip Resurfacing: Lessons from a Lifetime of Experience; Treatment of Failed Hip Resurfacing; The Future of Hip Resurfacing

Scott T. Ball, MD
Assistant Professor, Department of Orthopaedic Surgery, University of California, San Diego; Assistant Professor and Adult Reconstruction Specialist, Department of Orthopaedic Surgery, University of California, San Diego, Medical Center and Thornton Hospital, and Veterans Administration Medical Center, San Diego, San Diego, California
Treatment of Failed Hip Resurfacing

Paul E. Beaulé, MD, FRCSC
Associate Professor, University of Ottawa; Head of Adult Reconstruction, The Ottawa Hospital, Ottawa, Ontario, Canada
Femoral Head Vascularity and Hip Resurfacing

Ahmad Bin Nasser, MBBS, FRCSC
Fellow, Orthopedics, University of Ottawa; Fellow, Surgery, The Ottawa Hospital, Ottawa, Ontario, Canada
Femoral Head Vascularity and Hip Resurfacing

Paul D. Boitano, BS
Long Beach, California
Osteonecrosis of the Hip

Patricia A. Campbell, PhD
Associate Professor, Orthopaedic Surgery, David Geffen School of Medicine at UCLA; Director, Implant Retrieval Lab, J. Vernon Luck Sr. MD Orthopaedic Research Center, Orthopaedic Hospital, Los Angeles, California
Modes of Failures: Fractures and Loosening; Reaction to Wear Products

Frederick J. Dorey, PhD
Research Professor, Pediatrics, Keck School of Medicine of USC, Los Angeles, California
Outcome Studies and Data Collection

Richie H. S. Gill, BEng, DPhil
University Lecturer in Orthopaedic Engineering, Nuffield Department of Orthopaedic Surgery, University of Oxford, Oxford, United Kingdom
The Mechanics of the Resurfaced Hip

Thomas A. Gruen, MS
Consultant, Zonal Concepts, Wesley Chapel, Florida
Imaging of Hip Resurfacing

Michel J. Le Duff, MA
Clinical Research Lead, Joint Replacement Institute, St. Vincent Medical Center, Los Angeles, California
Evolution of Hip Resurfacing; Outcome Studies and Data Collection; Results of Conserve®Plus Hip Resurfacing; Primary Osteoarthritis; Osteonecrosis of the Hip; Childhood Disorders; Post-Traumatic Arthritis; Rheumatoid Arthritis and Related Disorders; Hip Resurfacing for Other Conditions and Etiologies; Rehabilitation and Activity Following Total Hip Resurfacing

J. Paige Little, PhD, BEng
Oxford Orthopaedic Engineering Collaboration, University of Oxford, Oxford, United Kingdom
The Mechanics of the Resurfaced Hip

William Lundergan, BA
Medical Student, Keck School of Medicine of USC, Los Angeles, California
Modes of Failures: Fractures and Loosening

John B. Medley, PhD, Peng
Professor, Mechanical and Mechatronics Engineering, University of Waterloo, Waterloo, Ontario, Canada
Tribology of Bearing Materials

Thomas P. Schmalzried, MD
Associate Medical Director, Joint Replacement Institute, St. Vincent Medical Center, Los Angeles; Physician Specialist, Orthopaedic Surgery, Harbor-UCLA Medical Center, Torrance, California
Rehabilitation and Activity Following Total Hip Resurfacing

David J. Simpson, BEng, PhD
Nuffield Department of Orthopaedic Surgery, University of Oxford, Oxford, United Kingdom
The Mechanics of the Resurfaced Hip

Edwin P. Su, MD
Assistant Professor of Clinical Orthopaedic Surgery, Orthopaedic Surgery, Weill Medical College of Cornell University; Assistant Attending Orthopaedic Surgeon, Orthopaedic Surgery, Hospital for Special Surgery, New York, New York
Childhood Disorders

Karren Midori Takamura, BA
Medical Student, UCLA, Los Angeles, California
Reaction to Wear Products

Foreword

I first met Harlan Amstutz, Professor Harlan Amstutz as he was later to become, in 1966 at a Biomechanics Course in Manchester run by Professor Sir John Charnley. At that time Professor Amstutz was a Fellow at the Royal National Orthopaedic Hospital in London and I was setting up the Biomechanics Unit in the Department of Mechanical Engineering at Imperial College with Professor S.A.V. Swanson. Thus Professor Amstutz and I have had a long friendship during which we have worked in the fields of biomechanics and joint replacement. It therefore now gives me a special pleasure to be able to write a foreword for this volume.

The history of resurfacing arthroplasty is outlined in Chapter 1. As the reader will see I happened to be involved in the design of one of the first metal/polyethylene cemented implants: Trentani employed such a device early in 1972 and I followed later in the same year. In the 1980s I wrote in the Journal of Arthroplasty that I thought the operation should be abandoned until better materials were available. All the other originating designers took the same view. All, that is, save for Amstutz who displayed the greatest tenacity of purpose, remained with the concept, and changed the materials.

The materials to which Professor Amstutz changed were, as everyone knows, cobalt chrome articulating with cobalt chrome. The combination had been used for the first total hip replacement in the 1960s by McKee. In the context of resurfacing joint replacement it was used by McMinn in Birmingham at about the same time as by Amstutz.

Because of his enormously long continuous experience of this operation, longer by far than that of anyone else worldwide, Professor Amstutz is ideally suited to produce a book of this kind. It covers all aspects of the subject and details the fact that in hip terms this operation is now a successful competitor for conventional prostheses. That this is so, is a tribute to Professor Amstutz' work.

One area of uncertainty remains, the biology of the wear debris produced from cobalt chrome on cobalt chrome articulating surfaces. It is as yet too early to know how this topic will evolve: ironically improvements in manufacturing techniques may again have made polyethylene a competitor. The subject is fully covered in Chapter 11 and the reader can be certain that Professor Amstutz and his team give as informed and objective a description of the facts as is available today.

I am delighted to be able to write this foreword for such a valuable book produced by such an old friend. I wish both the book and the friend all possible success.

Michael A. R. Freeman, BA, MB, BCh, MD, FRCS
Visiting Professor
Biomedical Engineering
University College London
Honorary Consultant Orthopaedic Surgeon
Royal London Hospital
London, United Kingdom

Preface

Today, younger and more active patients seek total hip replacement in an attempt to restore a lifestyle lost to the debilitating effect of hip arthritis. With this change in patient population, the likelihood of revision and replacement surgery increases even though the durability and complication rates of THR for the older population decreases with the advent of better performing devices. The need to develop more conservative methods, improve component fixation and bearing couple performance, and to enhance physiologic designs with biocompatible materials stimulated our interest 35 years ago in developing an anatomic and physiologic surface arthroplasty. By being less invasive, a revision from resurfacing when necessary could be carried out more simply with improved results.

While surface arthroplasty with polyethylene was largely abandoned because of wear problems, modern metal-on-metal hip resurfacing's mid-term results already show greater durability, especially when the bone quality is good. With minimal wear issues even those implanted with early surgical techniques are stable beyond 10 years. Now with improvements in technique, even patients with substantial bone defects can be resurfaced with promising results although to establish efficacy longer follow-up is necessary. With hip resurfacing being today the fastest growing hip procedure, it is quite appropriate to analyze the state of its art.

The purpose of this text is to assess the materials, designs, and surgical techniques of modern hip resurfacing so that they can be compared with the long-term results of the conventional total hip stem-type systems not only to put into perspective the field's developments, but also hopefully to stimulate further advancement. It is our hope that this text will provide students, residents, radiologists, and practitioners of joint replacement, as well as engineers, materials scientists, and biology researchers, with a comprehensive reference on hip resurfacing.

The inter-relationships of surgical demands and material capabilities have long shaped my approach to hip replacement. To compile a text that clearly and cohesively presents this approach, I have assembled contributions from colleagues with whom I have been closely associated at the Joint Replacement Institute (now in its new location at the St. Vincent Medical Center in Los Angeles). Chapter 1 details the history and evolution of hip resurfacing including some of the more available designs. The contributions of several authors from other institutions are also included, who have special expertise and experience with fundamental basic science on vascularity (my former associate Paul Beaulé), on biomechanics (Richie Gill) and tribology (John Medley). The chapter on imaging is authored by my long-time associate Tom Gruen who carefully analyzed standardized x-ray examinations of our Conserve®Plus Series and designed the data collection tools for x-ray analysis. There is also a chapter detailing the techniques used for data collection and outcome analysis in our Clinical Evaluation Unit, authored by Michel Le Duff and by our statistician, Fred Dorey.

A major portion of this book contains our experience with the Conserve®Plus including: Indications and results of our carefully followed first 1000 hips and our current recommended technique; Modes of Failure, presented in a comprehensive analysis by long-time collaborator Pat Campbell on retrievals from failed cases from all investigators of the FDA Conserve®Plus FDA IDE trial, as well as from outside submissions from around the world with all types of devices and finally some from our will joint program. Her analysis led to operative technique refinements and improved durability. Reaction to wear products information includes what is known today and what is yet to be determined. The remainder of the book deals with specific evaluation and treatment implications for various etiologic groups with pertinent literature review as well as the results of treatment compared to the overall series (cohort) and evaluation of poorly performing or failed resurfacing and treatment thereafter. To conclude, there is a chapter dealing with post-op rehabilitation and activity, and finally one questioning "What is the future of resurfacing?"

During the preparation of this book, chapters have been restructured and revised many times. I wish particularly to acknowledge the contributions of Michel Le Duff, my wife, Patti, and past fellows who provided valuable proofreading. And finally, I wish to acknowledge the important contributions over the years of my many mentors, teachers and associates, the members of the North American and International Hip Societies who have provided the educational stimulus for this endeavor.

Harlan C. Amstutz

Contents

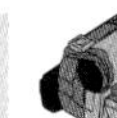

CHAPTER 1

Evolution of Hip Resurfacing

Harlan C. Amstutz

Michel J. Le Duff

Introduction

Hip resurfacing with metal-on-metal bearings is currently emerging as a major evolution of hip arthroplasty in the beginning of the 21st century. The popularity of this procedure in Europe and Australia is already undeniable, and the United States is most likely soon to follow. This notoriety was illustrated by the importance hip resurfacing took at the 2007 American Academy of Orthopaedic Surgeons, which featured more than 15 podium presentations, an instructional course lecture, and multiple scientific exhibits and poster presentations devoted to this topic. Already seen by many surgeons as the solution of choice for young patients with end-stage osteoarthritis,[1-5] hip resurfacing is not, however, a new concept, and previous attempts to replace arthritic hip joints without resecting the femoral head and neck have been made with various levels of success. The history of hip resurfacing has previously been described in the literature,[6-8] but the continued study of the early results of the current prosthetic solutions has provided probable explanations for some of the most common modes of failure associated with the successive resurfacing designs.

History of Resurfacing

The origin of hip resurfacing is generally attributed to Smith-Petersen,[9] whose mold arthroplasty was not intended as a hip replacement originally but as a mold for cartilage regeneration, with the intention of removing the mold when the femoral head and acetabulum would have become smooth and congruent (Fig. 1-1). This concept was abandoned because the regenerated surfaces were incomplete, mainly composed of fibrous cartilage and not optimal for weight bearing in most patients. The molds were never removed. However, the concept inspired several subsequent designs (cup arthroplasty) based on the interposition of a cup between the femoral head and acetabular cartilage with varying degrees of freedom between the cup and the femoral head and neck (illustrated here by the Luck cup [Fig. 1-2]). The main criticism associated at the time with these designs was that avascular necrosis developed under the cup, leading to a necessary revision. In fact, osteonecrosis was not present in most of those cases of collapse of the reshaped femoral head, but the confusion between necrosis and erosion of the femoral head due to lack of fixation of the component continued. Later, the double-cup arthroplasty (surface arthroplasty per se) was developed, in which weight bearing was provided by a double cup in an attempt to limit the friction between the bone or cartilage and a foreign material. A few pioneers made unsuccessful attempts (like Charnley with Teflon bearings in the 1950s, Müller and Boltzy[10] with metal-on-metal in the 1960s [Fig. 1-3], and Gerard[11] in the 1970s, also with metal-on-metal and later metal on polyethylene [PE][12]), but with components allowing mobility between the bone and the prosthetic cups. These prostheses were cementless designs, but the surfaces were smooth, unlike today's components designed to obtain rigid fixation. In the early 1970s, however, the consensus was that fixed cemented components with the entire joint mobility located at the interface between femoral and acetabular component would provide the best pain relief and durability. All polyethylene cemented cups and cobalt-chromium (CoCr)–cemented femoral components were used almost simultaneously in five different countries. Wagner in Germany (Fig. 1-4); Paltrinieri and Trentani in Italy (Fig. 1-5); Freeman (Fig. 1-6) in the United Kingdom; Tanaka, Furuya and Nishio in Japan; Gerard in France; and Eicher and Capello (Fig. 1-7), and Amstutz in the United States were among the pioneers of this technique. The successive prosthetic designs referred to as double-cup arthroplasty are summarized in Table 1-1.

Because the target age was younger than total hip replacement (THR), the majority of the results from these early designs exhibited poor long-term performance compared with THR,[13-15] and these high, early failure rates were later explained by the effects of increased polyethylene wear debris generated by large femoral heads articulating with ultra-high-molecular-weight polyethylene (UHMWPE),[16] even though

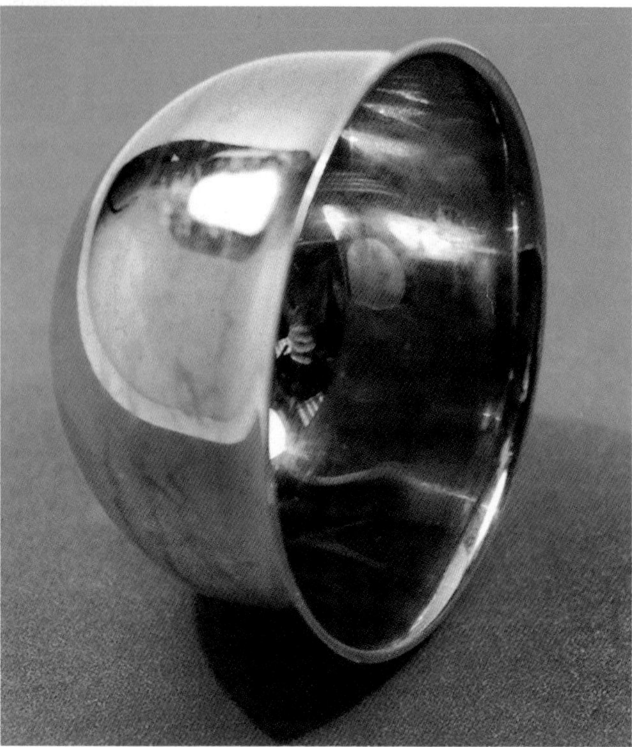

Figure 1-1 Smith-Petersen's mold arthroplasty. The Vitallium (cobalt-chromium-molybdenum alloy) component (1938) replaced the original molds, which were made of glass and were too brittle for use in the procedure. The device was designed to restrict motion between the reshaped femoral head and the component.

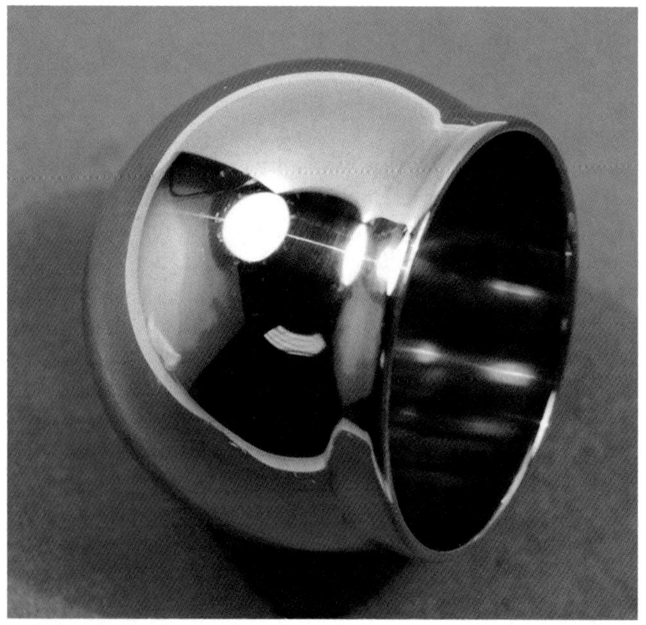

Figure 1-2 The Luck cup (1948) featured a collar and, although it was cementless, it did not allow as much motion between the reshaped femoral head and the component.

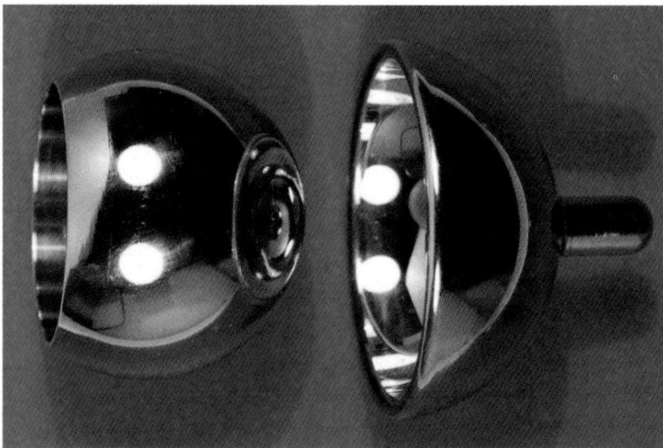

Figure 1-3 The very first surface replacement with metal-on-metal bearing was developed by Müller and Boltzy,[10] who implanted 18 of these press-fit devices and reported their results in 1968. Note the presence of Teflon pads on the bearing surface of the acetabular component.

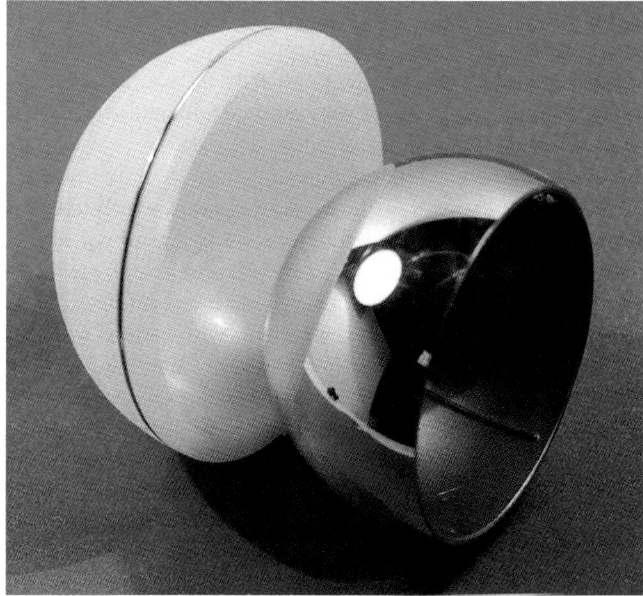

Figure 1-4 Wagner (1974) double-cup design using cemented polyethylene acetabular components and cemented cobalt-chromium-molybdenum femoral components.

acrylic fragmentation contributed to the osteolysis. In the meantime, the procedure had been largely abandoned and the resurfacing concept itself rejected by the larger orthopaedic community. As an example of the performance of one of the devices used during this era, the results of the cemented components articulating with polyethylene bearings and implanted by the senior author are discussed later.

An Example of All-Cemented Metal-Polyethylene Device: The THARIES

In 1973, the Total Hip Articular Replacement Using Internal Eccentric Shells (THARIES) was developed at the University

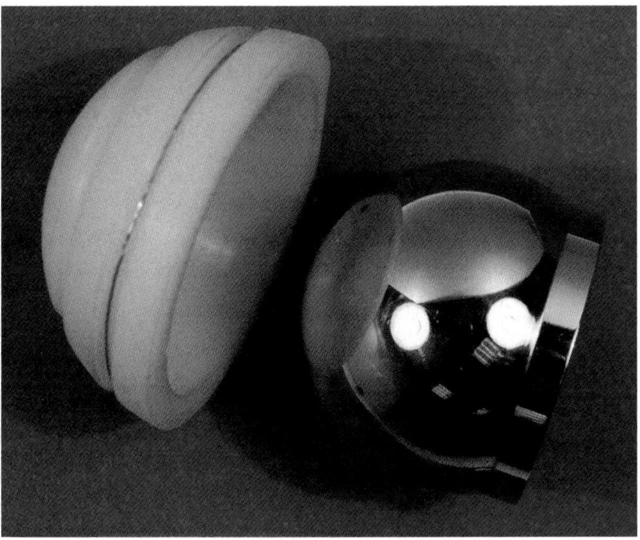

Figure 1-5 Paltrinieri and Trentani (1971) hip resurfacing device.

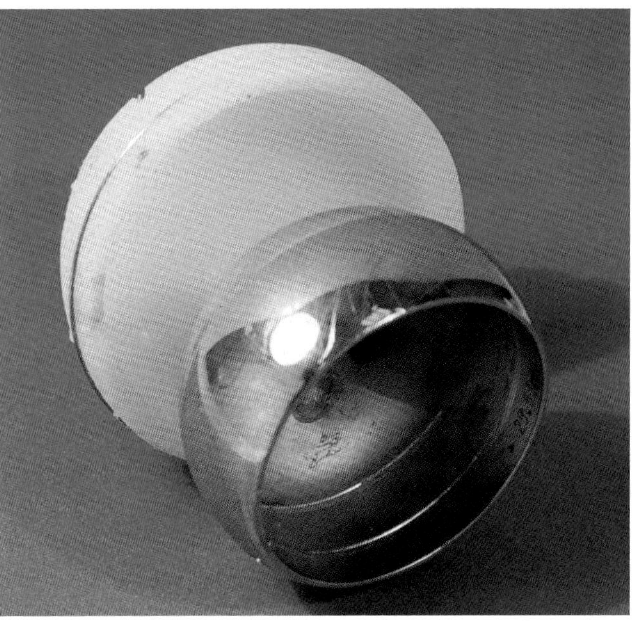

Figure 1-6 Imperial College-London Hospital (ICLH) hip resurfacing device developed by Freeman and Swanson (1976).

Table 1-1 Double-Cup Arthroplasty Designs

Surgeon	Date of First Implantation	Implant Fixation	Inner Shape of the Femoral Component	Bearing Material
Charnley	Early 1950s	Cementless	Cylindrical	Polytetrafluoroethylene (Teflon)
Townley (TARA)	1964	Cemented	Cylindrical	Polyurethane then UHMWPE
Muller	1968	Cementless	Cylindrical + hemispherical dome	Metal-on-metal (CoCr) + Teflon spacers
Patrinieri and Trentani	1971	Cemented	Hemispherical	UHMWPE cup and stainless steel head
Furuya	1971	Cemented	Cylindrical	Steel cup and UHMWPE head, then UHMWPE cup and steel head, then Al/Al
Freeman (ICLH)	1972	Cemented	Cylindrical	Metal cup and UHMWPE head, then UHMWPE cup and CoCr head
Eicher and Capello (ICH)	1973	Cemented, then porous coated on femoral side	Hemispherical	UHMWPE cup and CoCr head
Wagner	1974	Cemented	Hemispherical	UHMWPE cup and CoCr head, then alumina head
Amstutz (THARIES)	1975	Cemented	Chamfered cylinder	UHMWPE cup and CoCr head
Amstutz (PSR)	1983	Cementless chamfered cylinder with mesh, then hemispherical with beads, then hybrid	Chamfered cylinder then tapered cylinder	UHMWPE liner and CoCr head, then alumina head

Al, Alumina; CoCr, cobalt-chromium; ICH, Indiana Conservative Hip; ICLH, Imperial College-London Hospital; PSR, porous-coated surface replacement; TARA, Total Articular Replacement Arthroplasty; THARIES, Total Hip Articular Replacement Using Internal Eccentric Shells; UHMWPE, ultra-high-molecular-weight polyethylene.

of California-Los Angeles (UCLA) Medical Center by Amstutz and Clarke and commercialized in 1975. The femoral component was cemented, made of Co-Cr-Mo, and articulated with an all-polyethylene acetabular component, which was also cemented (Fig. 1-8). Both components were eccentric to minimize the thickness of the components and bone removal. The three polyethylene components had a maximum wall thickness of 3.5 to 5.5 mm in the weight-bearing areas. Femoral head diameters ranged from 36 to 54 mm, in 3- and 4-mm increments. The THARIES was the design that introduced the chamfered cylinder design (CCD, now adopted by most current designs) as the optimal reshaping of the head to ensure resection of the diseased bone but to maintain as much femoral head and neck bone as possible. Following is a summary of

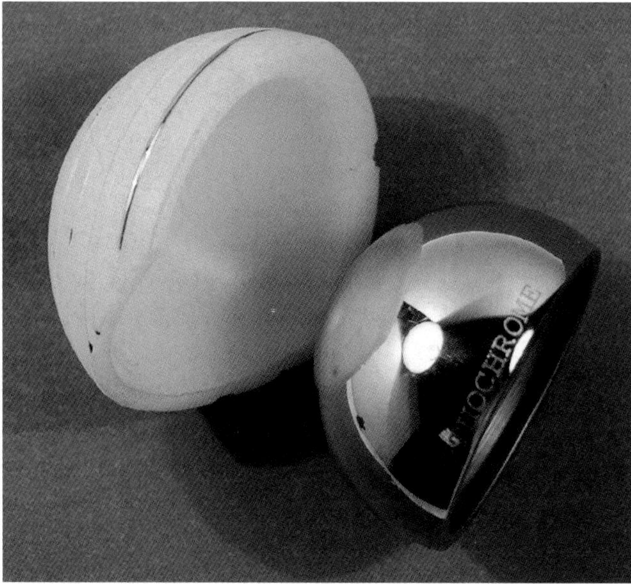

Figure 1-7 Indiana Conservative Hip (ICH; DePuy, Warsaw, IN) developed by Eicher and Capello (1973).

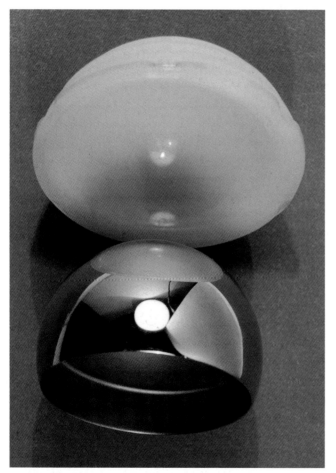

Figure 1-8 First generation of the metal-on-polyethylene resurfacing system: The Total Hip Articular Replacement with Internal Eccentric Shells (THARIES, Zimmer, Warsaw, IN) developed by Amstutz and Clarke (1975). Both components were cemented, and the femoral head was reamed with a chamfer, which is a pattern now adopted by most current resurfacing devices.

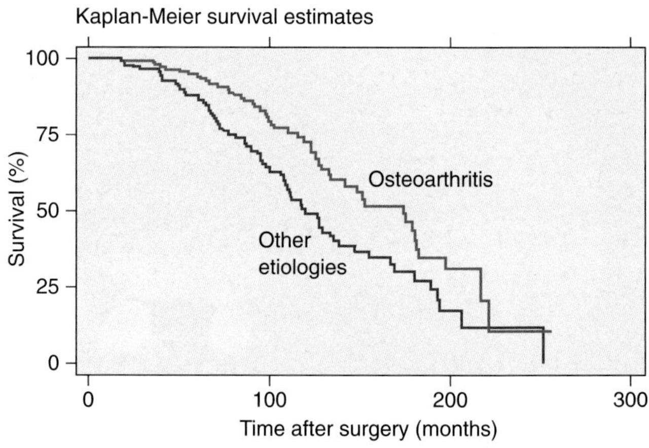

Figure 1-9 Kaplan-Meier survivorship curve of the THARIES devices implanted by the senior author, illustrating the greater implant durability for patients with a diagnosis of primary osteoarthritis versus other etiologies.

the results of our experience with THARIES, which has been previously published.[17,18]

Three hundred and twenty-two THARIES were implanted between 1975 and 1984 by the senior author using a transtrochanteric approach. The mean patient age at the time of surgery was 51 years (range 20 to 67 years), and 55% were men. The primary diagnoses were: osteoarthritis (53%), osteonecrosis (16%), developmental dysplasia (10%), rheumatoid arthritis (7%), post-trauma (5%), slipped capital femoral epiphysis (SCFE 4%), and other diagnoses (5%) and were consistent with the etiology of arthritis in a young population. The average follow-up was 117 months, with 172 patients older than 10 years at the last review. Survivorship data shown in Figure 1-9 included 189 revisions. Only 4 were consecutive to femoral neck fracture. Aseptic loosening of one or both components was the main mode of failure and accounted for 97% of the failures, with a higher incidence of acetabular failures compared with femoral failures at revision surgery. With any revision as the endpoint, the 5-, 10-, and 16-year survivorship for the entire group was 88%, 48%, and 26%, respectively. The best survivorship of hips was in men with osteoarthritis, who had larger component sizes than women. Survivorship was 91% at 5 years, 66% at 10 years, and 43% at 15 years. There was a significant difference between the etiologies (see Fig. 1-9, Log rank test: $P = 0.011$), and the 10-year estimated survivorships were osteoarthritis, 51%; rheumatoid disease, 50%; osteonecrosis, 33%; and developmental dysplasia, 28%.

Despite these disappointing survivorship results, the patients benefited from good functional outcomes (Fig. 1-10), and whenever revision became necessary, newer and more advanced implants were available (including cementless acetabular and femoral stem-type components) to be implanted into a virgin femoral canal, resulting in the probability of securing long-term function for these patients, most of whom were still young and active.

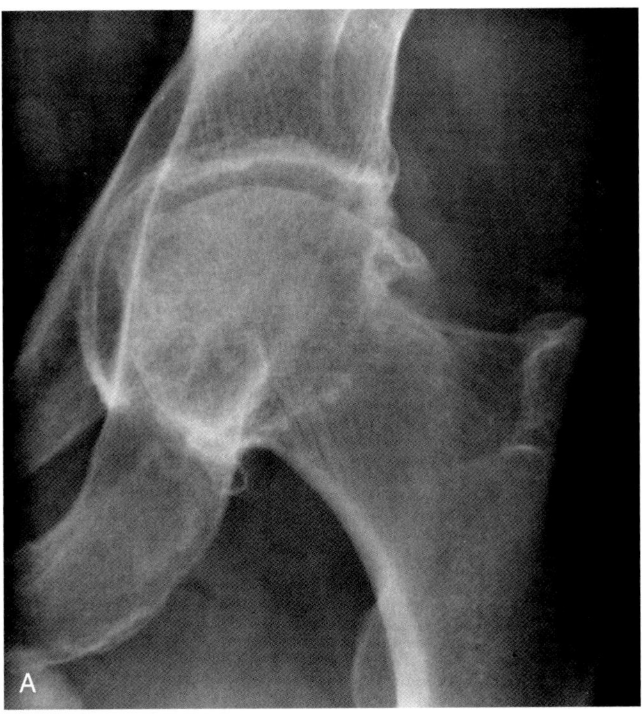

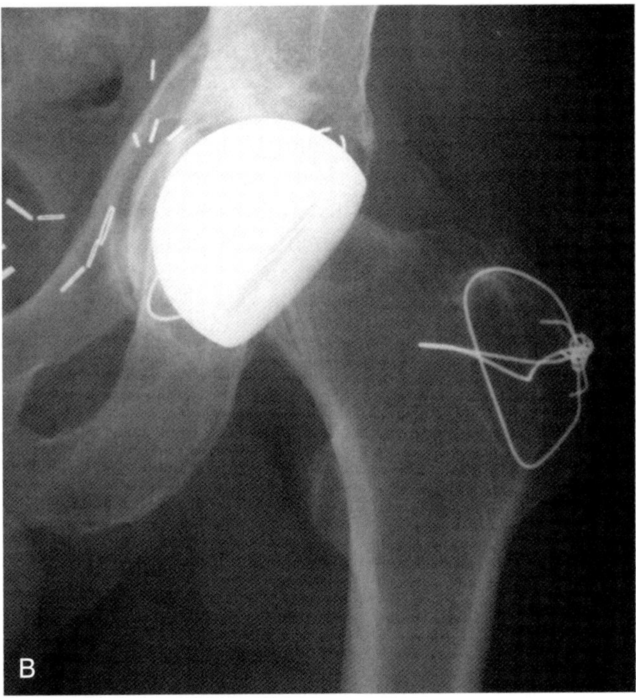

Figure 1-10 A, Anteroposterior pelvic radiograph of a 46-year-old man with osteoarthritis of the right hip. **B,** Twenty-two and a half years after resurfacing with THARIES, the femoral head eventually wore through the cemented polyethylene acetabular component, leading to a necessary revision of otherwise well fixed components. *(Reprinted with permission from Amstutz H, Le Duff M: Background of metal-on-metal resurfacing. Proc Inst Mech Eng [H] 2006;220:85-94.)*

Cementless Metal-Polyethylene Hip Resurfacing: The Porous-Coated Surface Replacement

Although other innovators abandoned resurfacing, the development of cementless fixation for resurfacing devices in our laboratories was driven by the belief that cement was the main cause of implant failure in 1981, just as it was believed to be the problem in conventional stem-type devices. The role of polyethylene debris was still unknown in the component loosening process. Also, the absence of additional reaming of the acetabulum to provide space for the cement mantle was a major factor in the adoption of porous coating or titanium mesh for the fixation of hip resurfacing components. These modifications to resurfacing devices were made in conjunction with the evolution of stem-type devices during the early 1980s. Although the acetabular durability improved considerably, the overall survivorship performance of these devices did not improve compared with the THARIES because the rapid wear rate of UHMWPE remained the dominant cause of failure. Two consecutive designs of the acetabular components–the CCD (Fig. 1-11) and the hemispherical design (Fig. 1-12) provided important information for the development of future prostheses. Because the CCD was press fit without screw holes, debris penetration into the acetabulum was prevented but the femoral component mesh-bone interface showed greater vulnerability with more extensive femoral osteolysis, and fracture of the femoral neck occurred earlier and with much greater frequency than in our cemented THARIES, illustrating the hypothesis that the debris travels a path of least resistance.[19] The gain in acetabular bone preservation associated with the CCD was large enough to outweigh the difficulty of positioning of these components but we changed to a hemispherical socket design to facilitate insertion. However, the acetabulum became vulnerable to osteolysis due to debris penetration through the screw holes into the

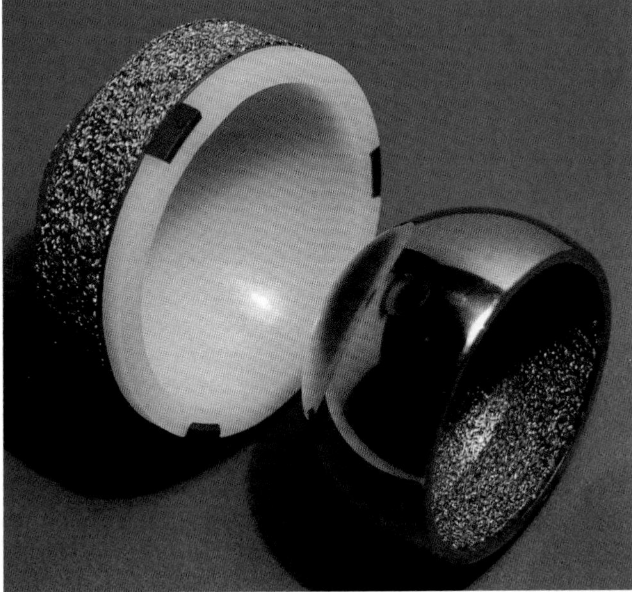

Figure 1-11 Zimmer chamfered cylinder Porous Surface Replacement.

superior acetabulum even when screws were not used in our later experience. On the femoral side, the cementless components almost without exception became fixed despite some malposition and incomplete bone ingrowth (whether titanium alloy/commercially pure titanium mesh or the later beaded cobalt-chrome porous was used) and the fixation remained good until osteolysis, facilitated by the gaps under the femoral component, ultimately undermined the stability of the component. The CCD design of the porous-coated surface replacement (Zimmer, Warsaw, IN) with mesh remained, but the side walls of the porous-beaded version (DePuy, Warsaw, IN) was changed in 1990 to a gentle 3-degree taper to facilitate seating of the component without tilting.

However, for patients with low, or in a few cases, moderate activity level, some of those prostheses are still functioning nearly 20 years later (Figs. 1-13 and 1-14).

The Role of Hemiresurfacing

During the era of metal-on-polyethylene resurfacing beginning in 1981, a series of patients with Ficat stage III or early stage IV osteonecrosis, in which the acetabular cartilage damage was not severe, were implanted with a type of hemiresurfacing in which a resurfaced femoral head articulates directly with the host acetabular cartilage. In this procedure, aseptic loosening of the device is extremely rare and no such adverse outcome was observed in the 25-year experience in the senior author's series.[20,21] Revision of the femoral component became necessary mainly when the acetabular cartilage wore out (Fig. 1-15). This observation supported our resurfacing concept and suggested that a low wear-bearing material was the likely key to the success of total resurfacing.

Although long-term durability was unlikely for the young and active patient implanted with a conventional polyethylene device, the resulting lessons of this early era of hip resurfacing were useful in designing the present generation systems.

Those lessons from the era 1973 to 1992 include

1. The preservation of femoral bone stock
2. The increased stability due to the large ball size was associated with a markedly reduced prevalence of dislocation compared with THA[17]
3. The procedure did not cause femoral head necrosis[22] because the blood supply in the arthritic hip is primarily intraosseous from the metaphysis and there is an associated hyperemia present in the arthritic hip.[23] The extraosseous retinacular vessels, which enter the posterior head-neck junction in the normal hip, are compromised by the growth of osteophytes at the head-neck junction in the osteoarthritic disease process.
4. There were some short-term neck fracture failures, but these appeared to be related to bone stock and technique.
5. Although acrylic fragmentation was a factor, the majority of the failures were due to component loosening secondary to polyethylene debris–induced osteolysis because the wear of polyethylene was increased 4 to 10 times with large femoral heads compared with the smaller sizes used at that time in total hip arthroplasty. Additionally, a reduction in incidence and severity was not obtained by the introduction of a smoother alumina, femoral component.

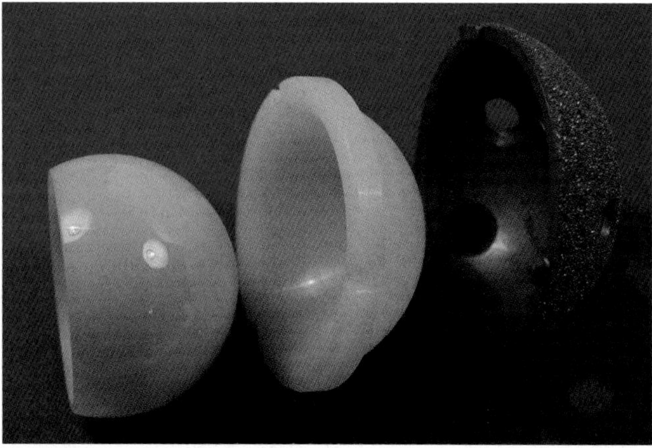

Figure 1-12 DePuy Hemispherical Porous Surface Replacement. Shown here in a hybrid combination (1990 to 1992) with a cemented alumina femoral component (Kyocera, Kyoto, Japan), to reduce polyethylene wear. The acetabular porous coating is provided by beads that replaced the titanium mesh of the chamfered cylinder design.

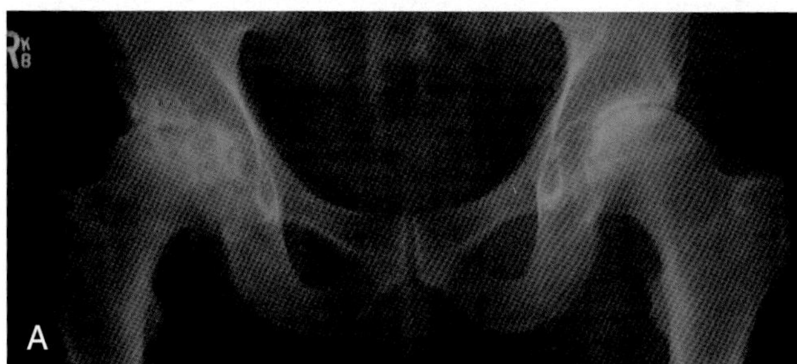

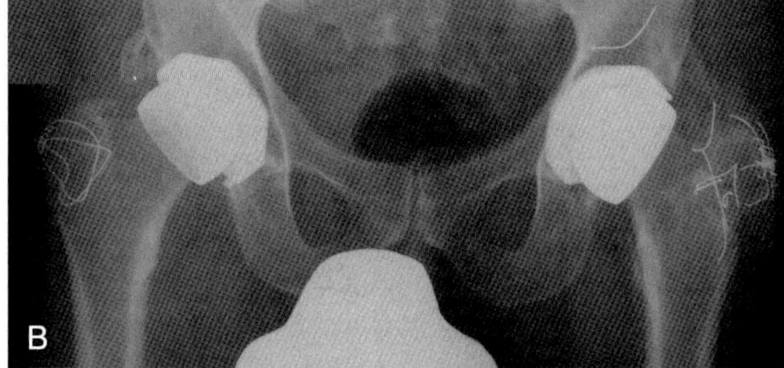

Figure 1-13 **A,** Anteroposterior (AP) pelvic radiograph of a 54-year-old man with bilateral osteoarthritis. **B,** AP radiograph showing the patient 19 years after resurfacing on the right and 18 years on the left. The patient is still pain free and the components well fixed, although the polyethylene is thin laterally on the left hip. *(Reprinted with permission from Amstutz H, Le Duff M: Background of metal-on-metal resurfacing. Proc Inst Mech Eng [H] 2006;220:85-94.)*

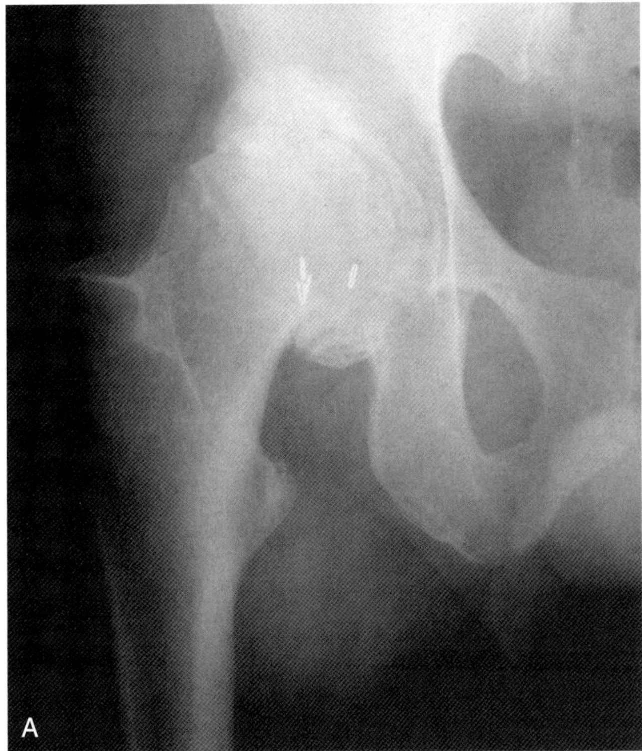

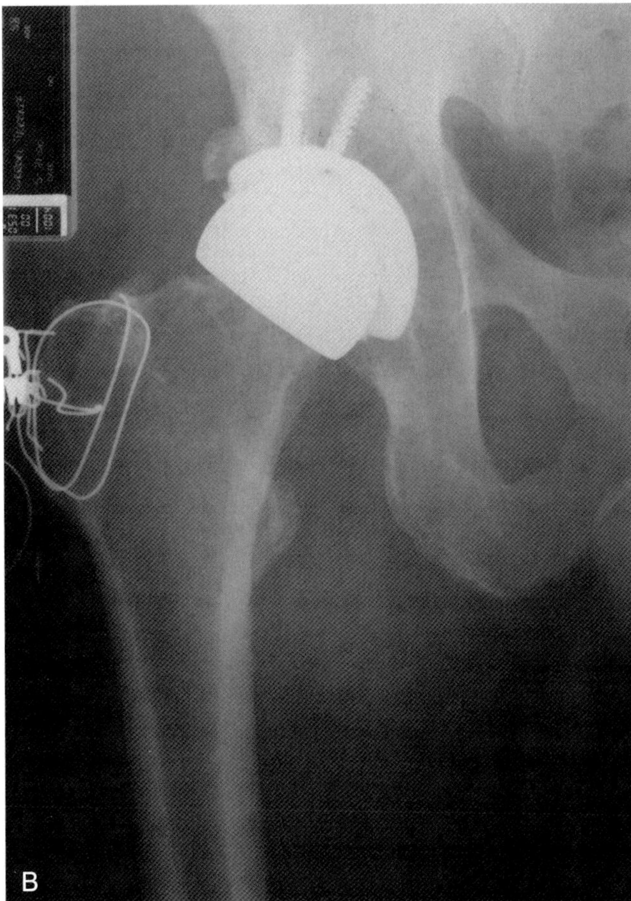

Figure 1-14 A, Anteroposterior (AP) pelvic radiograph of a 48-year-old man with osteoarthritis secondary to an old slipped capital femoral epiphysis. **B,** AP radiograph showing the patient 14 years after resurfacing. A small area of bone erosion at the superolateral junction of the neck and femoral component, and radiolucent zones around the socket suggest the presence of osteolysis. *(Reprinted with permission from Amstutz H, Le Duff M: Background of metal-on-metal resurfacing. Proc Inst Mech Eng [H] 2006;220:85-94.)*

6. Femoral fixation was critical due to a small fixation area, with larger diameter components characterized by a better survivorship.[24]
7. The revision to a conventional stem-type device for the femoral component was easy because the femoral canal was left intact by the resurfacing procedure. However, there was often extensive acetabular bone loss due to osteolysis, especially with cemented components in patients who were not followed regularly.

Although socket loosening was dramatically reduced with cementless components, the device did not conserve acetabular bone stock because of the thickness of the two-component system (a metallic shell and a liner insert). The PSR was, however, the first system (1983) with both femoral and acetabular components available in 3-mm increments in order to increase the surgical technique flexibility and to minimize bone resection of the acetabulum. Later, in 1990, hemispherical components with porous-beaded surfaces became available in 2-mm increments, which is necessary for optimal flexibility.

Despite the limitations of this era in the history of resurfacing, in the late 1980s, Heinz Wagner and Harlan Amstutz discussed the possibility of resurfacing using metal-on-metal bearings. We both still believed in continuing the pursuit of resurfacing because of its conservative and more physiologic basis and the appeal expressed to us by our previous generation of patients.

Why Metal-on-Metal Bearings?

In the late 1980s, Hardy Weber in Switzerland and independently Harlan Amstutz in Los Angeles observed remarkable durability in some patients with metal-on-metal total hip arthroplasty (MM THA) implanted in the 1960s. One of my patients from a series of McKee-Farrar prostheses (Howmedica Limited, London, UK) implanted in 1967 had come to Los Angeles to have a contralateral Charnley prosthesis (DePuy International, Leeds, United Kingdom) revised for polyethylene wear after 19 years, whereas the Mckee-Farrar prosthesis on her other side continued to perform well, and in fact, continues after 40 years (Fig. 1-16).

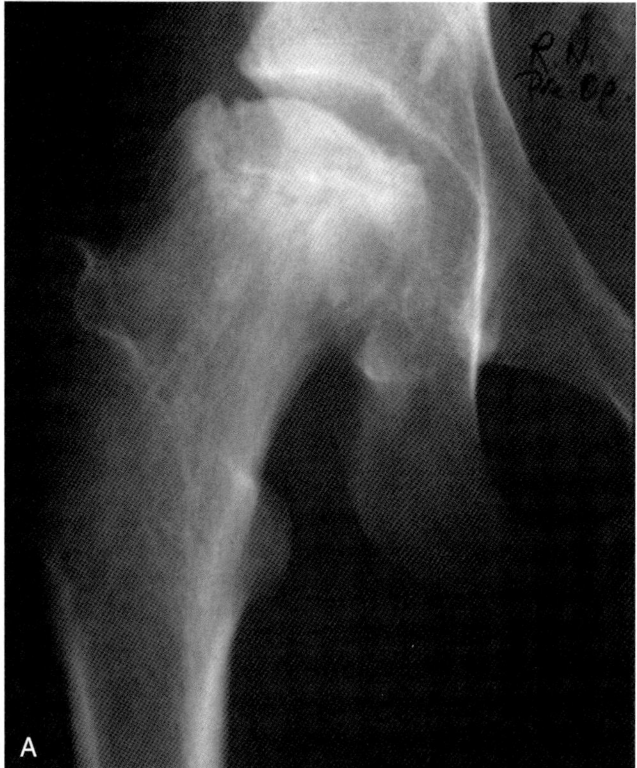

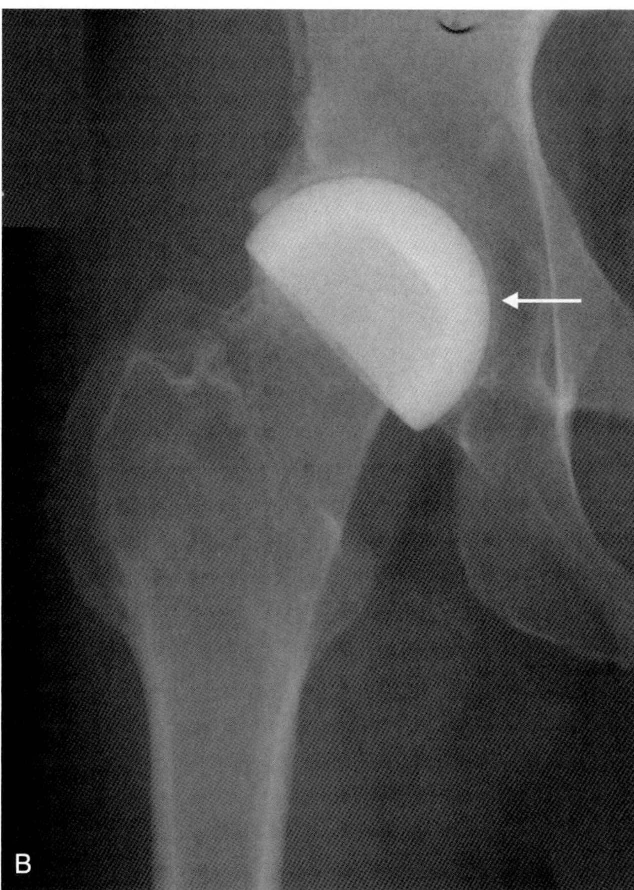

Figure 1-15 **A,** Eighteen-year-old man with post-trauma–induced osteonecrosis, Ficat stage III. **B,** Sixteen years after hemiresurfacing, the cementless Alumina femoral resurfacing component shows excellent fixation. There is preservation of some articular space. Note the formation of new bone in the acetabular fossa (*arrow*), which has uniformly prevented a protrusion of the hemiresurfacing component into the acetabulum. The component was eventually revised 18 years after surgery as the result of complete acetabular cartilage wear. *(Reprinted with permission from Amstutz H, Le Duff M: Background of metal-on-metal resurfacing. Proc Inst Mech Eng [H] 2006;220:85-94.)*

This was one of three components that I had implanted with a contralateral Charnley prosthesis. In each case, the metal-on-metal bearing outperformed the Charnley prosthesis in durability. Weber, having made similar observations with the Müller and Huggler devices (Sulzer, Wintertur, Switzerland), was able to persuade Sulzer in 1988 to conceive a new design of MM THA with 28-mm heads. However, all types of metal-on-metal total hip arthroplasties (McKee-Farrar, Ring, Müller, and Huggler) widely used in the 1960s and 1970s had large-diameter heads similar to the sizes used in surface replacements.[25-27] Wagner also began with Sulzer with a MM resurfacing design. However, until 1992, I was less successful in convincing the device manufacturers in the United States to pursue MM resurfacing despite the potential advantages over earlier metal-PE designs.

Besides the poor results of the early resurfacing designs, one of the main criticisms directed toward resurfacing was that the procedure did not conserve bone on the acetabular side compared with a conventional THA because of the need to accommodate for a femoral head of a larger diameter. Today among the potential bearing materials available to provide a satisfactory alternative to the conventional UHMWPE radiated in air, both cross-linked polyethylene (which was not commercially available until 1999) and ceramics require too thick an acetabular system (because of the two-part components) to be optimal for a bone-conserving resurfacing. At present, only metallic devices can be manufactured with sufficient strength for a thin, one-piece shell that combine a low wear-bearing quality with an outside rough surface such as sintered porous beads or other suitable coating for cementless fixation. In addition, the excellent wear properties of large femoral heads,[28,29] the self-healing capacity of metal-on-metal bearings,[30] and the absence of runaway wear confirm that metal-on-metal is currently the optimal bearing of choice for resurfacing.

Modern Generation of Resurfacing

The current generation of hip resurfacing devices uses exclusively cobalt-chromium-molybdenum alloy (CoCrMo) metal-on-metal bearings. The first two designs to appear were introduced in the early 1990s by Heinz Wagner[31] in Germany

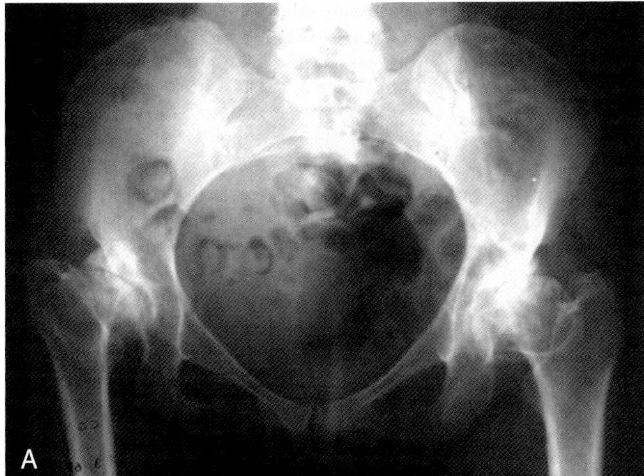

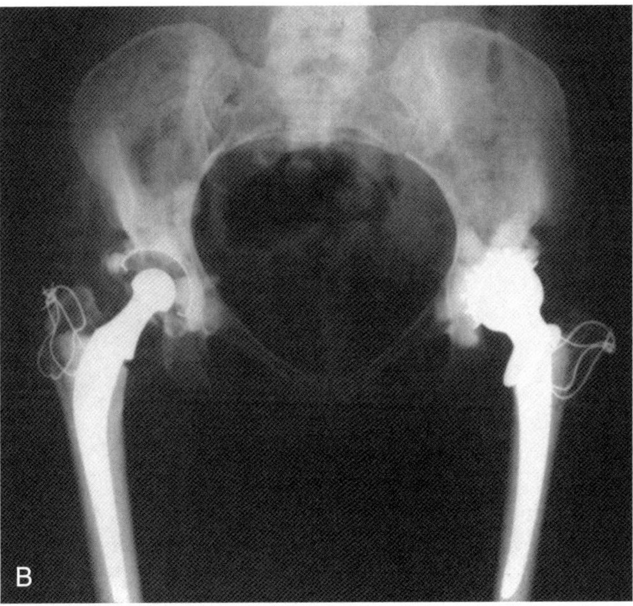

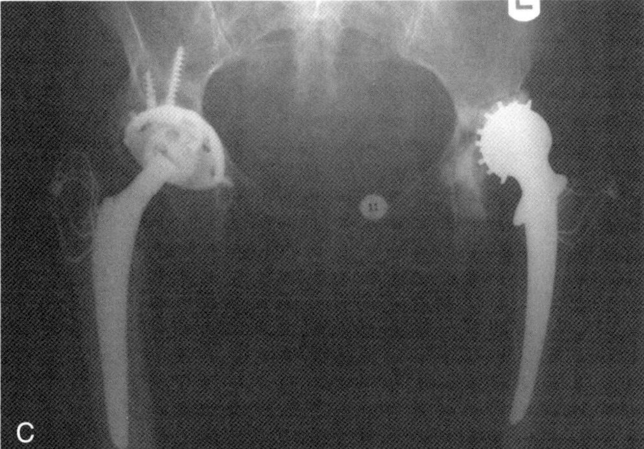

Figure 1-16 **A,** Anteroposterior radiograph of a 46-year-old woman with developmental dysplasia of the hip. **B,** Postoperative radiograph showing a Charnley prosthesis in place on the right hip and a McKee-Farrar device on the left hip. **C,** The Charnley low-friction arthroplasty was revised 19 years after initial surgery to a cemented ATH stem and a cementless acetabular component. The McKee-Farrar metal-on-metal device is still in place 40 years after primary surgery.

and Derek McMinn[32] in England. Initially, both systems were all cementless. The Wagner design (Fig. 1-17) used forged cobalt-chrome (CoCr) alloy (F799 with a high carbon content) as a bearing surface and a grit-blasted, titanium alloy shell with macro features for fixation to the bone. The long-term results of this design were recently reported in a series of 54 hips implanted between 1991 and 2004.[33] Of these 54 hips, 46 used cementless femoral components and eight used cemented components in cases in which bone quality was judged improper for cementless reconstruction. There were 17 revisions performed, but no dominant mode of failure could be determined from this early experience. However the authors concluded that the prosthesis would have been a viable solution had it been implanted with a more rigorous patient selection process. This conclusion was based in part on information revealed by a study of more recent designs.[3,34] The initial McMinn resurfacing (Fig. 1-18) used a cast, high-carbon CoCrMo alloy, uncoated, and press fitted (cementless fixation) both on the femoral and the acetabular side. The preparation of the femoral head was similar to that of the total hip articular replacement by internal eccentric shells (THARIES, Zimmer, Warsaw, IN) with a CCD using the same 4-mm increments. Both components were cementless and hydroxyapatite (HA)

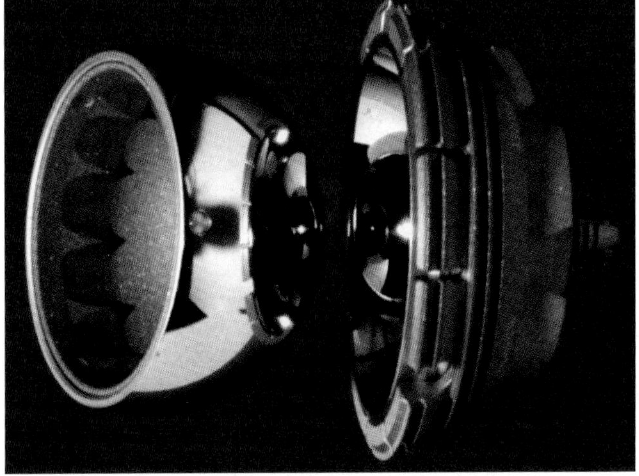

Figure 1-17 Wagner metal-on-metal cementless resurfacing design (1991).

coated, but the geometry did not provide enough interference with the bone for initial and enduring fixation. The femoral component had peripheral, antirotation ridges and a short metaphyseal stem to assist with the alignment of the femoral component and its initial stability. The acetabular component

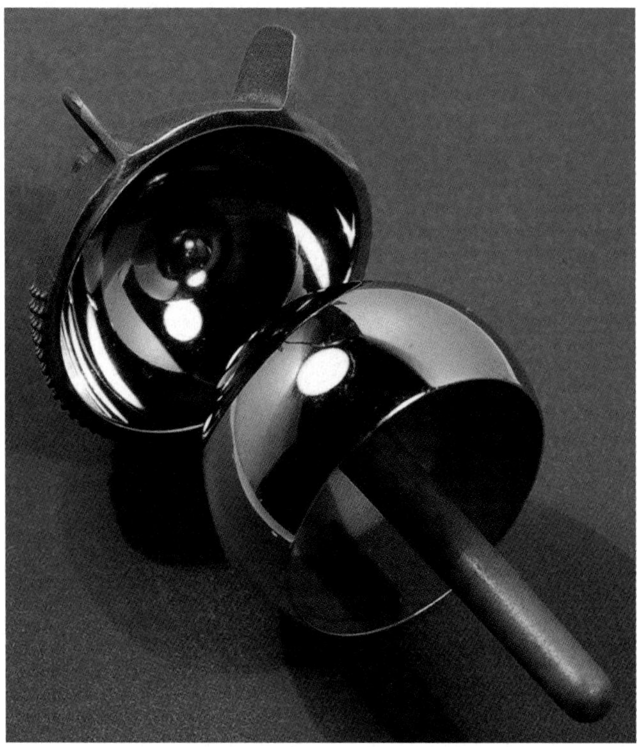

Figure 1-18 Original McMinn metal-on-metal cementless resurfacing design (1991).

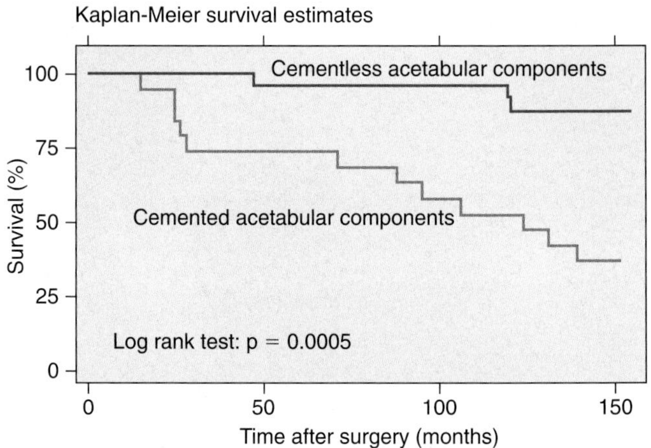

Figure 1-19 Kaplan and Meier survivorship curves of the acetabular components used in the Joint Replacement Institute pilot study. The cementless acetabular components largely outlived the cemented ones.

also had a short stem to assist in initial stability by penetrating the inner wall of the pelvis. The failure rates were high, and both components were modified for acrylic fixation. Subsequently McMinn modified his component further for cementless fixation on the acetabular side using a series of sharp fins, and he reintroduced HA coating on macro-size beads.

In October 1993, we began a pilot program with metal-on-metal resurfacing using four Wagner resurfacing devices and 42 McMinn cemented femoral components, articulating with four different socket systems (two cemented and two cementless). These devices were implanted over a 3-year period. We reported on the assessment of technique, initial fixation, and early results of 21 hips.[35]

The fixation of the cementless Wagner acetabular components was satisfactory at 11 to 12 years despite their difficulty of insertion. Only one prosthesis was revised at 8 years for late hematogenous sepsis. That femoral component was retrieved and sectioned, and it revealed metallosis associated with weaknesses in the bond between the femoral head itself and the porous-coated inlay interfacing with the bone.

The mid-term results of the experience with the McMinn components has been reported.[4] The average age was 47.5 years (range 16 to 64 years), with only eight patients older than 60 years. The porous-beaded double sockets and six of seven HA-coated McMinn sockets also showed enduring fixation. The McMinn socket was used in its original cemented design in 11 hips, but the short-term radiographic analysis revealed radiolucencies in a large percentage of these sockets, which were then customized (eight hips) by the senior author (HCA) by shortening the central stud and adding grooves and rounded depressions for better acrylic keying. At 12 to 13 years of follow-up, only one of these original sockets remains. Nine have been revised for either socket cement disassociation or bone cement loosening, and one was retrieved after the patient died of causes unrelated to the surgery. Of the eight HCA modified cemented acetabular components, three were revised for acetabular loosening and one was removed secondary to a femoral neck fracture. Four (50%) of these components are still in place at a follow-up ranging from 11 to 12 years.

In contrast, the acetabular components with a porous bone-socket interface showed greater durability, as illustrated in Figure 1-19. The Kaplan and Meier survival estimate for the cemented acetabular components was 52.6% at 10 years (95% confidence interval, 29% to 72%), whereas the estimate for the cementless acetabular components was 91.7% at 10 years (95% confidence interval, 71% to 98%).

This experience strongly suggested the need for cementless fixation to provide predictable durable fixation of the acetabular component. Although cement added versatility, the inability to consistently obtain a dry and bloodless acetabular field decreased the ability to obtain optimal initial fixation, which jeopardized long-term fixation.

Although the Wagner socket system remained unchanged, there were several femoral changes resulting ultimately in his practice of using acrylic fixation. The McMinn prosthesis underwent a series of evolutions starting in 1997, leading to the development of the current Cormet 2000 (Corin Medical Ltd., Cirencester, UK) and the Birmingham Hip Resurfacing (BHR-Midland Medical Technologies Ltd., Birmingham, UK) prostheses. Meanwhile, Amstutz conceived the design for the Conserve®Plus with improved instrumentation, and the first prototypes were developed in 1993, initially with Orthomet in Minneapolis, MN and subsequently with Wright Medical

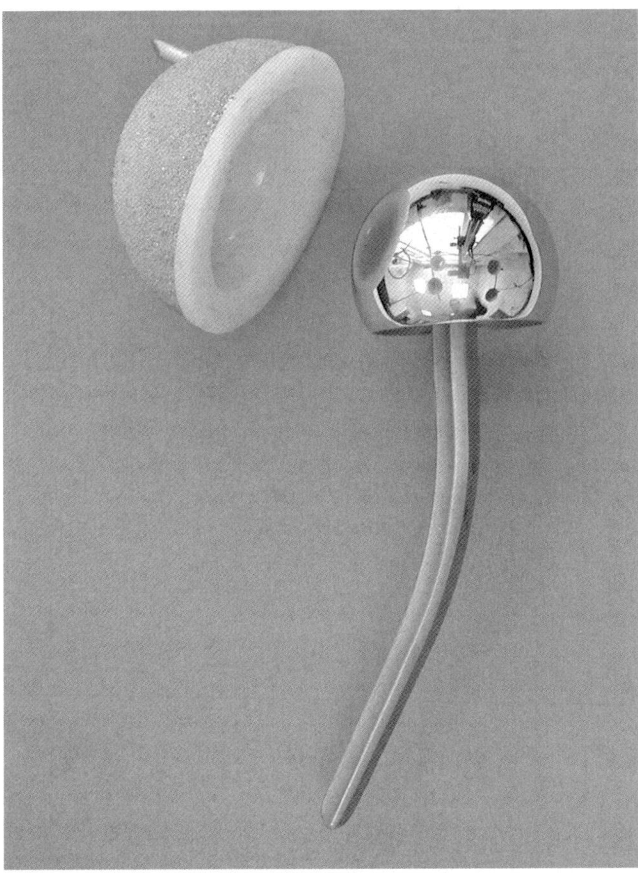

Figure 1-20 Total Articular Replacement Arthroplasty (TARA, DePuy, Warsaw, IN) designed by Townley (1977).

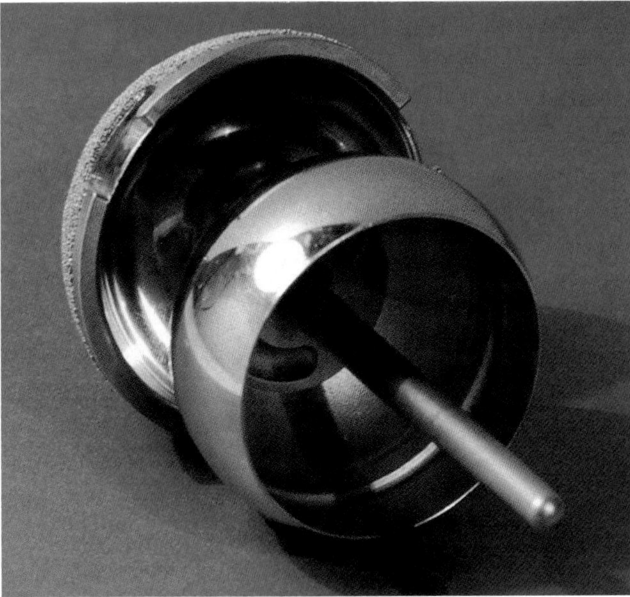

Figure 1-21 Conserve®Plus resurfacing system (Wright Medical Technology Inc., Arlington, TN). The acetabular component has 50- to 150-μm sintered beads, with a coverage of 170 degrees. The metaphyseal stem was designed to facilitate the alignment of the component during insertion and to ensure a constant cement mantle.

Technology Inc., Arlington, TN, when that company purchased Orthomet. The first Conserve® was implanted as a hemiresurfacing system (available in 1-mm increments) in 1995 and the Conserve®Plus in November of 1996. The metaphyseal stem was inspired by the Total Articular Replacement Arthroplasty (TARA, DePuy, Warsaw, IN) designed by Townley[36] (Fig. 1-20). The senior author had the opportunity to review the serial radiographs of large series of TARAs used as both a hemisurface and a full resurfacing system with PE, and he believed that there was an advantage in improving instrumentation guidance by straightening and shortening the stem, which could also potentially aid with component fixation. There did not appear to be any definitive evidence of stress shielding due to the stem, although long-term follow-up was not available either from the series reviewed or in the literature. Thus, benefits for more precision reaming and fixation seemed to outweigh any potential disadvantages that is, long-term stress shielding.

The Conserve®Plus (Wright Medical Technology, Arlington, TN), became the subject of a U.S. Food and Drug Administration (FDA) Investigational Device Exemption multicenter trial in August 2000 (Fig. 1-21). The Conserve®Plus acetabular shell is hemispherical (170 degrees) with a sintered porous coating of 75 to 150 microns for cementless fixation. The design of the femoral component is similar to the Conserve® used for hemiresurfacing. A short stem facilitates both the alignment of the component and the uniformity of the cement mantle around the prepared femoral head. Only the roundness and surface finish tolerances were different to allow the articulation with the acetabular component and to permit hydrodynamic lubrication.[28,37] Now all of the components are superfinished for bearing wear whether used as a hemisurface or full surface system. That change was accompanied by the introduction in November 2003 of a thin shell acetabular component with a reduction in wall thickness to 3.5 mm. Femoral component sizes range from 36 to 58 mm in 2-mm increments. The difference between the outside diameter of the acetabular component (range 46 to 64 mm) and the femoral component was 10 mm for the original socket, and the difference between the outside diameters of the femoral and acetabular components is actually 7.5 mm with the thin shell that is now used in more than 98% of hips. The thin shell facilitates saving both acetabular and femoral bone and lessening the risk of reaming too closely to the femoral neck (Fig. 1-22). All components were made of a cast F-75 CoCrMo, but in late 2006, a forged (or hardened) femoral component was introduced to further reduce the wear of the components.

With more than 11 years of experience worldwide, it is now possible to enumerate the advantages of metal-on-metal resurfacing over THRs as well as the risk factors. It must be emphasized that risk factors will vary according to the reported experience of a specific device, its instrument package, and the surgeon's experience.

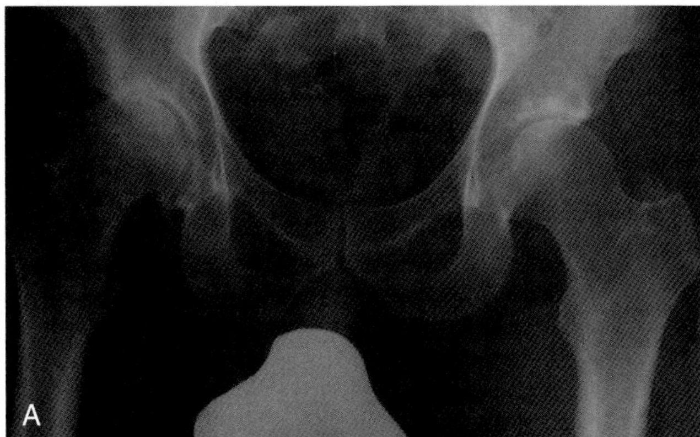

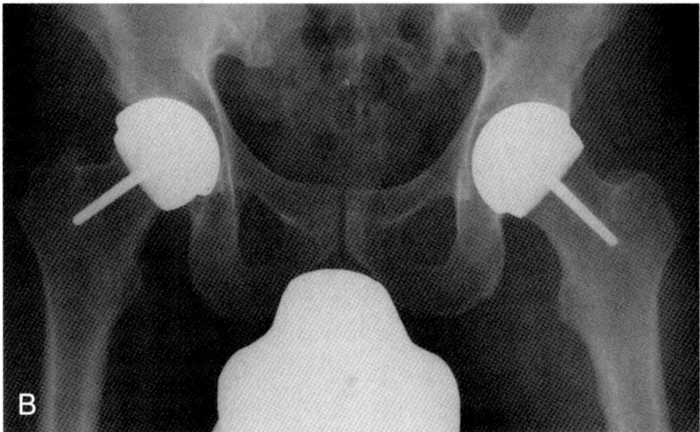

Figure 1-22 **A,** Forty-seven-year-old man with end-stage osteoarthritis of the right hip and showing early degenerative changes on the left side. **B,** The patient underwent staged bilateral resurfacing procedures 7.5 years apart. The radiograph shows a Conserve®Plus resurfacing system featuring the original (5-mm thick) acetabular component 7.8 years after surgery on the right side, and a Conserve®Plus with the new thin shell (3.5 mm) 6 weeks after surgery. The femoral component had a 50-mm outside diameter on the right side and a 52-mm diameter on the left side. Note the slight neck remodeling on the right side. *(Reprinted with permission from Amstutz H, Le Duff M: Background of metal-on-metal resurfacing. Proc Inst Mech Eng [H] 2006;220:85-94.)*

Biologic Bone Preservation and More Normal Joint Physiology

A. The technique preserves the anatomic femoral head and neck, and normalizes the biomechanics of the hip joint, provided that the acetabular shell is thin enough and low profile (e.g., Conserve®Plus thin shell) to minimize the medialization (shift of the center of the joint towards the central axis of the body) that was necessary with the thicker shells.

1. Only the pathologic bone is removed.
2. Although the femoral head subchondral bone is partially removed during the femoral head preparation, the femoral trabecular bone is preserved so that the femoral neck, greater trochanter, lesser trochanter, and subtrochanteric areas are essentially normally loaded from a biomechanical stand point.

B. With the Thin Acetabular Shell Conserve®Plus resurfacing system, acetabular bone stock is preserved. No more acetabular bone is removed than for a conventional THR. Normal anatomic relationships are restored. The proper offset is normalized, and in general, leg lengths are equalized. There is less concern about making the legs of equal length as there is with a THR.

Tribology and Response to Wear Products

A. The metal-on-metal bearing itself is self-healing, with no instances of runaway wear being observed, although opening the socket greater than 55 degrees has been associated with higher wear with the BHR. This association has not been verified to date with the Conserve®Plus device.

B. The inflammatory response to metal debris is considerably reduced compared with polyethylene debris. Incidence and magnitude of osteolysis appear insignificant at 11 years.

Stability of the Hip Joint

Stability has improved significantly compared with conventional stem-type devices using conventional head sizes:

A. Component orientation is anatomic, with excellent initial component stability.

B. Anatomic restoration and stability permits early capsular stretching to maximize range of motion

C. Range of motion is restored and occasionally increased compared with the normal hip.

D. Dislocation risk is minimal in postoperative period and beyond.

E. Recurrent subluxation is rare, and recurrent dislocations have not been observed.

Revisability

A. Because there have been no socket problems, removal is unnecessary and revision to conventional stem-type replacement, if necessary, is relatively simple and much like a primary joint replacement. A unipolar ball with similar metal-on-metal bearing tolerances can be attached to a femoral stem-type device to mate with the existing socket, preserving comparable stability and range of motion to the original resurfacing.

B. Socket loosening with the Conserve®Plus is unlikely because the porous-beaded surface is very stable. However, if it is ever necessary, removal of the socket is relatively simple with minimal bone loss because the socket has no prominent appendages, which are not necessary for initial stability as in most other resurfacing systems.

Component Design

The majority of hip resurfacing systems now are hybrids (cementless acetabular and cemented femoral components) and very similar to the Conserve®Plus with a thin-walled one-piece acetabular component and a femoral component that features a short metaphyseal stem designed for component alignment during insertion. There are many differences in the designs, including component size and increment range, factors influencing both tribology and component fixation as reported in Table 1-2.

Component Size Increments

Femoral and acetabular components in 2-mm increments compared with 4-mm increments enable the surgeon maximum flexibility to optimize bone preparation for different anatomic and pathologic conditions facilitating minimal bone removal of the acetabulum or femoral head. The larger femoral surface area potentially enhances long-term durability. However, in very young patients, it is recommended to remove minimal acetabular bone to save bone stock if the acetabular walls are thin.

Femoral Design and Bone Preparation

The Conserve®Plus femoral bone preparation technique permits fine tuning and optimizing the pin placement before final reaming and subsequent hole preparation for the stem. Other systems require optimal initial pin placement because the stem hole is made before reaming. If it is not optimally positioned it is difficult to alter the direction of reaming.

Cement Mantel Thickness

The designs that allow for a 1-mm cement mantle facilitate a more uniform penetration of doughy acrylic with hand pressurization into all of the reamed areas of the bone and full component seating with light mallet taps if needed. The systems (such as the BHR and the Cormet designs) that have a tighter fit of the femoral component to the prepared bone permit only a very thin or no cement mantle, and a low-viscosity cement must be used that cannot be hand pressurized into the cylindrical reamed bone, reducing penetration. Only a minimal amount of acrylic will penetrate this area because of the shear force generated on the component as it is inserted. In addition, because of the tight fit, it is difficult for cement to extrude between the component and the bone, and there is a danger of overpenetration of cement into the proximal femoral head. Further seating of the component is more difficult with a minimal cement mantle, which often requires hammer blows that could injure the femoral neck. A femoral component tapered geometry also predisposes to a similar difficulty in component seating as compared with a CCD. Long-term follow-up studies will be needed to determine the significance and effects on survivorship of these differing techniques.

Socket Design

Profile

A lower profile of 165 to 170 degrees versus 180 degrees facilitates a more anatomic and conservative approach. Reaming to the floor of the acetabular fossa is generally not necessary. All but one of the designs are spherical. The eccentric socket with

Table 1-2 Comparative Features of Current Metal-on-Metal Hip Resurfacing Designs

System	Year of introduction	Coverage (o)	Clearance (mm)	Shape	Surface	Shell thickness (mm)	Size increments (mm)	Cement Mantle (mm)	Stem
Conserve®Plus	1996	170	100 to 220	Truncated hemisphere	Sintered cobalt-chromium beads (50–150 mm) +/– HA	3.5 or 5	2	1	Tapered, proportional to size
BHR	1997	160 in, 180 out	260 (Size 54 only)	Hemisphere	Cobalt-chromium beads (0.9–1.3 mm) cast-in + HA	3 rim, 6 dome	4	0	Tapered
CORMET	1997	180	250	Equatorial expansion	Ti-VPS + HA	3 and 4 (2 cups per head)	4	0	Slight taper
DUROM	2001	165	150	Truncated hemisphere	Ti-VPS	4	2	1	Tapered
ASR	2003	156 in, 170 out	100	Truncated hemisphere	Sintered cobalt-chromium beads (200–300 mm) + HA	3-5	2	0-1	Tapered, short
ReCap	2004	180	?	Hemisphere	Ti-VPS +/– HA	3	2	0.5	Cylindrical

ASR, articular surface replacement; BHR, Birmingham Hip Resurfacing; HA, hydroxyapatite; Ti-VPS, titanium-vacuum plasma sprayed.

additional 2 mm at the equator may make socket seating more difficult.

Socket Fixation

The plasma spray surfaces and especially small porous beads facilitate optimal initial socket stability in comparison to those sockets with much larger macro beads, which require fins and careful technique to avoid a socket spin out. With the Conserve®Plus, it is feasible to leave the socket uncovered approximately 1 to 2 cm laterally or posteriorly in cases with acetabular dysplasia because the stability attained at insertion is excellent (see Chapter 7). Pelvic adjunct screws are necessary with the BHR and Cormet Designs in Crowe class II developmental dysplasia of the hip (DDH) cases. In addition, those systems that have a simple spherical geometry without adjunct fixation are more simply extracted and reinserted at surgery to optimize component positioning at surgery, or removed with minimal bone loss should they have to be exchanged later after ingrowth.

Wear

There are insufficient data and clinical retrievals to compare the in-service wear of the differing designs. This factor will be difficult to quantify because of the multifactorial nature of wear and there are few comparative simulator studies in which all the variables are controlled. Wear can be minimized by optimizing the clearance and roundness tolerances, and the surface finish of the components to facilitate lubrication. Although this result is somewhat controversial, wear is similar in simulator studies whether the components are made from CoCr or heat treated and solution annealed or forged, which reduces grain and carbide size. Retrieval and simulator data have determined that 80% of the bearing wear occurs on the femoral side. WMT has gathered unpublished simulator data using a bearing with differential hardness making the femoral component harder by forging, which reduces the bearing couple wear by as much as 50%.

Stem Design

The importance of size and shape of the stem is yet to be determined. The Conserve®Plus metaphyseal stem is thinner than that of the BHR and Cormet designs, and the length is proportional to the size of the component. It occupies a smaller portion of the femoral neck, which may decrease the potential for stress shielding, especially in patients with a small femoral head. Long-term analysis will be required to evaluate the true significance of these differences.

Results of Modern Generation Resurfacing Devices

The most recent reports from series with up to 10 years of follow-up (BHR and Conserve®Plus) are extremely encouraging[1,2,5,34,38,39] and illustrate the importance of instrumentation, patient selection and especially surgical technique as the key elements for the success of resurfacing.[3,40-42] In addition short-term follow-up of series of more recently introduced implants are confirming the validity of the concept of resurfacing itself.[43-45]

Today hip resurfacing, once abandoned, has emerged worldwide as a viable option for young and active patients who require a prosthetic solution. This has been possible primarily because of the wear reduction of improved metal-on-metal bearings, and improvements in design and technique. The safety and efficacy of the procedure, and consequently its future popularity, will now rely heavily on the quality of the training programs, emphasizing prevention of femoral neck fractures and component loosening, and ultimately, future efforts to further reduce component wear.

References

1. Back D, Dalziel R, Young D, Shimmin A: Early results of primary Birmingham hip resurfacings. An independent prospective study of the first 230 hips. J Bone Joint Surg 2005;87B:324-329.
2. Amstutz H, Beaulé P, Dorey F, Le Duff M, Campbell P, Gruen T: Metal-on-metal hybrid surface arthroplasty: two to six year follow-up. J Bone Joint Surg 2004;86A:28-39.
3. Beaulé P, Dorey F, Le Duff M, Gruen T, Amstutz H: Risk factors affecting early outcome of metal on metal surface arthroplasty of the hip in patients 40 years old and younger. Clin Orthop 2004;418:87-93.
4. Beaulé P, Le Duff M, Campbell P, Dorey F, Park S, Amstutz H: Metal-on-metal surface arthroplasty with a cemented femoral component: A 7-10 year follow-up study. J Arthroplasty 2004;19:17-22.
5. Daniel J, Pynsent PB, McMinn D: Metal-on-metal resurfacing of the hip in patients under the age of 55 years with osteoarthritis. J Bone Joint Surg 2004;86B:177-188.
6. Amstutz HC, Sparling EA, Grigoris P, Campbell PA, Dorey FJ: Surface replacement: the hip replacement of the future. Hip International 1998;8:187-207.
7. Grigoris P, Roberts P, Panousis K, Bosch H: The evolution of hip resurfacing arthroplasty. Orthop Clin North Am 2005;36:125-134.
8. Amstutz H, Le Duff M: Background of metal-on-metal resurfacing. Proc Inst Mech Eng [H] 2006;220:85-94.
9. Smith-Petersen M: Evolution of mould arthroplasty of the hip joint. J Bone Joint Surg 1948;30 B:59-75.
10. Müller M, Boltzy X: Artificial hip joints made from Protasul. Bull Assoc Study Probl Internal Fixation 1968;1-5.
11. Gerard Y: Hip arthroplasty by matching cups. Clin Orthop Rel Res 1978;134:25-35.
12. Gerard Y, Chelius P, Legrand A: Hip arthroplasty using non-cemented paired cups. 14-year experience. Rev Chir Orthop Reparatrice Appar Mot 1985;71(Suppl):82-85.
13. Bell RS, Schatzker J, Fornasier VL, Goodman SB: A study of implant failure in the Wagner resurfacing arthroplasty. J Bone Joint Surg Am 1985;67A:1165-1175.
14. Head WC: Wagner surface replacement arthroplasty of the hip. Analysis of fourteen failures in forty-one hips. J Bone Joint Surg Am 1981;63:420-427.
15. Jolley M, Salvati E, Brown G: Early results and complications of surface replacement of the hip. J Bone Joint Surg Am 1982;64:366-377.

16. Kabo J, Gebhard J, Loren G, Amstutz H: In vivo wear of polyethylene acetabular components. J Bone Joint Surg 1993;75B:254-258.
17. Amstutz H: Hip Arthroplasty. New York, Churchill Livingstone, 1991, p 975.
18. Amstutz H, Grigoris P, Dorey F: Evolution and future of surface replacement of the hip. J Orthop Sci 1998;3:169-186.
19. Schmalzried TP, Jasty M, Harris WH: Periprosthetic bone loss in total hip arthroplasty. Polyethylene wear debris and the concept of the effective joint space. J Bone Joint Surg 1992;74A:849-863.
20. Beaulé P, Amstutz H, Le Duff M, Dorey F: Surface arthroplasty for osteonecrosis of the hip: Hemiresurfacing versus metal-on-metal hybrid resurfacing. J Arthroplasty 2004;19:54-58.
21. Beaulé P, Schmalzried T, Campbell P, Dorey F, Amstutz H: Duration of symptoms and outcome of hemiresurfacing for hip osteonecrosis. Clin Orthop Rel Res 2001;385:104-117.
22. Campbell P, Mirra J, Amstutz HC: Viability of femoral heads treated with resurfacing arthroplasty. J Arthroplasty 2000;15: 120-122.
23. Freeman M: Some anatomical and mechanical considerations relevant to the surface replacement of the femoral head. Clin Orthop Rel Res 1978;134:19-24.
24. Mai MT, Schmalzried TP, Dorey FJ, Campbell PA, Amstutz HC: The contribution of frictional torque to loosening at the cement-bone interface in Tharies hip replacements. J Bone Joint Surg Am 1996;78:505-511.
25. Muller ME: The benefits of metal-on-metal total hip replacements. Clin Orthop Rel Res 1995;54-59.
26. McKee GK, Watson-Farrar J: Replacement of arthritic hips by the McKee-Farrar prosthesis. J Bone Joint Surg 1966;48B:245-259.
27. Ring PA: Complete replacement arthroplasty of the hip by the Ring prosthesis. J Bone Joint Surg 1968;50B:720-731.
28. Smith S, Dowson D, Goldsmith A: The effect of femoral head diameter upon lubrication and wear of metal-on-metal total hip replacements. Proc Inst Mech Eng [H] 2001;215:161-170.
29. Rieker C, Schon R, Konrad R, Liebentritt G, Gnepf P, Shen M, Roberts P, Grigoris P: Influence of the clearance on in-vitro tribology of large diameter metal-on-metal articulations pertaining to resurfacing hip implants. Orthop Clin North Am 2005;36:135-142.
30. Sieber HP, Rieker CB, Kottig P: Analysis of 118 second-generation metal-on-metal retrieved hip implants. J Bone Joint Surg Br 1999;81:46-50.
31. Wagner M, Wagner H: Preliminary results of uncemented metal on metal stemmed and resurfacing hip replacement arthroplasty. Clin Orthop Rel Res 1996;329(Suppl):S78-S88.
32. McMinn D, Treacy R, Lin K, Pynsent P: Metal on metal surface replacement of the hip. Experience of the McMinn prothesis. Clin Orthop Rel Res 1996;329(Suppl):S89-S98.
33. Bohm R, Schraml A, Schuh A: Long-term results with the Wagner metal-on-metal hip resurfacing prosthesis. Hip International 2006;16:58-64.
34. Schmalzried T, Silva M, de la Rosa M, Choi E, Fowble V: Optimizing patient selection and outcomes with total hip resurfacing. Clin Orthop Relat Res 2005;441:200-204.
35. Schmalzried TP, Fowble VA, Ure KJ, Amstutz HC: Metal on metal surface replacement of the hip. Technique, fixation, and early results. Clin Orthop Rel Res 1996;S106-S114.
36. Townley C: Hemi and total articular replacement arthroplasty of the hip with the fixed femoral cup. Orthop Clin North Am 1982;13:809-894.
37. Dowson D, Hardaker C, Flett M, Isaac G: A hip joint simulator study of the performance of metal-on-metal joints—Part II: Design. J Arthroplasty 2004;19:124-130.
38. Treacy R, McBryde C, Pynsent P: Birmingham hip resurfacing arthroplasty. A minimum follow-up of five years. J Bone Joint Surg Br 2005;87:167-170.
39. De Smet K: Belgium experience with metal-on-metal surface arthroplasty. Orthop Clin North Am 2005;36:203-213.
40. Amstutz H, Campbell P, Le Duff M: Fracture of the neck of the femur after surface arthroplasty of the hip. J Bone Joint Surg 2004;86A:1874-1877.
41. Beaulé P, Lee J, Le Duff M, Amstutz H, Ebramzadeh E: Orientation of the femoral component in surface arthroplasty of the hip: a biomechanical and clinical analysis. J Bone Joint Surg 2004;86-A:2015-2021.
42. Amstutz H, Le Duff M, Campbell P, Dorey F: The effects of technique changes on aseptic loosening of the femoral component in hip resurfacing. Results of 600 Conserve Plus with a 3-9 year follow-up. J Arthroplasty 2007;22:481-489.
43. Siebel T, Maubach S, Morlock M: Lessons learned from early clinical experience and results of 300 ASR hip resurfacing implantations. Proc Inst Mech Eng [H] 2006;220:345-353.
44. Vendittoli P, Lavigne M, Roy A, Lusignan D: A prospective randomized clinical trial comparing metal-on-metal total hip arthroplasty and metal-on-metal total hip resurfacing in patients less than 65 years old. Hip International 2006;16: 873-881.
45. Grigoris P, Roberts P, Panousis K: The development of the Durom metal-on-metal hip resurfacing. Hip International 2006;16: 65-72.

CHAPTER 2

Femoral Head Vascularity and Hip Resurfacing

Ahmad Bin Nasser

Paul E. Beaulé

Introduction

Hip resurfacing is regaining popularity among orthopedic surgeons as an alternative to conventional total hip arthroplasty for the young active patient with symptomatic hip arthritis.[1]

Thus far, survival rates at 5 years have ranged from 94% to 99%,[2,3] which is a significant improvement over the first generation of metal on polyethylene[4,5] resurfacings. These improved results are for the most part due to the introduction of metal on metal bearings and cementless acetabular fixation.[1] However long-term follow-up will be critical to confirm its place in the treatment of hip arthritis as well as minimizing early failures secondary to femoral neck fracture, which is unique to hip resurfacing. Femoral neck fracture after hip resurfacing is multifactorial in origin with both mechanical and biological components.[6] In terms of mechanical causes, varus positioning of the femoral component and notching of the femoral neck have been implicated.[7,8] Although the risk of neck fracture with varus positioning relates to abnormal mechanical stresses on the femoral neck,[9] notching may also compromise the blood flow to the femoral head[10] with a possible subsequent osteonecrotic event. The occurrence of femoral neck fracture as well as femoral loosening in the presence of osteonecrotic lesions within retrieved femoral heads[11,12] have fostered the ongoing concern that disruption of the vascularity to the femoral head after resurfacing may lead to premature failure of the femoral component.[6]

There are multiple factors to be considered when one is evaluating the vascularity of the arthritic femoral head and its impact on the clinical performance of metal on metal hip resurfacing. These would include the surgical anatomy of the extraosseous blood supply and its importance to the choice of surgical approach as well as implantation technique and type of femoral fixation.

Although a complete understanding of the impact of compromising femoral head vascularity while performing hip resurfacing is yet to be reached, knowledge of these variables should aid the surgeon in making an informed decision on how to proceed with this surgical procedure.

Extraosseous Blood Supply to the Normal Femoral Head

The ascending branch of the medial femoral circumflex artery (MFCA) is the most important vascular nutrient vessel to the femoral head,[13] although its role in the arthritic hip has been questioned.[14,15] In the majority of people, the medial femoral circumflex artery originates from the profunda femoris artery but occasionally it branches off the superficial femoral artery. One of its branches, the ascending branch, runs to the intertrochanteric crest between the pectineus medially and the iliopsoas laterally at the level of the inferior border of the obturator externus. It gives off a trochanteric branch at the proximal border of the quadratus femoris then passes posterior to the obturator externus and anterior to the gemelli muscles and obturator internus (Fig. 2-1). Then it perforates the capsule at the caudal edge of piriformis and divides into two to four retinacular branches that run deep to the synovial sheath on the posterior superior aspect of the femoral neck to enter the bone through vascular foramina located 2 to 4 mm lateral to the cartilage bone junction[13] (Fig. 2-2). Eighty percent of the vascular foramina are located on the superior aspect of the neck/head junction mostly posterosuperiorly and to a lesser extent anterosuperiorly.[16] Finally, one in five hips has an inferior retinacular branch entering the femoral head along the inferior neck, which could compensate for damage to the superior vessels.[6]

With this knowledge, it is clear that the integrity of the ascending branch of MFCA will be compromised by an approach that involves detachment of the short external rotators, more specifically the obturator externus tendon. This would be the case for the posterior approach to the hip which

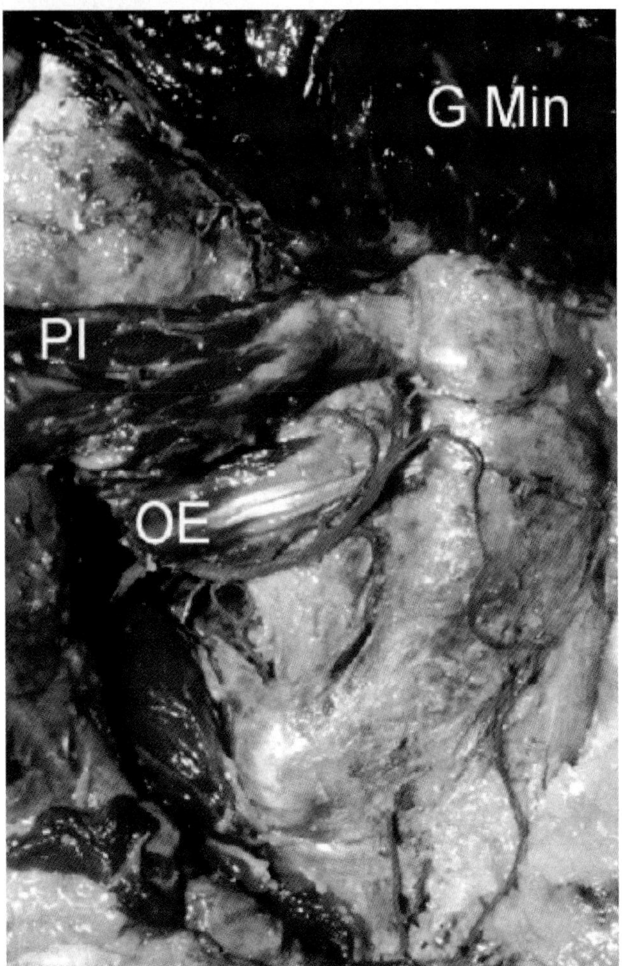

Figure 2-1 Dissection of the posterior part of the hip. The medial femoral circumflex artery follows the inferior border of the obturator externus (OE), overcrosses its tendon, and undercrosses the short external rotators and piriformis muscle (PI) before entering the posterior capsule (the gluteus minimus nuscle [G Min]). *(Reprinted with permission from The Journal of Bone and Joint Surgery, Inc., Beaule PE, Campbell P, Lu Z, et al: Vascularity of the arthritic femoral head and hip resurfacing. J Bone Joint Surg Am 2006;88A (Suppl 4):85-96, Fig 4.)*

is the most common approach for hip resurfacing for the arthritic hip.[2,3,17,18]

Blood Supply to the Arthritic Femoral Head

Freeman[14] introduced the concept that the blood supply in the arthritic hip is different based on intraoperative observation of osteophytes at the head-neck junction compressing the retinacular vessels, and leading to the development of an intraosseous collateral circulation. Whiteside and associates[19] tested this concept on a dog model and found that stripping the retinaculum and reaming the femoral head in normal nonarthritic hips stopped femoral head blood flow, whereas in six arthritic hips (three secondary to developmental dysplasia of the hip [DDH] and three secondary to "induced" arthritis), the femoral heads were still vascular although flow was significantly decreased. Although the degree of arthritis was not stated or illustrated, he cautioned surgeons against destruction

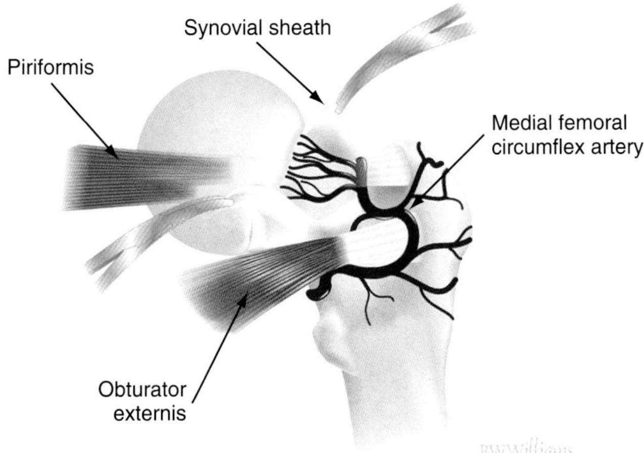

Figure 2-2 Illustration of the posterior aspect of the hip showing the relationship of the ascending of the medial circumflex artery to the obturator externus and short external rotators. *(Reprinted with permission from The Journal of Bone and Joint Surgery, Inc., Beaule PE, Campbell P, Lu Z, et al: Vascularity of the arthritic femoral head and hip resurfacing. J Bone Joint Surg Am 2006;88A (Suppl 4):85-96, Fig 5.)*

of the retinacular vessels in the arthritic head, because the intraosseous channels may not be sufficiently developed to protect against diffuse osteonecrosis.

There are several studies that have confirmed a significant acute reduction in blood flow to the arthritic femoral head intraoperatively[10,11,20-22] and extremes of hip positioning. Khan and associates[21] reported cefuroxime levels in retrieved arthritic femoral heads in patients undergoing total hip replacement through either a lateral approach or a posterior approach were significantly lower in the group that underwent the posterior approach, suggesting an impairment in blood flow to the femoral head. Similarly, Steffen and associates[20] looked at oxygen concentration using a gas electrode system at the superolateral aspect of the femoral head before and after completion of the posterolateral approach in patients undergoing hip resurfacing, and found a 60% drop in oxygen tension, with an additional 20% drop after implant insertion. Most of the drop in the oxygen tension occurred with the detachment of the short external rotators and the posterior capsulotomy.

These findings have led some surgeons to pursue alternative approaches for hip resurfacing as well as maximizing the preservation of the soft tissue envelope around the femoral head neck junction in order to avoid impairing the vascularity of the femoral head and minimize the incidence of femoral component failure due to osteonecrosis.[23,24] Based on the anatomy of the extraosseous blood supply to the femoral head, a disruption can occur at the level of the medial femoral circumflex artery or its ascending branch when approaching the posterior aspect of the proximal femur, or at the level of the retinacular branches on the superior aspect of the femoral neck.[6] One such example of potential damage to the vasculature can occur with notching of the femoral neck. De Waal Malefijit and Huiskes[25] found that hips that had notching

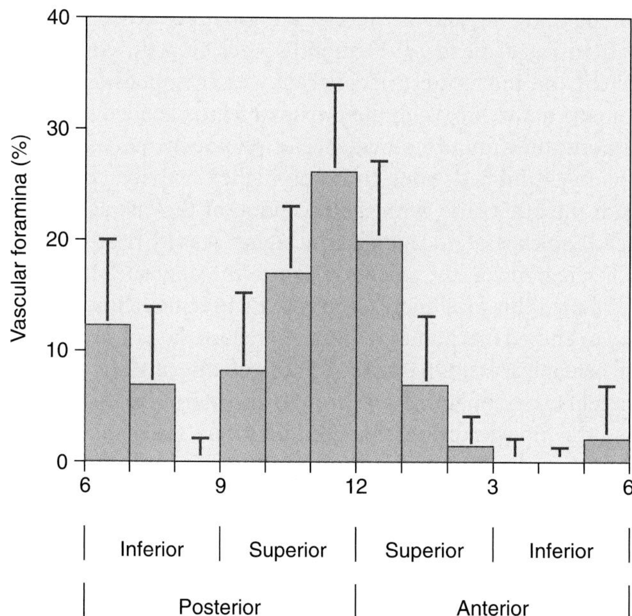

Figure 2-3 Simulation of femoral head after reaming for hip resurfacing as it relates to the blood supply. *(Reprinted with permission from British Journal of Bone and Joint Surgery, Sevitt S, Thompson RG. The distribution and anastomoses of arteries supplying the head and neck of the femur. J Bone Joint Surg Br 1965;47:560–573, Fig 10.)*

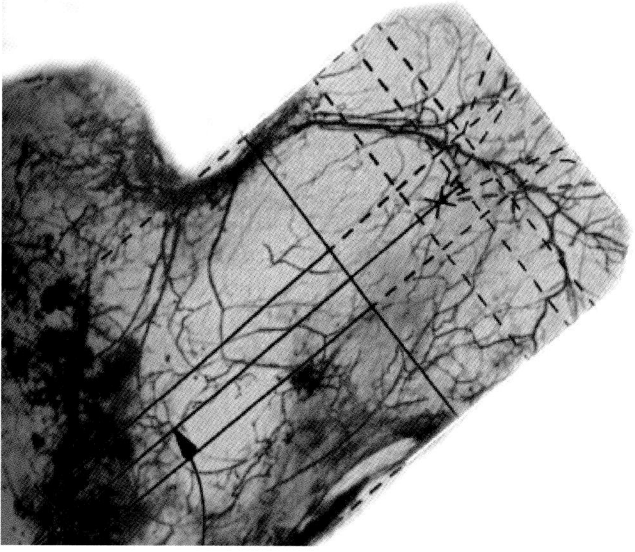

Figure 2-4 Distribution of the vascular foramina at the femoral head neck junction using a clock face. *(Reprinted from Orthopedic Clinics of North America, Lavigne M, Kalhor M, Beck M, et al: Distribution of vascular foramina around the femoral head and neck junction: relevance for conservative intracapsular procedures of the hip. Orthop Clin North Am 2005;36:171–176, with permission from Elsevier.)*

during resurfacing had a higher rate of femoral loosening than those without notching, which is somewhat contrary to the concept that notching leads to femoral neck fracture by means of mechanically weakening the superior subcapital region.[8] To examine the impact of femoral neck notching on femoral head blood flow, Beaulé and associates[10] using laser Doppler flowmetry evaluated patients undergoing total hip replacement through a lateral approach. Using an osteotome to notch the femoral neck superiorly at the level of the retinacular vessels in order to mimic the cylindrical reamer engaging the femoral neck, 10 out of 14 hips showed a drop in femoral head blood flow of more than 50%. The fact that not all the hips experienced the same degree of blood flow may be explained by the variable distribution of the foramina around the neck in relation to the entry point of the osteotome where some of the retinacular vessels may have been spared (Fig. 2-3). In another study, Beaulé again using laser Doppler flowmetry in patients undergoing hip resurfacing through a surgical dislocation as described by Ganz,[26] the use of the cylindrical reamer on the head without breaching the femoral neck cortex caused a 70% drop in femoral head blood flow in nine out of 10 patients. Based on these data, they recommended directing the reamer superolaterally and staying as close as possible to the inferomedial neck because damage to the retinacular vessels can occur without penetrating the femoral neck (Fig. 2-4).

Although it is known that a decrease in blood flow can result in osteonecrosis,[27] the relationship of failure of the femoral component secondary to osteonecrosis is controversial.[12,15,17] The disruption of the femoral head blood supply may play a role in the occurrence of femoral neck fracture, but the exact pathogenesis is unknown.[6,11] Thus, although disruption of the femoral head blood supply inevitably plays a role in the occurrence of femoral neck fracture,[6,11] the actual incidence of femoral neck fracture after resurfacing is relatively low at less than 2%.[3,15,28] A more common mode of failure shown in multiple studies such as those by Pollard[29] and Amstutz[2] has been aseptic loosening of the femoral component. Although surgical technique in terms of femoral head preparation is paramount (see Chapter 9), the presence or absence of femoral head cysts has been demonstrated to be a major factor influencing durability of femoral fixation, and an osteonecrotic event within the femoral head followed by the reparative phase could compromise the fixation area to permit implant micromotion and ultimately loosening of the femoral component.[30] Unfortunately, it is not clear from retrieval analysis what the respective roles of potential thermal or vascular insult in the loosening process (see Chapter 10).

One explanation might be that an osteonecrotic event actually occurred, but the necrotic bone is no longer present, having been either resorbed during the reparative phase or with implant micromotion.[12] Another likely explanation is that for osteonecrosis to occur, a certain threshold must be reached,[6] and other factors come into play such as the presence or absence of an intraosseous blood supply, extent of cement penetration, as well as bone quality. Unfortunately, we have yet to determine what that threshold might be for each individual patient. Consequently, it would appear preferable to preserve as much of the blood supply to the femoral head as possible by minimizing the dissection around the retinacular vessels as well as its main nutrient artery, especially in relatively early cases of arthritis.

Assessment of Viability of Femoral Heads After Failed Hip Resurfacing

A review of the literature on retrieval analysis of metal-on-polyethylene resurfacing designs is complex and difficult to correlate to the metal-on-metal designs.[6] The massive osteolysis associated with the polyethylene debris complicated the analysis of the failed specimens as well as the frequent lack of differentiation between generalized osteonecrosis and more focal disease and thermal necrosis from cement polymerization.[31] There was also a wide variability in the actual definition of histologic osteonecrosis.[32-34] Howie and associates[32] performed a detailed retrieval analysis of 72 failed hip resurfacings, differentiating between diffuse and localized osteonecrosis, and attempted to correlate the degree of loosening with the histologic appearance. They found that diffuse necrosis was rare, with patchy necrosis present in four of 64 cases of loosening. Campbell and associates[12] performed an analysis of 98 failed modern hybrid metal-on-metal designs, including 28 that failed from neck fracture and 23 from femoral loosening. Five femoral loosening cases had complete loss of the cement-bone interface and resorption of proximal bone. Histologic analysis noted the presence of healed osteonecrosis in many of the femoral failures, although whether the initial cause was mechanical, chemical, thermal, or vascular could not be determined. Although the role of vascular damage in the majority of femoral failures was unclear, five cases that failed from late (median 15 months) fracture, and two that were revised for unexplained pain, were found to have large proximal segments of avascular necrotic bone, and the lack of remodeling was consistent with devascularization occurring at the time of surgery.

Little and associates[11] reported that 12 of 13 hips that had a fractured neck out of 377 consecutive hip resurfacing procedures performed through a posterior approach had a variable degree of osteonecrosis both central and peripheral. They concluded that hip resurfacing can cause osteonecrosis of the subcapital region and that this could lead to failure of the procedure, although this was only seen in 1.9% of their cases.

As mentioned earlier, the extent of cement penetration within the femoral head may influence bone viability due to thermal necrosis during cement polymerization.[12] Campbell and associates[12] found that femoral failures due to loosening had significantly more total cement than those revised for other modes of failure. At present, in order to minimize the risk of thermal necrosis, it is recommended to use copious irrigation on the metal shell during the curing process as well as suction in the lesser trochanter.[35]

Assessment of Vascularity of the Femoral Head After Resurfacing in Well-Functioning, Asymptomatic Patients

Two recent studies have studied femoral head viability after hip resurfacing using nuclear imaging technology.[36,37] Forest and associates,[36] using [18F] fluoride positron emission tomography, looked at a selected group of asymptomatic patients at a mean of 20 months after surgery, comparing activity on the hip resurfacing side with the opposite asymptomatic native hip. With the proximal femur divided into four regions, they found no evidence of photopenic areas, and all regions exhibited nonsignificant higher activity compared with the other side, with the exception of the lateral femoral head, which showed significantly higher activity relative to the other regions on the same hip and to the opposite side. They attributed this focal increase in activity to remodeling secondary to altered mechanics rather than reperfusion of small areas of osteonecrosis. One critical point of this study is that all patients were operated on through an anterolateral approach and the hip was dislocated anteriorly. Thus, the main nutrient artery to the retinacular vessels was preserved. In another study by McMahon and associates,[37] Tc 99m bone scan/single-emission computed tomography was used on 32 asymptomatic patients, who were compared with 36 patients whose hips were resurfaced through a posterior approach at a mean of 26 months' follow-up. The result of the scans showed 60% to 85% activity in the resurfaced hips compared with the normal contralateral hips, and the resurfaced hips were considered normal. They concluded that all femoral heads were vascular but could not comment on their viability. More specifically, little is known of the bone viability at the interface as well as presence or absence of a reparative process secondary to an osteonecrotic event.

From the current available data, the importance of the extraosseous blood supply in maintaining overall femoral head viability has yet to be fully determined. Sophisticated imaging techniques such as that reported by McMahon and associates[37] need to be pursued in order to evaluate the three-dimensional aspects of femoral head vascularity as a function of different surgical techniques and approaches, as well as prosthetic survival.

Surgical Technique

Finally, careful surgical technique in terms of minimizing the damage to the femoral head vasculature has a direct impact on the different variables discussed earlier. Avoiding excessive dissection of the posterosuperior neck and careful reaming of the femoral head will help maintain the retinacular vessels. Finally, the choice of surgical approach will also have an impact on femoral head vascularity[20,21] and choosing an approach that dislocates the hip anteriorly, maintaining the attachment of the obturator externus tendon, has the potential for preserving more femoral head vascularity.[23,24] The need for these measures in an arthritic hip that has increased blood flow remains controversial. The lateral approach offers adequate exposure, preserves the blood supply, but risks abductor weakness. Also, in cases of larger femoral heads, acetabular exposure can be difficult. In 2001, Ganz and associates[26] described a technique of surgically dislocating the nonarthritic hip joint without causing osteonecrosis, which was reproduced by others. This approach involves a trochanteric slide osteotomy exiting proximally, leaving a cuff of the gluteus medius attached to the greater trochanter as well as all the short external rotators. The gluteus medius and minimus are mobilized anterosuperiorly and a z-capsulotomy is performed, permitting an anterior hip dislocation. This approach allows excellent exposure of the proximal femur and the acetabulum while preserving the blood supply to the femoral head. However, this approach carries a risk of nonunion of the osteotomy site as well as increased incidence of trochanteric bursitis, which can require removal of internal fixation later. The senior author has had extensive experience with this approach for hip resurfacing. In a consecutive series of 119 hips, there were three cases of fibrous union and six nonunions, with three cases of nonunion requiring a reoperation. An alternative approach, preserving the blood supply without the need for a trochanteric osteotomy, is the Hueter anterior approach.[6,38] Although not commonly used in North America, this method has been used more extensively in Europe for total hip replacements and hip resurfacing. It involves minimal soft tissue trauma, allowing early rehabilitation, but requires a specialized operating table that allows a wide range of motion of the hip during the surgery. It is not an extensile approach, and proper patient selection for this approach is recommended, such as avoiding cases of protrusio and short varus necks.

Controversy remains as to which approach is best suited for hip resurfacing, and although the posterior approach is currently the most commonly used, long-term studies comparing the durability of components inserted through different approaches will be required to determine the optimal approach. Until then, we recommend the surgeon who is starting hip resurfacing to use the approach he or she is most comfortable with.

Summary

Hip resurfacing arthroplasty is increasingly being performed, and techniques to increase its durability to match the results of total hip replacement need to continue to be pursued. The vascularity of the proximal femur after resurfacing plays a role in the femoral failures and can be minimized by careful surgical technique. Finally, although osteonecrosis does occur, a certain threshold must be reached; thus, the surgeon should attempt to preserve as much as possible of the vascularity to the femoral head.

References

1. Beaule PE: Surface arthroplasty of the hip: a review and current indications. Semin Arthroplasty 2005;16:70-76.
2. Amstutz HC, Beaule PE, Dorey FJ, Campbell PA, Le Duff MJ, Gruen TA: Metal-on-metal hybrid surface arthroplasty: two to six year follow-up. J Bone Joint Surg 2004;86A:28-39.
3. Treacy R, Pynsent P: Birmingham Hip Resurfacing arthroplasty. A minimum follow-up of five years. J Bone Joint Surg 2005; 87B:167-170.
4. Howie DW, Campbell D, McGee M, Cornish BL: Wagner resurfacing hip arthroplasty. The results of one hundred consecutive arthroplasties after eight to ten years. J Bone Joint Surg 1990; 72A:708-714.
5. Amstutz HC, Dorey F, OCarroll PF: THARIES resurfacing arthroplasty. Evolution and long-term results. Clin Orthop Rel Res 1986;213:92-114.
6. Beaule PE, Campbell PA, Lu Z, Leunig-Ganz K, Beck M, Leunig M, et al: Vascularity of the arthritic femoral head and hip resurfacing. J Bone Joint Surg 2006;88A(Suppl 4):85-96.
7. Shimmin A, Back D: Femoral neck fractures following Birmingham hip resurfacing. A national review of 50 cases. J Bone Joint Surg 2005;87B:463-464.
8. Markolf KL, Amstutz HC: Mechanical strength of the femur following resurfacing and conventional total hip replacement procedures. Clin Orthop Rel Res 1980;147:170-180.
9. Beaule PE, Lee J, LeDuff M, Dorey FJ, Amstutz HC, Ebramzadeh E: Orientation of femoral component in surface arthroplasty of the hip: A biomechanical and clinical analysis. J Bone Joint Surg 2004;86A:2015-2021.
10. Beaule PE, Campbell PA, Hoke R, Dorey FJ: Notching of the femoral neck during resurfacing arthroplasty of the hip. A vascular study. J Bone Joint Surg 2006;88:35-39.
11. Little CP, Ruiz AL, Harding IJ, McLardy-Smith P, Gundle R, Murray DW, et al: Osteonecrosis in retrieved femoral heads after failed resurfacing arthroplasty of the hip. J Bone Joint Surg 2005;87B:320-323.
12. Campbell PA, Beaule PE, Ebramzadeh E, LeDuff MJ, De Smet KA, Lu Z, et al: The John Charnley Award: A study of implant failure in metal-on-metal surface arthroplasties. Clin Orthop Rel Res 2006;453:35-46.
13. Gautier E, Ganz K, Krugel N, Gill TJ, Ganz R: Anatomy of the medial circumflex artery and its surgical implications. J Bone Joint Surg 2000;82B:679-683.
14. Freeman MAR: Some anatomical and mechanical considerations relevant to the surface replacement of the femoral head. Clin Orthop Rel Res 1978;134:19-24.
15. Amstutz HC, Le Duff MJ, Campbell PA: Fracture of the neck of the femur after surface arthroplasty of the hip. J Bone Joint Surg 2004;86A:1874-1877.
16. Lavigne M, Kalhor M, Beck M, Ganz R, Leunig M: Distribution of vascular foramina around the femoral head and neck junction: relevance for conservative intracapsular procedures of the hip. Orthop Clin North Am 2005;36:171-176.
17. Daniel J, Pynsent PB, McMinn DJW: Metal-on-metal resurfacing of the hip in patients under the age of 55 years with osteoarthritis. J Bone Joint Surg 2004;86B:177-184.
18. Back DL, Dalziel R, Young D, Shimmin A: Early results of primary Birmingham Hip Resurfacings. An independent prospective study of the first 230 hips. J Bone Joint Surg 2005;87B:324-329.
19. Whiteside LA, Lange DR, Capello WN, Fraser B: The effects of surgical procedures on the blood supply to the femoral head. J Bone Joint Surg 1983;65A:1127-1133.
20. Steffen RT, Smith SR, Urban JP, McClardy-Smith P, Beard DJ, Gill HS, et al: The effect of hip resurfacing on oxygen concentration in the femoral head. J Bone Joint Surg 2005;87:1468-1474.
21. Khan A, Yates P, Lovering A, Bannister GC, Spencer RF: The effect of surgical approach on blood flow to the femoral head during resurfacing. J Bone Joint Surg 2007;89B:25.
22. Beaule PE, Campbell PA, Shim P: Femoral head blood flow during hip resurfacing. Clin Orthop Rel Res 2006;456:148-152.

23. Beaule PE: A soft tissue sparing approach to surface arthroplasty of the hip. Oper Tech Ortho 2004;14:16-18.
24. Nork SE, Schar M, Pfander G, Beck M, Djonov V, Ganz R, et al: Anatomic considerations for the choice of surgical approach for hip resurfacing arthroplasty. Orthop Clin North Am 2005;36: 163-170.
25. de Waal Malefijt MC, Huiskes R: A clinical, radiological and biomechanical study of the TARA hip prosthesis. Arch Orthop Trauma Surg 1993;112:220-225.
26. Ganz R, Gill TJ, Gautier E, Ganz K, Krugel N, Berlemann U: Surgical dislocation of the adult hip. A new technique with full access to the femoral head and acetabulum without the risk of avascular necrosis. J Bone Joint Surg 2001;83B:1119-1124.
27. Nishino M, Matsumoto T, Nakamura T, Tomita K: Pathological and hemodynamic study in a new model of femoral head necrosis following traumatic dislocation. Arch Orthop Trauma Surg 1997;116:259-262.
28. Shimmin AJ, Black D: Femoral neck fractures following Birmingham hip resurfacing. A national review of 50 cases. J Bone Joint Surg 2005;87B:463-464.
29. Pollard TCB, Baker RP, Eastaugh-Waring SJ, Bannister GC: Treatment of the young active patient with osteoarthritis of the hip. Two to seven year comparison of hybrid total hip arthroplasty and metal-on-metal resurfacing. J Bone Joint Surg 2006; 88B:592-600.
30. Mjoberg B: Theories of wear and loosening in hip prostheses. Wear-induced loosening vs loosening-induced wear-a review. Acta Othop Scand 1994;65:361-371.
31. Howie D, Cornish B, Vernon-Roberts B: Resurfacing hip arthroplasty. Classification of loosening and the role of prosthetic wear particles. Clin Orthop Rel Res 1990;255:144-159.
32. Howie DW, Cornish BL, Vernon-Roberts B: The viability of the femoral head after resurfacing hip arthroplasty in humans. Clin Orthop Rel Res 1993;291:171-184.
33. Campbell PA, Mirra J, Amstutz HC: Viability of femoral head treated with resurfacing arthroplasty. J Arthroplasty 2000;15: 120-122.
34. Bell RS, Schatzker J, Fornasier VL, Goodman SB: A study of implant failure in the Wagner resurfacing arthroplasty. J Bone Joint Surg 1985;67A:1165-1175.
35. Gill HS, Campbell PA, Murray DW, De Smet KA: Reduction of the potential for thermal damage during hip resurfacing. J Bone Joint Surg 2007;89B:16-20.
36. Forrest N, Murray AD, Schweiger L, Hutchison J, Ashcroft SA: Femoral head viability after Birmingham resurfacing hip arthroplasty: assessment with use of [18F] fluoride positron emission tomography. J Bone Joint Surg 2006;88A(Suppl 3): 84-89.
37. McMahon ST, Young D, Ballok Z, Badaruddin BS, Larbaiboonpong V, Hawdon G: Vascularity of the femoral head after Birmingham hip resurfacing. A technetium Tc 99m bone scan/single photon emission computed tomography study. J Arthroplasty 2006;21:514-521.
38. Judet J, Judet R: The use of an artificial femoral head for arthroplasty of the hip joint. J Bone Joint Surg 1950;32B: 166-173.

CHAPTER 3

The Mechanics of the Resurfaced Hip

J. Paige Little

David J. Simpson

Richie H. S. Gill

Introduction

One of the main quoted advantages of hip resurfacing is that it maintains normal mechanics as opposed to the abnormal cantilever loading of a conventional total hip replacement (THR). This chapter focuses on the mechanical effects of resurfacing, in terms of the immediate situation and possible longer term consequences.

The human hip joint is required to function in a very demanding mechanical environment, part of which is due to the way in which our joints work. The joints in the body allow mobility, and are both stabilized and activated by the action of muscles. Without the stabilizing effect of muscles, the skeleton would collapse. In order to move a given limb, an unbalanced joint moment is required to act at the joint connecting that limb to the rest of the body. Before delving further into this topic, a brief framework of terminology and background will be given.

Mechanics covers two fundamental fields of study, statics and dynamics. The names of these fields are very descriptive:

Statics: The science that deals with forces that balance each other to keep objects in a state of rest. *(Concise Oxford English Dictionary)*

Dynamics: The science of forces involved in movement. *(Concise Oxford English Dictionary)*

In this chapter, we are mostly going to cover statics, but will brush on dynamics. Both of the above-mentioned definitions include force, which deserves a definition of its own:

Force: An effect that causes objects to move in a particular way *(Concise Oxford English Dictionary)*. Units are newtons (N). The definition of 1 N is the force required to accelerate 1 kg of mass by 1 meter per second per second.

A more useful definition is "a disembodied push or pull," and forces generally act in a particular direction. The main concept is that we need only consider what a particular force does, the laws of mechanics do not care what gives rise to a given force. Forces act on objects (or bodies), and cause them to change their behavior; the direction in which a force acts is termed the line of action.

In statics, the concept of equilibrium is important. Consider the following situation (Fig. 3-1), in which an object is at rest on a level table. The object (of mass m) will feel the effect of gravity, producing a force W equal to its mass multiplied by the g, the acceleration due to gravity. This force will act downward. The table provides an equal and opposite force, R, acting upward, the reaction force. Because these two forces are equal and opposite and act at the same point, the net effect is of no forces acting and, therefore, no movement of the object. It is said to be in static equilibrium.

Moments are caused by forces acting on rigid bodies such that a rotary motion is induced. In Figure 3-2, we have a see-saw with an object of mass m_1 placed on one side of the see-saw, which generates a force W_1 ($= m_1 \times g$) acting at a certain distance from the pivot point. The important distance as far as moments are concerned has a very precise definition and is termed the moment arm. The moment arm of a given force is the perpendicular distance between the line of action of the force and the pivot point (or center of rotation). The amount of turning effect or magnitude of the moment generated is given by the product of the force and the moment arm. Thus, if M_1 is the moment generated by the force W_1, we can determine its magnitude from the following relationship:

$$M_1 = W_1 \times a$$

Therefore, the units of moments are newton meters (Nm). If the see-saw was originally level before the object m_1 was placed upon it, the effect of placing the object on the left-hand side of the see-saw is to give rise to an unbalanced moment tending to rotate the see-saw counterclockwise. Because the see-saw is not in equilibrium, it will rotate in a counter-clockwise direction (until the edge contacts the ground and provides a balancing reaction force). For a body to be in full

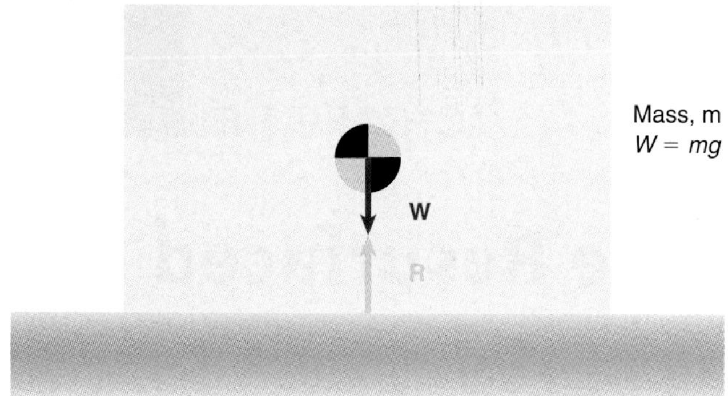

Figure 3-1 Static mass resting on a surface; reaction force is equal and opposite to the weight of the mass.

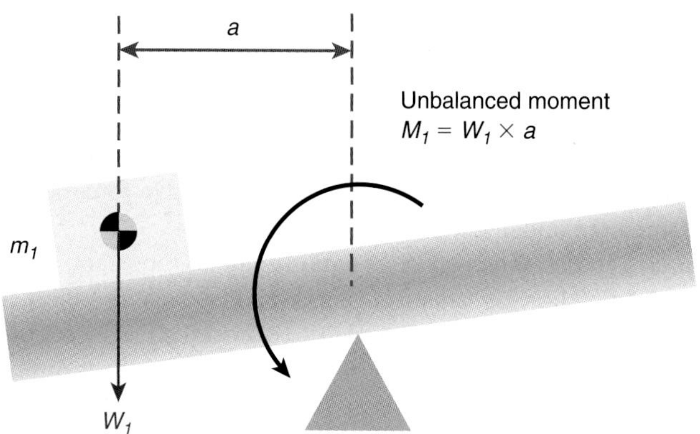

Figure 3-2 Unbalanced see-saw, mass gives rise to an unbalanced moment.

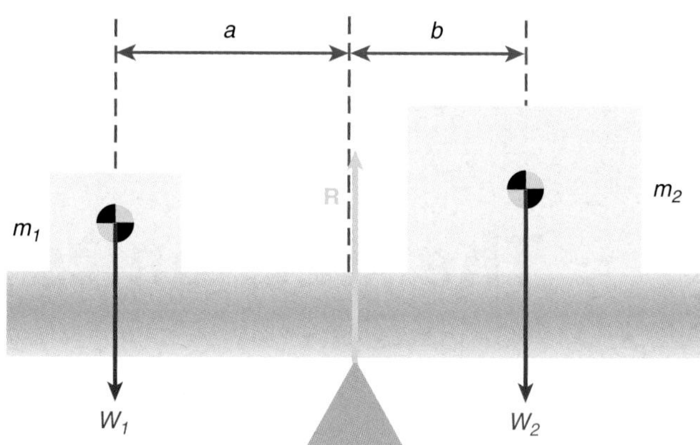

Figure 3-3 Balanced see-saw, the masses m_1 and m_2 give rise to equal and opposite moments because they are positioned at different distances from the pivot point.

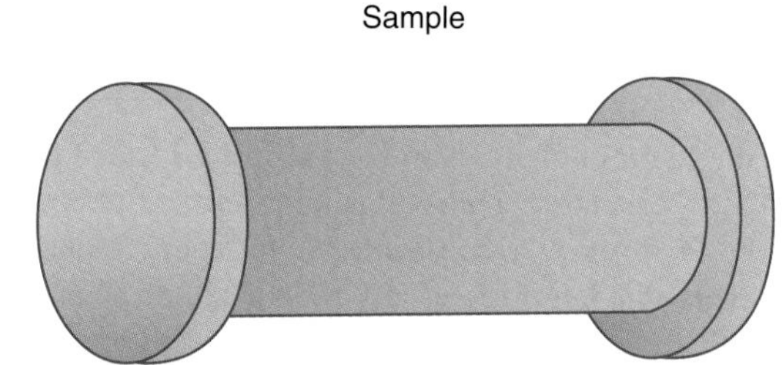

Figure 3-4 Typical tensile test sample.

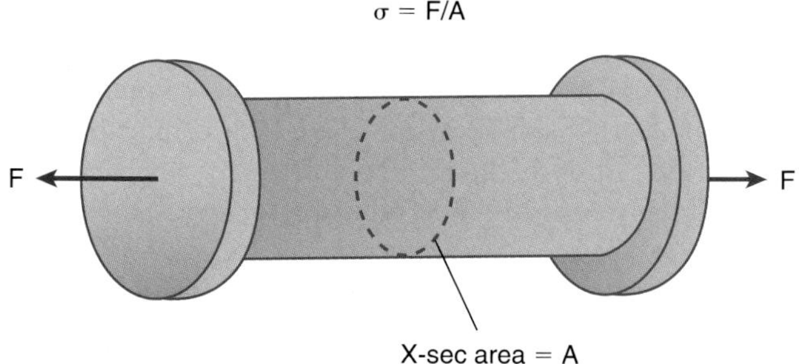

Figure 3-5 Definition of stress, σ.

equilibrium, both the forces and moments acting upon have to be in equilibrium; that is to say the sum of all forces acting must be zero and the sum of all moments acting must be zero.

In Figure 3-3, we have the same see-saw with additional object of mass m_2 placed on the right-hand side of the see-saw. In this case m_2 is equal to $2 \times m_1$. Therefore, balance is achieved if the moment arm of this mass is half of that of mass m_1. Then if:

$$b = a/2$$

$$W_1 \times a = W_2 \times b$$

Now there is a moment balance. There must also be a force balance. The two weight forces both act downward, and are balanced by the reaction force (R) acting upward at the pivot point:

$$R = W_1 + W_2$$

To summarize, for static equilibrium to be achieved, there must be a force and moment balance. The magnitude of a moment is dependent on the magnitude of the force giving rise to the moment and that of the moment arm.

We will now discuss some terms that are useful for examining how strong materials are and how forces are transmitted through objects. The two main concepts are those of stress and strain. These concepts have been developed from engineering practice and the testing of materials in standard material testing machines. These material tests typically use what are called standard samples, which are often cylindrical objects of a certain size (Fig. 3-4). The terms stress and strain are defined later.

Stress (σ): This is defined as the force per unit cross-sectional area. In the material testing machine, the standard samples are subject to either pulling (tensile) forces (Fig. 3-5) or pushing (compressive) forces. The units of stress are

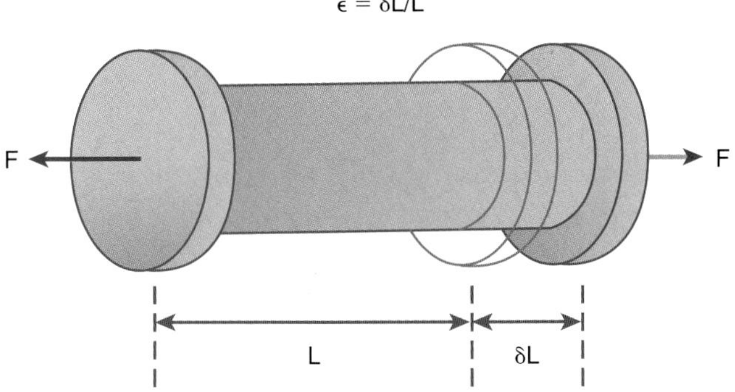

Figure 3-6 Definition of strain, ε.

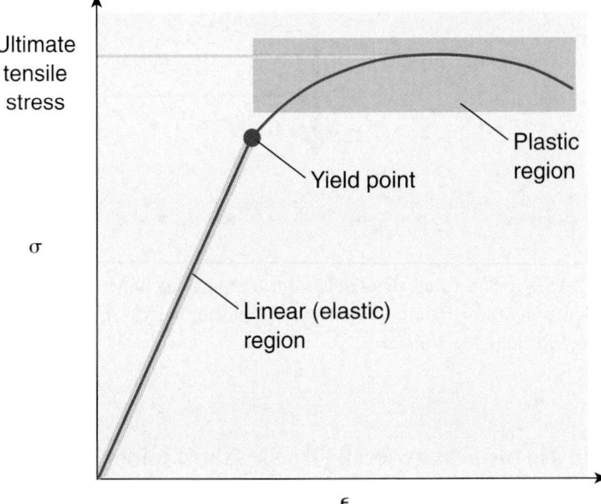

Figure 3-7 Typical tensile stress/strain curve for a metal.

newtons per meter squared (N/m^2), or pascals (Pa) with 1 N = 1 Pa.

Strain (ε): When an object has forces acting on it, it usually stretches (Fig. 3-6) or compresses, depending on what kind of force was applied. Strain is defined as the change in length divided by the original length of the object. Strain is unitless.

The concepts of stress and strain allow us to talk about the properties of the material itself, as opposed to a particular object that is made of a given material. Valuable information about the behavior of a particular material can be gained looking at the stress and strain in a sample subject to testing forces. Commonly, the stress is plotted against the strain, giving the stress/strain plot (Fig. 3-7).

The stress/strain curve shows how the material responds to being loaded by a force. The slope of the stress/strain curve is directly related to the stiffness of the material. A steep slope means that the material does not stretch much as increasing force is applied (stiff material), whereas a not so steep slope indicates that the material stretches significantly as force is increased. The slope is also called Young's modulus (E). Thus E = s/e. Young's modulus is used to quantify the stiffness of materials and has the same units as stress (N/m^2). The first

Table 3-1 Typical Material Properties for Some Biologic Materials, and for Steel

	E	Max Stress	Failure Strain
Bone	10-20 × 10^9 N/m^2	59-120 × 10^6 N/m^2	5-20 × 10^3
Tendon	~1 × 10^9 N/m^2		
Cartilage	~1 × 10^7 N/m^2		
Steel	206 × 10^9 N/m^2	600 × 10^6 N/m^2	100 × 10^3

part of the curve for most materials is linear, that is, there is a direct relationship between the amount of stress and strain. If the force is removed while the test is performed in this region, then the sample returns to its original size; this is termed elastic behavior. At some point, the curve is no longer linear; the material starts to deform to a greater degree. The deformation at this stage now remains permanent, and this is called plastic behavior. Increasing the force further leads to the fracture of the sample; the value of stress at which this occurs is important, because it allows us to determine the maximum amounts of load that can be transmitted by objects made of a given material. The fracture stress for metals is usually somewhat less than the maximum stress recorded (the maximum is termed the ultimate stress); this is due to the necking of the material sample resulting from yielding before fracture.

Different biologic tissues have different values of E; for comparison, the values for a typical steel are also given in Table 3-1.

Mechanics of the Normal Hip Joint

The hip joint can be considered as a ball and socket joint, and allows a considerable range of movement. During many functional activities, such as walking and stair climbing, the hip joint is often involved in single leg support. If we consider the situation represented in Figure 3-8, where an individual is standing on one leg, it is possible to estimate some of the forces acting through and round the hip joint.

If we make some simplifying assumptions, we can perform some straightforward mechanics:

1. The weight force of the body (W, the mass of the body minus that of the support limb multiplied by the acceleration due to gravity) acts through the center of the pelvis.
2. The pelvis is a rigid body.
3. We are considering only the balance in the frontal plane.
4. Only the abductors act to support the body.

We can use the principle of free-body diagrams to simplify the analysis. In order to calculate the muscle force and the joint contact force, we need only concern ourselves with what is happening to the pelvis. So, as shown in Figure 3-9, we have the pelvis (which is considered to be a rigid body) acted upon by a number of forces.

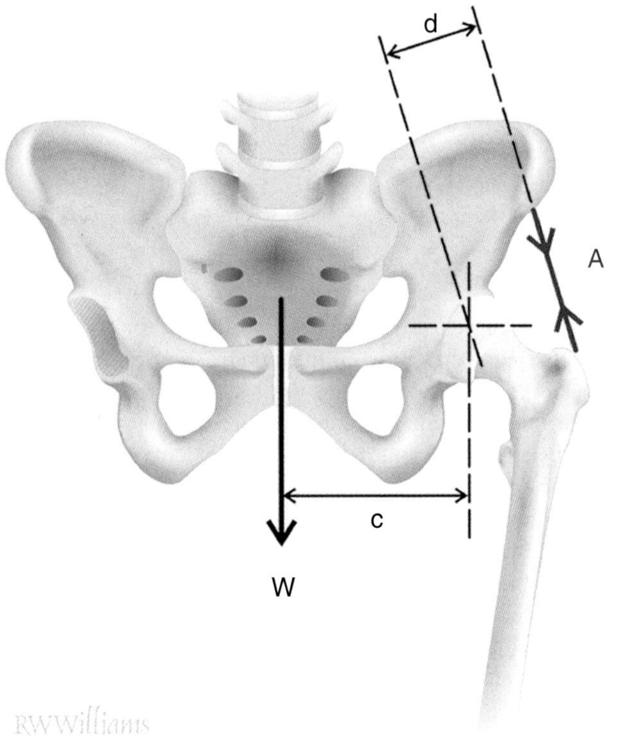

Figure 3-8 Forces acting around the hip joint during single-leg stance. *W*, weight force, *c*, moment arm of weight force, *A*, tension in abductor muscle, *d*, moment arm of abductor.

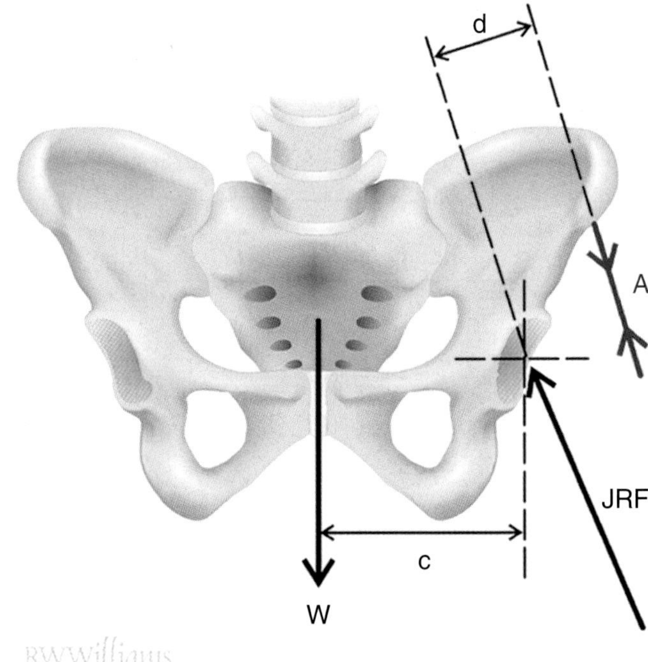

Figure 3-9 Free-body diagram of pelvis during single-leg stance. *W*, weight force, *c*, moment arm of weight force, *A*, tension in abductor muscle, *d*, moment arm of abductor, *JRF*, joint reaction force.

We are considering the pelvis to be stationary, so thus it must be in static equilibrium. We can think of the pelvis as a see-saw, pivoting about the hip joint center. In order for the pelvis to be in static equilibrium, the moments acting about the hip joint must be in balance. The moment arm of the weight force, *W*, is *c* and that of the abductor muscle force, *A*, is *d*. As the force representing the reaction between the pelvis and the femur, *JRF* or the joint reaction force, acts through the center of the joint, its moment arm is zero and consequently it produces zero moment about the hip joint. Therefore, for moment balance:

$$W \times c = A \times d$$

Putting some dimensions to the given example, we can calculate the magnitude of the abductor force. From Figures 3-8 and 3-9, we see that the moment arm of the weight force is greater than that of the muscle force:

$$c = 272 \text{ mm}$$

$$d = 140 \text{ mm}$$

So in this case, $A = W \times c/d = 1.94W$. The fact that the moment arms of the external forces (here we consider the forces acting as a consequence of gravity to be external) are greater than those available to the internal forces (in this case the muscle force) is generally true for most joints of the human body. The result of this is that there is force amplification experienced at the joints; the internal forces required to balance an external load are usually greater than the external forces.

In the current example, there must also be a force balance, which can be calculated geometrically. If a force acting on a body is represented in magnitude by the length of an arrow and the direction in which the force acts is the same as that of the arrow, we can perform some graphical vector addition, as in Figure 3-10.

If the vector representations of all forces acting on a body form a closed polygon, the body will be in static equilibrium. Therefore, the magnitude and direction of the remaining unknown force, *JRF*, can be calculated. The arrow closing the two sides of the triangle formed by the weight and muscle forces represents the magnitude and direction of the joint reaction force. In this particular example, we see that the force magnitude is $2.9W$.

This simple analysis shows that the consequences of standing on one leg are to give rise to large muscle and joint reaction forces. Of course, in the real case, many more muscles are present and will act. There are more complex reasons than pure balance for muscles to act, such as minimizing bending moment.[1] The main result to bear in mind is that muscle action is responsible for the majority of the joint reaction force, and the magnitude of the muscle is highly dependent on the moment arm of the muscle. As a joint is moved through its range of motion, the lines of action of the muscle forces and their moment arms will change.

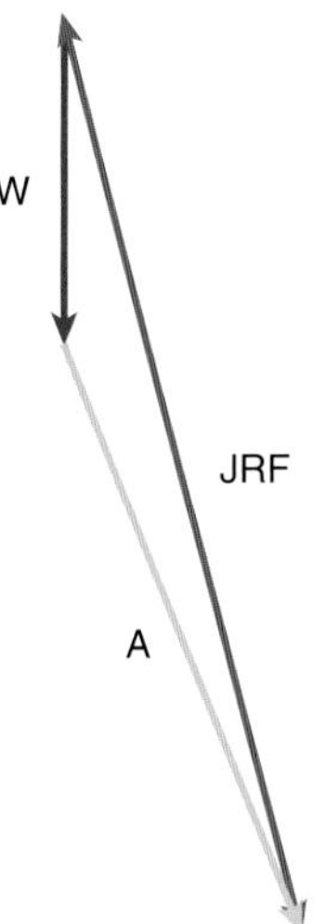

Figure 3-10 Triangle of forces acting on pelvis during single leg stance. *W*, weight force, *A*, tension in abductor muscle, *JRF*, joint reaction force.

The normal anatomic components of the hip are optimized for the normal geometry of the individual concerned. Bone is an adaptive material and becomes optimized for load carriage, the muscles are optimized for working at a particular length, and the soft tissues are optimized for their given envelope of movement. Articular cartilage is a biologic supermaterial that performs a number of demanding functions. It is extremely smooth, with a very low coefficient of friction. It can transmit the large forces placed upon it during the normal function of a given joint. Disease can alter the joint geometry and load-bearing capacity of the individual components. If the moment arms of the muscles are reduced by the joint degeneration, then greater muscle force will be required to generate the required moment for equilibrium.

The above-mentioned analysis allows us to estimate the muscle and joint reaction forces. The forces, or loads, applied to the muscloskeletal system are transmitted through the various tissues. In order to determine the effects of joint replacement, we need to examine the effect of loads applied to the muscloskeletal system. To get a more complete picture of the mechanical environment we need to determine the stress and strain distributions. As discussed earlier, stress and strain are simple to calculate for simple shaped materials testing samples. The above-mentioned discussion was also limited to uniaxial loading of samples. In reality, objects are three dimensional and are loaded with three-dimensional forces. There are components of stress and strain in all directions, and the calculation of these factors requires information of the object geometry and distribution of material within the object. The detailed description of the methods of calculation are beyond the scope of this chapter and the reader is referred to standard engineering texts for further details.[2]

If the geometry and material distribution of a given object are known and the loads placed on the object are known, the stress and strain distribution can be calculated. This process is relatively straightforward for objects with simple shapes such as rectangular cross-section beams, and analytical methods exist for such calculations. However, when the object considered is complex, analytical methods become cumbersome. Numeric methods have been developed for this purpose, and most commonly used is the Finite Element (FE) method. In essence, the FE method basically considers a complex object to be divided into a number of small (or finite) blocks; these are called elements. The process of dividing the object into these elements is termed meshing, and the resulting collection of elements is termed an FE mesh. These small blocks generally have simple geometry, and the normal analytical methods can be applied to each element. Summing the calculations for each element over the whole object allows a numeric estimate of the stress and strain distribution for the complex three-dimensional object. It must be borne in mind that the FE method provides a numeric solution that is dependent on many parameters. The description of the geometry, subdivision into elements and the material properties for a given object is called an FE model.

The material properties for models of biologic systems are an additional source of complication. For artificial materials, the material properties can be determined through testing of samples and the manufacturing quality control ensures that these properties will remain fairly constant. However, there is biologic variation for natural materials, and in addition, many biologic materials are not homogenous. Bones in particular have variable density, with cortical bone being considerably denser and stiffer than cancellous bone. In the region of the head and neck of the femur, the distribution of bone is complex. Modeling the individual trabecular structures is not currently feasible; however, considering the bone tissue to be divided into multiple subtypes with different material properties is an approach to representing its complexity.

In order to determine if a model is producing reliable predictions, validation needs to be performed. Validation usually requires that data from mechanical testing is compared with predictions from numeric simulations performed using the model. Identical loading conditions must be used in the mechanical testing of the actual object and in the simulation. Measuring stress directly is not usually possible; however, it is possible to measure strain. Strain gauges are placed on the surface of the object to be tested, and the measured surface strains are compared with those predicted for validation.

Effects of Surgery

Joint reconstruction performs two main functions, replacement of the joint articular surface and restoration of the joint geometry. The replacement of the joint articular surface addresses the pain caused by joint disease. To restore function, the geometry needs to be adequately restored. As mentioned previously, considering only one muscle to act at any one given instance is a gross simplification. The hip joint is crossed by many muscles, and their activity is coordinated. Antagonistic muscle activity can minimize bone bending moments but will generally increase the joint reaction force. The human body has a certain degree of redundancy, with several muscles able to fulfill similar mechanical functions. This is fortunate, because surgical approaches can compromise the function of some muscles. Reducing the force-generating capabilities of some muscles will result in others having to compensate. This will give rise to changes in the way the overall loads are transmitted through the bones and will ultimately cause the bone to remodel.

The implantation of a replacement device will also change the load transmission within the joint. The materials available for joint replacement are limited and generally have very different material properties to the natural tissues. The materials available are metals, ceramics, and plastics. Generally, metal components are implanted directly into bone and these are much stiffer than the bone, with Young's moduli at least an order of magnitude greater (see Table 3-1).

We will describe the effects of resurfacing surgery using the results obtained from validated FE models of an intact femur and the same femur after resurfacing. The validation of these two models is fully described by Taddei and colleagues.[3]

Finite Element Models

A fresh-frozen human cadaveric femur (male, aged 51 years; height, 175 cm; weight, 75 kg, right side) was scanned by computed tomography (CT). The geometry of the femur was derived from the CT dataset, and a finite element mesh of the intact femur was constructed that consisted of 76,026 elements. The CT numbers were converted into a realistic distribution of material parameters using the public domain software Bonemat_V2.[4] In total, 381 materials defined the femoral bone with an average Young's modulus of 12.9 GPa and a maximum of 19.8 GPa. This intact femur model will be referred to hereafter as the Intact model.

The Intact model validation gave an R^2 value of 0.91 between the experimentally measured strain and the predicted strain.[3]

After testing was completed on the intact cadaveric femur, a resurfacing femoral component (Conserve®Plus, size 48 mm, Wright Medical Technology Inc., Memphis, TN) was implanted. At the time of implantation, the bone on the anterosuperior femoral neck was over-reamed to create a notch (width 1.8 to 5 mm, Fig. 3-11A). The reamed bone topology was digitized using a three-dimensional digitizer (Micro Scribe Model 3DX, Immersion Corporation, San Jose, CA). The geometry for the implanted model, incorporating the digitized topology, was then developed using these measurements and computer-aided design models of the final reamer and the implant. The mesh consisted of 67,333 elements (implant, 11,540 elements; bone cement, 7,809 elements; bone, 47,984 elements, Fig. 3-11C).

The cement mantle thickness ranged between 1 and 3.8 mm, and the cement penetration into the bone was not

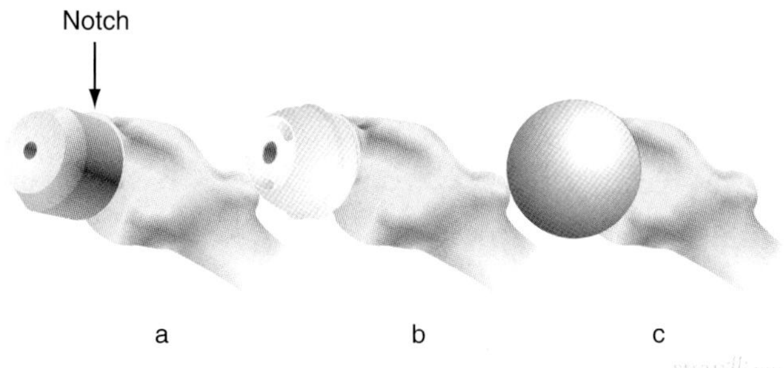

Figure 3-11 Construction of finite element model, showing **(A)** prepared bone with notch, **(B)** cement mantle in place, and **(C)** final implant/cement/bone construct.

modeled (see Fig. 3-11B). This approach will introduce some errors, because there is cement penetration into the bone in reality; however, a rigorous validation of this model was performed and the effect of this assumption was small.[3] A Coulomb friction model at the implant-cement interface was used ($\mu = 0.3$). The bond between the bone and cement was assumed to be rigid. This model will be hereafter referred to as the Implanted model.

Distributed material parameters for the reamed femoral bone were obtained using the same method as for the Intact model. The cement mantle and the cobalt chrome implant were modeled as linear elastic materials with a Poisson's ratio of 0.3 and Young's modulus of 2,700 MPa and 210,000 MPa, respectively.[5,6] The Implanted model validation gave an R^2 value of 0.94 between the experimentally measured strain and the predicted strain.

Effects of Physiologic Loading

The experimental loading gives valuable information for validating the model. However, if we wish to examine what happens during functional activity, a more complex loading scenario is needed. We applied a physiologic load case simulating an instant at 10% of the level walking gait cycle. During this instant in the gait cycle, both the abductors and adductors are active.[7] Magnitudes for the muscle forces were derived from the work of Brand and associates.[7,8] Data for the attachment origins and lines of action of the muscle and hip contact forces were based on the work of Duda[9] and Polgar and colleagues.[10] Muscle forces were scaled by the subject's body weight. Hip contact force was based on forces measured using telemetered hip replacements[11] and scaled by body weight of the femur donor.

This loading was applied to both the Intact and Implanted models, the FE models were solved using Ansys software (version 8.1, Ansys Inc., Canonsburg, PA).

We can now examine the effects of resurfacing in a very detailed way, first we will explain the variables used. As mentioned earlier, the stress and strain in a three-dimensional object is distributed in a three-dimensional manner. Principal

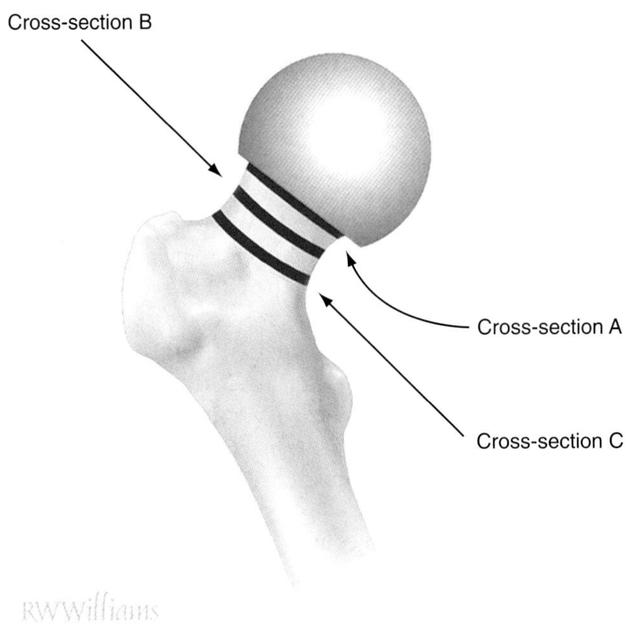

Figure 3-12 Cross-sections of interest in the femoral neck.

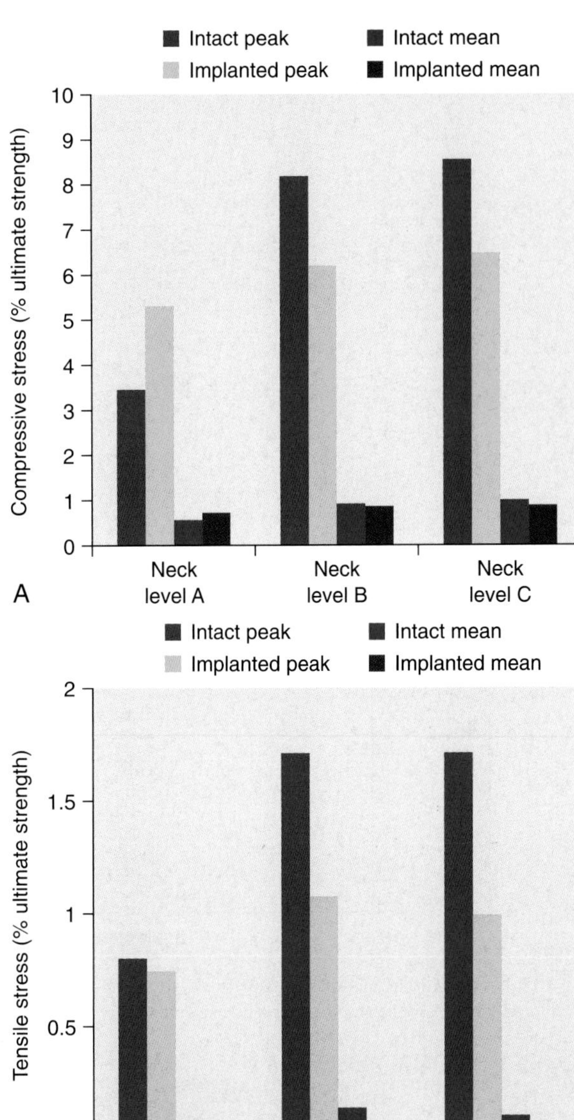

Figure 3-13 A, Peak and mean compressive stress at each cross-section of interest in the femoral neck for the intact and implanted femurs. B, Peak and mean tensile stress at each cross-section of interest in the femoral neck for the intact and implanted femurs.

stresses/strains are the maximum and minimum normal stresses/strains in a material; the word normal means that they are orthogonal to each other. These stresses are commonly either tensile or compressive; and are oriented in directions of zero shear stress/strain. The first principal stress/strain (σ1/ε11) is predominately tensile and will hereafter be referred to as tensile stress/strain; similarly, the third principal stress/strain (σ3/ε33) is predominately compressive and will hereafter be referred to as compressive stress/strain. There is concern about femoral neck fracture, so we will look in particular at three cross-sections of the neck, defined in Figure 3-12A, B, and C.

Looking first at the values of compressive stress, expressing these as percentages of the ultimate compressive strength of bone (145 MPa for cancellous bone and 193 MPa for cortical bone [12, 13]), we see that this level of loading actually gives very low values of compressive stress in the femoral neck. The highest peak compressive stress is approximately 9% of the ultimate compressive strength (Fig. 3-13A). As a result of implantation of the resurfacing, we can see that there is very little change in compressive stress; the peak stress changes in Sections A, B, and C are 1.8%, –2.0%, and –2.1%, respectively. The peak tensile stresses are even lower, with the maximum of 1.7% of ultimate tensile strength occurring in cross-section B for the *Intact* model (Ultimate tensile strength taken as 100 MPa for cancellous bone and 133 MPa for cortical bone[12,13]). The peak changes due to resurfacing are –0.1%, –0.6% and –0.2% in Sections A, B, and C, respectively (see Fig. 3-13B). Average stresses are low in comparison to the peak stress (see Fig. 3-13), and do not differ greatly between the Intact and Implanted models.

To determine the potential for femoral bone fracture under this physiologic loading condition, a risk of fracture (RF) scalar can be calculated as the ratio between the Von Mises stress* and the ultimate strength of bone.[3,14,15] An RF value greater than 1 indicates a potential fracture site. The median RF value for the neck volume of the Intact model is

*Stress is a three-dimensional vector quantity (σ_1, σ_2, σ_3); the Von Mises stress (σ_v) reduces it to a single scalar, by $\sigma_v = \sqrt{\frac{(\sigma_1 - \sigma_2)^2 + (\sigma_2 - \sigma_3)^2 + (\sigma_3 - \sigma_1)^2}{2}}$. Von Mises stress is commonly used for finite element analysis because it represents the overall stress state for complex loading conditions.

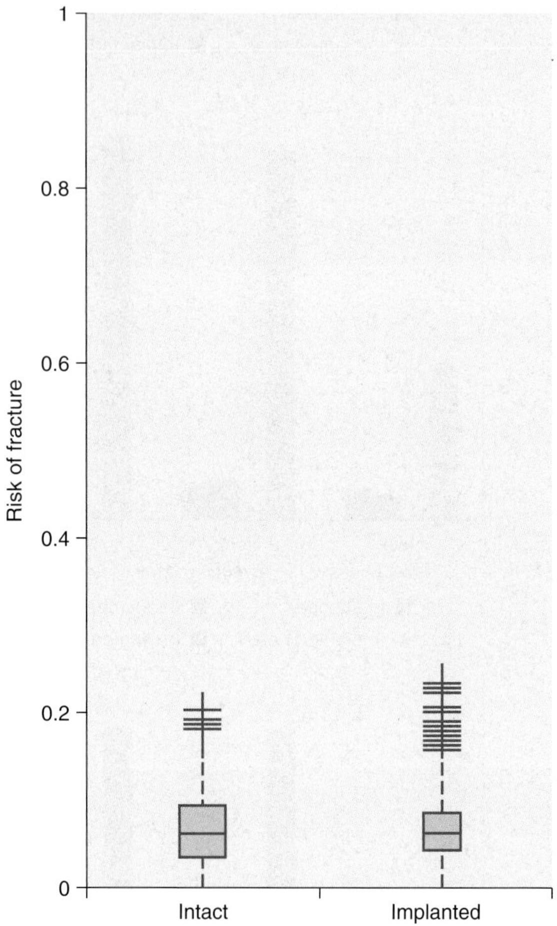

Figure 3-14 Box and whisker plot showing the risk of fracture index (RF) distribution in the neck volume for the intact and implanted femurs.

0.1 and this is not changed greatly as a consequence of resurfacing (Fig. 3-14). Even with the presence of a notched femur, the maximum values of RF are 0.23 in the femoral neck region.

The differences between resurfacing and THR can also be shown using FE models. In addition to modeling a resurfacing, a finite element model of the femur implanted with a generic uncemented Zweymuller-type stem was developed; this model was termed *THR*. Again, the same physiologic loading condition was applied. Now if we compare the compressive strains along a path on the medial outer cortex, we can see some differences between the various models (Fig. 3-15). The Intact and Implanted (implanted with a resurfacing) models have similar strains along the medial cortex; however the THR model has a lower amount of strain along the same path. This is indicative of the stress shielding due to the presence of the THR.

There are some changes in strain energy that some authors consider important for remodeling of bone. After resurfacing, there is a small amount of stress shielding under the femoral component; this is mostly located under the superior medial part of the implant. The decrease in strain energy in the cancellous bone beneath the inferior rim of the implant may be sufficient to cause bone remodelling.[16,17] To our knowledge, the model presented is the only validated FE model of hip resurfacing. There have been numerous other FE studies,[18-20] but they have not been validated. They have used either simplified representations of the bone, considering only two material properties,[18,20] or applied only simplified loading.

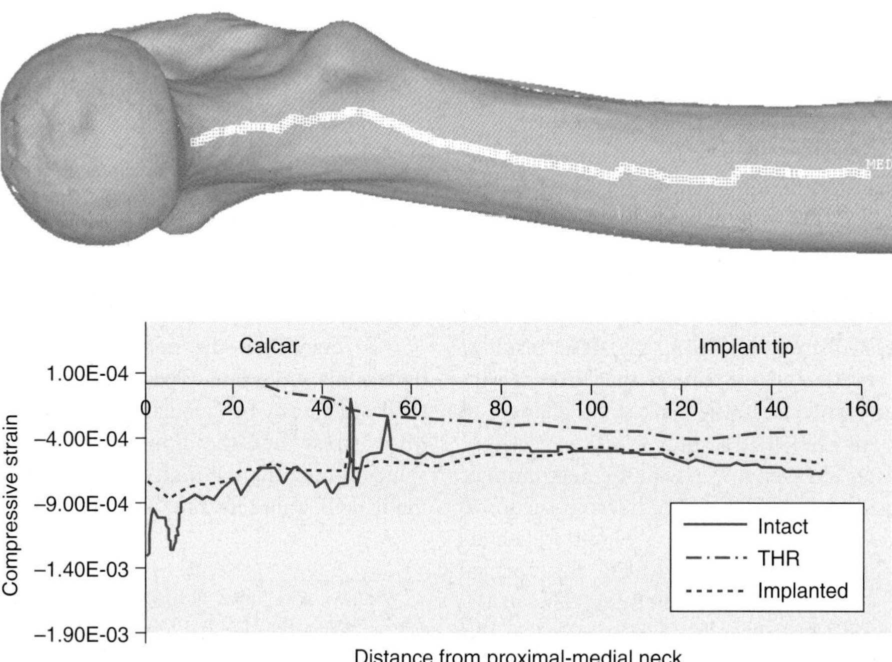

Figure 3-15 Comparison of compressive strain distribution on the outer surface of the bone for an intact femur, a femur implanted with a surfacing and a femur implanted with a total hip replacement (THR).

Summary

Normal hip mechanics are dominated by the effect of muscle forces. The forces in the hip joint for even relatively sedate functional activities are multiples of body weight. After hip resurfacing, validated finite element models show that the stress and strain in the femoral head and neck are close to normal. The changes in tensile stress predicted by the Implanted model as a consequence of hip resurfacing are less than 2% of the ultimate tensile stress in the region of the neck. Stress in the femoral head decreases after resurfacing; for this physiologic load case, this decrease is not large enough to result in stress shielding.[21] The peak observed in the medial cortex in the intact femur reduces—some of the load transfer after resurfacing, occurs directly between the stem and the bone—but overall, the stress distribution in the neck is similar after resurfacing. The decrease in strain energy in the cancellous bone beneath the inferior rim of the implant, may be sufficient to cause bone remodelling.[16,17] The simulated notch in the Implanted model gave rise to only small increases in stress in this region of the neck. Over the remainder of the femur, when compared with published values for changes in tensile strain due to total hip arthroplasty, hip resurfacing gives rise to considerably smaller deviations from the intact condition. Total hip replacement by contrast is reported to give up to an 80% change in compressive strain around the region of the calcar.[22]

A major concern associated with hip resurfacing is early femoral neck fracture. On average, this would seem to occur in 1% or 2% of patients and most commonly, between 1 and 2 months following surgery. Fractures tend to occur during activities of daily living rather than when the hip is subject to major load. This would suggest that a fracture can only occur if the neck has been substantially weakened. The finite element modeling indicates that both the tensile and compressive stresses in the neck region remain virtually normal. Therefore, it is likely that some other process is weakening the bone and causing fracture. Leaving uncovered reamed bone, as a result of inadequate seating of the femoral component, will result in a weaker construct and may contribute to neck fracture. Some studies have shown that during hip resurfacing surgery, blood flow to the femoral head is decreased,[23,24] and histologic studies have shown that fractures are associated with avascular necrosis.[25] Necrotic bone has been shown to have substantially lower mechanical properties[26]; avascular necrosis may substantially weaken the bone and may be the cause of the observed fractures. From the current available data, sufficient femoral head viability is generally preserved based on McMahon's study and Cambell's retrieval analysis (see Chapter 10) after hip resurfacing arthroplasty; there are patchy areas of necrosis in some retrievals with associated remodeling and rare cases of whole head necrosis. However, further longitudinal studies using both intra-operative blood flow or oxygenation measurements and post-operative measurements with techniques such as positron emission scanning are needed to determine the long-term consequences of blood vessel transaction/occlusion at the time of surgery.

Acknowledgments

The authors thank Marco Viceconti, Fulvia Taddei, and Luca Cristofolini of the Istituti Ortopedici Rizzoli, Bologna, Italy, who were instrumental in the development and validation of the models described in this chapter.

References

1. Pauwels F: Biomechanics of the Locomotor Apparatus. Berlin, Springer-Verlag, 1980.
2. Cook RD, Young WC: Advanced Mechanics of Materials. Upper Saddle River, NJ, Prentice Hall, 1998.
3. Taddei F, Cristofolini L, Martelli S, Gill HS, Viceconti M: Subject-specific finite element models of long bones: an in vitro evaluation of the overall accuracy. J Biomech 2006;39: 2457-2467.
4. Taddei F, Pancanti A, Viceconti M: An improved method for the automatic mapping of ct numbers onto finite element models. Med Eng Phys 2004;26:61-69.
5. Lewis G: Properties of acrylic bone cement: State of the art review. J Biomed Material Res 1997;38:155-182.
6. Black J, Hastings G (eds): Handbook of Biomaterial Properties. New York, Springer, 1998.
7. Brand RA, Pederson DR, Friederich JA: The sensitivity of muscle force predictions to changes in physiologic cross-sectional area. J Biomech 1986;19:589-596.
8. Brand RA, Pedersen DR, Davy DT, Kotzar GM, Heiple KG, Goldberg VM: Comparison of hip force calculations and measurements in the same patient. J Arthroplasty 1994;9:45-51.
9. Duda GN: Influence of Muscle Forces on the Internal Loads in the Femur During Gait. Aachen, Germany, Technical University Hamburg-Harburg, 1996.
10. Polgár K, Gill HS, Viceconti M, Murray DW, O'Connor JJ: Strain distribution within the human femur due to physiological and simplified loading: finite element analysis using the muscle standardized femur model. Proc Inst Mech Eng [H] 2003;217:173-189.
11. Kotzar GM, Davy DT, Goldberg VM, Heiple KG, Berilla J, Heiple KG Jr, et al: Telemeterized in vivo hip joint force data: a report on two patients after total hip surgery. J Orthop Res 1991; 9:621-633.
12. Bayraktar HH, Morgan EF, Niebur GL, Morris GE, Wong EK, Keaveny TM: Comparison of the elastic and yield properties of human femoral trabecular and cortical bone tissue. J Biomech 2004;37:27-35.
13. Reilly DT, Burstein AH: The elastic and ultimate properties of compact bone tissue. J Biomech 1975;8:393-405.
14. Keller TS: Predicting the compressive mechanical behaviour of bone. J Biomech 1994;19:583-586.
15. Ford CM, Keaveny TM, Hayes WC: The effect of impact direction on the structural capacity of the proximal femur during falls. J Bone Mineral Res 1996;11:377-383.
16. Van Rietbergen B, Huiskes R, Weinans H, Sumner DR, Turner TM, Galante JO: ESB Research Award 1992. The mechanism of bone remodeling and resorption around press-fitted THA stems. J Biomech 1993:26:369-382.

17. Kerner J, Huiskes R, van Lenthe GH, Weinans H, van Rietbergen B, Engh CA, et al: Correlation between pre-operative periprosthetic bone density and post-operative bone loss in tha can be explained by strain-adaptive remodelling. J Biomech 1999;32: 695-703.
18. Huiskes R, Strens P, Vroemen W, Slooff TJ: Post-loosening mechanical behavior of femoral resurfacing prostheses. Clin Mater 1990;6:37-55.
19. Taylor M: Finite element analysis of the resurfaced femoral head. Proc Inst Mech Eng [H] 2006;220:289-297.
20. Watanabe Y, Shiba N, Matsuo S, Higuchi F, Tagawa Y, Inoue A: Biomechanical study of the resurfacing hip arthroplasty: finite element analysis of the femoral component. J Arthroplasty 2000;15:505-511.
21. Beaupré GS, Orr TE, Carter DR: An approach for time-dependent bone modelling and remodeling—application: a preliminary remodelling simulation. J Orthop Res 1990;8:662-670.
22. Kleemann RU, Heller MO, Stoeckle U, Taylor WR, Duda GN: THA loading arising from increased femoral anteversion and offset may lead to critical cement stresses. J Orthop Res 2003;21:767-774.
23. Steffen RT, Smith SR, Urban JP, McLardy-Smith P, Beard DJ, Gill HS, et al: The effect of hip resurfacing on oxygen concentration in the femoral head. J Bone Joint Surg (Br) 2005;87: 1468-1474.
24. Khan A, Yates P, Lovering A, Bannister GC, Spencer RF: The effect of surgical approach on blood flow to the femoral head during resurfacing. J Bone Joint Surg (Br) 2007;89:21-25.
25. Little CP, Ruiz AL, Harding IJ, McLardy-Smith P, Gundle R, Murray DW, et al: Osteonecrosis in retrieved femoral heads after failed resurfacing arthroplasty of the hip. J Bone Joint Surg (Br) 2005;87:320-323.
26. Brown TD, Way ME, Ferguson AB Jr: Mechanical characteristics of bone in femoral capital aseptic necrosis. Clin Orthop Relat Res 1981;156:240-247.

CHAPTER 4

Tribology of Bearing Materials

John B. Medley

Friction, lubrication, and wear are the unavoidable consequences of allowing a load to be transmitted through two interacting surfaces in relative motion while in the presence of a lubricant. Surface replacement arthroplasty (SRA) of the hip is essentially an approach that provides a less invasive implant by simply replacing the natural bearing surfaces, but as a consequence, these implants articulate large diameter heads in rather thin-walled cups. So far, only medical grade cobalt-based alloys have provided bearing surfaces with the strength and fatigue resistance to avoid in situ damage and the wear resistance needed to avoid osteolysis.[1] The present chapter concentrates exclusively on metal-on-metal (MM) bearings using these alloys. The typical compositions of the cobalt-based alloys are similar except for small but significant differences in carbon (C) content (Table 4-1).

As discussed by Brown et al,[2] recent concerns/issues with MM SRA of the hip include elevated metal-ion levels in the blood of patients caused by the dissociation of the wear particles, the reported toxic/necrotic or hypersensitive[3] tissue response to wear particles and the possibility of a delayed osteolytic response to the wear particles. In addition, there are concerns regarding acetabular fixation that may be related to poor design of the cup geometry that causes elevated friction levels.[4-8] Furthermore, flaws in alloy metallurgy[9] and surface damage caused by microseparation[10] have been suggested as potential problems. Despite these concerns, MM SRA remains a widely practiced and successful operation. All of the issues mentioned earlier can be related to the implant tribology and can be addressed to some extent by specific features of lubrication, geometry and alloy microstructure.

There are ongoing attempts to introduce new tribological innovations to MM hip bearings. For example, there have been efforts to mix higher hardness with lower hardness surfaces. In many engineering applications, the more easily replaced component is made from a material of significantly lower hardness and, usually, it sustains more wear (producing more wear particles) and does less damage to the mating higher hardness component that is more difficult to replace. Thus, if one component in an articulating pair can be replaced more easily and the amount of wear debris is not a problem, it is beneficial to make it from a lower hardness material.

It is not clear which component of MM SRA is more easily replaced. However, it may be possible to make heads from medical-grade ceramics, and hip simulator studies[4,11] have shown remarkably low wear rates and ion levels for this pairing. It seems that the higher hardness ceramic retains a smooth enough surface to avoid causing elevated wear of the cobalt alloy cup. A similar approach can also be achieved by attaching layers of chromium nitride to cobalt alloy surfaces, and in hip simulator testing, this has been shown to reduce wear rate and blood ion levels.[12,13] A more conventional approach to "differential hardness" design is to use existing approved cobalt-based alloys.[14] The largest differential hardness here may be to combine a high hardness head (F1537 HC) with a low hardness cup (F75 subject to various heat treatments), as suggested by Carroll.[15]

A discussion of new tribological innovations is not complete without mentioning the idea that not just the head but the cup can also have chromium nitride surface layers, and in hip simulator testing,[16] this gives perhaps the lowest recorded wear rates, as noted by Isaac et al.[4]

The ultimate clinical success in SRA of the above-mentioned novel approaches is not known, and eventual wear damage to the harder surfaces (perhaps by fatigue mechanisms) may release hard, highly abrasive particles that may act to produce an undesirable acceleration in total wear rates.

The present chapter provides an overview of the tribology of MM SRA with a focus on designs and materials used in current clinical practice. Efforts are made to consolidate and simplify without losing a factual perspective. Thus, key technical details are presented in appendices, leaving the main body free for concise overall discussion.

Lubrication and Geometry

During repetitive activities such as walking, MM implants for SRA can entrain lubricant films (Fig. 4-1) that protect the surfaces,[17,18] and simulator wear has been shown to decrease with increasing estimated lubricant film thickness.[19] A simple elastohydrodynamic lubrication (ehl) analysis for transient conditions was developed by Chan et al[20] that predicted the

Table 4-1 Typical Chemical Composition of Cobalt-Based Alloys (in wt%) Run-in Used in Metal-on-Metal Surface Replacement Arthroplasty[24]

Alloy (ASTM grade)	Cr	Mo	C	Fe	Si	Mn	Co
F1537 LC	28	5.7	0.051	0.18	0.66	0.57	Bal
F1537 HC	27	5.7	0.23	0.36	0.66	0.57	Bal
F75 HIP + SA*	29	5.7	0.27	0.38	0.59	0.50	Bal
F75 As-Cast	as above						

ASTM, American Society for Testing and Materials; Cr, chromium; Mo, molybdenum; C, carbon; Fe, iron; LC, low carbon; HC, high carbon; Si, silicon; Mn, manganese; Co, cobalt.
**The F75 grade is cast but usually includes subsequent heat treatments to produce a more uniform microstructure, such as hot isostatic pressing (HIP) in which the component is heated in an argon atmosphere to 1200 °C for 4 hours while a pressure of 103 MPa is applied, with a slow cooling in an argon atmosphere, followed by solution annealing (SA) in which the component is heated to 1200 °C for 4 hours in a vacuum with a rapid gas-fan quenching in nitrogen.*[40]

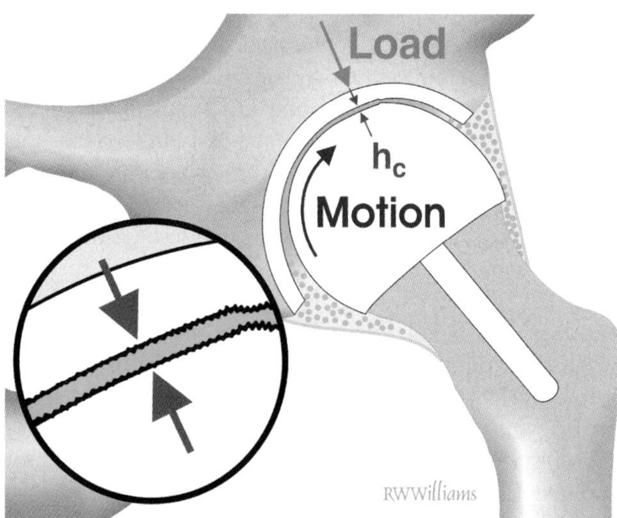

Figure 4-1 Fluid film lubrication (created by elastohydrodynamic mechanisms) of metal-on-metal implants in surface replacement arthroplasty. Note that the thickness of the fluid film, the amount of surface deformation, the faint suggestion of surface roughness, and deformation in the contact zone plus the relative component radii are all exaggerated for the purposes of schematic representation. Also, it is suggested that the film has a higher density of large molecules than the bulk fluid in the capsule. However, although this is perhaps plausible, this is not known to be true. In classic fluid film lubrication, the influence on flow of the chemical interactions within the lubricant (rheology) is considered, and the lubricant directly adjacent to a moving surface is expected to have the same velocity (no slip condition), but any chemical interaction of elements in the lubricant with the surface is classified as boundary lubrication and is not considered.

time-varying central film thickness (h_C) during various activities (Appendix 4A).

Although there were many limitations to this simple approach,[20,21] a very important finding emerged. As mentioned in Appendix 4A and documented by Chan et al,[19,20] the average central film thickness of the lubricant during walking (the most common representative in vivo activity) could be calculated from the steady entraining action formula using the average load and velocity acting over the walking cycle. Thus, the central film thickness depended on the head radius (R_H) and the cup radius (R_C), combined in a geometric parameter known as the effective radius (R) in the following manner

$$h_C \propto R^{0.767}$$

where $R \approx \dfrac{R_H^{\,2}}{R_C - R_H}$ and the radial clearance is $R_C - R_H$

Because the head size in MM SRA is chosen depending on the individual patient, changing the effective radius, R, through selection of an appropriate clearance is the most effective way for a manufacturer to use lubricant film protection to reduce implant wear. In addition, increasing R causes an increase in the radius of the contact area (a) under transient conditions (Appendix 4A), and so the average contact stress of the implant decreases with increasing R. Lower contact stress may permit the protein elements of the synovial fluid that form after arthroplasty to be more effective in protecting the surface through boundary lubrication mechanisms.[22,23] Furthermore, a lower contact stress can perhaps reduce the strain-induced transformation of the alloy microstructure[24] that is associated with higher wear, as discussed subsequently in the present chapter. Therefore, it was considered beneficial to show the influence of R on the wear rates found in both simulator testing and in implant retrieval analysis.

In Appendix 4B, a considerable amount of data from published (peer-reviewed) studies involving wear simulators and implant retrievals from various groups was correlated with the above-mentioned R parameter. Simply put, as R increased, the wear rate decreased. A similar result was found by Dowson,[25] who correlated wear rate with a representative calculation of the minimum elastohydrodynamic film thickness (h_{MIN}) acting over the walking cycle, rather than the R used in the present study. Also, Dowson separately correlated run-in and steady state wear rates with h_{MIN}, showing even more dramatic effects for run-in compared with steady state wear. In the correlation of Appendix 4B, the issue of run-in wear was ignored and overall wear rates were used as determined by simply dividing volumetric wear by years in the patient or, for simulators, using 2 million cycles (Mc) as equivalent to 1 year in vivo following Silva et al.[26] In this manner, both simulator and retrieval wear were included in the correlation and could be compared in an approximate fashion. It was considered significant that both the simulator and the retrieval studies indicated similar behavior and suggested that, as stated by Dowson[25]:

> "For minimum wear and wear rate the diameter of the femoral component should be as large as possible, while the clearance should be as small as practicable."

This advice promoted SRA implants with large diameters (40 to 56 mm) and low diametral clearances (120 to 200 μm) or, essentially, implants with high values for R (4 to 13 m).

Because implants are subject to wear in vivo, Lui et al[7] examined the issue of how the change in surface shape during simulator wear influenced the predicted lubricant film thickness, using a sophisticated numerical analysis. They found a three-fold increase in the predicted minimum film thickness of a 28-mm diameter implant using the surface shape that developed in simulator testing after 1 Mc, that persisted until 5 Mc, and they attributed the lower wear rates in this test interval, in part, to better lubrication. However, they did not report any deep scratches in the surface, as found by Paré et al,[27] that had developed as simulator wear proceeded and could act to drain lubricant films, thus allowing direct surface contact (and probably more wear). Also, they warned that an increase in wear depth beyond a certain limit was shown to cause a constriction of the lubricant film at the edges and thus a decrease in film thickness. Interestingly, a patent had been filed that advocated the preshaping of implant surfaces to improve conformity and, at the same time, to remove edge constriction.[28]

Whether in vivo changes to the implant geometry increased lubricant film thicknesses or not, there remained a strong rationale for using implants with high R values to promote better lubrication conditions from the start.

Cup Fixation and Clearance

The issue of what was "practicable" in terms of clearance was discussed by McMinn and Daniel[9] who stated that progressive acetabular radiolucent lines were found in a low-clearance patient group, suggesting the possibility of peripheral loosening of the cup. They attributed this problem to equatorial contact/interference caused by cup shape distortion during implantation, which was made worse by the low clearance. This apparently led to increased frictional torque, micromotion, and thus, a compromised fixation. Unfortunately, there was a lack of detail provided regarding the low-clearance patient group and, as yet, no information on whether the patients did go on to develop acetabular component loosening. Thus, the sequence of events proposed by McMinn and Daniel remained without compelling evidence. However, equatorial contact under conditions of low clearance was recognized as a problem for the early McKee-Farrar MM implants[29] and had been shown to cause high wear (and friction) in a simulator study of MM hip implants.[30]

The issue of cup deformation was considered experimentally[5] and analytically.[6] In both studies, it was noted that a thin-walled cup could distort enough during surgical insertion to have equatorial contact, and thus the researchers advocated a stiffer cup to allow the smaller clearance. However, they did warn against too stiff a cup that could cause stress/strain shielding of the subchondral bone and thus impair fixation. Also, Yew et al[6] noted that the bone would gradually relax and the cup distortion would decrease after surgery to some extent. This process might well be encouraged by the articulation of the head in the cup as patient activities resume. Overall, it is not clear from the literature whether low clearances did actually cause clinical problems, and the lower wear with increased R (corresponding to decreased clearances) that was noted in Appendix 4B suggested otherwise.

Contacting Surfaces

All MM hip bearings initially had carbides protruding from the surface, but after the surfaces were subjected to wear, the carbides were either fractured or pulled out and the asperity tips (composed of both carbides and matrix material) were worn down.[23,27,31] Consequently, the implant surfaces sustained abrasive wear, as illustrated in Figure 4-4 of Park et al.[32] Surface scratches were found and attributed to the original manufacturing process and to the ongoing abrasive wear. Paré et al[27] found that root mean square roughness (when deep surface scratches were avoided) remained about the same.

The boundary lubrication behavior at the surfaces was also very interesting. Brockett et al[18,22] noted that increased protein concentration in the lubricant reduced friction. However, Wimmer et al[33] reported that the organic elements of the lubricant (proteins) combined with the surface material to form tribochemical reactions films. These films seemed to increase friction in implants after resting periods under load and, perhaps, sheared in preference to the substrate, thus acting as boundary lubricants to protect against wear.[34]

Thus, it seemed that adhesive wear was suppressed by the tribochemical reaction films but abrasive wear (made slightly worse by carbide pull-out and fracture) and a mild "corrosion" wear associated with the formation of these reaction films did occur at the surfaces. In the tissue surrounding implants[35] and in the fluid from simulator testing,[36] round nanometer-sized wear particles, composed of chromium and oxygen, were found and their likely source was the tribochemical reaction films. Needle-shaped particles were also found, as discussed in the next section.

Alloy Microstructure

The cobalt-based alloys used in MM SRA were composed mainly of cobalt, chromium, and molybdenum (CoCrMo) with either high carbon (HC) or low carbon (LC) and classifications according to the American Society for Testing and Materials (ASTM), as described in Table 4-1 and in Appendix 4C. Despite the previously mentioned abrasive wear caused by the carbides, the LC (F1537 LC) alloys, with fewer surface carbides, tended to have higher wear in most wear simulator studies.[37]

All of the cobalt-based alloys used in MM hip implants had a combination of two crystal structures; hexagonal close packed (HCP) and face-centered cubic (FCC). The regions with an HCP structure were hard, brittle, and susceptible to fatigue wear,[38] whereas the regions with an FCC structure were more ductile and wear resistant.[39] Under the influence of deformation in the wear process,[24] the FCC structure could undergo a strain-induced transformation to the less desirable HCP structure. However, as explained and demonstrated in Appendix 4C, the amount of dissolved carbon in the matrix could suppress this transformation.[24]

Because the F75 As-Cast material had the highest amount of carbon dissolved in the matrix (as opposed to residing in the carbides), it had the lowest wear in linear reciprocating pin-on-plate wear tests.[24,39] This dependence of wear on dissolved carbon provided an interpretation of the simulator wear testing of Firkins et al,[11] who found much higher wear for wrought F1537 LC alloys compared with wrought F1537 HC alloys, because the F1537 LC alloys had been shown by Varano et al[24] to have less carbon dissolved in the matrix.

However, in the simulator testing of Bowsher et al,[40] there was no difference detected between implants made from F75 hot isostatic pressing (HIP) + solution annealing (SA) material and those made from F75 As-Cast material, despite their likely differences[39] in dissolved carbon. Bowsher et al tested under normal walking conditions and more extreme fast jogging conditions that showed significant and similar increases in wear rate for implants made from both materials. Bowsher et al suggested that the choice of alloy (F75 As-Cast versus F75 HIP + SA) was clinically irrelevant, in contrast to the assertions of McMinn and Daniel.[9] Furthermore, there were no obvious alloy microstructure effects in the simulator and retrieval wear rates presented in Appendix 4B.

One explanation for the findings of Varano et al,[24] as summarized in Appendix 4C, can be developed from a consideration of the contact stress. Varano et al suggested that a controlling factor for wear seemed to be the "presence and formation of the HCP phase due to surface deformation," as explained by Buscher et al.[38] The HCP phase tended to form beneath the surface of implants because of strain and was subject to fatigue wear, giving the needle-shaped wear particles that were detected in tissues surrounding SRA implants by Catelas et al.[35] So, in the pin-on-plate experiments of Varano et al, the initial contact stress was much higher than that found in implants, such as those used by Bowsher et al[40] in simulator wear testing. Consequently, the reduced amount of dissolved carbon in the F75 HIP + SA material allowed a transformation to the higher wearing HCP phase, and thus, Varano et al found somewhat higher wear for the F75 HIP + SA alloy compared with the F75 As-Cast alloy.

The extent to which an implant in vivo would be subjected to higher contact stresses and direct surface contact, thus needing the higher levels of dissolved carbon, such as that found in the F75 As-Cast material, to avoid the transformation to the higher wearing HCP phase, remained a concern and a subject for future research. However, implants with highly effective radii appeared to avoid this problem. Also, even the rigorous hip simulator testing described by Bowsher et al,[40] that had implants all with relatively low effective radii (~ 3 m), did not show any difference in the wear of F75 HIP + SA compared with F75 As-Cast alloy. Thus, low-wearing MM SRA implants apparently could be made from F75 As-Cast, F75 HIP + SA, wrought high carbon alloy (F1537 HC) or a combination of the two (as advocated by Carroll[15]).

Concluding Remarks

The case for MM SRA implants with a low clearance and thus a large effective radius (R) follows from a consideration of transient elastohydrodynamic lubrication (Appendix 4A) and the correlation of simulator and retrieval wear rates (Appendix 4B). In addition, a case can be made for developing alloys with high levels of dissolved carbon in the matrix (Appendix 4C).

Broader, more detailed discussion of the literature suggests that it may be necessary to provide cups that are stiff enough to allow low clearances to be maintained. It is noted that surface carbides tend to cause some abrasive damage at the same time as tribochemical reaction films form that may help protect the surfaces, while causing a mild corrosive wear. Unfortunately, methods to influence these processes in a significant manner and thus further reduce wear and blood ion levels have not been developed, with the exception of the possibility of using surface layers (and this may introduce other concerns at the surfaces). Provided contact stresses remain low, it may not be necessary to use alloys with high levels of dissolved carbon, but heat treatments and further testing to explore this possibility should be undertaken.

References

1. Amstutz HC, Le Duff MJ: Background of metal-on-metal resurfacing. Proc Inst Mech Eng [H] 2006;220:85-94.
2. Brown C, Fisher J, Ingham E: Biological effects of clinically relevant wear particles from metal-on-metal hip prostheses. Proc Inst Mech Eng [H] 2006;220:355-369.
3. Davies AP, Willert HG, Campbell PA, Learmonth ID, Case CP: An unusual lymphocytic perivascular infiltration in tissues around contemporary metal-on-metal joint replacements. J Bone Joint Surg 2005;87A:18-27.
4. Isaac GH, Thompson J, Williams S, Fisher J: Metal-on-metal bearing surfaces: materials, manufacture, design optimization and alternatives. Proc Inst Mech Eng [H] 2006;220:119-133.
5. Jin ZM, Meakins S, Morlock MM, Parsons P, Hardaker C, Flett M, Isaac G: Deformation of press-fitted metallic resurfacing cups. Part 1: experimental simulation. Proc Inst Mech Eng [H] 2006;220:299-309.
6. Yew A, Jin ZM, Donn A, Morlock MM, Isaac G: Deformation of press-fitted metallic resurfacing cup. Part 2: finite element simulation. Proc Inst Mech Eng [H] 2006;220:311-319.
7. Liu F, Jin ZM, Hirt F, Rieker C, Roberts P, Grigoris P: Effect of wear of bearings surface on elastohydrodynamic lubrication of metal-on-metal hip implants. Proc Inst Mech Eng [H] 2005; 219:319-328.
8. Liu F, Jin Z, Roberts P, Grigoris P: Importance of head diameter, clearance, and cup wall thickness in elastohydrody-

namic lubrication analysis of metal-on-metal hip resurfacing prostheses. Proc Inst Mech Eng [H] 2006;220:695-704.
9. McMinn D, Daniel J: History and modern concepts in surface replacement. Proc Inst Mech Eng [H] 2006;220:239-251.
10. Williams S, Jalai-Vahid D, Brockett CL, Jin Z, Stone MH, Ingham E, Fisher J: Effect of swing phase load on metal-on-metal hip lubrication, friction and wear. J Biomechanics 2006:30:2274-2281.
11. Firkins PJ, Tipper JL, Ingham E, Stone MH, Farrar R, Fisher J: A novel low wearing differential hardness, ceramic-on-metal hip joint prostheses. J Biomech 2001a;34:1291-1298.
12. Fisher J, Hu XQ, Tipper JL, Stewart TD, Williams S, Stone MH, Davies C, Hatto P, Bolton J, Riley M, Hardaker C, Isaac GH, Berry G, Ingham E: An in vitro study of the reduction in wear of metal-on-metal hip prostheses using surface-engineered femoral heads. Proc Inst Mech Eng [H] 2002;216:219-230.
13. Williams S, Isaac G, Hatto P, Stone MH, Ingham E, Fisher J: Comparative wear under different conditions of surface-engineered metal-on-metal bearings for total hip arthroplasty. J Arthroplasty 2004;19(suppl 3):112-117.
14. Firkins PJ, Tipper JL, Saadatzadeh MR, Ingham E, Stone MH, Farrar R, Fisher J: Quantitative analysis of wear and wear debris from metal-on-metal hip prostheses tested in a physiological hip joint simulator. Biomedical Mater Eng 2001b;11: 143-157.
15. Carroll ME: Metallic bearings for joint replacement. US Patent 20,060,085,079, April 20, 2006.
16. Fisher J, Hu X, Stewart T, Williams S, Tipper J, Ingham E, Stone M, Davies C, Hatto P, Bolton J, Riley M, Hardaker C, Isaac GH, Berry G: Wear of surface engineered metal on metal hip prostheses. J Mater Sci Mater Med 2004;15:225-235.
17. Dowson D, McNie CM, Goldsmith AAJ: Direct experimental evidence of lubrication in metal-on-metal total hip replacement tested in a joint simulator. Proc Inst Mech Eng [C] 2000;214: 75-86.
18. Brockett C, Harper P, Williams S, Isaac G, Dwyer-Joyce R, Jin Z, Fisher J: Direct measurement of lubrication in large diameter metal-on-metal hi implants. Trans Orthopaedic Research Society 2007;32:Poster 1653.
19. Chan FW, Bobyn JD, Medley JB, Krygier JJ, Tanzer M: Wear and lubrication of metal-on-metal hip implants. Clin Orthop 1999;369:10-24.
20. Chan FW, Medley JB, Bobyn JD, Krygier JJ: Time-varying fluid film lubrication of metal-metal hip implants in simulator tests. ASTM STP 1346, American Society for Testing and Materials, West Conshohocken, PA, 1998, pp 111-128.
21. Medley JB, Bobyn JD, Krygier JJ, Chan FW, Tanzer M, Roter GE: Elastohydrodynamic lubrication and wear of metal-on-metal hip implants. World Tribology Forum in Arthroplasty. Hans Huber, Bern, Switzerland, 2001, pp 125-135.
22. Brockett C, Williams S, Jin Z, Isaac G, Fisher J: Friction of total hip replacements with different bearings and loading conditions. J Biomed Mater Res 2007;81:508-515.
23. Vassiliou K, Elfick APD, Scholes SC, Unsworth A: The effect of 'running-in' on the tribology and surface morphology of metal-on-metal Birmingham hip resurfacing device in simulator studies. Proc Inst Mech Eng 2006;220:269-277.
24. Varano R, Bobyn JD, Medley JB, Yue S: The effect of microstructure on the wear of cobalt-based alloys used in metal-on-metal hip implants. Proc Inst Mech Eng [H] 2006;220:145-159.
25. Dowson D: Tribological principles in metal-on-metal hip joint design. Proc Inst Mech Eng [H] 2006;220:161-171.
26. Silva M, Shepherd EF, Jackson WO, Dorey FJ, Schmalzried TP: Average patient walking activity approaches 2 million cycles per year: pedometers under-record walking activity. J Arthroplasty 2002;17:693-697.
27. Paré P, Medley JB, Chan F, Young S, Bobyn JD, Krygier J: The role of the lambda parameter on the simulator wear of metal-metal hip implants. Tribology Series 41, Elsevier, 2003, pp 281-290.
28. Lippincott AL, Medley JB: Low-wear ball and cup joint prosthesis. WIPO 9716138, May 9, 1997. US patent 6,059,830, May 9, 2000.
29. Walker PS, Gold BL: The tribology (friction, lubrication and wear) of all-metal artificial hip joints. Wear 1971;17:285-299.
30. Farrar R, Schmidt MB: The effect of diametral clearance on wear between head and cup for metal on metal articulations. 43rd Annual Meeting of the Orthopaedic Research Society, San Francisco, CA, 1997.
31. Wang A, Yue S, Bobyn JD, Chan F, Medley JB: Surface characterization of metal-on-metal hip implants tested in a hip simulator. Wear 1999;225-229:708-715.
32. Park S-H, McKellop H, Lu B, Chan F, Chiesa R: Wear morphology of metal-metal implants: hip simulator tests compared with clinical retrievals. ASTM STP 1346, American Society for Testing and Materials, West Conshohocken, PA, 1998, pp 129-143.
33. Wimmer MA, Sprecher C, Hauert R, Täger G, Fischer A: Tribochemical reaction on metal-on-metal hip joint bearings—a comparison between in-vitro and in-vivo results. Wear 2003; 255:1007-1014.
34. Wimmer MA, Nassutt R, Sprecher C, Loos J, Täger G, Fischer A: Investigation on stick phenomena in metal-on-metal hip joints after resting periods. Proc Inst Mech Eng [H] 2006;220: 219-227.
35. Catelas I, Campbell PA, Bobyn JD, Medley JB, Huk OL: Wear particles from metal-on-metal total hip replacements: effects of implant design and implantation time. Proc Inst Mech Eng [H] 2006;220:195-208.
36. Catelas I, Medley JB, Campbell PA, Huk OL, Bobyn JD: Comparison of in vitro with in vivo characteristics of wear particles from metal-metal hip implants. J Biomed Mater Res 2004;70B: 167-178.
37. Dowson D, Hardaker C, Flett M. Isaac GH: A hip joint simulator study of the performance of metal-on-metal joints. Part 1: the role of materials. J Arthroplasty 2004;19(Suppl 3):118-123.
38. Buscher R, Tager G, Dudzinski W, Gleising B, Wimmer MA, Fischer A: Subsurface microstructrue of metal-on-metal hip joints and its relationship to wear particle generation. J Biomed Mater Res 2004;72B:206-214.
39. Varano R: Wear behaviour of CoCrMo alloys used in metal-on-metal hip implants. PhD Thesis, McGill University, Montreal, QC, 2004.
40. Bowsher JG, Nevelos J, Williams PA, Shelton JC: 'Severe' wear challenge to 'as-cast' and 'double heat-treated' large-diameter metal-on-metal hip bearings. Proc Inst Mech Eng [H] 2006b; 220:135-143.
41. Dowson D, Jin ZM: Metal-on-metal hip joint tribology. Proc Inst Mech Eng [H] 2006;220:107-118.
42. Medley JB, Pare PE, Bobyn JD, Krygier J, Chan F, Aust SK: Can metal-metal surface replacement implants generate thick enough elastohydrodynamic films to protect the surfaces effectively? 4th International Biotribology Forum and 24th Biotribology Symposium "Compliant and Hard Bearing Surfaces for Artificial Joints,

Alternative Solutions and Future Directions," Kyushu University, Fukuoka, Japan, Session 1, 1-4, 2003.
43. Hamrock BJ, Dowson D: Elastohydrodynamic lubrication of elliptical contacts for materials of low elastic modulus: 1 fully flooded conjunction. Trans ASME J Lubric Technol 1978;100:236-245.
44. Medley JB, Krygier JJ, Bobyn JD, Chan FW, Lippincott A, Tanzer M: Kinematics of the MATCOJ hip simulator and issues related to wear testing of metal-metal implants. Proc Inst Mech Eng [H] 1997;211:89-99.
45. Medley JB, Dowson D, Wright V: Transient elastohydrodynamic lubrication models for the human ankle joint. Eng Med 1984; 13:137-151.
46. Smith TJ, Medley JB: Development of transient elastohydrodynamic models for synovial joint lubrication. Tribology Series 11, Elsevier, 1987, pp 369-374.
47. Gaman IDC, Higginson GR, Norman R: Fluid entrapment by a soft surface layer. Wear 1974;28:345-352.
48. Higginson GR: Squeeze films between compliant surfaces. Wear 1978;46:387-395.
49. Chan FW, Bobyn JD, Medley JB, Krygier JJ: Simulator wear of metal-metal hip implants under adverse loading conditions. Trans Orthopaedic Research Society 1999;24:310.
50. Bowsher JG, Hussain A, Williams PA, Shelton JC: Metal-on-metal hip simulator study of increased wear particle surface area due to 'severe' patient activity. Proc Inst Mech Eng [H] 2006; 220:279-287.
51. Rieker CB, Schon R, Kottig P: Development and validation of a second-generation metal-on-metal bearing. Laboratory studies and analysis of retrievals. J Arthrop 2004;9:5-11.
52. Medley JB, McGarry W, Campbell P, De Smet K, Amstutz HC: Well-positioned large diameter surface replacement implants can have low wear in vivo. Trans Orthopaedic Research Society 2007;32:Poster 1696.
53. Medley JB, Chan F, Krygier J, Bobyn JD: Comparison of alloys and designs in a hip simulator study of metal on metal implants. Clin Orthop 1996;329S:S148-S159.
54. Medley JB, Dowling JM, Poggie RA, Krygier J, Bobyn JD: Simulator wear of some commercially available metal-on-metal hip implants. ASTM Symposium on Alternative Bearing Surfaces in Total Joint Replacement, ASTM STP 1346, American Society for Testing and Materials, West Conshohocken, PA, 1998, pp 92-110.
55. Willert HG, Buchhorn GHH, Gobel D, Koster G, Schaffner S, Schenk R, Semlitsch M: Wear behavior and histopathology of classic cemented metal on metal hip endoprosthesis. Clin Orthop 1996;329S:S160-S186.
56. McKellop H, Park S-H, Chiesa R, Doorn P, Lu B, Normand P, Grigoris P, Amstutz H: In vivo wear of 3 types of metal on metal hip prostheses during 2 decades of use. Clin Orthop 1996;329(suppl):S128-S140.

APPENDIX 4A

A Simple Transient Elastohydrodynamic Lubrication Analysis for Metal-on-Metal Hip Implants

Deriving a Governing Equation

Lubrication analysis for metal-on-metal (MM) surface replacement arthroplasty (SRA) of the hip requires a full consideration of the fluid flow and the deformation of the surfaces as shown by Liu et al.[8] Such analysis cannot be performed without a high level of expertise in tribology, and requires advanced numerical methods. Even with such levels of expertise, the solutions can be questionable. For example, the analysis of Liu et al shows a larger central film thickness during the stance phase than the swing phase, despite the higher load, and attributes this to an out-of-phase "squeeze-film effect." Later, in a review paper by Dowson and Jin,[41] a somewhat similar case (but with higher viscosity and a smaller diameter) gives a slightly higher swing phase film thickness as expected. The non-intuitive behavior noted by Liu et al may be a consequence of the ripples that develop in the relatively compliant surfaces of MM SRA under conditions of time-varying loads and surface velocities. During the stance phase, the central film thickness may no longer be a good representation of the average lubricant film thickness over the contact.

In any case, it is possible to develop an approximate analysis that captures much of the essential nature of elastohydrodynamic lubrication (ehl) behavior under transient conditions, and this analysis can be implemented with an elementary knowledge of numerical methods.[20,21,42] This approximate analysis combines well-supported correlations for pure steady entraining action and pure squeeze action in a single nonlinear ordinary differential equation that represents transient ehl.

The analysis begins with a formula for the central lubricant film thickness (h_C) under conditions of pure steady entraining action is based on the numerical analysis of Hamrock and Dowson[43] as adapted by Medley et al[44] as follows:

$$h_C = 5.083\frac{(\eta u)^{0.660} R^{0.767}}{(E')^{0.447} F^{0.213}} \tag{A1}$$

where $u = \dfrac{\omega R_H}{2}$, $E' = \dfrac{E}{1-\nu^2}$ and $R = \dfrac{R_H R_C}{R_C - R_H} \approx \dfrac{R_H^{\,2}}{R_C - R_H}$

In the above-mentioned formula, the surface properties are represented by the elastic modulus (E) and Poisson's ratio (ν) that are combined to give the effective elastic modulus (E') for the contact. The lubricant is represented by viscosity (η) and hip implant geometry is included as the radius of the head (R_H) and the cup (R_C) but conveniently combined in the effective radius (R), a term that includes the radial clearance ($R_C - R_H$). The resultant angular velocity of the hip (ω) can be used to calculate the entrainment velocity (u) and the resultant load (F) completes the conditions imposed on the implant. This formula (equation A1) is well supported by experimental data and some numerical analysis of metal-on-metal hip implants subject to pure steady entraining action as described by Medley et al.[42]

Equation A1 can be rearranged algebraically in terms of the load (F) as follows:

$$F = 8.9259\frac{(\eta u) R^{0.4848} a^{2.030}}{h_C^{\,1.5152}}$$

Note that $a = \left(\dfrac{1.5FR}{E'}\right)^{\frac{1}{3}}$ is identified and incorporated because it provides a good estimate of the radius of the essentially circular contact zone of hip implants. Under transient conditions, it is assumed that the contact area geometry is determined by the total load acting at an instant in time. It is further assumed that the load carried by the entraining action (F_E) can be expressed by the right hand side of the above equation. This pair of assumptions attempts to decouple the entraining action from the surface shape and is based on similar assumptions made in the lubrication analysis of Medley et al[45] and Smith and Medley.[46]

Next, an expression for the load (F) carried by the contact under pure squeeze action is considered using a simple analytical expression[47,48] as follows:

$$F = -\frac{3\pi\eta a^4}{2h_C^{\,3}}\frac{dh_C}{dt}$$

where once again the estimated radius of the contact zone (a) appears. This expression is supported by some experimental data and some numerical analysis of metal-polyethylene hip implants subject to pure squeezing action as described by Medley et al.[42] Once again and for the same reasons, it is assumed that under transient conditions, the contact area geometry is determined by the total load acting at an instant and thus the load carried by the squeeze action (F_S) can be expressed by the right hand side of the above equation.

Following the above-mentioned assumptions, the total load carried during both entraining and squeezing action ($F = F_E + F_S$) can be represented as

$$F = 8.9259\frac{(\eta u)R^{0.4848}a^{2.030}}{h_C^{1.5152}} - \frac{3\pi\eta a^4}{2h_C^3}\frac{dh_C}{dt}$$

By algebraically rearranging this expression, a single nonlinear ordinary differential equation can be derived as follows:

$$\text{(A2)} \qquad \frac{dh_C}{dt} = C1\frac{R^{C2}(h_C)^{C3}u}{a^{C4}} - C5\frac{(h_C)^3 F}{\eta a^4}$$

where $a = \left(\frac{1.5FR}{E'}\right)^{\frac{1}{3}}$ and $C1 = 1.8941$ $C2 = 0.48485$ $C3 = 1.4848$ $C4 = 1.9700$ $C5 = 0.21221$

Both the entrainment velocity (u) and the total resultant load (F) are functions of time.

Some Results

Equation A2 was solved using a 4th order Runge-Kutta algorithm with natural cubic spline interpolation for the time-varying entrainment velocity and load functions. Global (rather than local) step-size halving was performed to find a solution with minimal truncation error and about fourteen significant digits were carried in the calculations to discourage round-off errors.

The solutions of equation A2 for the central film thickness (h_C) variation with time were an approximate representation of transient ehl of metal-metal hip implants. It was best suited to thick solidly backed acetabular cups and thus became less accurate for the large thin-walled SRA cups. The predicted

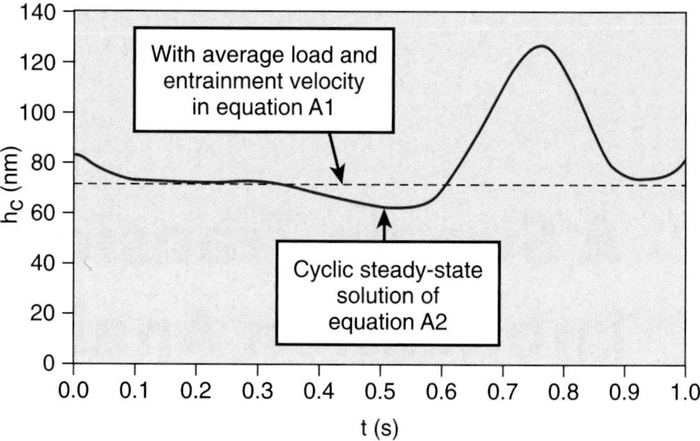

Figure A1 An example of the present simple analysis for a head radius (R_H = 25 mm), a cup radius (R_C = 25.075 mm), a viscosity (η = 0.0025 Pa s), elastic modulus (E = 230 GPa) and a Poisson's ratio (ν = 0.3). The load and entrainment velocity were as presented by Medley et al.[42] The average value of the load (F_{AVG} = 1208 N) and the average value of the entrainment velocity (u_{AVG} = 22.91 mm/s) were used in equation A1 to provide an estimate for the central film thickness (h_C) that avoided performing a transient solution.

film thickness values for SRA implants of low clearance were 5-10 times larger than the root mean square surface roughness, thus suggesting significant surface protection from ehl films. This protection might be compromised by stop-dwell-start motion,[49] severe patient activity,[50] microseparation,[10] progressive surface damage,[27] and interference from tribochemical reaction films.[33] However, even compromised film protection could reduce wear.

A very important concept did emerge from the simple analysis described in the present appendix. Equation A1 for the steady entraining action applied with the average load and entrainment velocity over the walking cycle gave a fairly accurate estimate of the average film thickness at cyclic steady state as shown in Figure A1 and this occurred in all cases analyzed by Chan et al[20] and Medley et al,[21,42] as well as in the more rigorous analysis presented by Lui et al[8] and by Dowson and Jin.[41] As a final note, Lui et al found considerable increase in the predicted film thickness for MM SRA because of the relatively compliant cup surface as a result of its thin walls and subchondral bone backing. Thus, the present simple analysis would require an effective elastic modulus for cup and supporting structures in MM SRA to give an accurate film thickness value representing the average over the contact at an instant in time.

APPENDIX 4B

A Correlation of Retrieval and Simulator Wear Rates with the Effective Radius

Both the radius of the implant head (R_H) and the clearance (R_C–R_H) influence the transient elastohydrodynamic lubrication of metal-on-metal (MM) surface replacement arthroplasty (SRA).[25] The decision to have large heads (and thus large R_H) has already been proscribed in SRA by the patient anatomy and ranges from about $R_H = 20\text{-}28$ mm. However, the clearance can be set during the manufacturing process, thus determining the effective radius (R)

$$R = \frac{R_H R_C}{R_C - R_H} \approx \frac{R_H^{2}}{R_C - R_H}$$

and this quantity directly influences lubrication. The R of MM SRA implants can vary over a wide range of about 2.5 to 8 m. Thus, it is expected that an influence of R on in vivo and simulator wear can be demonstrated. To allow simulator wear rates to be included with in vivo wear rates, the simulator wear rates were converted by assuming 2 million cycles was equal to 1 year in vivo, following Silva et al.[26]

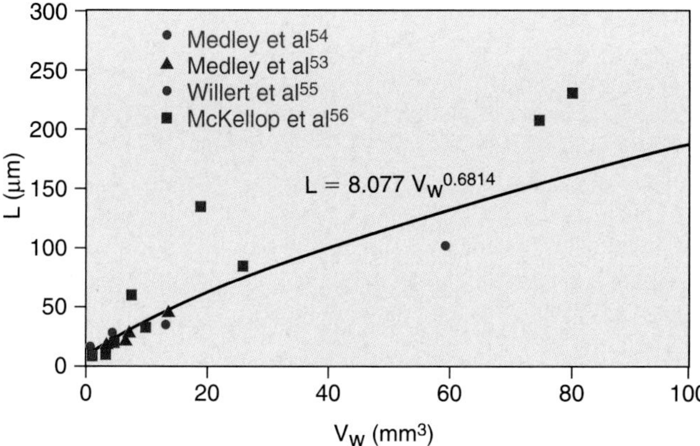

Figure B1 An expression for relating linear (L) to volumetric (V_W) wear. Note that L was assumed to have the most scatter and thus the curve fit was of L vs V_W. This curve fit expression was then manipulated to give an expression of the form $V_W = 0.0466\ L^{1.47}$ for converting linear to volumetric wear when examining clinical data. The formula was developed from calculated values from Medley et al[53,54] and from Willert et al,[55] along with measured retrieval wear, both L and volumetric wear of the head only (V_{WH}) with the assumption that $V_W = 1.5\ V_{WH}$, from McKellop et al.[56] The wear rates (V) in mm^3/yr were simply volumetric wear (V_W) divided by implantation time. A similar expression was found by Paré et al.[27]

Unfortunately, most of the retrieval wear data are presented as total linear wear (i.e., the sum of the maximum wear depth on the head and on the cup) and, thus, a conversion formula was developed (Fig. B1). With this conversion formula, retrieval data from Rieker et al[51] and retrieval data

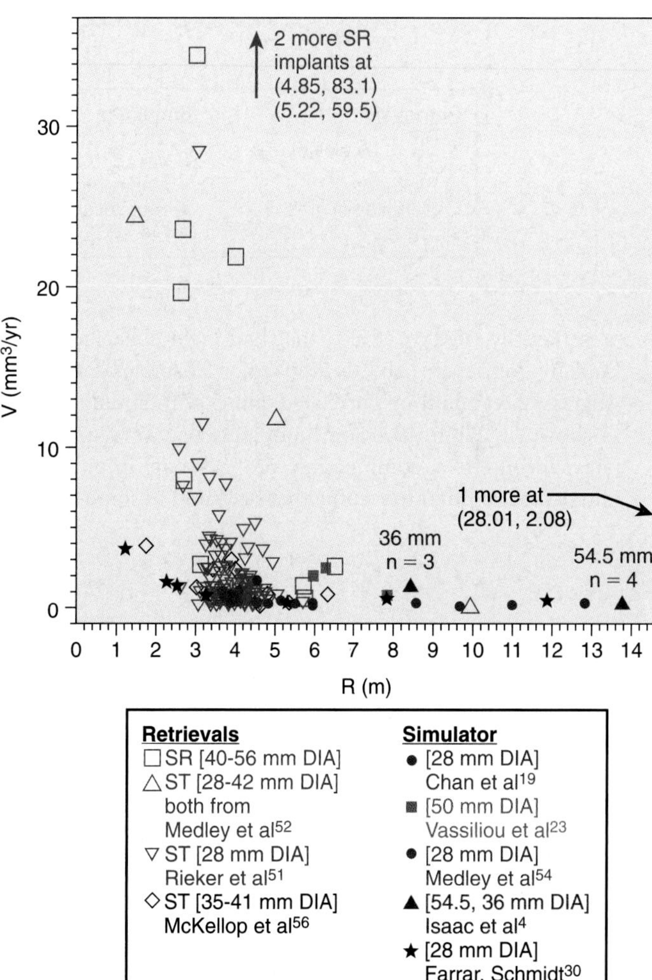

Figure B2 Volumetric wear rate versus effective radius where the simulator data was included by assuming that 2 Mc as equivalent to 1 year in vivo following Silva et al.[26] The higher wear was caused by micro-separation, impingement and/or loosening that occurred in some patients. (SR = MM SRA implants; ST = MM, stem-type implants.)

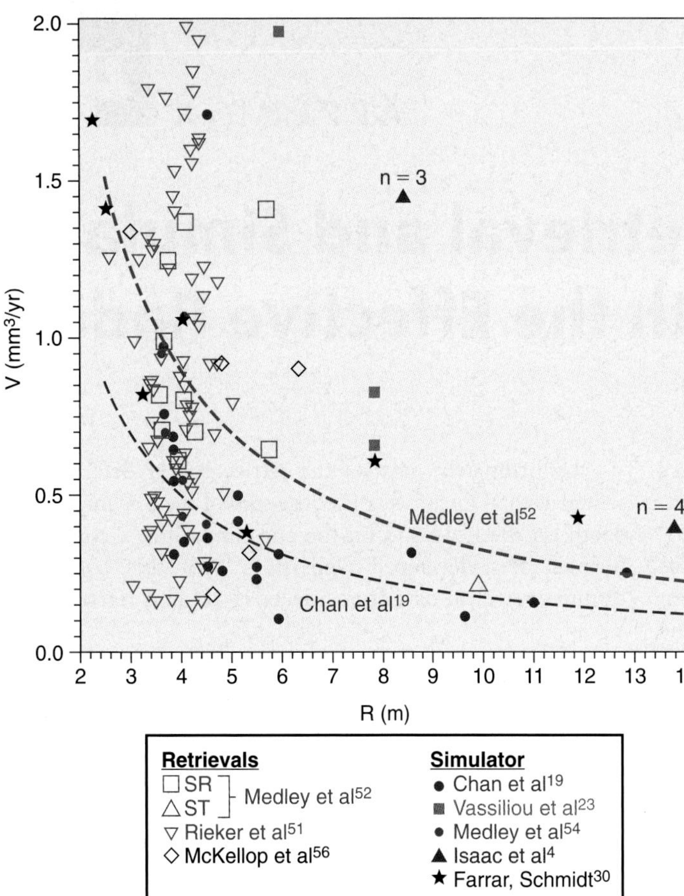

Figure B3 A close-up view of the volumetric wear rate (V) versus effective radius (R) taken from Figure B2 for V < 2 mm^3/yr.

presented by Medley et al[52] (that had been collected by the Implant Retrieval Lab, Orthopaedic Hospital/UCLA, Los Angeles, CA) could be correlated, along with simulator data, as shown in Figure B2. Some implants had very high wear rates, owing to a combination of neck-cup impingement, micro-separation or loosening that occurred in some patients; these implants did not have large R values. As R increased, there was a powerful reduction in the wear rate found in simulator testing and found in implant retrievals, many of which were SRA with implants made from either F75 As-Cast or F75 HIP + SA alloys as clearly shown in the close-up view of Figure B3.

An Effect of Microstructure on Wear

A study of the fundamental wear behavior of cobalt-based alloys was performed by Varano[39] using a multistation pin-on-plate apparatus (Fig. C1) in the presence of a 25% bovine serum lubricant. The pin had a spherical tip, but the conditions were not conducive to elastohydrodynamic lubrication. Thus a combination of boundary lubrication and direct surface interaction occurred.[24] Such conditions were not considered likely to occur at all times in metal-on-metal (MM) surface replacement arthroplasty (SRA), but such conditions were considered possible during stop-dwell-start motion[49] and at some local sites in the contact.

Various cobalt-based alloys (Table 4-1), composed mainly of cobalt, chromium, and molybdenum (CoCrMo) pairs, were tested in the pin-on-plate apparatus, including alloys that were wrought (ASTM F1537 HC) with a high-carbon (HC) level of about 0.23%, wrought (ASTM F1537 LC) with a low-carbon (LC) level of about 0.05%, cast followed by a hot isostatic pressing (HIP) and solution annealing (SA) heat treatments (ASTM F75 HIP + SA), with about 0.27% carbon and simply cast (ASTM F75 As-Cast) also with about 0.27% carbon. The HIP and SA procedures were very similar to those described in Table 4-1, based on information provided in Bowsher et al.[40] After 1 million cycles (Mc) of testing, the F75 As-Cast pairs had the lowest wear (Fig. C2). The morphology of the wear tracks of the F75 HIP + SA compared with the F75 As-Cast clearly showed the difference in the amount of wear (Fig. C3). Also, metallographic presentation (Fig. C3) showed that the carbides had a "depleted" lamellar structure in the F75 HIP + SA compared with the F75 As-Cast, but quantitative analysis[39] showed that the amount of carbon contained in the carbides was increased for the F75 HIP + SA because the heat treatments caused carbide precipitation.

The search for a mechanism involved a consideration of the face centered cubic (FCC) and hexagonal close packed (HCP) crystal structures, both of which occurred in this class of cobalt-based alloys. The FCC phase was more wear resistant but a strain-induced transformation to HCP could occur at the surface. Dissolved carbon in the matrix (as opposed to in the carbides) could suppress the tendency of the FCC to undergo the transformation. Thus, the total carbon residing in the carbides (estimated using carbide chemistry and the volume fraction of carbides determined from image analysis of the specimen surfaces) was subtracted from the total carbon content to estimate the dissolved carbon in solid solution. The wear was reduced for the higher amounts of dissolved carbon (Fig. C4). The F75 As-Cast alloy had the highest amount of dissolved carbon and, thus, the lowest wear. However, Varano[39] had some success in heat treating wrought alloys to increase their dissolved carbon and reduce the wear (Fig. C4).

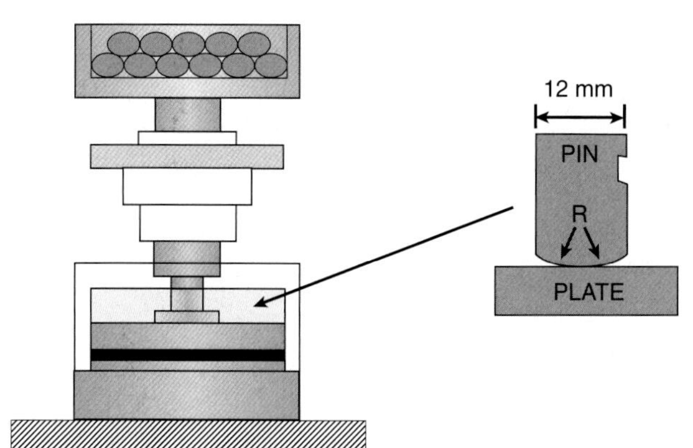

Figure C1 A single station of the linear reciprocating pin-on-plate apparatus used by Varano[39] showing the 12-mm diameter pin with a 100-mm radius spherical tip.

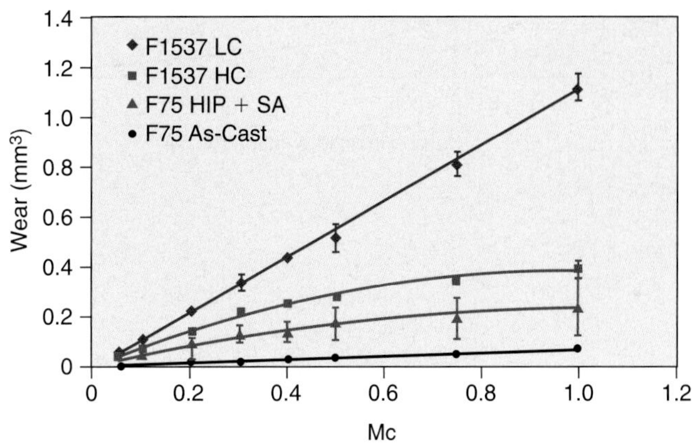

Figure C2 The wear of various cobalt-based alloy pairs (n = 3) in a linear reciprocating pin-on-plate apparatus.[39] For F75 As-Cast, the standard deviation scatter bars were within the data points. Also, because wear amounts at zero Mc cycles were not actually measured, they were not included.

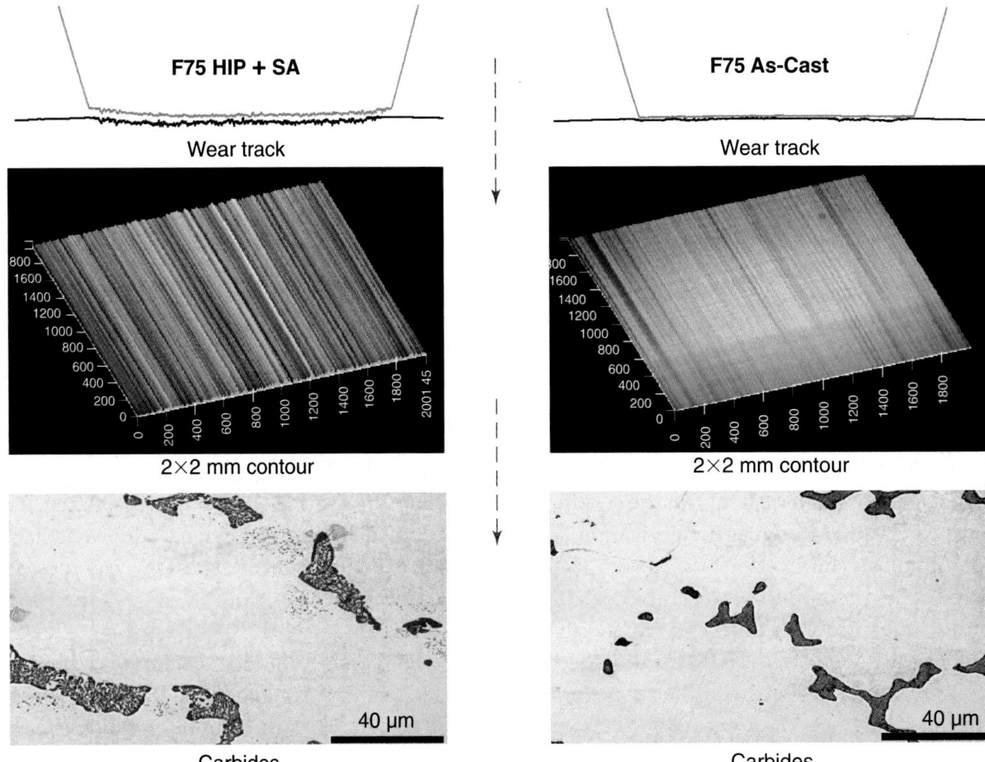

Figure C3 Details of the wear tracks and carbide morphology for the F75 HIP + SA compared with the F75 As-Cast materials. The track width for the F75 HIP + SA was about 4.9 mm, whereas for the F75 As-Cast it was about 4.5 mm. The peak-to-peak roughness of the F75 HIP + SA plate was about 2 μm. A metallographic presentation at the bottom of the figure shows the carbide morphology (all from Varano[39]).

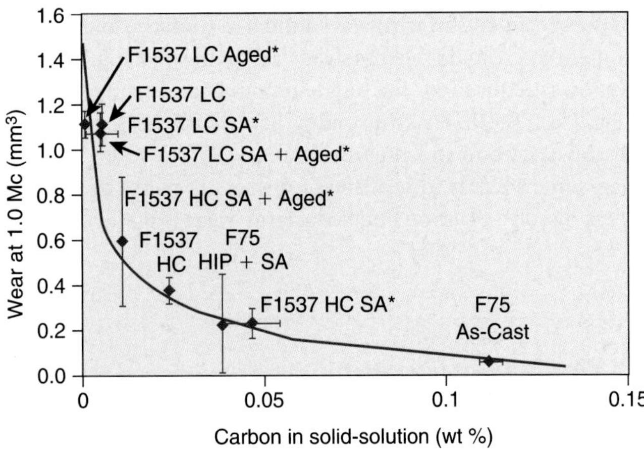

Figure C4 Wear at 1.0 Mc versus the carbon in solid-solution (dissolved in the matrix). Data values were taken from Varano et al.[24,39]

* The wear tests that generated these data points were not shown in Figure C2.

CHAPTER 5

Imaging of Hip Resurfacing

Thomas A. Gruen

Introduction

Evolutionary changes are vital to the advancement of surgical treatment options for patients with musculoskeletal disorders of the hip joint. Total hip arthroplasty (THA) is acknowledged to be one of the most successful surgical procedures and is continuing to expand into patients with select indications, for example, younger and more active patients, who had historically inferior results with THA.[1-3] One such recent option is the current generation of metal-on-metal (MM) articulation hip resurfacing arthroplasty. This represents a resurgence from the previous generation of hip resurfacing based on metal-on-polyethylene articulation surfaces, which had a high failure rate related to polyethylene particle–mediated osteolysis[4,5] and long-term resorptive changes of the femoral head or femoral neck.[3,6] It was after numerous successful clinical experiences with the use of MM in conventional total hip arthroplasty using intramedullary stem-type femoral components that this technology of MM was extended to hip resurfacing prosthetic components starting in the 1990s.[7,8]

Nevertheless the surgical expertise needed for preoperative planning, particularly the epiphyseal and metaphyseal parts of the proximal femur, demand careful assessment of the wide variation, both normal and pathologic, of the femoral anatomy.[9] Proper planning is usually made with the use of plain radiographs during preoperative clinical evaluation; however, each radiographic image, being a two-dimensional representation of a complex three-dimensional structure, often is not very accurate, owing to substantial projective distortion and superimposition of anatomic structures. It is very important to know and understand the limitations of such two-dimensional diagnostic information.

To date, most short- and intermediate term results have been promising, but detailed assessments of clinical outcomes on the effectiveness of MM hip resurfacing are relatively scarce because it is a relatively new technique.[1,2,10-12] Because current systems of MM hip resurfacing have been introduced within the past 10 years,[10,13] it is only within the past 3 years that a small number of published results, with detailed radiographic outcomes associated with these procedures in general patient populations, have appeared in peer-reviewed literature.[14-18]

The objective of this chapter is to update the state on the art of radiographic outcomes assessment related to MM hip resurfacing as evaluated from conventional medical imaging, that is, plain radiography. It is intended to review radiologic protocol, as well as discuss radiographic parameters with appropriate terminologies, as used in a clinical setting, in patients with hip resurfacing and to summarize their relevance and clinical significance.

Radiologic Protocol

Plain radiography is the conventional imaging method for preoperative and postoperative assessment of patients who undergo hip arthroplasty.[19,20] No consensus currently exists, however, regarding which radiographic views reproducibly and reliably predict clinical outcomes. For all hip arthroplasty procedures, including hip resurfacing, it is required to have at least two (ideally if truly orthogonal) standardized antero-posterior (AP)-pelvis and lateral projections, which can realistically elucidate on the complex three-dimensional structural implant-hip relationships of the reconstructed hip joint and allow for more accurate diagnosis and treatment planning, treatment monitoring, and radiographic outcomes analysis in heterogeneous patient populations. Furthermore, variations in radiologic techniques often make a valid comparison of serial radiographs obtained during the postoperative course almost impossible. Subtle variations in radiologic technique from one examination to the next may render serial evaluation inadequate for obtaining reliable measurements to detect radiographic changes at the interface or within the surround supportive bone structures.

The AP-pelvis view should be centered over the pubic symphysis, with the patient in the supine position and having the toes pointing upward or slightly internally rotated. Ideally, when two diagonal lines from opposite corners of the film are superimposed on the AP-pelvis image, the intersection of the two diagonals would be at or very near the pubic symphysis (Fig. 5-1A). The profile of both obturator foramina, particularly the horizontal and vertical dimensions, should be symmetric to minimize measurement errors associated with

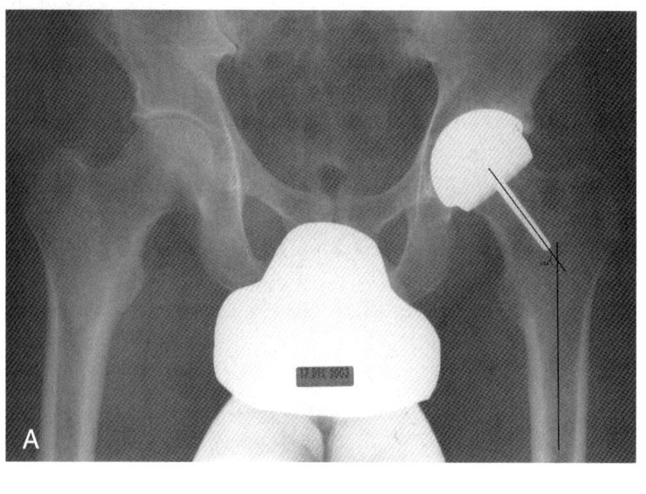

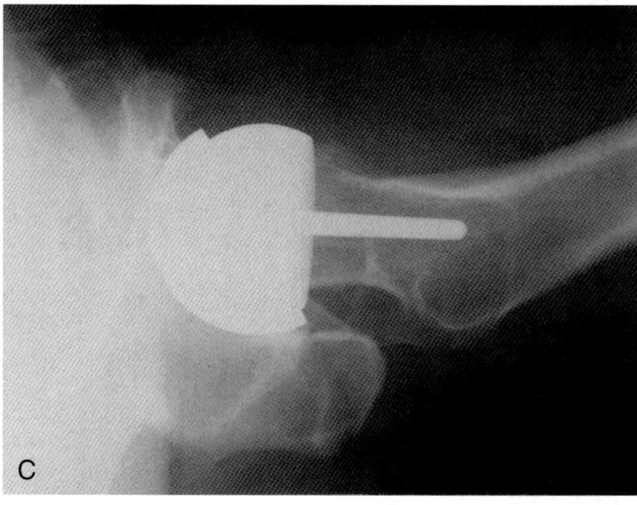

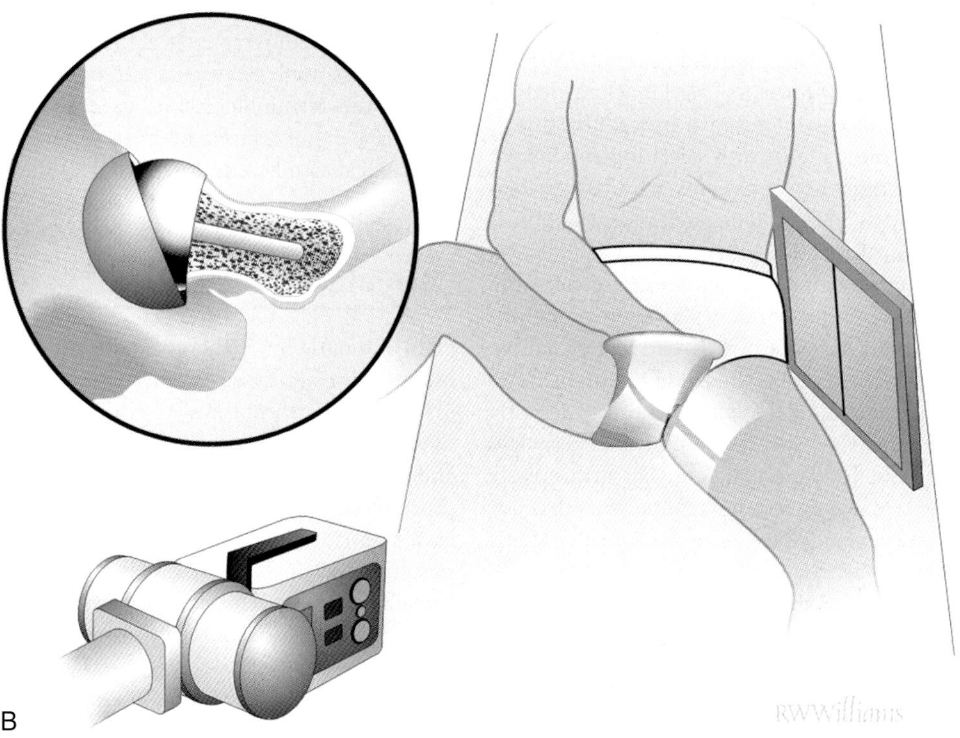

Figure 5-1 Exemplary anteroposterior (AP) and lateral postoperative radiographs following metal-on-metal hip resurfacing. The measurement of the stem-shaft angle is shown. **A,** "Low," that is, centered at pubic symphysis, AP-pelvis view with hip prosthesis in place. The assessment of femoral component positioning in the frontal plane (stem-shaft angle) is shown. **B,** Schematic of the positioning of the patient's hip, X-ray tube and cassette, to provide a high quality True-lateral (Johnson or cross-table lateral) view. The long axis of the left femoral neck is localized by imaging a line drawn between the anterosuperior iliac spine and the superior border of the symphysis pubis, determining the midpoint of the line, and then palpating the greater trochanter and imaging a point 1 inch distal to it. A line drawn between these two points parallels the long axis of the femoral neck. The cassette is placed in the vertical position with its cephalad border in contact with the body at the level of the iliac crest; it is parallel with the long axis of the femoral neck. The central ray is perpendicular to the long axis of the femoral neck and cassette and is centered 2.5 inches below the point of intersection of the localization lines. **C,** Cross-table lateral view with hip prosthesis in place. The anterior osteophyte present on the anterior aspect of the femoral neck was preserved at surgery.

variations in pelvic tilt or rotation. It would be convenient to add an AP-hip centered view that would be the preferred tangential AP projection of the hip joint rather than with the AP-pelvis view.

Owing to the fact that few, if any, published studies have reported on the use of true lateral projection, it is essential to use this view to provide a more realistic, as well as reliable and reproducible, spatial assessment of the reconstructed hip joint following hip resurfacing. Conventionally the "standard" frog-leg lateral has been used to evaluate patients postoperatively after hip replacement; however, the projection of this view has been acknowledged to be inconsistent over the course of time and to be of some discomfort to the patient.

The cross-table (axiolateral) projection, a "shoot-through view" initially described by Johnson,[21] to view the neck of the femur tangentially is essential to adequately evaluate bone changes after hip resurfacing in that plane. Ideally the entire neck should be visible up to the neutrally orientated component face without overlap of anterior and posterior rims. The correct positions of the patient and the orientation of the x-ray beam with a cone to provide better image quality are illustrated in Figure 5-1B. It is important to flex the hip enough so that the femoral component-neck junction is observed. The more the acetabular component is anteverted, the more the hip will have to be flexed to be able to view this area of the neck. This view has also been helpful for estimating acetabular version (Fig. 5-1C), but it is not as accurate as other methods because evaluation criteria based on reliable bony landmarks have not been clearly delineated.[22] Although difficult, the technologist should strive to reproduce the same flexion and rotation at each visit. Therefore, it is vital that the previous radiographs are available for viewing and comparison. Unfortunately in many clinics the image quality of the proximal femur obtained in the cross-table lateral view has often been suboptimal, and in these cases, the interpretation of periprosthetic changes was not reliable at or near the femoral component. A more reproducible lateral view is the modified frog lateral view, that is, the mediolateral projection as described by Lauenstein, which is often referred to as the "table-down" lateral view.[22,23] Many, if not most, radiologic technicians probably are not familiar with this technique, making request of this view difficult unless it is recognized that this is a more practical lateral view of the proximal femur. From the supine position, the patient is asked to flex the affected knee and maintain both the knee and ankle of the affected leg touching the table top. This is more feasible for consistent positioning at each serial follow-up examination. Sometimes the patient needs to have the opposite hip extended or abducted to avoid superimposition of the affected side. The x-ray beam is centered perpendicular over the hip joint. The evaluation criteria for a good lateral projection should include: (1) clear demonstration of the femoral neck overlapped by the greater trochanter; (2) a small amount of the greater trochanter on the anterior and posterior surfaces of the proximal femur when the femur is properly inverted, that is, about 15 to 20 degrees; (3) slight extension of the lesser trochanter on the posterior surface of the femur; and (4) a clear, radiodense, curvilinear profile of the true calcar femorale.[24] This view is helpful preoperatively, but it is less valuable for hip resurfacing follow-up examinations.

Radiographic Protocol

In addition to the detailed preoperative radiographic assessments used in the diagnostic evaluation of the patient's appropriate musculoskeletal status for the resurfacing arthroplasty procedures, the patient is advised to follow-up periodically during the postoperative course at the recommended intervals of 6 weeks, 3 or 6 months, 1 year, 2 years, and annually thereafter, especially at milestone postoperative examinations including at every fifth postoperative interval with both detailed clinical and radiographic outcomes assessment. It is essential that the first return postoperative examination include a set of both AP-pelvis and lateral hip radiographs, which will serve as the "baseline" view from which all subsequent serial radiographs will be compared for any periprosthetic or other radiographic changes. It is essential that the baseline postoperative views be investigated to corroborate the predictions from preoperative templating to validate the appropriate size selection of the implant components and their respective achieved anatomic positioning and orientation, for example, operative technical aspects such as component seating, variation from the preoperative neck-shaft angle, and biomechanical restoration of hip joint mechanics including femoral and acetabular offsets and radiographic leg-length discrepancy.

Intraoperative findings are recommended to be documented, such as the extent (dimensions in millimeter units) and location of lesions present at the prepared bone surfaces before component insertion and the location and extent of neck notching (Fig. 5-2). It is also important to note the presence, if any, of residual intra-articular or juxta-articular pelvic cystic lesions from the radiographic features associated with primary osteoarthrosis[25-28] or avascular necrosis because these features should not be misinterpreted as radiographic evidence of apparent early onset of periprosthetic osteolysis.

Radiographic Evaluation of Baseline Views

Radiographic outcomes parameters to be determined from the baseline views are summarized in Table 5-1. Most of these measurement parameters, either linear or angular measurements, are not only clinically relevant but are also affected significantly by variations in the radiologic protocol, which, in turn, rely on proper selection of reference structural landmarks whether they are associated with the supportive hip bone structure or of the hip implant itself. Hence, it is imperative to follow consistent radiologic protocol for the initial baseline views and for all subsequent serial postoperative examinations. As an example, a situation unique with hip resurfacing implants relates to the measurement of the neck-shaft angle preoperatively and of the postoperative assessment of the stem-shaft angle subtended by the stem (or pin) of the femoral component to the longitudinal axis of the proximal femur, which can have measurement errors associated with the internal or external rotational position of the femur. This appears to be corroborated by the lack of published data of such measurements across the entire spectrum of hips evaluated in the peer-reviewed literature. The difficulty with reliable measurement of the metaphyseal femoral angle measurements from a single AP radiograph is related to the considerable wide

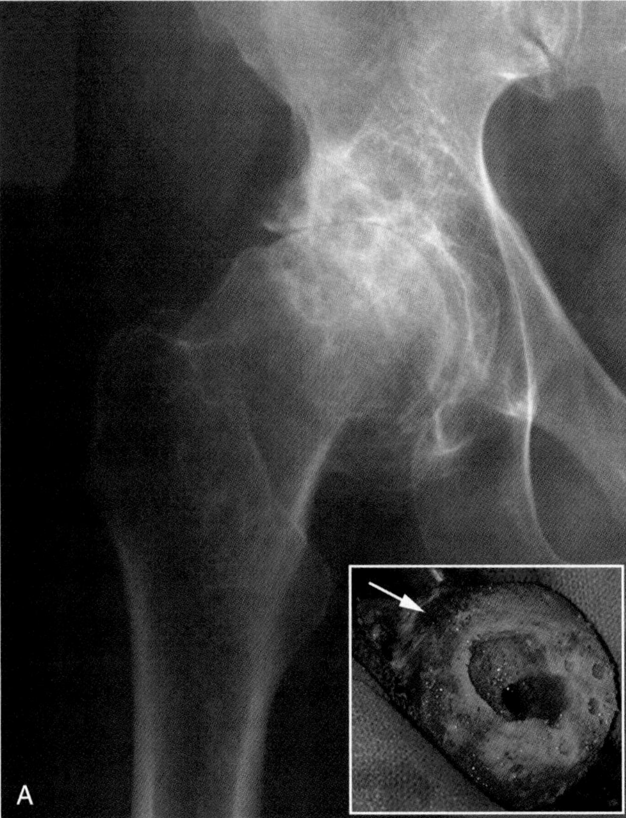

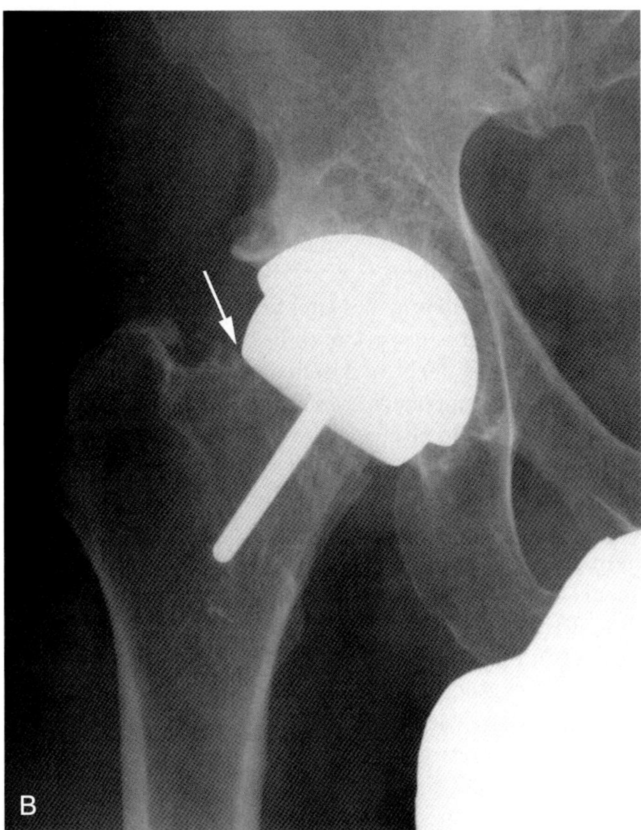

Figure 5-2 Neck notching as noted intraoperatively and postoperatively. **A,** Preoperative anteroposterior radiograph of a 40-year-old man who underwent metal-on-metal hip resurfacing for osteoarthritis secondary to slipped capital femoral epiphysis. The femoral head is flattened and the neck extremely wide, yielding a characteristic low head-neck ratio. As noted in the insert, a notching of the neck is visible in the intra-operative photograph *(arrow)*. There is a large cystic defect. **B,** Five years after surgery, the notch is still evident on the lateral aspect of the femoral neck *(arrow)*. The patient has done well clinically.

variability both within and between human (normal and patient) populations.[29-32] Consequently, femoral rotation relative to the film cassette has a significant effect on radiographic measurements of the neck-shaft angle, to which this would apply also to assessment of stem-shaft angle measurements for most, if not all, metaphyseally fixed femoral hip components.[33–36] One recent study demonstrated that external rotation of the proximal femur, which should be avoided during patient positioning, as little as 7 degrees can simulate a change of more than 10 degrees in the apparent neck-shaft angle.[34] Similarly a quantitative study on position-related errors in measuring femoral neck anteversion using computed tomography (CT) scans demonstrated measurement errors of the projected anteversion angle of up to 10 degrees.[37] Other studies have noted an apparent change in the valgus/varus orientation of stem-type femoral components on AP radiographs, and it was observed that external rotation caused pseudovalgus orientation and internal rotation caused pseudovarus orientation.[38,39]

Radiographic Evaluation of Serial Postoperative Views

Radiolucent Lines and Implant Stability

Although the above-mentioned is applicable to the study of similar hip views of different patients, similar concerns are to be heeded in temporal, that is, serial, assessment of similar views taken during the postoperative course of each individual patient in the study cohort. This pertains to the radiographic assessment of changes, if any, with interface radiolucent lines associated with stable (osseointegrated) implants or changes with unstable (fibrous fixation) implant components having diaphyseal intramedullary stem fixation, as evidenced by migration in conjunction with progressive widening and extension of the interface radiolucent lines. Traditionally, thin radiolucent lines with adjacent thin sclerotic lines within interface zones indicate the formation of a fibrous membrane about the prosthesis. Hence, fibrous fixation rather than osseointegration has apparently occurred in this region. This radiographic appearance may remain stable or progress to implant loosening. Clinical outcomes with hip implants having fibrous fixation may be less optimal than with bone ingrowth fixation.

To recapitulate, it is this author's experience that all loose prosthetic components with measurable radiographic evidence of unstable, loose, migrating components always have had concurrent evidence of progressive extension or widening of interface radiolucent lines. This agrees with the earlier discussion on the significance of interface radiolucency:

Table 5-1 Radiographic Outcomes Parameters in Evaluating Metal-on-Metal Hip Resurfacing

Postoperative Examination	Parameter	Femoral Component	Acetabular
Baseline (AP)	Initial orientation	Stem-shaft angle (in degrees)	Abduction/inclination angle (in degrees)
		Femoral offset	—
	Implant seating	Proud/shortened	Lateralized/medialized
	Technical aspects	Neck notching	Acetabular fracture
		Uncovered reamed bone	Socket protrusion
	Interface status	Radiolucent gap (oversized drilling)	Radiolucent gap (incomplete seating)
	Bone morphometry	Neck width (superoinferiorly)	—
Baseline (lateral)	Initial orientation	Relative to neck version	Anteversion/neutral/retroversion
	Bone morphometry	Neck width (anteroposteriorly)	—
Serial (AP)	Interface status	Radiolucent lines (RLLs)	RLLs
	Interface zones[14]	Three zones (Fig. 5-3A)	Three zones (Fig. 5-3B)
	Component migration	≥5 mm (vertical)	≥5 mm (superior/medially)
		≥5 degree tilt (varus/valgus)	≥5-degree tilt (abduction or adduction)
		Tip sclerosis (pedestal)	—
	Fixation scoring system[14]	Ten-tiered (see Table 5-2)	Ten-tiered (see Table 5-2)
	Periprosthetic osteolysis	5 mm (minimum size criterion)	5 mm (minimum size criterion)
	Adaptive bone remodeling	Neck narrowing (minimum 10% change)	—
		Corticocancellization of medial neck	—
Serial (lateral)	Interface status	RLLs	RLLs
	Interface zones	Three zones (Fig. 5-3)	Three zones (Fig. 5-3)
	Component migration	≥5 mm (vertical)	≥5 mm (superior/medially)
		≥5-degree tilt (anteverted/retroverted)	≥5-degree tilt (anteverted/retroverted)
		Tip sclerosis	—
	Fixation scoring system	Ten-tiered (see Table 5-2)	Ten-tiered (see Table 5-2)
	Periprosthetic bone remodeling	Neck narrowing (?)	

> . . . a radiolucent zone of any size at this interface elicits concern about the longevity of fixation. The greater the width and extent of the radiolucency, the greater the concern. Therefore, both the width and extent of a . . . radiolucency should be recorded.[40]

That is, until the recent advent of third-generation MM hip resurfacing systems that all have a short, straight, axial, metaphyseal stem serving not only "to facilitate alignment of the component during insertion"[41] but also to be a reliable reference "antenna" structure to monitor the quality of its fixation stability, as determined from serial radiographs. This represents a modern version of the short (metaphyseal), stainless steel rod used to reinforce the so-called press-fit stem of the original Judet acrylic femoral head prosthesis implanted more than 50 years ago,[42] which was reported to help identify a tilt or varus shift of the femoral implant.[43,44]

The absence of the metaphyseal stem from all second generation, femoral hip resurfacing implants made the radiographic assessment of component stability very difficult for early determination of implant migration because the primary fixation surface within the femoral cup was completely shielded by the radiodense metallic or ceramic femoral component.

As a result of numerous reviews of component fixation stability with third-generation MM hip resurfacing, a 10-tiered radiographic scoring system of zero to nine points was designed, indicative of the absence or presence of radiolucencies in the three zones around each of the short, metaphyseal femoral stems as well as three zones for the acetabular component (Table 5-2) in the AP-pelvis view.[14] The three equal acetabular zones, each extending 60 degrees, are slightly modified from the right-angle designation by DeLee and Charnley.[45] Note that the zones of the femoral component are to be reported in Arabic numbers, and those for the acetabular component are reported in Roman numerals for consistent reporting of interface radiolucencies.

For the corresponding lateral view, the three femoral zones around the metaphyseal stem, in accordance with the

Table 5-2 Ten-Tiered Implant Fixation Scoring System for the Metaphyseal Femoral Component and Acetabular Component; Refer to Figure 5-3 for Delineation of Interface Zones

Grade	Femoral Component	Acetabular Component
0	No radiolucent line (RLL)	No radiolucent line (RLL)
1	RLL in zone 2 (tip only)	RLL in zone I (superior)
2	RLL in zone 1 (superior)	RLL in zone II (central)
3	RLL in zone 3 (inferior)	RLL in zone III (inferior)
4	RLL in both zones 1 & 2	RLL in both zones I and II
5	RLL in both zones 2 & 3	RLL in both zones I and III
6	RLL in both zones 1 & 3	RLL in both zones II and III
7	RLL in zones 1-3 (incomplete)	RLL in zones I-III (incomplete)
8	RLL in zones 1-3 (complete)	RLL in zones I-III (complete)
9	Migration	Migration

zones delineated for stem-type intramedullary designs, are delineated in Figure 5-3.

The assessment of interface radiolucencies with MM hip resurfacing is evaluated with two cohorts:

The first cohort consists of patients with hips having radiographic evidence of interface gaps, as evidenced by early radiolucencies typically with press-fit, metal-backed, acetabular components, observed in the first postoperative baseline film, which need to be followed up for any of the following subsequent radiographic changes: (1) persistent interface radiolucent lines, (2) apparent slight settling of the socket into narrow (i.e., less than 2 mm in width) gaps, or (3) apparent filling-in with new bone into the wide (i.e., 2 mm or more in width) gaps associated with stable cementless acetabular components. On a rare occasion, a thin incomplete radiolucent gap has been noted adjacent to the metaphyseal stem, which would be indicative of over-drilling of the centering hole.

The second cohort involves patients with hips having initially intact implant-bone interface with no interposing radiolucent lines, which later then develops new radiolucencies in one or more zones in subsequent postoperative examinations and that were not discernible in the corresponding baseline view. The 10-tiered implant fixation scoring system is a convenient way to grade the variability of the extent of radiolucent lines as well as being able to simplify by stratification according to the number of interface zones involved. For example, grades 1 through 3 would signify any one zone with a radiolucency (Fig. 5-4), grades 4 through 6 would signify any two zones involved with a radiolucency, and grades 7 and 8 with all three zones involving a thin (<2 mm), linear radiolucency signifying stable fibrous fixation. Grade 9, that is, measurable migration associated with unstable fibrous fixation, typically was manifested by radiographic evidence of sclerotic lines and/or divergent radiolucent lines around the metaphyseal stem that often appeared 2 or more years before failure (Fig. 5-5).[46] In the study published in 2004, fixation scores of 7 through 9 were used as endpoint criterion. It was noted that

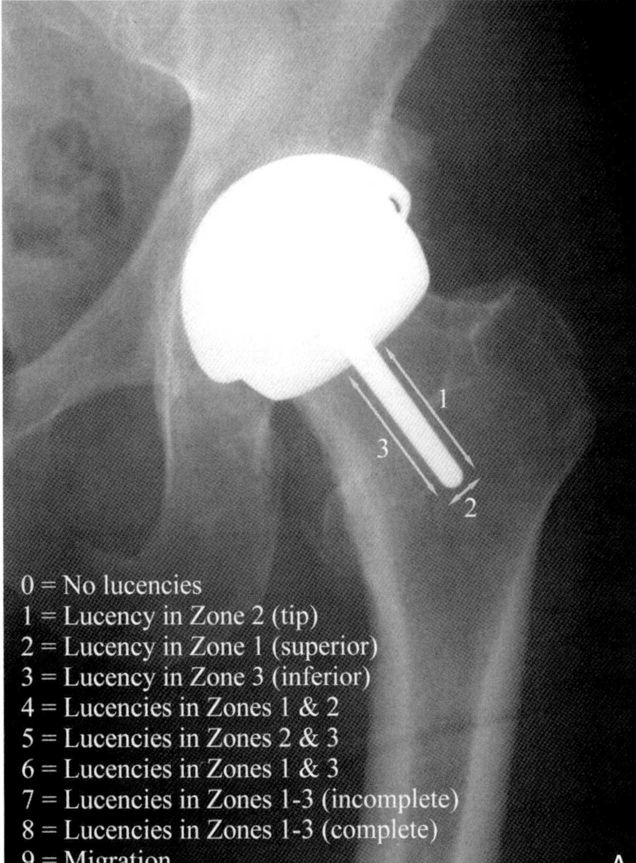

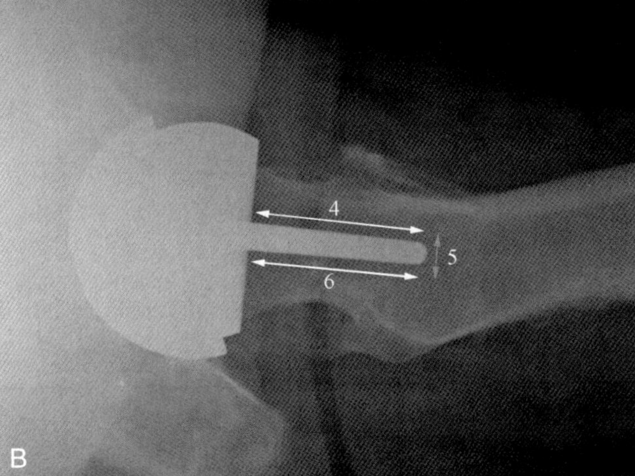

Figure 5-3 **A,** Metaphyseal stem zones 1, 2, and 3 defined on anteroposterior view. **B,** Metaphyseal stem zones defined from the Johnson cross-table lateral view. Zone 4 represents the anterior portion of the neck adjacent to the stem, zone 5 the tip of the stem, and zone 6 the posterior aspect of the neck adjacent to the stem. *(Reprinted with permission from Amstutz HC, Beaule PE, Dorey FJ, LeDuff MJ, Campbell PA, Gruen TA: Metal-on-metal hybrid surface arthroplasty: Two to six-year follow-up study. J Bone Joint Surg 2004;86A:28-39.)*

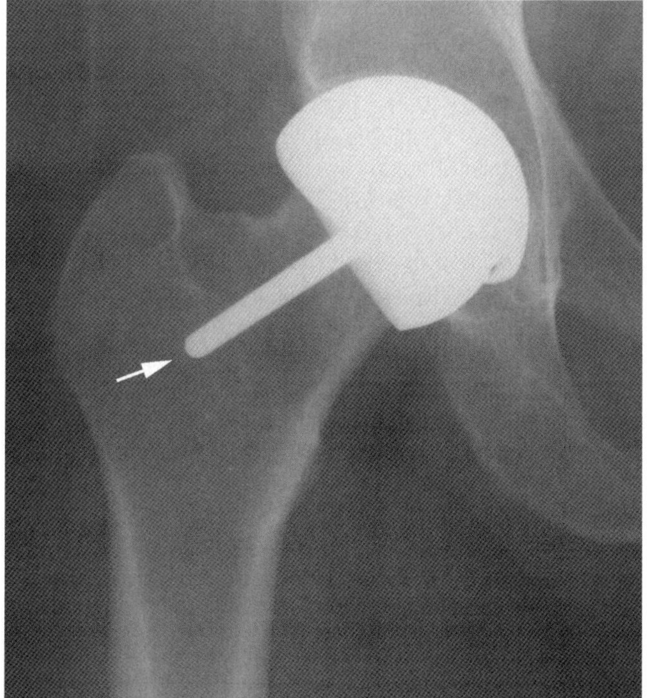

Figure 5-4 Six-year postoperative anteroposterior radiograph illustrating onset of a new femoral interface radiolucency demarcated by a thin sclerotic line situated at the distal tip of the metaphyseal stem, which represents grade 1 femoral fixation. This sign is not representative of a "pedestal" as alluded to in other published reports on hip resurfacing replacements.

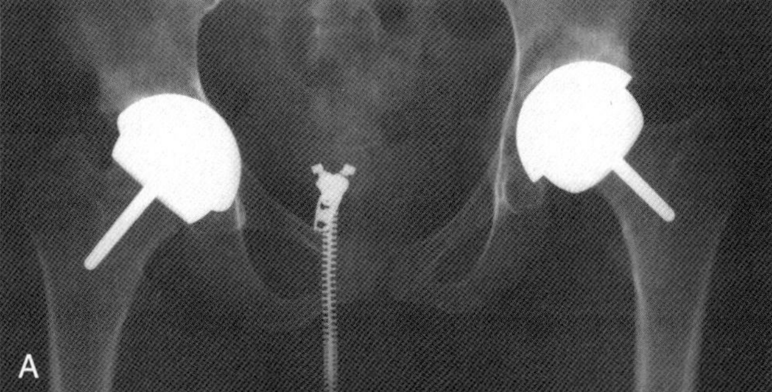

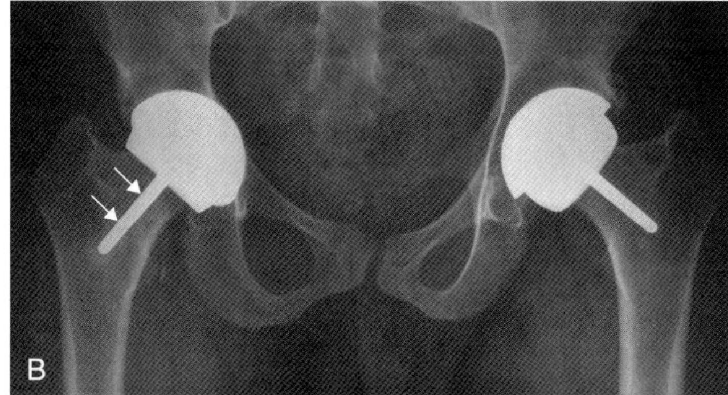

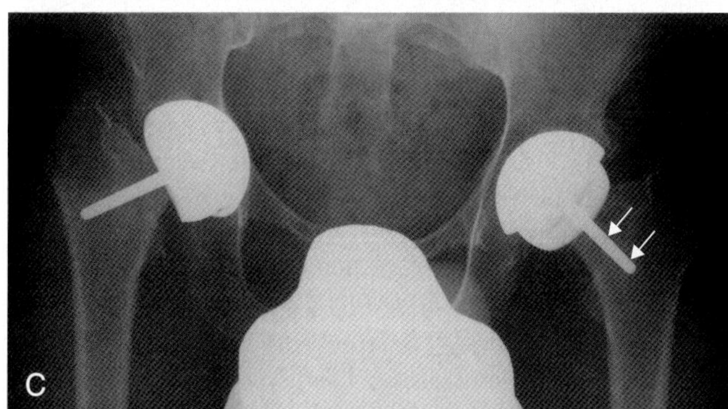

Figure 5-5 Serial postoperative anteroposterior radiographs illustrating evidence of progressive changes of interface radiolucent lines and tilting of the femoral hip resurfacing component. **A,** Immediate postoperative radiograph of a 31-year-old man after bilateral one-stage resurfacing for osteoarthritis secondary to Legg-Calvé-Perthes disease. He had extensive cystic defects and had first-generation bone preparation technique (see Chapters 7 and 14). **B,** Two years after surgery, a wide and extensive interface radiolucency is evident around the entire metaphyseal stem (right hip) and a narrower incomplete radiolucency around the contralateral femoral implant. The patient had returned to competitive mountain biking. **C,** Four and a half years after surgery, the right femoral component has tilted into varus (estimated as a change of 25 degrees from its initial orientation) with continued divergence of the wide circumferential metaphyseal radiolucency with the stem on the left hip. The left hip demonstrated grade 8 loosening. Both hips were converted to total hip replacement in a one-stage bilateral revision procedure. *(Reprinted with permission from Amstutz H, Ball S, Le Duff M, Dorey F: Hip resurfacing for patients under 50 years of age. Results of 350 Conserve Plus with a 2-9 year follow-up. Clin Orthop Rel Res 2007;460:159-164.)*

23 hips of 384 (6.0%) were identified with this group; 6 (1.6%), 5 (1.3%), and 12 (3.9%) were identified with a score of 7, 8, and 9, respectively. Of the 12 hips with a score of 9, seven had already been converted to total hip replacement (THR), four hips were asymptomatic, and one was symptomatic but the patient was deported and lost to follow-up.[14]

Regarding the score of 9, that is, implant migration with unstable fibrous fixation, it remains to be seen if the proposed criteria for the magnitude of linear and angular migration are acceptable for consideration as reliable radiographic outcomes measure because to date there have yet to be sufficient detailed assessments of radiographic measurements from failed MM hip resurfacing cases needing (and pending or at risk for) revision for aseptic component loosening or from implant retrieval analysis.[46] Such assessments would have to include a test for the comparability of serial films, that is, consistency of following the radiologic protocol as evidenced by reasonable superposition of the different projections at various reference bony and implant landmarks as commonly performed in research settings using sophisticated computerized implant micromotion analysis of stem-type femoral hip components with reported accuracy of 1 mm of migration (95% confidence interval) using digital analysis, for example, Ein Bild Roentgen Analyse-Femoral Component Analysis (EBRA-FCA)[47] or accuracy between 0.1 mm and 0.8 mm for translation movement and 1 to 2 degrees for rotation (at the 99% significance level) when using roentgen-stereophotogrammetry (RSA) methods.[48,49] The problem with this technique is that each radiograph must be taken precisely with identical hip positioning and beam centering, otherwise the sensitivity is diminished dramatically. The reader should be aware that very recently, the concern for a consensus of reporting comparative results in clinical RSA studies from different research centers has been strongly advocated owing to issues related to patient positioning, follow-up intervals, length of follow-up, and patient selection.[50] Although RSA is currently the optimal research tool for assessing implant stability, it is not practical to be used for every patient.

Periprosthetic Osteolysis

At this time, only incidental cases of osteolytic lesions have been reported for early and intermediate follow-up of patients with contemporary MM hip replacements, for example, 10 of 171 hips with total hip replacements (5.8%)[51] compared with two of 94 hips (2.1%)[52] and one of 52 (1.9%)[18] in younger patients with MM hip surface replacements. The first study is of concern not only because the early lesions were all associated with stable hip implants, but that the lesions were demonstrably visible (as evidenced by the average lesion size of 132.5 mm^2 [range, 54.0 to 299.5 mm^2]) and that the lesions may signify hypersensitivity reactions to elements of the MM bearing surfaces[53-57] and previously for metal-on-polyethylene bearing couples.[58] Owing to the concern about these osteolytic lesions, it is recommended to implement standardized criteria for reliable assessment of these radiographic observations.

It is paramount to recognize that an osteolytic lesion is typically first evident as a focal area of cavitary, resorptive bone loss that was not present at or near the implant-bone interface on the immediate postoperative radiograph (Fig. 5-6). The minimum size criteria for recording its presence would be 5 mm so to discriminate these signs from linear and divergent implant-bone radiolucent lines associated with implant loosening or from other artifacts such as neck notching or lesions associated with synovial plication leading to bone erosion at or near the superior head-neck junction of the femoral neck due to femoral-acetabular impingement.[59-61]

For each zone in which a lesion is situated, two dimensional measurements are made, the first along the length (l) of the interface and the second measurement (w) taken perpendicular to the first measurement. These two dimensions are then used for a real size determination using the formula for a semi-ellipse, that is, $1/4\ \pi$ (length × width) or 0.785 (length × width). As an example for a small (i.e., 5 × 5 mm) lesion, the corresponding areal size would be 19.6 mm^2. With additional radiographic follow-up, the lesion may remain the same or either increase in length along the implant-bone interface (extensile) or increase in its width perpendicular to the interface (expansile) into the surrounding cancellous bone. Hip prostheses can remain stable in the presence of progressive loss of bone stock from wear-related osteolysis. Clinical symptoms have not correlated well with the radiographic appearances of such osteolytic lesions.

Periprosthetic Adaptive Bone Remodeling

Owing to the sparseness of radiographic outcomes criteria for periprosthetic bone structural changes, it would appear that there are several parameters relevant to MM hip resurfacing implants. This would include corticocancellization of the medial neck, a radiographic feature evidential of localized decreased loading of the proximal-medial neck cortex,[20,62] neck narrowing,[3,63,64] and healing of neck notches. Radiographic evidence of narrowing of the neck, as manifested in 21 cases by a reduction of at least 10% of the initial neck dimension, was noted to have had its onset ranging from the first to the fourth postoperative year. At last follow-up from 3 to 8 years, progressive narrowing of at least an additional 10% was noted in 10 hips in nine patients (Fig. 5-7). These cases merit continuous radiographic assessment because a recent study of late failure mechanisms of the first-generation of total hip resurfacing mentioned that "all late femoral failures (greater than 10 years postoperatively) showed narrowing of the femoral neck secondary either due to stress-shielding" or compromised vascularity of the femoral head[3,6] or due to osteolytic destruction from the debris-induced osteolysis. Neck narrowing has not been observed in any of our hemiresurfacing follow-ups. There is an incidence of 2.3% in our Conserve®Plus series of MM hip resurfacing, and the etiology is unknown. However, the incidence is lower in more recent hips, possibly due to a larger retained head circumference due to the use of thin sockets. In two hips, the femoral component loosened, one after 9 years (but the head was very abnormal prior to resurfacing) and the other after 4 years, but radiographic follow-up was not good, and we did not receive the specimen; thus, the actual mode of failure is unknown. The reported incidence of neck narrowing in the literature with other devices is higher. Beaulé and colleagues[63] reported a 20% incidence in our McMinn implantations. Cossey and associates[64] reported 27% with the Birmingham hip resurfacing (BHR), and Lilikakis and coworkers also reported 27% with the press-fit Cormet.[65] The BHR incidence was higher in women, who had smaller component sizes. With both of these devices, the stem circumference is larger than that of the Conserve®Plus, especially in smaller sizes because the stem size is not proportional to the component size, and perhaps this could support a hypothesis for stress shielding. The Conserve®Plus is anthropometric and graduates in length and diameter with component size. A possible explanation for the high incidence with the cementless Cormet component relates to the fact that the proximal stem is partially coated with hydroxyapatite. The observed phenomenon may be similar to those observed when a porous-coated resurfacing stem was used in a canine resurfacing model. In those hips, there was a rapid ingrowth into the stem, with stress shielding of the head peripherally.[66]

Adaptive neck remodeling changes often appear to be the result of neck-socket impingement due either to a malpositioned component or, if component orientation is ideal, to a patient's extreme range of motion. The latter has been observed in ballet dancers and those who regularly practice Yoga; for example, remodeling from component malorientation can occur when the socket is excessively anteverted (Fig. 5-8) or lacks abduction angle horizontal (Fig. 5-9).

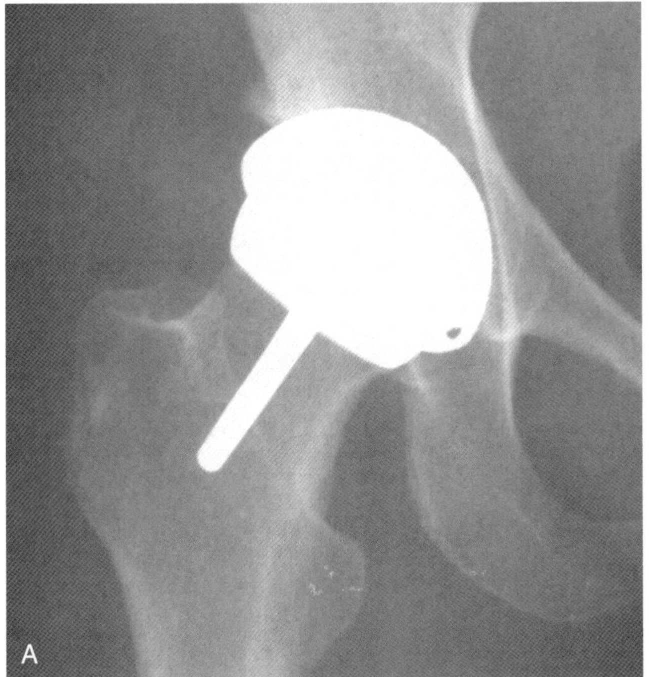

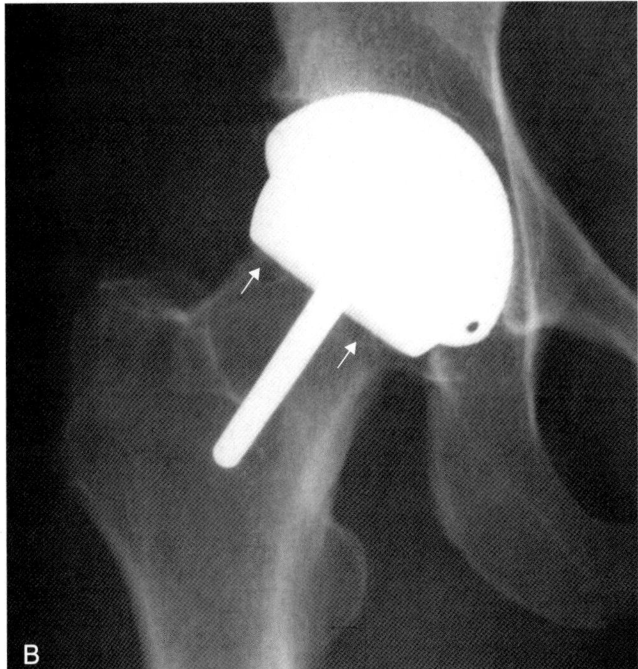

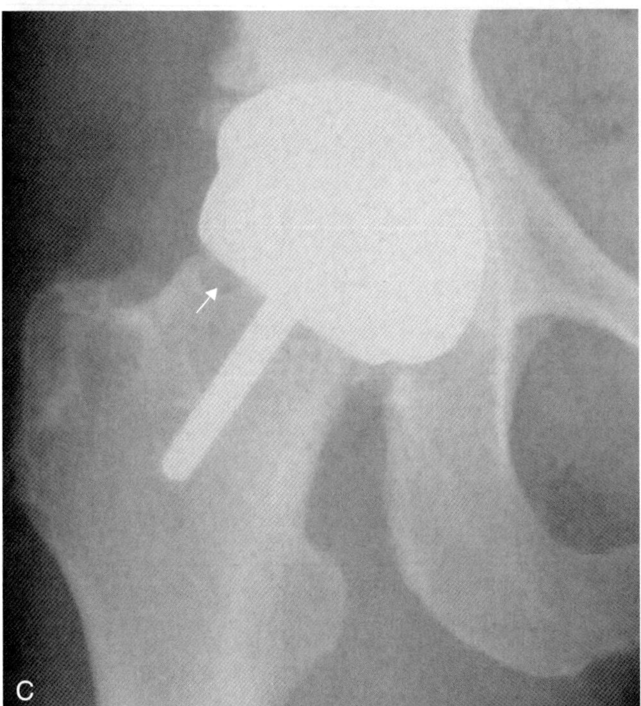

Figure 5-6 Serial radiographs of a case with femoral periprosthetic osteolysis. **A,** Immediate postoperative anteroposterior view showing an intact femoral neck. **B,** One-year postoperative anteroposterior view showing a new focal lesion situated at the superior aspect of the femoral neck; the lesion's area I size is estimated to be 26.3 mm^2. **C,** Three years after surgery, the lesion shows an apparent slight increase in area I size estimated as 48.2 mm^2.

The Use of Computed Tomography and Magnetic Resonance Imaging in Evaluating Resurfacing Patients

CT has been valuable in assessing the exact dimensions of the acetabulum and the width of neck to determine the component size for resurfacing. This has been particularly true in cases of developmental dysplasia of the hip, using existing off-the-shelf components, or when custom precise sizing is necessary. Because it is difficult to lengthen the leg, custom sockets have been used to add length.

Magnetic resonance imaging (MRI) scans have not been particularly useful in evaluating patients with osteonecrosis. Generally, Ficat staging can be determined from AP, frog, and modified table-down lateral views on plain radiographs, and defect size could be best assessed at surgery. Our experience is limited to evaluating patients who have symptoms following

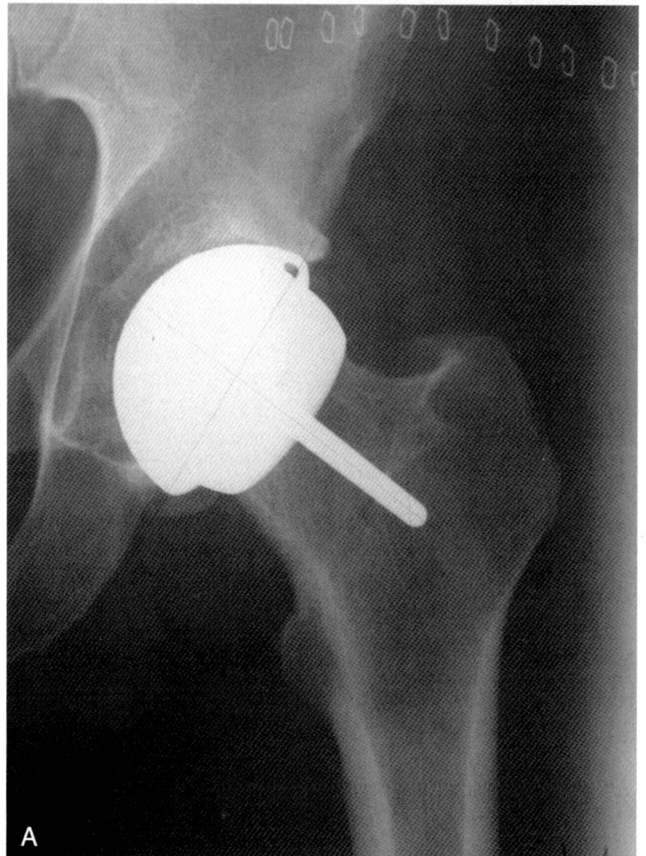

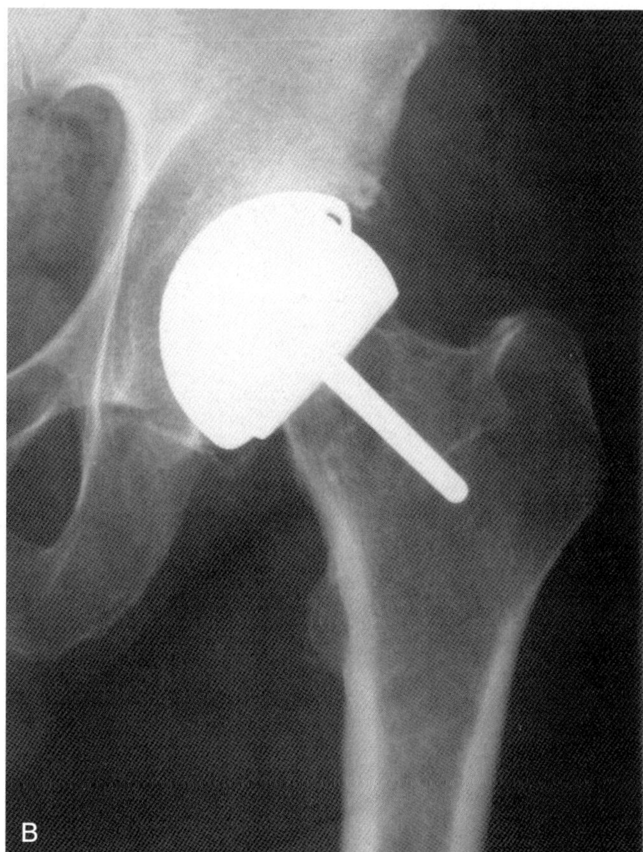

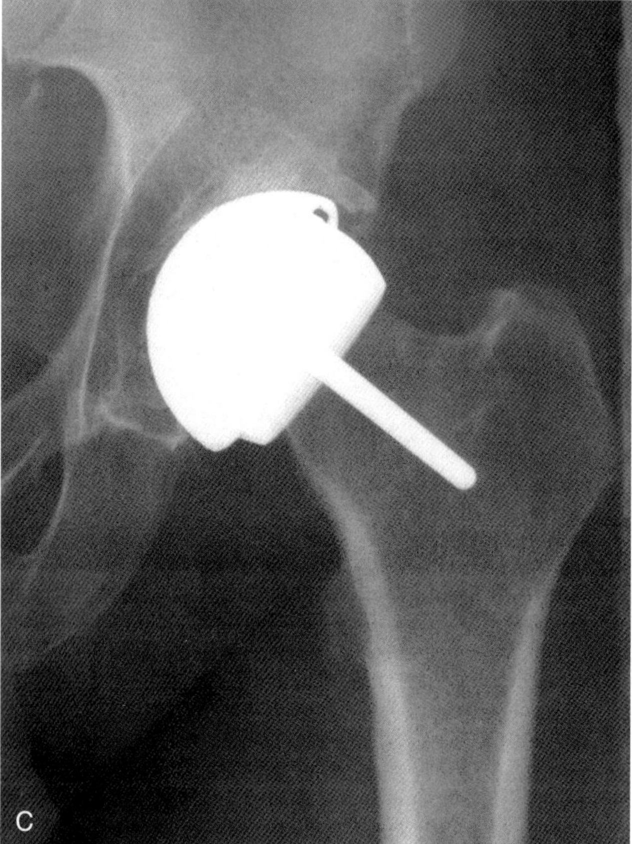

Figure 5-7 Serial postoperative anteroposterior radiographs illustrating temporal changes of narrowing of the femoral neck after metal-on-metal hip resurfacing. **A,** Immediate postoperative view of a 46-year-old man who underwent surgery for "primary" osteoarthritis. **B,** Two years after surgery, the femoral neck has narrowed by 10%. **C,** Six years after surgery, progressive narrowing is evident with a 17% decrease of the width of the neck. The patient has only occasional discomfort (pain 9, walking and function 10, and activity 8).

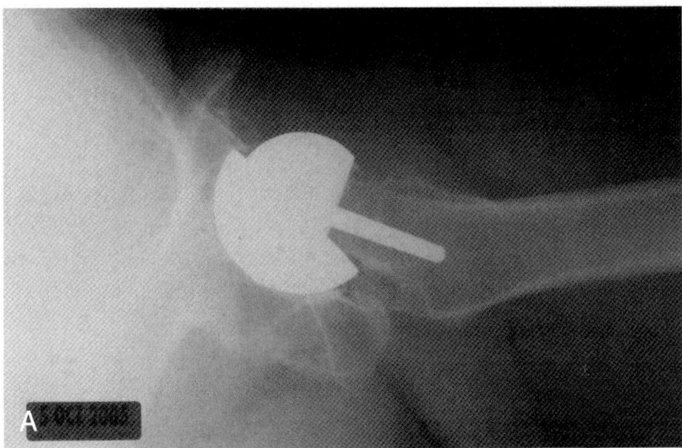

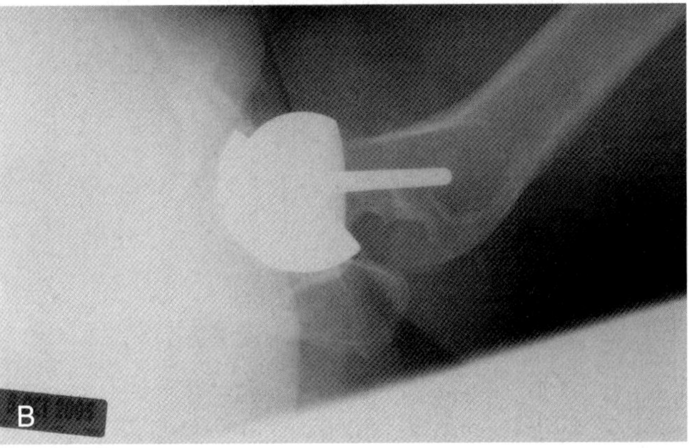

Figure 5-8 Two Johnson cross-table lateral views taken consecutively but with a different flexion angle of the hip on the same follow-up visit (4 years) in a 54-year-old woman who underwent surgery for "primary" osteoarthritis. Note the relationship between the cup posterior impingement in full extension **(A)** and the location of the neck remodeling **(B)**.

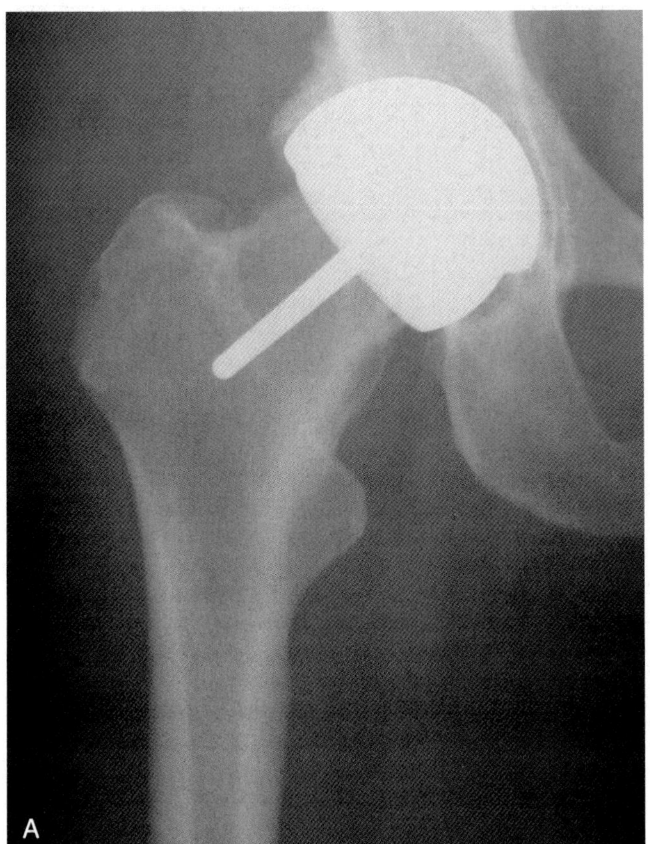

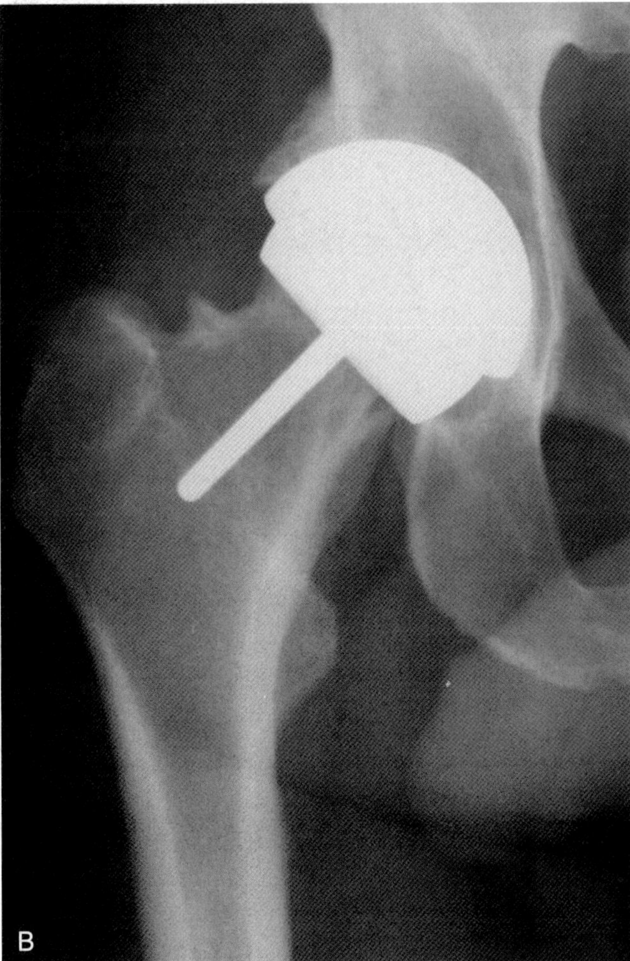

Figure 5-9 Serial anteroposterior x-ray studies of a 48-year-old man who underwent surgery for "primary" osteoarthritis. The abduction angle of the acetabular component is 33 degrees with lateral neck remodeling due to impingement. Patient is an avid surfer and rower and is asymptomatic. His 9-year abduction is 40 degrees; pain score is 10. **A,** Immediate post-operative film. **B,** Two-year follow-up film.

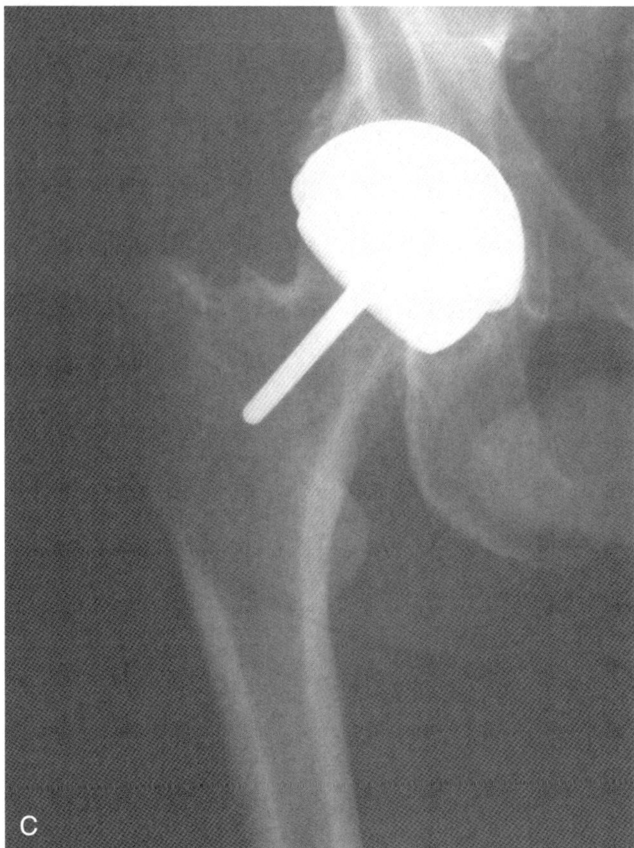

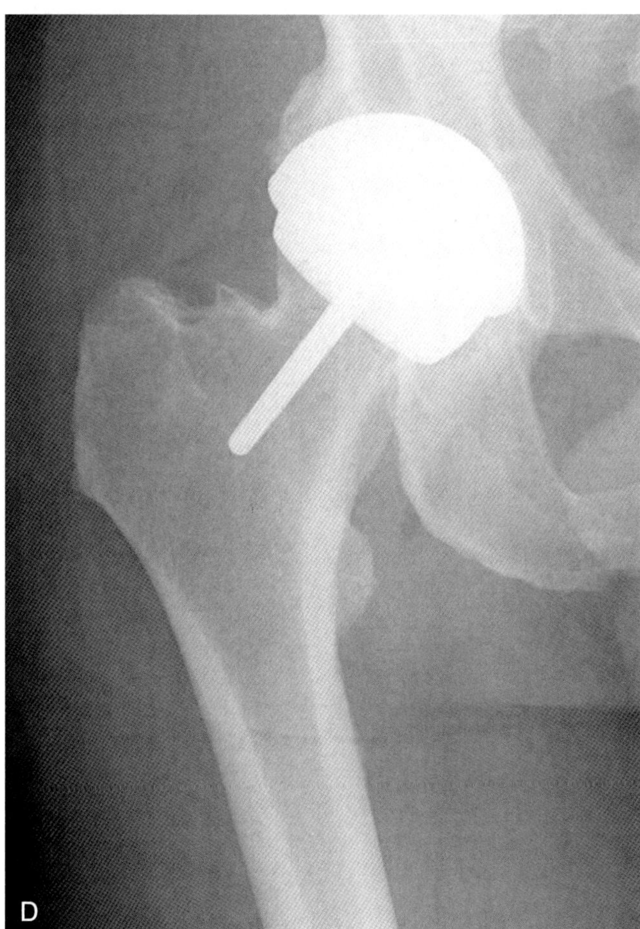

Figure 5-9, cont'd **C,** Five-year follow-up film. **D,** Nine-year follow-up film.

resurfacing, for example, if one suspects iliopsoas bursitis. This has not been documented in any of our patients perhaps because of the low-profile socket and because we have been carefully making certain that the socket is below the anterior rim of the pubis.

We have begun to evaluate patients with neck narrowing to determine if there may be a soft tissue mass pressing on the neck. This has not been verified so far beyond two hips that presented severe neck narrowing after resurfacing with McMinn hip devices.

Discussion

To date, most series of patients undergoing MM hip resurfacing have had good to excellent clinical outcomes, and the procedure is said to be an attractive alternative to conventional (stem-type) total hip replacements. Generally, the best clinical results are achieved when it is performed on large men with good quality bone stock. Nevertheless, the criteria for patient selection for hip resurfacing needs to be continuously reassessed. Also, it is important to assess the surgical techniques and accurate placement and orientation of both the acetabular and femoral components to ensure the implants' longevity. Recently, this procedure has been performed with increasingly advanced surgical technologies such as fluoroscopy-guided surgery, computer-assisted surgery, CT-based planning, and imageless navigation systems, in an attempt to improve safety and precision in hip resurfacing procedures.

Nevertheless, it is essential to reiterate the need for proper radiologic techniques for preoperative planning and postoperative radiographic outcomes assessments; this is particularly true for hip resurfacing in which the femoral component is oriented relative to the femoral neck axis, either in neutral or slight valgus, unlike the stem-type femoral prosthesis which is oriented relative to the femoral shaft axis and is approximately parallel to the x-ray film cassette. The assessment of femoral component orientation in hip resurfacing, whether relative to the neck-shaft angle or to the femoral anteversion, requires strict consistency in both the AP and lateral radiographic views. This consistency is also needed for the subsequent serial postoperative radiographic assessments and efforts need to be emphasized for identifying appropriate comparability of serial films based on reference anatomic landmarks for the pelvis and the proximal femur.

Various landmarks have been identified for the pelvis and the acetabulae within it, for example, the often-cited reference of Massin et al.[67] and other recent publications.[68-71] Multiple horizontal and vertical reference lines have been used as described in EBRA studies of implant migration following THRs[72,73] and recently following hip resurfacing.[74] However a major limitation to the use of EBRA for evaluation of component migration in resurfacing is that EBRA measures two-dimensionally a phenomenon that is three-dimensional in nature and is thus very sensitive to differences in femoral rotation between radiographs. Another option is to refer to the lesser trochanter as a reference landmark not only for implant migration[75] and leg-length discrepancy but also for monitoring the variance in the extent of femoral rotation related to patient positioning during serial radiographs.[76]

In the meantime, a consensus in proper reporting of radiographic outcomes with a radiographic atlas featuring the relevant and unique observations associated with any hip resurfacing procedure is essential to provide consistency among different radiographic observers reviewing the appropriate views in understanding the three-dimensional behavior of this promising hip procedure.

Further radiographic outcomes will be required to establish the prevalence of femoral neck fractures and, if possible, avascular necrosis of the remaining femoral head within the metallic femoral component. It is essential to obtain a better understanding of implant failure from clinical outcomes assessment and implant retrieval analysis. Intermediate and long-term outcome assessments with detailed radiographic observations may provide a realistic answer to the orthopaedic community regarding the future of MM hip resurfacing arthroplasty.

References

1. Schmalzried TP, Fowble VA, Ure KJ, Amstutz HC: Metal on metal surface replacement of the hip. Technique, fixation, and early results. Clin Orthop Rel Res 1996;329(suppl):S106-S114.
2. Schmalzried TP, Silva M, de la Rosa MA, Choi ES, Fowble VA: Optimizing patient selection and outcomes with total hip resurfacing. Clin Orthop Rel Res 2005;441:200-204.
3. Ritter MA, Lutgring JD, Berend ME, Pierson JL: Failure mechanisms of total hip resurfacing: implications for the present. Clin Orthop Rel Res 2006;453:110-114.
4. Mai MT, Schmalzried TP, Dorey FJ, Campbell PA, Amstutz HC: The contribution of frictional torque to loosening at the cement-bone interface in THARIES hip replacements. J Bone Joint Surg 1996;78A:505-511.
5. Howie DW, Cornish BL, Vernon-Roberts B: Resurfacing hip arthroplasty. Classification of loosening and the role of prosthesis wear particles. Clin Orthop Rel Res 1990;255:144-149.
6. Duijsens AW, Keizer S, Vliet-Vlieland T, Nelissen RG: Resurfacing hip prostheses revisited: failure analysis during a 16-year follow-up. Int Orthop 2005;29:224-228.
7. Dumbleton J, Manley M: Metal-on-metal total hip replacement: what does the literature say? J Arthroplasty 2005;20:174-188.
8. Isaac GH, Siebel T, Schmalzried TP, Cobb AG, O'Sullivan T, Oakeshott RD, Flett M, Vail TP: Development rationale for an articular surface replacement: a science-based evolution. Proc Inst Mech Eng [H] 2006;220:253-268.
9. Kudrna JC: Femoral version: definition, diagnosis, and intraoperative correction with modular femoral components. Orthopaedics 2005;28(suppl):s1045-s1047.
10. Amstutz HC (ed): Metal on metal hip prostheses: past performance and future directions. Clin Orthop Rel Res 1996;329: S2-S306.
11. Wyness L, Vale L, McCormack K, Grant A, Brazzelli M: The effectiveness of metal on metal hip resurfacing: a systematic review of the available evidence published before 2002. BMC Health Servs Res 2004;4:39.
12. Mont MA, Ragland PS, Etienne G, Seyler TM, Schmalzried TP: Hip resurfacing arthroplasty. J Am Acad Orthop Surg 2006;14: 454-463.
13. McMinn DJW, Treacy RBC, Lin K, Pynsent PB: Metal on metal surface replacement of the hip. Experience of the McMinn prosthesis. Clin Orthop Rel Res 1996;329S:S89-S98.
14. Amstutz HC, Beaule PE, Dorey FJ, LeDuff MJ, Campbell PA, Gruen TA: Metal-on-metal hybrid surface arthroplasty: Two to six-year follow-up study. J Bone Joint Surg 2004;86A1:28-39.
15. De Smet KA: Belgium experience with metal-on-metal surface arthroplasty. Orthop Clin North Am 2005;36:203-213.
16. Shimmin AJ, Bare J, Back DL: Complications associated with hip resurfacing arthroplasty. Orthop Clin North Am 2005;36: 187-193.
17. Treacy RBC, McBryde CW, Pynsent PB: Birmingham hip resurfacing arthroplasty. A minimum follow-up of five years. J Bone Joint Surg 2005;87B:167-170.
18. Pollard LCB, Baker RP, Eastaugh-Waring SJ, Bannister GC: Treatment of the young active patient with osteoarthritis of the hip. A five- to seven-year comparison of hybrid total hip arthroplasty and metal-on-metal resurfacing. J Bone Joint Surg 2006;88-B: 592-600.
19. Gruen TA (ed): Imaging, vol. 3. Rosemont, IL, American Academy of Orthopaedic Surgeons, 2006, pp 257-262.
20. Gruen TA: Radiographic criteria for the clinical performance of uncemented total joint replacements. In Lemons JE (ed): Quantitative Characterization and Performance of Porous Implants for Hard Tissue Applications, vol. ASTM STP 953. Philadelphia, American Society for Testing and Materials, 1987, pp 207-218.
21. Johnson CR: A new method for roentgenographic evaluation of the upper end of the femur. J Bone Joint Surg 1932;14:859-866.
22. Ballinger PW, Frank ED: Merrill's Atlas of Radiographic Positions and Radiologic Procedures, Vol 1. St. Louis, Mosby, 1999, pp 332-347.
23. Engh CA, Bobyn JD (eds): Biologic Fixation in Total Hip Arthroplasty. Thorofare, NJ, Slack, Inc., 1985, pp 45-48.
24. Hansson LI, Hagglund G, Ordeberg G, Sandstrom S: The calcar femorale as a landmark in hip physiolysis. Acta Orthopa Scand 1988;59:134-138.
25. Freeman MAR: The pathogenesis of primary osteoarthrosis: an hypothesis. In Apley AG (ed): Modern Trends in Orthopaedics, Volume 6. New York, Appleton-Century-Crofts, 1972, pp 40-94.
26. Kitamura N, Naudie DD, Leung SB, Hopper RH Jr, Engh CA Sr: Diagnostic features of pelvic osteolysis on computed tomography: the importance of communication pathways. J Bone Joint Surg 2005;87A:1542-1550.
27. Resnick D, Niwayama G, Coutts RD: Subchondral cysts (geodes) in arthritic disorders: pathologic and radiographic appearance of the hip joint. Am J Roentgenol 1977;128:799-806.

28. Schmalzried TP, Akizuki KH, Fedenko AN, Mirra J: The role of access of joint fluid to bone in periarticular osteolysis. A report of four cases. J Bone Joint Surg 1997;79-A:447-452.
29. Anderson JY, Trinkaus E: Patterns of sexual, bilateral and inter-populational variation in human femoral neck-shaft angles. J Anat 1998;192(Pt 2):279-285.
30. Clark JM, Freeman MA, Witham D: The relationship of neck orientation to the shape of the proximal femur. J Arthroplasty 1987;2:99-109.
31. Mills HJ, Horne JG, Purdie GL: The relationship between proximal femoral anatomy and osteoarthrosis of the hip. Clin Orthop Rel Res 1993;288:205-208.
32. Sugano N, Noble PC, Kamaric E: Predicting the position of the femoral head center. J Arthroplasty 1999;14:102-107.
33. West JD, Mayor MB, Collier JP: Potential errors inherent in quantitative densitometric analysis of orthopaedic radiographs. A study after total hip arthroplasty. J Bone Joint Surg 1987; 69-A:58-64.
34. Kay RM, Jaki KA, Skaggs DL: The effect of femoral rotation on the projected femoral neck-shaft angle. J Pediatr Orthop 2000; 20:736-739.
35. Reikeras O, Hoiseth A, Reigstad A: Evaluation of the Dunlap/Rippstein method for determination of femoral neck angles. Acta Radiol Diagn 1985;26:177-179.
36. Lindgren J, Rysavy J: Restoration of femoral offset during hip replacement. A radiographic cadaver study. Acta Orthop Scand 1992;63:407-410.
37. Muller O, Martini F, Haller M, Schaich M, Sell S: [Quantification of position-related errors in measurement of antetorsion of the femur with computerized tomography—introduction of a method for positional correction]. Z Orthop Ihre Grenzgeb 2001;139:317-325.
38. Albert TJ, Sharkey PF, Chao W, Hume EL, Rothman RH: Rotation affects apparent radiographic positioning of femoral components in total hip arthroplasty. J Arthroplasty 1991;6(suppl 6): S67-S71.
39. Goodman S, Rubenstein J, Schatzker J, Kadish L, Fornasier V: Apparent changes in the alignment of the femoral component in hip arthroplasties associated with limb positioning. Clin Orthop Rel Rese 1987;221:242-245.
40. Johnston RC, Fitzgerald RH Jr, Harris WH, Poss R, Mueller ME, Sledge CB: Clinical and radiographic evaluation of total hip replacement. A standard system of terminology for reporting results. J Bone Joint Surgery 1990;72-A:161-168.
41. Amstutz HC, Le Duff MJ: Background of metal-on-metal resurfacing. Proc Inst Mech Eng [H] 2006;220:85-94.
42. Judet J, Judet R: The use of an artificial femoral head for arthroplasty of the hip joint. J Bone Joint Surg 1950;32B: 166-173.
43. Buxton SJD, Waugh W: Radiographic bone changes at the hip after insertion of an acrylic prostheses. J Bone Joint Surg 1954;36B:50-56.
44. Merle d'Aubigne R, Postel M: Functional results of hip arthroplasty with acrylic prosthesis. J Bone Joint Surg 1954;36A: 451-475.
45. DeLee JG, Charnley J: Radiological demarcation of cemented sockets in total hip replacement. Clin Orthop Rel Res 1976;121: 20-132.
46. Campbell PA, Beaule PE, Ebramzadeh E, LeDuff MJ, DeSmet K, Lu Z, Amstutz HC: A study of implant failure in metal-on-metal surface arthroplasties. Clin Orthop Rel Res 2006;453:35-46.
47. Wilkinson JM, Hamer AJ, Elson RA, Stockley I, Eastell R: Precision of EBRA-digital software for monitoring implant migration after total hip arthroplasty. J Arthroplasty 1997;17:910-916.
48. Karrholm J, Herberts P, Hultmark P, Malchau H, Nivbrant B, Thanner J: Radiostereometry of hip prostheses. Review of methodology and clinical results. Clin Orthop Rel Res 1997;344: 94-110.
49. Nilsson KG, Karrholm J: Editorial. RSA in the assessment of aseptic loosening. J Bone Joint Surg 1996;78B:1-3.
50. Valstar ER, Gill R, Ryd L, Flivik G, Borlin N, Karrholm J: Guidelines for standardization of radiostereometry (RSA) of implants. Acta Orthop 2005;76:563-572.
51. Park Y-S, Moon Y-W, Lim S-J, Yang J-M, Ahn G, Choi Y-L: Early osteolysis following second-generation metal-on-metal hip replacement. J Bone Joint Surg 2005;87A:1515-1521.
52. Beaule PE, Dorey FJ, LeDuff MJ, Gruen TA, Amstutz HC: Risk factors affecting outcome of metal-on-metal surface arthroplasty of the hip. Clin Orthop Rel Res 2004;418:87-93.
53. Leopold SS: Commentary and perspective on "Early osteolysis following second-generation metal-on-metal hip replacement." J Bone Joint Surg 2005;87A:1515.
54. Willert HG, Buchhorn GH, Fayyazi A, Lohmann CH: Histopathological changes in tissues surrounding metal/metal joints—signs of delayed type hypersensitivity? (DTH). In Rieker C, Oberholzer S, Wyss U (eds): World Tribology Forum in Arthroplasty. Bern, Switzerland, Hans Huber, 2001, pp 147-66.
55. Willert HG, Buchhorn GH, Fayyazi A, Flury R, Windler M, Koster G, Lohmann CH: Metal-on-metal bearings and hypersensitivity in patients with artificial hip joints: a clinical and histomorphological study. J Bone Joint Surg 2005;87A:28-36.
56. Davies AP, Willert HG, Campbell PA, Learmonth ID, Case CP: An unusual lymphocytic perivascular infiltration in tissues around contemporary metal-on-metal joint replacements. J Bone Joint Surg 2005;87:18-27.
57. Baur W, Honle W, Willert HG, Schuh A: [Pathological findings in tissue surrounding revised metal/metal articulations]. Orthopaede 2005;34-3:225, 8-33.
58. Evans EM, Freeman MAR, Miller AJ, Vernon-Roberts B: Metal sensitivity as a cause of bone necrosis and loosening of the prosthesis in total joint replacement. J Bone Joint Surg 1974;56B: 626-642.
59. Beaule PE, Zaragoza E, Motamedi K, Copelan N, Dorey FJ: Three-dimensional computed tomography of the hip in the assessment of femoroacetabular impingement. J Orthop Res 2005;23:1286-1292.
60. Helenon C, Bergevin H, Aubert JD, Lebreton C, Helenon O: [Plication of the hip synovium above the femur neck]. J Radiol 1986;67:737-740.
61. Leunig M, Beck M, Kalhor M, Kim Y-J, Werlen S, Ganz R: Fibrocystic changes at anterosuperior femoral neck: prevalence in hips with femoroacetabular impingement. Radiology 2005;236: 237-246.
62. Carlsson AS, Rydberg J, Onnerfalt R: A large collar increases neck resorption in total hip replacement: 204 hips evaluated during 5 years. Acta Orthopaedica Scandinavica 1995;66:339-342.
63. Beaule PE, Amstutz HC, LeDuff MJ, Dorey FJ: Surface arthroplasty for osteonecrosis of the hip: hemiresurfacing versus metal-on-metal hybrid resurfacing. J Arthroplasty 2004; 19(suppl 3):54-58.
64. Cossey AJ, Back DL, Shimmin A, Young D, Spriggins AJ: The nonoperative management of periprosthetic fractures associated

with the Birmingham hip resurfacing procedure. J Arthroplasty 2005;20:358-361.
65. Lilikakis AK, Vowler SL, Villar RN: Hydroxyapatite-coated femoral implant in metal-on-metal resurfacing hip arthroplasty: minimum of two years follow-up. J Bone Joint Surg 2005;36: 215-222.
66. Hedley AK, Clarke IC, Kozinn SC, Coster I, Gruen TA, Amstutz HC: Porous ingrowth fixation of the femoral component in a canine surface replacement of the hip. Clin Orthop Rel Res 1982;163:300-311.
67. Massin P, Schmidt L, Engh CA: Evaluation of cementless acetabular component migration. An experimental study. J Arthroplasty 1989;4:245-251.
68. Foss OA, Klaksvik J, Benum P, Anda S: Pelvic rotations: a pelvic phantom study. Acta Radiol 2007;48:650-657.
69. Foss OA, Klaksvik J, Benum P, Anda S: Validation of the rotation ratios method. Acta Radiologica 2007;48:658-664.
70. Tannast M, Langlotz F, Siebenrock KA, Wiese M, Bernsmann K, Langlotz F: Anatomic referencing of cup orientation in total hip arthroplasty. Clin Orthop Rel Res 2005;436:144-150.
71. Tannast M, Murphy SB, Langlotz F, Anderson SE, Siebenrock KA: Estimation of pelvic tilt on anteroposterior x-rays—a comparison of six parameters. Skel Radiol 2006;35:149-155.
72. Biedermann R, Krismer M, Stoeckl B, Mayrhofer P, Ornstein E, Franzen H: Accuracy of EBRA-FCA in the measurement of migration of femoral components of total hip replacement. Einzel-Bild-Roentgen-Analyse-femoral component analysis. J Bone Joint Surg 1999;81B:266-272.
73. Krismer M, Tschupik JP, Bauer R, Mayrhofer P, Stoeckl B, Fischer M, Biedermann R: Einzel-Bild-Roentgen-Analyse (EBRA) zur Messung der Migration von Hueftendoprothesen. Orthopaede 1997;26:229-236.
74. Beaule PE, Krismer M, Mayrhofer P, Wanner S, LeDuff MJ, Mattesich M, Stoeckl B, Amstutz HC, Biedermann R: EBRA-FCA for measurement of migration of the femoral component in surface arthroplasty of the hip. J Bone Joint Surg 2005;87B: 741-744.
75. Malchau H, Karrholm J, Wang YX, Herberts P: Accuracy of migration analysis in hip arthroplasty. Digitized and conventional radiography, compared to radiostereometry in 51 patients. Acta Orthop Scand 1995;66:418-424.
76. Hananouchi T, Sugano N, Nakamura N, Nishii T, Miki H, Yamamura M, Yoshikawa H: Preoperative planning of femoral components on plain X-rays: Rotational evaluation with synthetic X-rays on ORTHODOC. Arch Orthop Trauma Surg 2007:127:381-385.

CHAPTER 6

Outcome Studies and Data Collection

Michel J. Le Duff
Frederick J. Dorey

Introduction

In this chapter, we give an overview of how we believe data should be collected by an institution where hip resurfacing is being performed, with examples drawn from our own practice at the Joint Replacement Institute in Los Angeles, California.

But first, why collect data when performing hip arthroplasty?

Systematic data collection can aid the surgeon with the following aspects of his or her practice:

- Formulation of a diagnosis and surgical decision-making process.
- Evaluation of the clinical results after surgery for each patient individually.
- Evaluation of the clinical results from a series of surgeries and comparison of these results to other surgical populations such as other devices and other approaches.
- Evaluation of the effect of selected independent variables on the clinical outcome within the same resurfacing patient population (for example, the changes in surgical technique or the importance of risk factors).
- Contribution of the results from this data to the orthopaedic community.

A second question that arises is related to the nature of the data to collect. Here we can distinguish between data that pertains to routine clinical evaluations of a patient and data related to a given research project driven by a specific research question at a given point in time. In this latter case, the nature of the data will dictate the means of collection and a new instrument (survey or data collection sheet) will often be designed.

Patient-Completed Surveys

The data drawn from a routine clinical evaluation should provide information on the disease-specific progress of the patient as well as the overall quality-of-life outcome, and should be collected not only preoperatively but also at every follow-up visit.

Disease-Specific Outcome Surveys

The most important aim of the disease specific outcome survey is to provide answers to the basic question: "How much better or different is the patient after surgery compared to before?" There are numerous hip surveys available to the surgeon to track the patients' progress from pre-operative to postoperative status. The Harris Hip Score (HHS),[1] the Western Ontario and McMaster University Osteoarthritis Index (WOMAC),[2] and the University of California, Los Angeles (UCLA)[3] hip scores are among the most widely used in the United States. In Europe, the Merle-D'Aubigné[4] and the Oxford[5] hip scores seem to be the most popular.

All these scoring systems present some common characteristics, among which is an assessment of pain, walking, and function. However, the UCLA hip scoring system is the only one to take patient activity into consideration. This addition proves to be even more useful when it comes to evaluating a young patient population as is the case with patients seeking the resurfacing procedure. The UCLA hip scoring system is presented in four separate scores (pain, walking, function, and activity), which gives the advantage of providing a more specific representation of the important parameters to evaluate in the patient's status compared with a single score lumping all categories together as is the case with the other surveys. It is for these particular reasons that the UCLA hip score is being used as the primary disease specific outcome measurement at our institution (Box 6-1). However, because the Harris Hip Score is the most widely used in the United States, we added its specific questions (sitting, public transportation, climbing stairs, ability to put on shoes and socks, and limp) to our already existing hip survey as of January, 2000. Thus we were able to compare the clinical outcome of our surgeries with a large portion of the existing literature related to hip arthroplasty in the United States.

BOX 6-1 University of California-Los Angeles Hip Scoring System

PAIN

Score	Description
10:	No pain
8:	Slight pain occasionally.
6:	Pain after *certain activities*, which requires light medication occasionally / aspirin, Motrin, and so on
4:	Pain with *most activities*, but no pain or minimum pain at rest. Light medication, frequently.
2:	Pain *all of the time*, but it is bearable. Strong medication occasionally / acetaminophen and hydrocodone (Vicodin) or codeine, and lighter medication frequently.
1:	Pain *all of the time*, which is unbearable. Strong medication frequently.

WALKING

Score	Description
10:	Unrestricted. No support, and no limp.
8:	Limp with no support *or* no limp with 1 support
6:	No support for 1 block, *or* 1 support up to six blocks, *or* unrestricted with bilateral support.
4:	No support about house *or* 1 support for less than 1 block, *or* bilateral support for short distances.
2:	Wheelchair bound, *or* transfer activities with a walker.
1:	Bedridden.

FUNCTION

Score	Description
10:	Normal activities
8:	Work on feet with a little restriction.
6:	Perform most of the housework / shopping. Desk-type work.
4:	Perform limited housework / some shopping.
2:	Partially dependent on others.
1:	Completely dependent and confined.

ACTIVITY

Score	Description
10:	Regular participation in impact sports.
9:	Sometimes participation in impact sports such as jogging, tennis, and heavy labor.
8:	Regular participation in bowling and/or golf.
7:	Regular participation in bicycling.
6:	Regular participation in moderate activities such as swimming and/or shopping, unlimited work around the house.
5:	Sometimes participation in moderate activities such as swimming and/or shopping, unlimited work around the house.
4:	Regular participation in mild activities such as walking, limited housework and limited shopping.
3:	Sometimes participation in mild activities such as walking, limited housework and limited shopping.
2:	Mostly inactive, very restricted to minimum activities of daily living.
1:	Wholly inactive, dependant on others; cannot leave residence.

Quality-of-Life Outcome Surveys

A quality-of-life outcome survey is the necessary complement to the disease-specific assessment because it will provide elements to the answers of that basic question: "How well is the patient after surgery when compared with the general population?" The quality-of-life survey we chose at the Joint Replacement Institute is the Short Form-12 (SF-12),[6] a condensed version of the SF-36 developed by Ware and Sherbourne.[7] Our choice for the SF-12, compared with the SF-36, was dictated by the shortened overall time required to complete all forms and, consequently, an improvement in patient compliance with a negligible loss of information.[8]

Surgeon-Generated Data

Range of Motion

A protractor-monitored assessment of range of motion is performed during the preoperative, the 3-month, and every annual follow-up visit as an assessment of patient status preoperatively, his recovery after the procedure, and for the evaluation of the proper functioning of the device. The range-of-motion assessment itself will not tell you how well the patient is doing overall, but it can often reveal the need to stretch out a flexion contracture, for example, or be an indicator of suboptimal component positioning or even the presence of heterotopic bone. The clinical value of range of motion testing is enhanced by a correlation with radiographic findings. Range-of-motion testing is a minor part of the Harris Hip Score but needs to be accurately performed should you elect to use this outcome tool in your practice.

A complete range-of-motion assessment of the hip joint should include the use of a protractor, which adds precision and minimizes errors. An assistant should record the measurements.

- Flexion
  We prefer to flex up both hips at the same time with the patient on a firm examining table. This will flatten the lumbar spine to a consistent endpoint for subsequent examinations, although it will add to the flexion due to the reduction of the lumbar lordosis. Then one hip is held in maximum flexion while the other hip is extended to determine the degree of flexion contracture (Fig. 6-1).
- Flexion Contracture
- Abduction both in flexion (with the hips resting comfortably in approximately 70 degrees of flexion and the feet resting on the table) and extension
- Adduction both in flexion and extension. The pelvis must be steadied with iliac crests as the reference.
- Internal rotation both in flexion (hips in 90 degrees of flexion) and extension (patient in prone position).
- External rotation both in flexion and extension

These measurements should be made on the affected hip and on the contralateral hip as an element of comparison because of

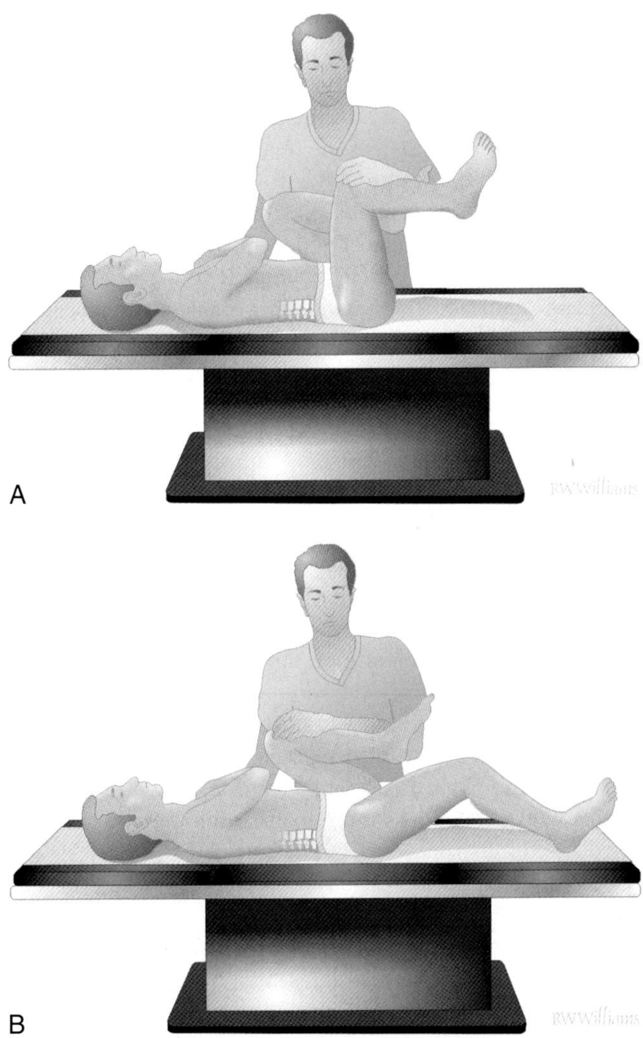

Figure 6-1 Assessment of flexion arc. **A,** The patient in supine position is instructed to bring the knees to the chest and maximum flexion is recorded. **B,** Then, with the contralateral knee held to the chest, the patient is instructed to extend the affected hip and flexion contracture is measured as the angle between the examination table and the femur.

the great variability in the values recorded among patients based on their natural flexibility. In their follow-up visits, fewer and fewer physicians include range-of-motion testing, and it seems to be becoming a little bit of a "lost art." Because our experience with the Conserve®Plus involved a large proportion of patients coming from out of state, we witnessed significant discrepancies in the readings of physicians whenever it was more convenient for the postoperative patient to consult with a local orthopaedist and forward the collected data to us. However, we have found that the range of motion rarely changes significantly after 1 year, so a complete range-of-motion test does not need to be recorded every year as long as it is done precisely on one occasion.

Surgical Data

Collecting surgical data serves two purposes:

1. To categorize implants or other surgical variables that can easily be used to create consecutive series of similar characteristics. For example, our database currently counts 1114 hips resurfaced with the Conserve®Plus prosthesis. This cohort can be studied as a whole and compared with other prosthetic designs, or it can be split into subsets based on a secondary variable (etiology, age at surgery, or implant size for example).
2. To record changes in the surgical technique and relate these changes to clinical, radiologic, or survivorship results.

When creating the surgical data collection tool, the most difficult task is to create fields of entry that will not only encompass all the various current possibilities but also foresee the possible evolution of a given variable. This process should not be underestimated because a well-designed data entry tool can save countless hours spent later on its modification or, even more cumbersome, modifications of the structure of the database itself. A safe way to avoid these problems is to create extra fields of answers and extra answer possibilities within the existing fields to allow for a subsequent expansion of the scope of research. In addition, an early and definitive decision needs to be made regarding the fields that include the possibility of multiple answers. When using a Microsoft Access database coupled with some kind of automated data entry system, the software development needed for these fields is of such complexity that later modifications require a deep knowledge of the program and the structure of the database (use of modules). Finally, even with a perfect design the surgical data entry tool is only as good as the person using it, and proper training of fellows or physician assistants who will collect the data is necessary if consistency in the data entry is to be achieved.

Patient Activity

As early as 1994, Wright and colleagues[9] highlighted that resuming recreational activities was the most important motivation for patients to undergo total joint replacement after the elimination of pain and the return to walking normally. Beaulé and coworkers have shown the need to integrate activity in all outcome measurements of hip arthroplasty.[10] Also, short of taking into consideration an assessment of patient activity in the survivorship analyses of joint arthroplasties, all comparisons between series are likely to be invalid. The value of accounting for patient activity in the outcome studies of hip arthroplasty has been explained in detail in an editorial article of the *Journal of Bone and Joint Surgery* by Dorey and Amstutz.[11] So far, the only disease-specific outcome survey geared toward hip patients following joint replacement that includes an evaluation of the patient activity is the UCLA hip scoring system, which presents a 10-point scale devised in 1981. The scale was designed to provide a simple assessment of patient activity for a wide variety of patients ranging from those that are wheelchair bound to those participating regularly in impact sports. However, our experience with patients who have undergone hip resurfacing is that the four levels (7 to 10) of the UCLA activity scale that refer to a participation in sporting activities may not be sufficiently sensitive to account for large differences in the volume of activity between patients.[11] For example, a patient playing doubles tennis for 2 hours, several times every week would be rated a 10 (regularly engages in impact sports) and receive the same score as a marathon runner who practices every day. There are methods of direct measurement of activity using devices able to record the number of hip cycles for a given amount of time. Nevertheless, if a relationship between a quantitative measure of patient activity and polyethylene wear has been established using these devices,[12,13] these methods are difficult to implement on a routine basis in a clinical setting. These observations led us to consider the need to collect specific data regarding the patient participation in sports, with a more precise assessment not only of the nature of the activity but also the frequency and duration of the sessions.

Data Forms

The forms used for data collection at the Joint Replacement Institute since 1998 are shown below as examples of a data collection tool. The most recent version of these forms are shown as some of them have undergone multiple modifications over time.

A. Patient completed, used by the surgeon during preoperative and follow-up visits:
  - **I.** Hip Survey form. Filled out by the patient before the physician's assessment (Fig. 6-2).
  - **II.** SF-12 Survey form. Filled out by the patient before the physician's assessment (Fig. 6-3).
  - **III.** Sports Activity Survey form. Filled out by the patient before the physician's assessment (Fig. 6-4).

B. Surgeon completed.
  - **I.** Preoperative/follow-up form. Includes physician analysis of patient completed forms and analysis. Filled out by the surgeon or the person conducting the follow-up visit (Fig. 6-5).
  - **II.** Surgery form. Filled out by the surgeon or a fellow or the physician's assistant (Fig. 6-6).

These forms were created using Design Expert software to be read by an optical scanner (Opscan 6) driven by Scantools software (all products of NCS Pearson, Inc., Bloomington, MN). The end product of this scanning process is a comma delimited text file (.txt), which is then imported into our Access database using a translation table and a series of specific queries developed to append the data to already existing tables.

From October 2000 until October 2004, the three patient-completed surveys were available online in particular for patients who live out of state or out of the country and could not be followed in a regular clinic setting. These patients would fill out the surveys on line and have a set of x-ray studies made at a local medical facility, which would then forward these to us. A telephone consultation with the surgeon would take place to complete the follow-up process. Beside the ability to reach patients who are out of the area, one of the advantages of online surveys resides in the quality of the data provided. Compared with the scantron-type forms, the online forms can be programmed to eliminate some of the user errors that are inherent to filling out a sheet of paper. For example, the use of a pen instead of a #2 pencil, incomplete filling of an answer field, and duplication of answers in a single-answer field are common errors that affect the accuracy of the data entered, and these problems are eliminated with the use of computerized means of entry. Nevertheless, this mode of data collection relies on the assumption that the patient is computer literate, which is not always the case in the hip replacement population. We have found that a combination of both data collection means (scantron and online) are necessity for our purpose. Unfortunately, the online data collection process had to be discontinued in 2004 when the U.S. Food and Drug Administration (FDA) inspected our center for compliance to the Conserve®Plus multicenter Investigational Device Exemption (IDE) protocol. The inspectors found that our setup was not compliant with Title 21, part 11 of the code of federal regulation, particularly item e of paragraph 11.10, even though this section of the Code of Federal Regulations (CFR) is dated April 1, 2002, which was more than a year after we had activated our online data collection system. Essentially, in our settings the records generated by the online systems needed to be deleted after their transfer into our access database to avoid a duplicate entry the next time we would use this macro. For the FDA, these records represented so-called source data and needed to be preserved for audit purposes. At the time, the simplest solution in this situation was to just remove the links from our website to these surveys and limit our data collection to the means accepted by the FDA. We do plan to reinstitute the online data collection forms because of the improved patient compliance and as a method of reducing errors in data transfer. This will happen as soon as the FDA study is over.

New Interfaces

With the advent of new technologies, the quest for a better interface for data collection has already seen major improvements and could be generalized to most physicians' offices once the regulatory hurdles are overcome or in a non–FDA-regulated setting. For patient-generated data, the most important feature of a system is that it is user friendly, and touch screen technology has already proven to be far more intuitive and natural for the user than a mouse- or keyboard-driven interface. This technology combines the advantages of computerized data collection systems (cleaner data; no "bubbling errors," better user guidance in terms of what fields need to be populated or the number of answers allowed for each field, electronic versus space-inefficient paper source data) with those of a paper-based survey (ease of use for anyone who can

Entered:

HIP SURVEY

Page 1 of 2

PATIENT NAME:____

Today's Date	Social Security #

1. In the past month, what has the intensity of your **HIP Pain** been like?
(Choose only ONE per hip)

Right Hip	Left Hip	
1	1	None/I have no pain in my hip. *(10)*
2	2	I have slight pain Occasionally. *(9)*
3	3	I have slight pain Frequently. *(8)*
4	4	I have significant pain after certain activities, which requires *light medication* Occasionally/Aspirin, Motrin, etc... *(6)*
5	5	I have significant pain with most activities, but No Pain or Minimum Pain at rest. I take *light medication*, Frequently. *(4)*
6	6	I have pain all of the time, but it is bearable. I take *strong medication* Occasionally/Vicodin, or Codeine, and *lighter medication* Frequently. *(2)*
7	7	I have pain all of the time, which is UNbearable. I take *strong medication* Frequently. (1)

2. The Pain that I am having in my Hip is located.... **(Choose ONE per hip)**

Right Hip	Left Hip	
1	1	In Front/Groin Region.
2	2	In the Back/Buttocks Region.
3	3	On the Side.
4	4	Any combination of the above.
5	5	I am Not having Pain.
6	6	Other:__________________

3. Do you have Thigh pain? **(Choose ONE)**

Right Hip	Left Hip	
1	1	No thigh pain. *(10)*
2	2	Some pain; No medication. *(8)*
3	3	A lot of pain; Some medication. *(6)*
4	4	Some pain standing, worse walking. *(4)*
5	5	Pain most of the time; limits activities. *(2)*

4. Currently, I am able to Walk.... **(Choose ONE)**

1. Without any sort of walking aid.
2. With (1) Cane.
3. With (1) Crutch.
4. With (2) Canes.
5. With (2) Crutches.
6. With a Walker.
7. I am unable to Walk.

5. Generally, how Far can you Walk comfortably, before you must stop to rest? **(Choose ONE)**

1. More than 6 Blocks.
2. About 4-6 Blocks.
3. About 1-3 Blocks.
4. Less than 1 Block.
5. Only from my bed to a chair or bathroom
6. I am unable to walk

6. The medication that I am taking for my Hip pain is...______________________

*Strength?*__________________ *How often?*__________________

Page 1

Figure 6-2 A, Page 1 of the hip survey filled out by the patients at each follow-up visit. This survey is composed of elements pertaining to the UCLA hip score, the Harris Hip scoring system, and other disease-specific independent questions.

HIP SURVEY

Page 2 of 2

PATIENT NAME:________________________________DATE:___/___/_____

7. Please ***Choose only ONE*** of the following statements that best describes your ability to **WALK**.

- (A) I am Unrestricted. I Do Not Use Support, and I Do Not Limp. *(10)*
- (B) I Do Not Use Support, but I do have a Limp, OR, I use (1) Support without a Limp. *(8)*
- (C) I Do Not Use Support for (1) Block, OR, I Use (1) Support up to six blocks, bilateral Support without restriction. *(6)*
- (D) I Do Not Use Support because I am house bound, OR, I use (1) Support Less than six blocks, bilateral support for a Short Distance. *(4)*
- (E) I am Wheelchair bound, OR, I transfer activities with a Walker. *(2)*
- (F) I am Bedridden. *(1)*

9. Stairs

- (A) Foot over foot without a bannister
- (B) Foot over foot using a bannister
- (C) Stairs in any manner
- (D) Unable to climb stairs

8. I can put on shoes and socks

- (1) With ease
- (2) With difficulty
- (3) I am unable to put on shoes or socks without assistance.

11. Able to enter Public Transportation

- (A) Yes
- (B) No

10. Sitting

- (A) Comfotable in any chair for one hour
- (B) Comfortable in a high chair for 1/2 hour
- (C) Unable to sit comfortably in any chair

12. Limp

- (1) None
- (2) Slight
- (3) Moderate
- (4) Severe
- (5) Unable to walk

13. If I had to, I could Sometimes......

- (1) Function Without Restriction. 8 hr work + sports *(10)*
- (2) Function with a little Restriction. 6 hr work + Occasional sport *(8)*
- (3) Do Most of the housework/Shopping. On feet 4 hours *(6)*
- (4) Do Limited housework/Shopping. *(4)*
- (5) None of the above. *(1)*

14. Please ***choose only ONE*** of the following statements which best describes your MAXIMUM Activity Level.

- (1) I Regularly participate in jogging, and/or tennis, skiing, aerobics, backpacking, heavy labor. (10)
- (2) I Sometimes participate in jogging, and/or tennis, skiing, aerobics, backpacking, heavy labor. (9)
- (3) I Regularly participate in bicycling. (8)
- (4) I Regularly participate in bowling and/or golf. (7)
- (5) I Regularly participate in swimming and/or shopping, unlimited work around the house. (6)
- (6) I Sometimes participate in swimming and/or shopping, unlimited work around the house. (5)
- (7) I Regularly participate in walking, limited work around the house/shopping. (4)
- (8) I Sometimes participate in walking, limited work around the house/shopping. (3)
- (9) I am VERY RESTRICTED and I am only able to do MINIMUM ACTIVITIES. (2)
- (10) I require assistance for most activities and generally do not leave the house. (1)

Page 2

Figure 6-2, cont'd B, Page 2 of the hip survey.

Entered:

SF 12 HEALTH SURVEY

(Standard)

This questionnaire asks for your views about your health. This information will help us keep track of how you feel and how well you are able to do your usual activities.

NAME:____

Date	Social Security #
0 1 2 3 4 5 6 7 8 9 (6 columns)	0 1 2 3 4 5 6 7 8 9 (9 columns)

1. In general, would you say your health is...

1 Excellent
2 Very good
3 Good
4 Fair
5 Poor

The following items are about activities you might do during a typical day. Does your health now limit you in these activities? If so, how much?

2. Moderate activities, such as moving a table, pushing a vacuum cleaner, bowling, or playing golf.

1 Yes, limited a lot.
2 Yes, limited a little.
3 No, not limited at all.

3. Climbing several flights of stairs.

1 Yes, limited a lot.
2 Yes, limited a little.
3 No, not limited at all.

During the past 4 weeks, have you had any of the following problems with your work or other regular daily activities as a result of your physical health?

4. Accomplished less than you would like?

1 Yes
2 No

5. Were limited in the kind of work or other activities?

1 Yes
2 No

During the past 4 weeks, have you had any of the following problems with your work or other regular daily activities as a result of your emotional problems (such as feeling depressed or anxious)?

6. Accomplished less than you would like?

1 Yes
2 No

6. Didn't do work or other activities as carefully as usual?

1 Yes
2 No

(s:\forms\SF12-97.DEW)

Page 1 of 2

Figure 6-3 A, Page 1 of the Quality-of-life Short Form-12 survey.

SF 12 HEALTH SURVEY

(Standard)

Page 2 of 2

NAME:______________________________ DATE:____/____/_____

8. During the past 4 weeks, how much did pain interfere with your normal work (including both work outside the home and housework)?

1 Not at all.
2 A little bit.
3 Moderately
4 Quite a bit
5 Extremely

These questions are about how you feel and how things have been with you during the past 4 weeks.
*For each question, please give the **ONE** answer that comes closest to the way you have been feeling.*

How much of the time during the past 4 weeks.......

9. .....have you felt calm and peaceful?

1 All of the time.
2 Most of the time.
3 A good bit of the time.
4 Some of the time
5 A Little of the time.
6 None of tho timc.

10. .....did you have a lot of energy?

1 All of the time.
2 Most of the time.
3 A good bit of the time.
4 Some of the time
5 A Little of the time.
6 None of the time.

11. .....have you felt downhearted and blue?

1 All of the time.
2 Most of the time.
3 A good bit of the time.
4 Some of the time
5 A Little of the time.
6 None of the time.

12. During the past 4 weeks, how much of the time has your physical health or emotional problems interfered with your social activities (like visiting friends, relatives, etc...)?

1 All of the time.
2 Most of the time.
3 A good bit of the time.
4 Some of the time
5 A Little of the time.
6 None of the time.

(s:\forms\SF12-97.DEW)

Page 2 of 2

Figure 6-3, cont'd B, Page 2.

Sport Activity Survey

PATIENT NAME: [ ]

Today's Date 2/26/2007

Social Security # [ ]-[ ]-[ ]

List the physical activities (up to 3) you have been participating in on a regular basis over the past 6 months.

ACTIVITY # 1 (Select one only)

Group 1	Group 2
Basketball ○	Badminton ○
European Handball ○	Ballet/Ballroom Dancing ○
Football ○	Baseball/Softball ○
Hockey ○	Handball ○
Rugby ○	Martial Arts ○
Soccer ○	Racquetball ○
	Aerobics ○
	Squash ○
	Tennis (singles) ○
	Volleyball ○

Group 3	Group 4
Cross-country skiing ○	Downhill skiing (groomed) ○
Cycling ○	Golf (walking between holes) ○
Downhill skiing (moguls) ○	Walking, Hiking, Backpacking ○
Ice skating ○	
Roller blading ○	
Running ○	
Water skiing ○	

Group 5	Group 6
Archery ○	Rock climbing ○
Bowling ○	Surfing ○
Golf (using a cart) ○	Swimming ○
Sailing ○	Scuba diving ○
Tennis (doubles) ○	OTHER: [ ] ○
Weight lifting ○	
Yoga ○	

Frequency (# of times per month)	Duration per session
1-4 times/month ○	0-30 minutes ○
5-8 times/month ○	30-60 minutes ○
9-12 times/month ○	60-120 minutes ○
>12 times/month ○	>120 minutes ○

Intensity (check one in each field)		Have you had a revision?
Competitive ○	Beginner ○	Yes ○
Recreational ○	Intermediate ○	No ○
	Advanced ○	
	Expert ○	

Figure 6-4 First page of the sports activity survey as it appeared on the Joint Replacement Institute website. The survey had two more similar pages, allowing the patient to enter information about up to three physical activities.

Entered:

PRE-OP/FOLLOW-UP FORM

Physician
(A) AMSTUTZ
(B) SCHMALZRIED
(C) BEAULE

PATIENT NAME:______________________

Social Security
(0)–(9) × 9

Date Seen
MO/DAY/YR
(0)–(9) × 6

Discrepancy
RIGHT LEFT
(A) (A) 0.0-1 cm
(B) (B) 1.1-2 cm
(C) (C) 2.1-3 cm
(D) (D) >3 cm

(A) REAL
(B) APPARENT ________ (actual)
(C) COMBINATION

Weight (kg) (0)–(9) × 3
Height (cm) (0)–(9) × 3

Follow-up Type
(A) Clinic
(B) Phone
(C) Survey

Charnley Class
(A) A
(B) B
(C) C

Range of Motion
RIGHT LEFT
(A) (A) >90 degrees of Flexion
(B) (B) >30 degrees of Internal Rotation
(C) (C) <15 degrees of Flexion Contracture

Complications

R		L
(A)	DISLOCATION	(A)
(B)	SUBLUXATION	(B)
(C)	LOOSE ACETABULAR COMPONENT	(C)
(D)	LOOSE FEMORAL COMPONENT	(D)
(E)	FRACTURED HEAD/NECK (bone)	(E)
(F)	FRACTURED ACETABULAR COMPONENT	(F)
(G)	FRACTURED FEMUR	(G)
(H)	FRACTURED PELVIS	(H)
(I)	HETEROTOPIC BONE FORMATION	(I)
(J)	NERVE PALSY	(J)
(K)	SEPSIS, Superficial	(K)
(L)	SEPSIS, Deep	(L)
(M)	MALIGNANCY	(M)
(N)	PEDAL EDEMA Over Pre-op Level	(N)
(O)	BROKEN WIRE	(O)
(P)	WIRE REMOVAL (local anesthesia)	(P)
(Q)	TENDER TROCHANTER	(Q)
(R)	TROCHANTERIC NON-UNION	(R)
(S)	TROCHANTERIC MIGRATION	(S)
(T)	Other ____________ (specify)	(T)

Trendelenberg
RIGHT LEFT
(A) (A) NEGATIVE
(B) (B) LEVEL
(C) (C) POSITIVE

Longer Extremity
(A) EQUAL
(B) RIGHT
(C) LEFT

Pain R		Pain L	Walk	Func	Activity
(10)	10	(10)	(10) 10	(10) 10	(10) 10
(9)	9	(9)	(9) 9	(9) 9	(9) 9
(8)	8	(8)	(8) 8	(8) 8	(8) 8
(7)	7	(7)	(7) 7	(7) 7	(7) 7
(6)	6	(6)	(6) 6	(6) 6	(6) 6
(5)	5	(5)	(5) 5	(5) 5	(5) 5
(4)	4	(4)	(4) 4	(4) 4	(4) 4
(3)	3	(3)	(3) 3	(3) 3	(3) 3
(2)	2	(2)	(2) 2	(2) 2	(2) 2
(1)	1	(1)	(1) 1	(1) 1	(1) 1

Figure 6-5 Preoperative/follow-up form. Used directly by the surgeon during patient visits or during phone consultations.

Entered:

SURGERY FORM

PATIENT NAME:______________________________

SURGEON:
Amstutz (A)
Schmalzried (B)
Beaulé (C)

Social Security #	Date of SX
0 1 2 3 4 5 6 7 8 9	0 1 2 3 4 5 6 7 8 9

SIDE: Right*(1)* (A)
Left*(2)* (B)

____
INCLUDING OUTSIDE MD REVISIONS

PRIMARY HIP ARTHROPLASTY

PROCEDURE
Total Hip Replacement*(A0)* (A)
Total Surface Replacement*(B0)* (B)
Hemiarthroplasty*(C0)* (C)
Surface Hemiarthroplasty*(xx)* (D)

ETIOLOGY
Osteoarthritis (OA)*(A0)* (A)
Osteonecrosis (ON)*(B0)* (B)
Developmental Dysplasia*(C0)* (C)
(e.g., RA, Ankylosing Spondylitis, Lupus Erythematosus) — Rheumatoid Disease*(D0)* (D)
Infection*(E0)* (E)
Post Trauma*(F0)* (F)
Fracture Acute*(H0)* (G)
Failed Other Procedure*(L0)* (H)
(e.g., Pagets, LC Perthes, SCFE, Otto Pelvis, Heterotopic Bone, Charcot, Ochronosis, Gout, Hemophilia, Gauchers, Osteoporosis, Renal Osteodystrophy, Other connective tissue disease.) — Developmental or Metabolic*(M0)* (I)
Anterior Impingement*(O0)* (J)
Other*(99)* (K)

____
(e.g., Arthrodesis, Arthrofibrosis, Mobile Pseudoarthrosis, etc...)

REVISION HIP ARTHROPLASTY

PROCEDURE
THR-Both components*(E2)* (A)
THR-Acetabular component ONLY*(E0)* (B)
THR-Femoral component ONLY*(E0)* (C)
SR-Both components*(E2)* (E)
SR-Acetabular component ONLY*(E0)* (F)
SR-Femoral component ONLY*(E0)* (G)
Hemi-SR*(E0)* (H)
Other*(D0)* (I)
____

DIAGNOSIS
Failed THR-Conventional*(O1)* (A)
Failed THR-Surface*(J0)* (B)
Failed Other Prosthesis*(KO)* (C)
____
(e.g., Hemiarthroplasty, Cup)

MODE OF FAILURE *(Check all that apply)*
Aseptic Loosening*(80)* (A)
Fracture*(D0)* (B)
Osteolysis*(99)* (C)
Sepsis*(A0)* (D)
Instability*(C0)* (E)
______________Other*(F0)* (F)

COMPLICATIONS LEADING TO REPEAT SURGERY
Greater Trochanter*(E0)* (A)
Heterotopic Bone, Leg Lengthening, Bone Cyst, Enigmatic Pain*(F0)* (B)
______________Other*(99)* (C)

Page 1 of 3

Figure 6-6 A, Page 1 of our hip surgery form. This form evolved over time as the surgical technique and components used in surgery changed.

SURGERY FORM

PATIENT NAME:________________________________ DATE:____/____/____

MISCELLANEOUS PROCEDURES

Removal of Hardware (A)
Bone Grafting (B)
Core Decompression (C)
Osteotomy (D)
Troch Wire Removal or Re-attachment (E)
H.O. Excision (F)
Arthrodesis (G)
__________ Other (H)

PREPARATION

ANESTHESIA *(Check all that apply)*
General (A)
Epidural (B)
Hypotensive Approach (C)
Normotensive (D)

APPROACH
No Osteotomy (A)
Osteotomy (B)

COMPONENTS

MANUFACTURER

Acetabular		Femoral
(A)	Depuy	(A)
(B)	Kinamed	(B)
(C)	Sulzer	(C)
(D)	Zimmer	(D)
(E)	Osteonics	(E)
(F)	Wright	(F)
(G)	Biomet	(G)
(H)	J&J	(H)
(I)	Other	(I)

DESIGN OF COMPONENTS

Acetabular
(A) Conserve+
(B) Thin Shell C+
(C) Double Socket
(D) Superfix
(E) Gap II
(F) Trilogy/Longevity
(G) Other

Femoral
(A) Conserve+
(B) Conserve
(C) ATH Standard GB
(D) ATH Long GB
(E) ATH Standard HA
(F) ATH Long HA
(G) Other

____________ ____________
OTHER ACETABULAR *OTHER FEMORAL*

ACET SIZE	STEM SIZE	NeckLen	HEAD SIZE
[ ][ ][ ]	[ ][ ].[ ]	[ ][ ][ ].[ ]	[ ][ ][ ]
(0)(0)(0)	(0)(0)(0)	(0)(0)(0)(0)	(0)(0)(0)
(1)(1)(1)	(1)(1)(1)	(1)(1)(1)(1)	(1)(1)(1)
(2)(2)(2)	(2)(2)(2)	(2)(2)(2)(2)	(2)(2)(2)
(3)(3)(3)	(3)(3)(3)	(3)(3)(3)(3)	(3)(3)(3)
(4)(4)(4)	(4)(4)(4)	(4)(4)(4)(4)	(4)(4)(4)
(5)(5)(5)	(5)(5)(5)	(5)(5)(5)(5)	(5)(5)(5)
(6)(6)(6)	(6)(6)(6)	(6)(6)(6)(6)	(6)(6)(6)
(7)(7)(7)	(7)(7)(7)	(7)(7)(7)(7)	(7)(7)(7)
(8)(8)(8)	(8)(8)(8)	(8)(8)(8)(8)	(8)(8)(8)
(9)(9)(9)	(9)(9)(9)	(9)(9)(9)(9)	(9)(9)(9)

Page 2 of 3

Figure 6-6, cont'd B, Page 2.

SURGERY FORM

PATIENT NAME:________________ DATE:___/___/___

CEMENT FIXATION

Acetabular		Femoral
A	None	A
B	Simplex	B
C	Other	C

OTHER ACETABULAR _OTHER FEMORAL_

ADJUNCT FIXATION

None	A
____Screws/#	B
______Other	C

BEARING MATERIALS
ACETABULUM ONLY

P.E. _(X-Linked)_	A
Metal/Metal	B
M/M Type A	C

BONE GRAFTING TECHNIQUE

Acetabular		Femoral
A	None	A
B	Autograft	B
C	Allograft-_Frozen_	C
D	Allograft-_Freeze dried_	D
E	Collagraft, Grafton, Pro-osteon	E
F	Other	F
	"Ling" Impaction Grafting	G

ACETABULAR _FEMORAL_

HOSPITAL COURSE

BLOOD LOSS
Estimated at surgery

One Unit	A
Two Units	B
Three Units	C
≥ Four Units	D

HEMOVAC DRAINAGE

One Unit	A
Two Units	B
Three Units	C
≥ Four Units	D

BLOOD REPLACEMENT

Autologous
(Surgery and Post op)

One Unit	A
Two Units	B
Three Units	C
≥ Four Units	D

Homologous
(Surgery and Post op)

One Unit	A
Two Units	B
Three Units	C
≥ Four Units	D

COMPLICATIONS

Sepsis	A
Dislocation/Subluxation	B
Nerve palsy	C
Thrombophlebitis	D
M.I.	E
Wound Healing	F
P.E.	G
Hematoma	H
G.I. Bleed	I
U.T.I.	J
Other	K

DATE OF DISCHARGE

0	0	0	0	0	0
1	1	1	1	1	1
2	2	2	2	2	2
3	3	3	3	3	3
4	4	4	4	4	4
5	5	5	5	5	5
6	6	6	6	6	6
7	7	7	7	7	7
8	8	8	8	8	8
9	9	9	9	9	9

PROPHYLAXIS:

Coumadin	A
Lovenox	B
Other	C

____

HETEROTOPIC OSSIFICATION

Indocin	A
Radiotherapy	B

Page 3 of 3

Figure 6-6, cont'd C, Page 3.

read). Also, touch screens are durable, cannot be stolen when used in public areas, are easy to clean, and can handle beverages being spilled on them. Various technologies can be used to produce the touch screen effect (including Resistive, Capacitive, Surface acoustic wave, or Infra-red), but all share these characteristics of durability. A waiting room could have several terminals, or even better, each examining room could be equipped with one of these devices, where the patients can fill out their surveys before their initial or follow-up visit starts. This investment can save countless hours of data verification and processing in the long run.

For surgeon-generated data, it seems that a portable device may be more appropriate. A Personal Digital Assistant (PDA) can provide the means to generate data during the interview with the patient or after the surgery. Other advantages of a PDA over a fixed terminal in the examination room are the greater privacy and the ability to review those notes instantly to support a dictation, for example.

Photographic Data

Long before the beginning of our series of metal-on-metal resurfacing, the senior author had included photographic intraoperative data collection to his surgical routine. Originally, this data collection was designed to provide case illustrations for manuscripts and presentations. However, a secondary use resulting from the review of these photographs in combination with the radiographic data and the retrieval analyses of failed components early in the series, led to the hypothesis that bone quality and femoral head preparation technique were associated with the survival of the prosthesis. This hypothesis was later confirmed from a statistical point of view.[14-16] The systematic measurement of femoral head defect size from the intraoperative photograph proved to be a key source of information for subsequent publications and can arguably be considered the most important covariate to adjust for in any survivorship analysis of modern resurfacing devices. The details and validation of our measurement method for femoral head defects were described in a recent article published in *Clinical Orthopaedics and Related Research*.[17] The most important intraoperative photograph for this purpose is one taken at the end of the femoral head preparation, just before cementing the femoral head. This is when an assessment can be made not only of the defect sizes but also the efficacy of the drying methods, the completeness of removal of cystic material and a count of the number of drilled holes. Examples of these important intra-operative photographs are shown in Figure 6-7.

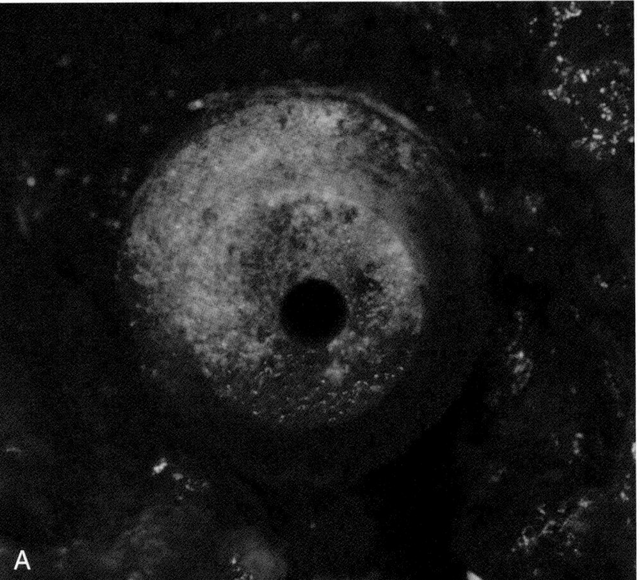

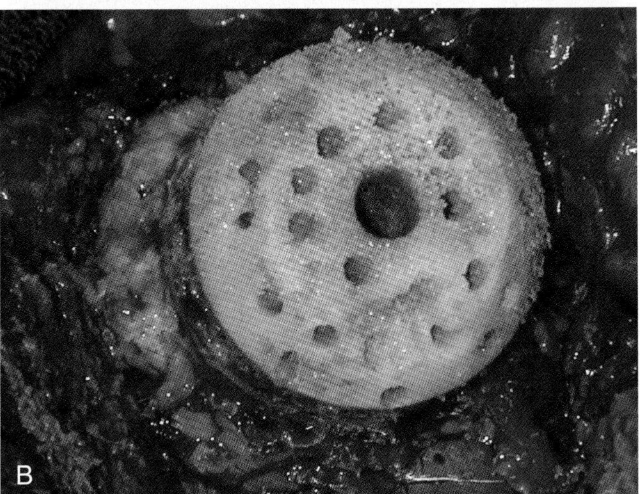

Figure 6-7 Examples of intraoperative photographs taken at the end of the femoral head preparation just before the femoral component was cemented. **A,** Hip #3 of our series (now 10.5 years postoperative). First-generation bone preparation technique before water picking and suction. Good bone quality (no cysts) with no drilled holes in the femoral head. **B,** Hip #760 of our series. The femoral cystic material was removed with a burr, numerous holes were drilled in the dome and sclerotic chamfer areas, the head was dried, and the stem was cemented.

Radiographic Data

Despite the increased use of more recent imaging technologies covered in the previous chapter, radiographs remain the orthopaedist's most important tool in the assessment of the interface between the bone and the prosthesis. The content of an x-ray analysis can vary greatly depending on the aim of the study. This is where the optical scanning data collection process keeps its value compared with the later, more sophisticated methods. Both the flexibility and the ease of creating a new data collection form with this system are definite advantages for projects with a limited duration. As the study of a new series progresses and the follow-up of early cases increases, new observations or findings are made from the radiographic assessments. Also, sometimes what seemed like an important change on an early x-ray can turn out to be insignificant clinically. In these situations, a modification to the data collection form is necessary. The x-ray data collection form used for the review of our first 400 cases[14] is shown in Figure 6-8.

SURFACE ARTHROPLASTY X-RAY FORM

Physician
(A) AMSTUTZ
(B) SCHMALZRIED
(C) BEAULE

PATIENT NAME:______________________________

Social Security
(0)–(9) × 9 digits

X-RAY Date
(0)–(9) × 6 digits

Side
(A) RIGHT
(B) LEFT

Visit type
(A) Pre-op
(B) Follow-up

Heterotopic ossification
None (A)
Grade I (B)
Grade II (C)
Grade III (E)
Grade IV (F)

Fixation Scores

	FEMORAL	ACETABULAR
(0)	None	None
(1)	2 (Tip)	I
(2)	1 (sup)	II
(3)	3 (inf)	III
(4)	1 and 2	I and II
(5)	2 and 3	I and III
(6)	1 and 3	II and III
(7)	1-3 (inc)	I-III (INC)
(8)	1-3 (C)	I-III (c)
(9)	Migration	Migration

Progressive (Femoral): No (A) Yes (B)
Progressive (Acetabular): No (A) Yes (B)

Osteolysis (AP) NONE (A)

FEMORAL
1 2 3
Yes (A) (A) (A)

ACETABULAR
I II III IV
(A) (A) (A) (A)

Progressive (Femoral): No (A) Yes (B)
Progressive (Acetabular): No (A) Yes (B)

Figure A: Antero-posterior view (Left Hip)

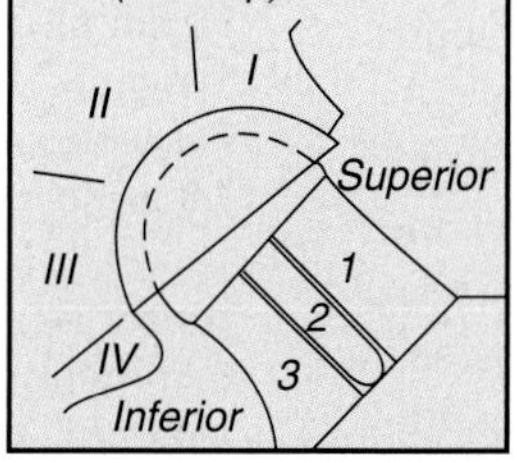

Neck Narrowing
(A) No
(B) Yes

Beads
(A) No
(B) Yes

Contralateral
(A) Nomal
(B) SA
(C) THA

Cem. stem
(A) No
(B) Yes

AP view

Neck or Stem Shaft Angle — (0)–(9) × 3 digits

Rotation
None (A)
Minor (B)
Major (C)

Cup Angle — (0)–(9) × 2 digits

Offset

Operated
Ab. Lev. Arm — (0)–(9) × 2 digits
Body — (0)–(9) × 3 digits

Contralateral
Ab. Lev. Arm — (0)–(9) × 2 digits
Body — (0)–(9) × 3 digits

Johnson Lat.

Positioning
(A) A to P
(B) Neutral
(C) P to A

Stem/Cortex
(A) Contact
(B) Through

Rotation
(A) None
(B) Minor
(C) Major

Figure 6-8 Form designed and used by our independent reviewer (TG) in the radiographic data collection for the initial report of our first 400 hips.

Data Processing

After global data collection and entry into our access database, the specific data for each of our studies are compiled into spreadsheets using Excel, which is a very powerful application for data treatment, particularly when calculations and sorting are needed within or between sets of data. These spreadsheets are updated regularly as new data are generated. This allows us to perform quick assessments of the status of a given study at any time. For an active study like our current research devoted to metal-on-metal resurfacing, we recommend updating a large spreadsheet that contains all the basic data stored in the database and creating subsets of this document, as needed, for specific research questions. A link from the cells of the subset that need regular update to the corresponding ones on the main spreadsheet creates an automatic update and avoids the redundancy of data entry. Special Excel files were also developed as tools to rapidly calculate clinical scores that require a complex algorithm like the SF-12 or the Harris Hip scores.

Statistics

The nature of the data collected for orthopaedic studies is such that a multiplicity of statistical tools is needed to establish the significance of a wide variety of variables. We generally use Excel to generate descriptive statistical summaries of the data such as averages, standard deviations, ranges, and percentages. Also, Excel allows us to perform simple correlation and differential statistical tests on parametric data (e.g., Pearson product moment coefficient of correlation or Student's t-tests). However, more complex analyses are often necessary and require the use of specialized statistical software packages. For all non-parametric data analyses (e.g., Mann-Whitney U test, Wilcoxon signed-ranks test), time-dependent analyses (e.g., Kaplan-Meier survival estimates, Log-rank test) or multivariate analyses (e.g., Cox proportional hazard ratio), we have been using Stata (Stata Corporation, College Station, TX).

Summary

Systematic data collection is an important part of the surgical practice because it allows not only the publication of the surgeon's results but also provides feedback conducive to technical improvement. The data collected should include disease-specific information, quality-of-life aspects, and activity assessments from the patients as well as from the surgeon, including information on surgical technique. A well-organized, user-friendly computerized data collection interface can save countless hours in the data processing phase.

References

1. Harris W: Traumatic arthritis of the hip after dislocation and acetabular fractures: treatment by mold arthroplasty. An end-result study using a new method of result evaluation. J Bone Joint Surg 1969;51A:737-755.
2. Bellamy N, Buchanan W, Goldsmith C, Campbell J, Stitt L: Validation study of WOMAC: a health status instrument for measuring clinically important patient relevant outcomes to antirheumatic drug therapy in patients with osteoarthritis of the hip or knee. J Rheumatol 1988;15:1833-1840.
3. Amstutz H, Thomas B, Jinnah R, Kim W, Grogan T, Yale C: Treatment of primary osteoarthritis of the hip. A comparison of total joint and surface replacement arthroplasty. J Bone Joint Surg 1984;66A:228-241.
4. Merle d'Aubiné R, Postel M: Functional results of hip arthroplasty with acrylic prostheses. J Bone Joint Surg Am 1954;36:451-475.
5. Dawson J, Fitzpatrick R, Murray D, Carr A: Comparison of measures to assess outcomes in total hip replacement surgery. Qual Health Care 1996;5:81-88.
6. Ware J, Kosinski M, Keller S: A 12-Item Short-Form Health Survey: construction of scales and preliminary tests of reliability and validity. Med Care 1996;34:220-233.
7. Ware JJ, Sherbourne C: The MOS 36-item short-form health survey (SF-36). I. Conceptual framework and item selection. Med Care 1992;30:473-483.
8. Jenkinson C, Layte R, Jenkinson D, Lawrence K, Petersen S, Paice C, Stradling J: A shorter form health survey: can the SF-12 replicate results from the SF-36 in longitudinal studies? J Public Health Med 1997;19:179-186.
9. Wright JG, Rudicel S, Feinstein AR: Ask patients what they want. Evaluation of individual complaints before total hip replacement. J Bone Joint Surg Br 1994;76:229-234.
10. Beaulé P, Dorey F, Hoke R, Le Duff M, Amstutz H: The value of patient activity level in the outcome of total hip arthroplasty. J Arthroplasty 2006;21:547-552.
11. Dorey FJ, Amstutz HC: The need to account for patient activity when evaluating the results of total hip arthroplasty with survivorship analysis. J Bone Joint Surg Am 2002;84A:709-710.
12. Feller J, Kay P, Hodgkinson J, Wroblewski B: Activity and socket wear in the Charnley low-friction arthroplasty. J Arthroplasty 1994;9:341-345.
13. Schmalzried TP, Shepherd EF, Dorey FJ, Jackson WO, dela Rosa M, Fa'vae F, McKellop HA, McClung CD: Martell J, Moreland JR, Amstutz HC: The John Charnley Award. Wear is a function of use, not time. Clin Orthop Rel Res 2000;381:36-46.
14. Amstutz H, Beaulé P, Dorey F, Le Duff M, Campbell P, Gruen T: Metal-on-metal hybrid surface arthroplasty: two to six year follow-up. J Bone Joint Surg 2004;86A:28-39.
15. Beaulé P, Dorey F, Le Duff M, Gruen T, Amstutz H: Risk factors affecting early outcome of metal on metal surface arthroplasty of the hip in patients 40 years old and younger. Clin Orthop Rel Res 2004;418:87-93.
16. Amstutz H, Le Duff M, Campbell P, Dorey F: The effects of technique changes on aseptic loosening of the femoral component in hip resurfacing. Results of 600 Conserve Plus with a 3-9 year follow-up. J Arthroplasty 2007;22:481-489.
17. Amstutz H, Ball S, Le Duff M, Dorey F: Hip resurfacing for patients under 50 years of age. Results of 350 Conserve Plus with a 2-9 year follow-up. Clin Orthop Rel Res (in press) Epub ahead of print.

CHAPTER 7

Surgical Technique

Harlan C. Amstutz

Introduction

The surgical technique of Conserve®Plus has been described in successive peer-reviewed articles,[1-4] reflecting its evolution since 1996. A new series of instruments (5803) have been developed for the Conserve®Plus prosthesis (Fig. 7-1), to improve the stability and accuracy of femoral head preparation while preserving maximum flexibility for the surgeon to adjust and fine tune pin placement before the final reaming, thereby enabling him or her to optimize the final position of the femoral component on the head and neck. Placing a larger bore spigot over the smaller pin improves the stability and accuracy of cylindrical and chamfer reaming while maintaining the ability of fine tuning the location of the smaller pin up to the final reaming in order to make certain that the component will be perfectly positioned on the neck to avoid notching and minimize impingement. Spigot-guided chamfering is more conservative, preserving more bone by reducing the chamfer reamer angle 10 degrees, lessening the cement mantle thickness. The system still maintains maximum flexibility for the surgeon to remove more abnormal bone if needed by reaming with a smaller chamfer without changing the cylindrical reaming size. The new system continues to provide for a 1-mm cement mantle, although a European system has a 0.5-mm mantle. We continue to believe that there should be a sufficient gap to allow excess acrylic to extrude rather than pressurize cement into the head.

Templating

Preoperative planning through the use of templates is essential. The surgeon should employ the same magnification templates he is accustomed to using. The 20% magnified templates is optimal for the anteroposterior (AP)-pelvis view of a patient of normal habitus (body mass index [BMI] < 30), but there will be a magnification variation of plus or minus 6% (one standard deviation) depending on whether the patient has a high or low BMI. Fifteen percent templates are available and are suitable for patients with thin body habitus (low BMI). The templates are used on analog film taken at a 40-inch tube to x-ray distance or a comparable printed out, plain paper or x-ray from a digital format. The AP template is oriented to provide an approximately 140-degree stem shaft angle. Note the series of hatch marks radiating from the center of the head with distance between each representing approximately 5 mm, which assist in locating the pin in the optimal position with respect to the observed superior indentation of the ligamentum teres (Fig. 7-2). In the example illustrated, the pin will be approximately 15 mm superior to the ligamentum teres. The hatch marks that are parallel to the neck indicate how much bone the reamer will take away for that templated size and how close the reamer will come to the femoral neck that will allow for a 1-mm cement mantle. A slightly superior placement is recommended, in which case the reaming cut will be closer to the neck. The template on the lateral view shows the position of the stem, which should be translated anteriorly and should be directed neutral to the neck axis unless there is an large anterior osteophyte, in which case it should be directed slightly posterior to anterior to avoid reaming into the osteophyte (Fig. 7-3). As the osteophyte grows in size, the underlying anterior cortex may be partially or completely replaced. In that case the osteophyte assumes an increasing structural role. Socket sizing is also done on the template in order to anatomically restore the offset and remove only the arthritic bone. For approximately 97% of patients, the thin shells are used. If there is a protrusio or more extensive erosion, then the thick 5.5-mm shells would be used. If there is still more erosion or leg-length descrepancy needs to be corrected, then the superfix socket may be indicated, which will replace a defect of 1 cm.

Patient Preparation

We recommend operating in a room with a high volume of air exchange and or laminar air flow. Alternatively, hood exhaust systems should be employed by the operating team. Most of our metal-on-metal surface arthroplasties are performed with the patient under epidural with an indwelling catheter or spinal supplemented with general hypotensive anesthesia. The epidural catheter is left in situ overnight and provides excellent pain relief. Prophylactic antibiotics are used until the Foley catheter is removed on the first postoperative day.

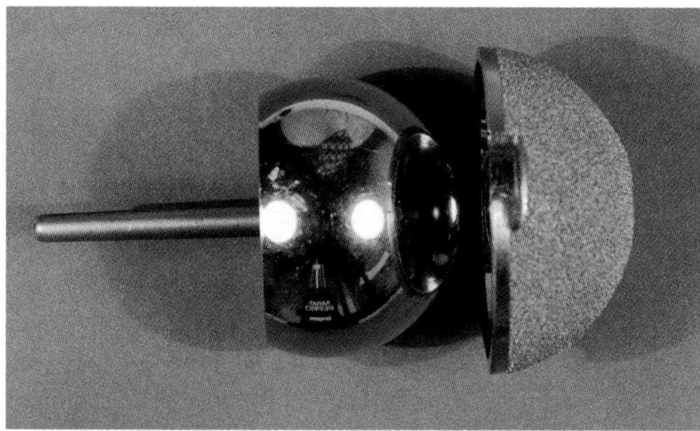

Figure 7-1 Conserve®Plus hip resurfacing prosthesis. Shown here with the thin (3.5-mm) shell.

The patient is positioned on the side in the lateral decubitus position, with the pelvis stabilized by a padded support on the pubis, the sacrum, the anterior and the posterior thorax, with the table tilted slightly anteriorly and the body perpendicular to the floor (Fig. 7-4). This table position will enable maximum roll back of the patient for more direct acetabular reaming and orientation. The pubic support is critical in location and fixation. The leg must allow at least 90 degrees of flexion and, preferably, 45 degrees of adduction, for the femoral head to be easily delivered through the gluteus maximus split after dislocation.

Approach

Although other approaches are possible, we recommend the posterior approach for the following reasons:

1. No important muscle groups are sectioned.
2. There is no release of the abductor muscles, which play the most important role in stabilizing the hip during walking and other activities.
3. The gluteus medius and minimus remain intact. The only muscle groups that are released are the short rotators that

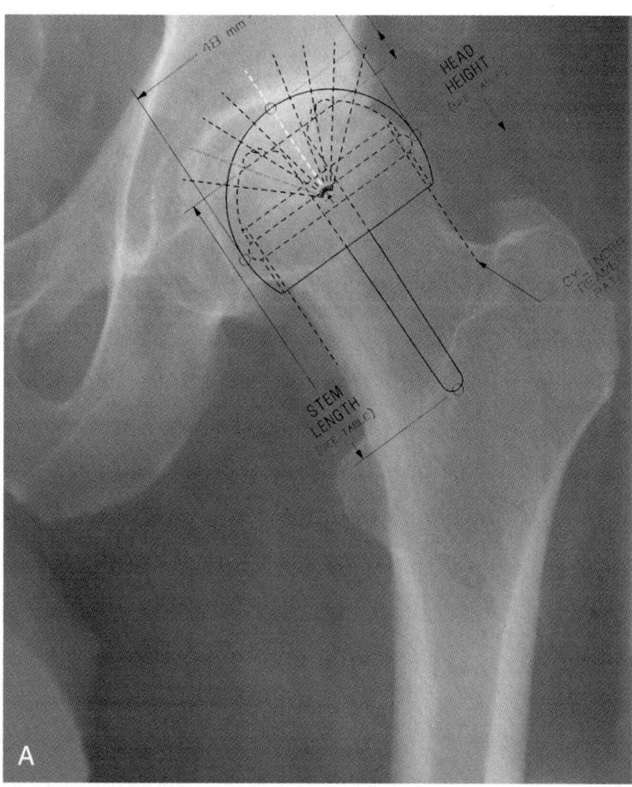

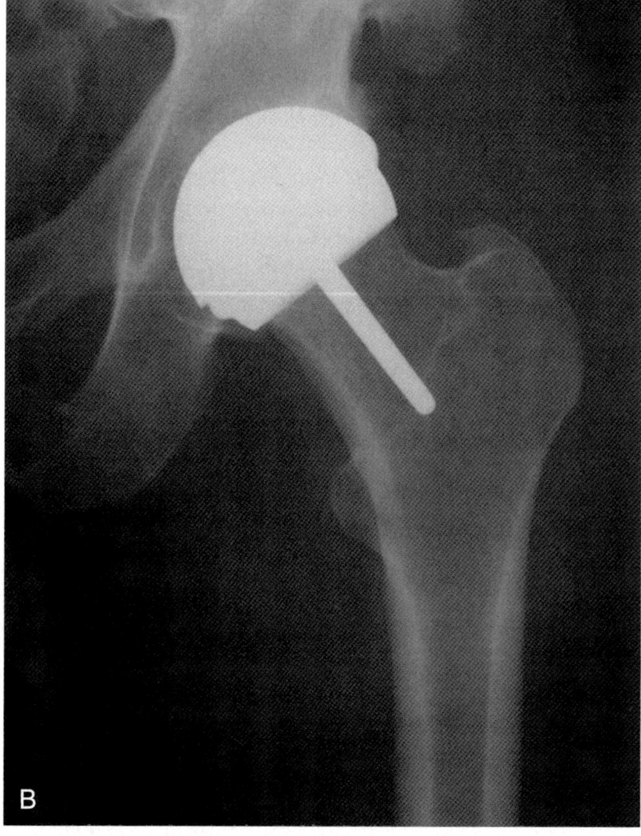

Figure 7-2 **A,** The template is placed on on the anteroposterior (AP) radiograph with a 140-degree stem-shaft angle and allows visualization of the entry point (*yellow dotted line*) of the pin with respect to the location of the ligamentum teres (*green dotted line*). Note how the stem is approximately parallel to the inferior cortex of the neck. **B,** Postoperative AP radiograph confirming the positioning of the femoral component.

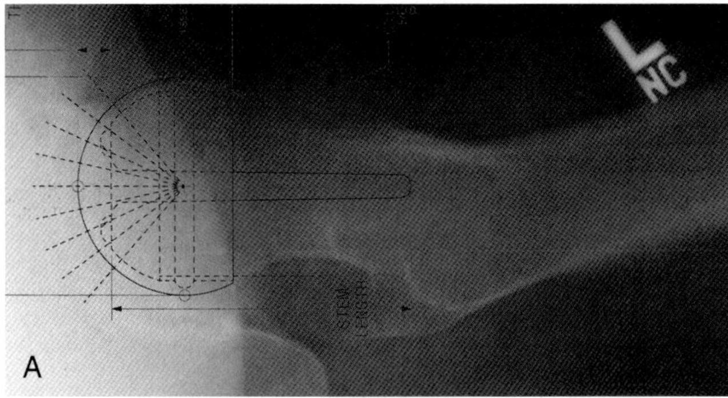

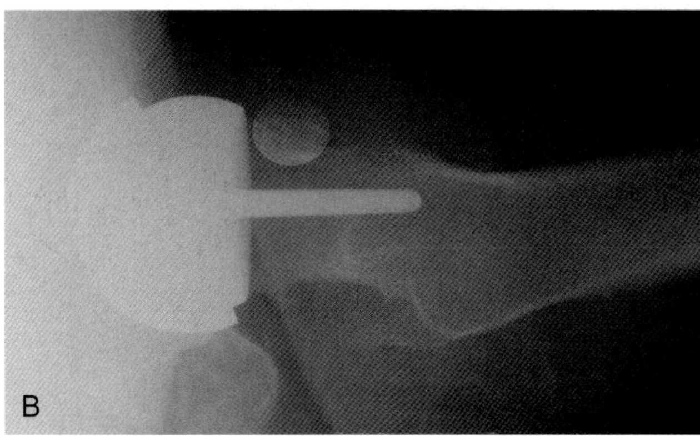

Figure 7-3 A, The template is positioned on the Johnson cross-table lateral film to assess the amount of anterior translation or posterior to anterior component shift needed to avoid reaming the anterior osteophyte. **B,** Postoperative Johnson cross-table lateral radiograph confirming the positioning of the femoral component. The region of interest highlights the anterior ostrophyte that was preserved.

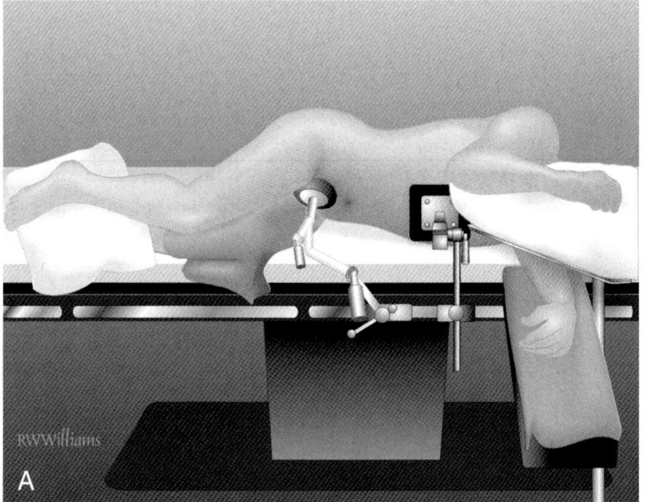

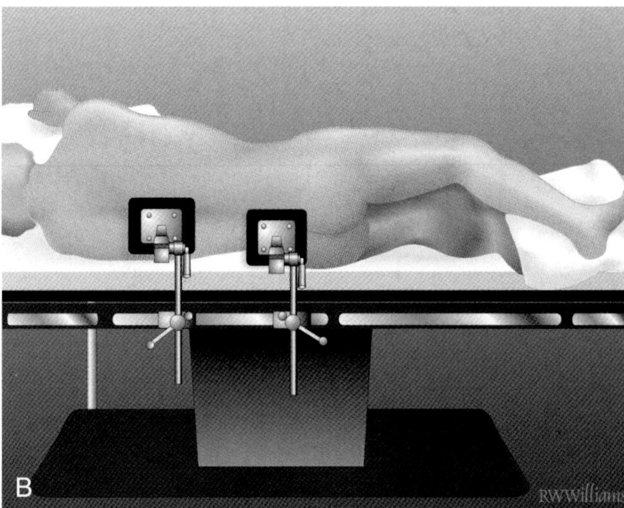

Figure 7-4 Positioning of the patient on the operating table. **A,** Note the location of the pubic support. The table is tilted forward and the patient is upright. **B,** Note the posterior pelvic and thorax support location.

are repaired at the conclusion of the procedure. However, there are no important gait or other disturbances resulting from a release even if they are not repaired because the rotation is accomplished by other muscles.

The incision starts 6 to 8 cm distal to the top of the greater trochanter, slightly posterior to the center of the shaft, and then angles posteriorly from the tip of the trochanter for about 4 to 6 cm (Fig. 7-5). With the hip flexed 90 degrees, the incision will be approximately straight. The length of the incision will vary with patient's size. Divide the fascia lateralis, then separate the gluteus maximus fibers. It is recommended that the gluteus maximus tendon be completely sectioned as it inserts into the linea aspera for the surgeons first cases. With experience, especially in thin patients and those with a small femoral head size (>48 mm), this step may not be necessary. However if any difficulty is encountered, then the leg can be returned to the lateral position and the tendon insertion sectioned. A self-retaining Charnley-type retractor is inserted. The short rotator muscle fibers are divided and may be tagged for reattachment. The capsule is then incised posteriorly from the intertrochanteric ridge to the the acetabulum, and a T incision is made superiorly toward the dome and inferiorly toward the base of the neck.

The hip is dislocated by flexion, adduction, and internal rotation. The major technical difference with a total hip replacement (THR) relates to the fact that the proximal femur head must be mobilized to prepare the head and acetabulum, and the entire capsule must be released. A superior capsulectomy is performed, and the capsule is released inferiorly. By adducting and internally rotating the leg beyond 90 to 100 or 110 degrees the interval between the head and neck and the acetabulum is widened first to incise and then to release the anterior capsule (Fig. 7-6). This anterior release is performed with a scalpel along the anterior neck in order to widen the neck-acetabulum interval to allow insertion of the neck elevator necessary for the placement of the pin-centering guide. The posterior capsule does not need to be excised and can be

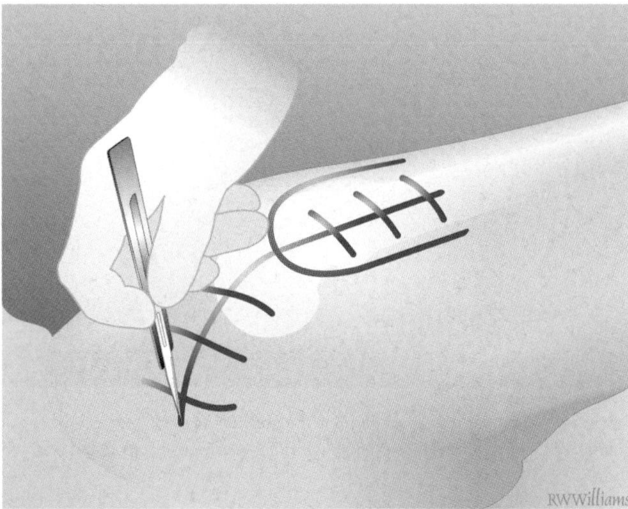

Figure 7-5 Skin incision for the posterior approach.

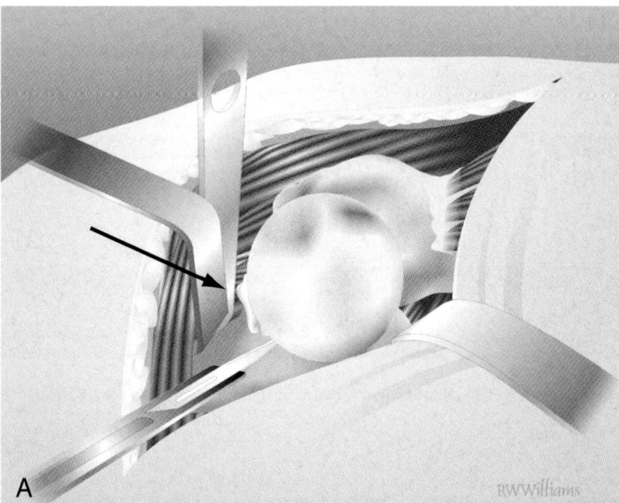

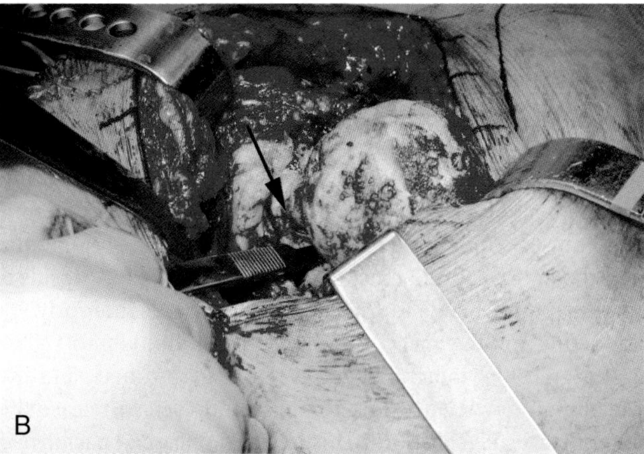

Figure 7-6 A, By rotating the hip in more internal rotation, the interval between the head and neck and the acetabulum is increased to release the anterior capsule from the anterior neck. B, Note the curved Homan device superiorly under the abductor muscles and the anterior osteophyte (*arrow*).

retracted later by a pin inserted into the ischium to facilitate acetabular preparation Proceed to debulk the femoral head as described later to facilitate capsular removal and to translocate the head superiorly and anteriorly for acetabular preparation and component implantation.

Pin Centering

The pin-centering guide is positioned using the angle finder (protractor), which has a range of 135 to 145 degrees so that the pin forms an angle of approximately 140 degrees[5] with the femoral shaft. The entry point of the pin is consistent with the position determined by templating. A cautery mark can be made on the head with the correct orientation through the protractor (Fig. 7-7). The pin should be centered in the middle of the neck, or if the head-neck ratio is greater than 1.2, just superior to the center in the frontal plane (AP view) to increase the lateral off-set (Fig. 7-8). Because the head is eccentrically positioned on the neck, more bone is removed from the posterior head than anterior as well as more from the inferior part of the head than superiorly. In the coronal plane, the pin is directed just anterior to the neck center and directed slightly posterior to anterior (see also cross-table lateral view in Fig. 7-3) to avoid reaming into the anterior osteophyte. A 3.2-mm Steinman pin is then inserted to a depth of 3 to 5 cm, using the guide to prevent the pin from moving offline during insertion. The cylindrical reamer gauge (or notch checker) for the anticipated final size (Fig. 7-9) is then used to check the positioning of the pin. The gauge should be close to the inferior cortex, with more room superiorly. It should be able to rotate freely with sufficient clearance around the neck to ensure that cylindrical reaming will not result in notching the femoral neck. A minimal amount of bone is removed from anterior portion of the head. If the cylindrical reamer gauge catches the neck at any location, the pin needs to be repositioned using the relocator guide (Fig. 7-10). With the relocator guide, it is possible to relocate the pin either one pin width (one reamer size so that the new pin will be juxtapositioned to the initial pin using the slot) or two pin widths using the hole and the slot (as illustrated) or even to change the angle in either the sagital plane (varus or valgus) or cornal plane (A to P or P to A). If three-dimensional changes are more difficult to make all at once and if not feasible, then make two serial pin changes to optimize the position. A quick-disconnect pin power driver is a most useful tool to facilitate pin relocation, which may have to be repeated for optimal reaming. Be sure to carefully consider the location and then check it again with the cylindrical reamer gauge. It is especially important to protect the superior or lateral cortex, which is thinner than on the inferior side and undergoes tensile loads to decrease the risk of femoral neck fracture. A small amount of bone is removed with the final reamer anteriorly so that this will ensure slight anterior displacement of the component which is desirable for maximum flexion without impingement. There are a variety of alternate methods of pin placement. One useful method

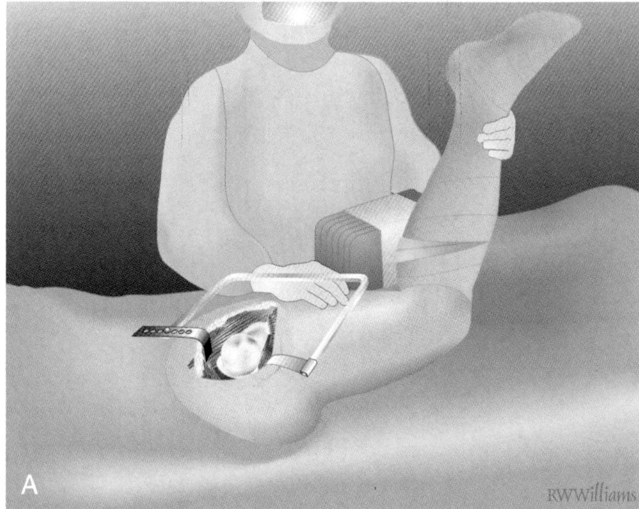

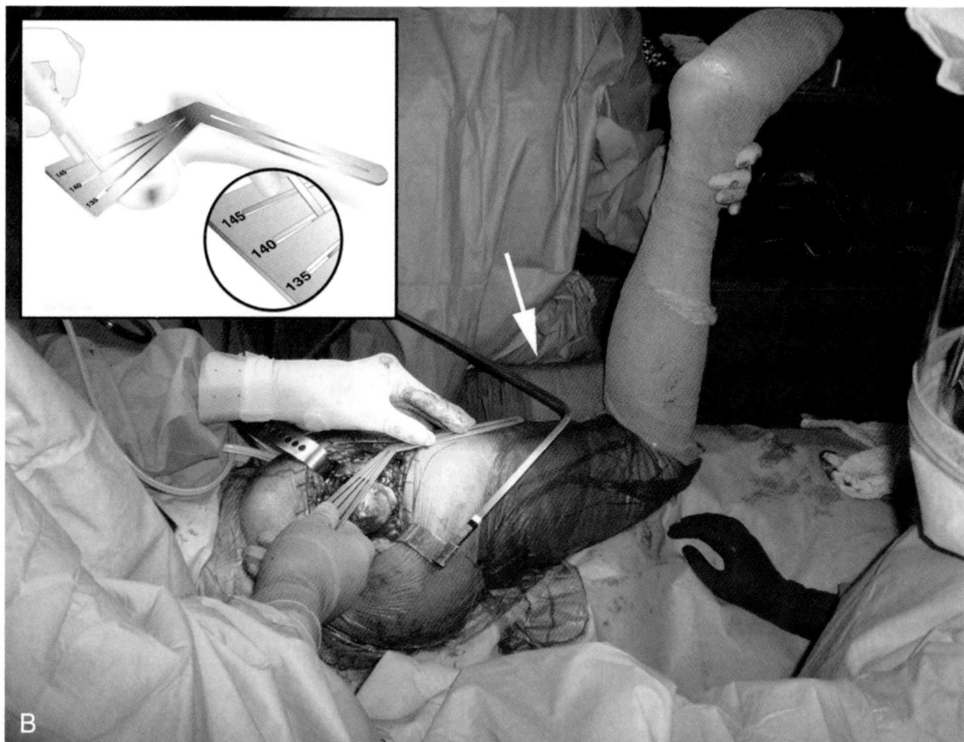

Figure 7-7 **A,** The leg should be perpendicular to the table. Note the towel pack, which helps the assistant to position the leg straight up to observe the neck-shaft angle. **B,** Place the protractor (angle finder) aligned with the neck-shaft angle, with the slots at 135, 140, or 145 degrees. Inset, Mark with the electrocautery. The stem-shaft angle generally used is 140 degrees.

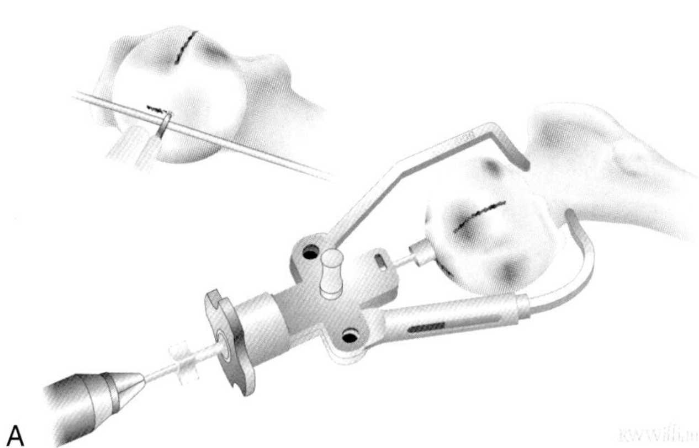

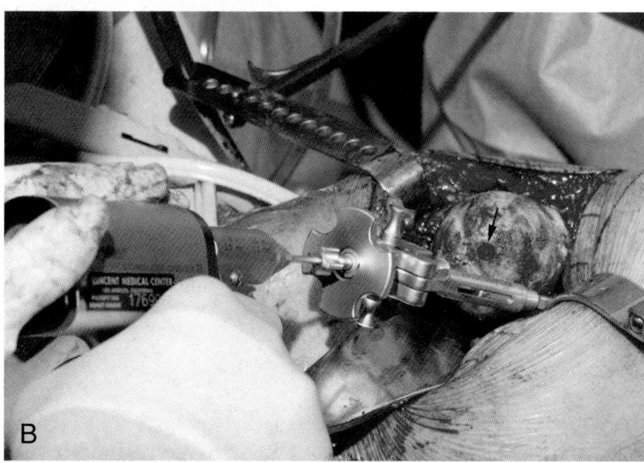

Figure 7-8 **A,** Upper left, mark the head with the electrocautery in the sagittal plane so that more bone will be removed inferiorly above the Steiman pin. Placement of the pin-centering guide with the telescoping arm to reach around osteophytes. **B,** As indicated, more bone will be removed from the posterior head than from the anterior portion. The ligamentum teres insertion is not clearly visible on this photograph but is represented by the highlighted area shown by the arrow.

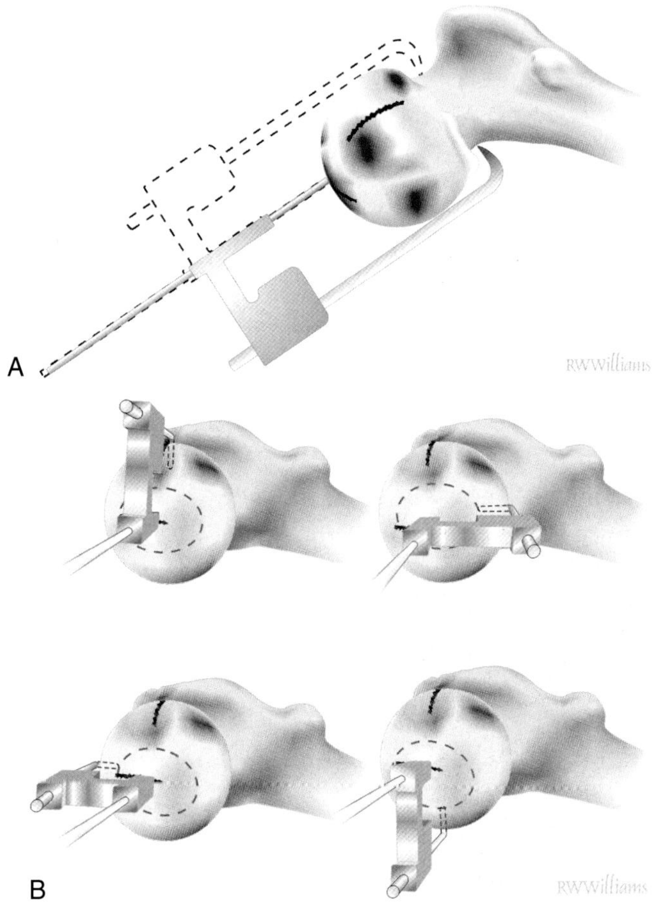

Figure 7-9 A, The cylindrical reamer gauge is used as templated to check the clearance of the same designated size reamer around the neck. **B,** Dotted lines indicate approximate neck outline. The reamer will remove more bone posteriorly and inferiorly.

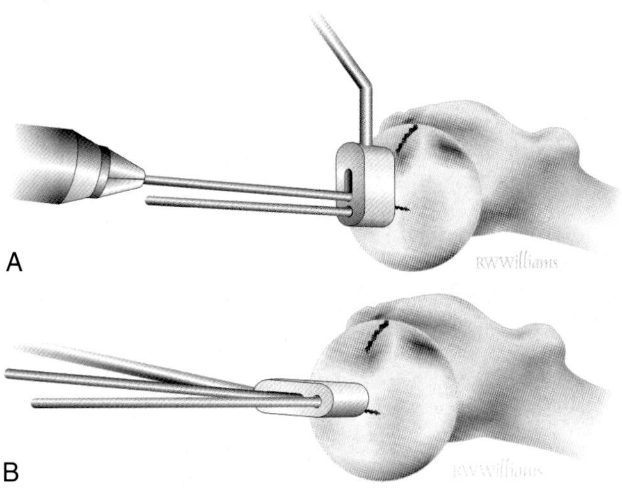

Figure 7-10 A, The pin-relocator guide allows the surgeon to modify the position of the pin in any direction. More posteriorly 2 pin widths as shown (each pin width equals to one reamer size so this move equals 2 reamer sizes). **B,** Moving the pin more superiorly in valgus using the slot.

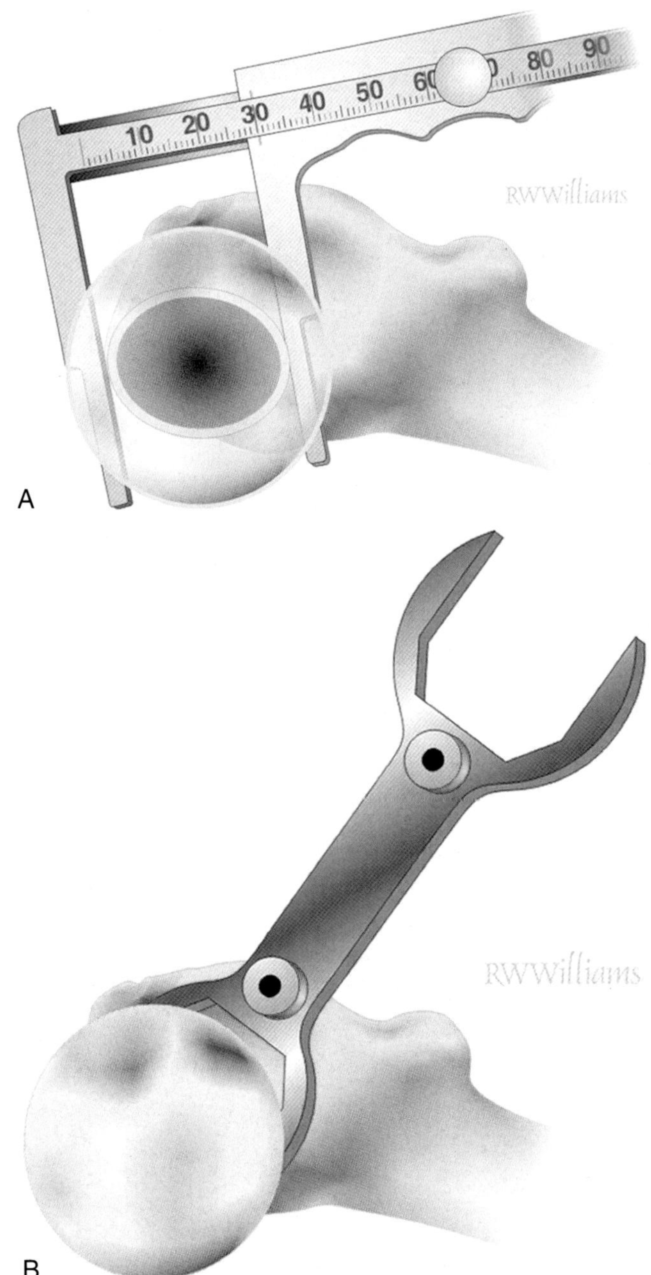

Figure 7-11 To asses minimum reamer size, use either (**A**) a caliper or (**B**) a "notch guide".

involves the use of the lollypop. Measure the maximum neck width with a caliper (Fig. 7-11) or notch guide and select the lollypop that fits snugly around the neck. A chart is available with the inside dimensions for each femoral component (Table 7-1). Align the device so that the angle subtends at a 140°-angle and mark the head with the electrocautery (Fig. 7-12). Rotate the hip 90 degrees in the other plane and make a similar mark. Insert the pin and check the alignment and orientation as above (with the protractor and cylindrical reamer gauge). This device (see Fig. 7-12) is helpful when there are very large osteophytes or when the patient is extremely obese or muscular, or when a very short incision is used.

Table 7-1 Dimensions of the Conserve®Plus Femoral Component for the Range of Sizes Available

		4802-20xx		
Conserve®Plus Femoral	Head OD (mm)	Head ID (mm)	Stem LengtH (mm)	Cylindric Reamer ID (mm)
38021036	36.0	29.5	50.0	27.5
38021038	38.0	31.5	53.0	29.5
38021040	40.0	33.5	56.0	31.5
38021042	42.0	35.5	59.0	33.5
38021044	44.0	37.5	62.0	35.5
38021046	46.0	39.5	65.0	37.5
38021048	48.0	41.5	68.0	39.5
38021050	50.0	43.0	71.0	41.0
38021052	52.0	45.5	74.0	43.5
38021054	54.0	45.5	74.0	43.5
38021056	56.0	48.5	77.0	46.5

		4803-00xx		
Conserve SF Femoral	Head OD (mm)	Head ID (mm)	Stem Length (mm)	Cylindric Reamer ID (mm)
38031036	36.0	29.5	50.0	27.5
38031038	38.0	31.5	53.0	29.5
38031040	40.0	33.5	56.0	31.5
38031042	42.0	35.5	59.0	33.5
38031044	44.0	37.5	62.0	35.5
38031046	46.0	39.5	65.0	37.5
38031048	48.0	41.5	68.0	39.5
38031050	50.0	43.5	71.0	41.5
38031052	52.0	45.5	74.0	43.5
38031054	54.0	47.5	74.0	45.5
38031056	56.0	49.5	77.0	47.5

OD, outer diameter; ID, inner diameter.

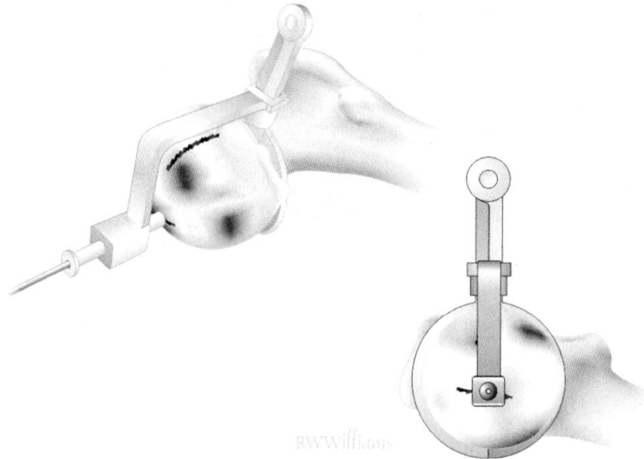

Figure 7-12 An alternate method of pin centering using the lollypop is to position the center where the cautery marks for stem-shaft angle intersect with the coronal plane mark, which is parallel to femoral axis, so that there will be more bone removed posteriorly and inferiorly.

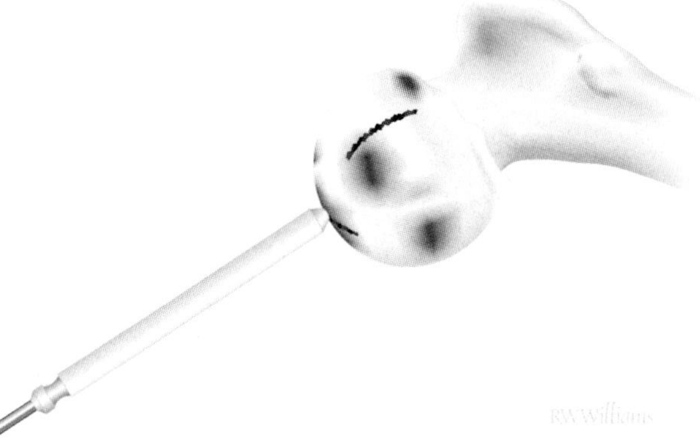

Figure 7-13 Place the canulated spigot over the pin.

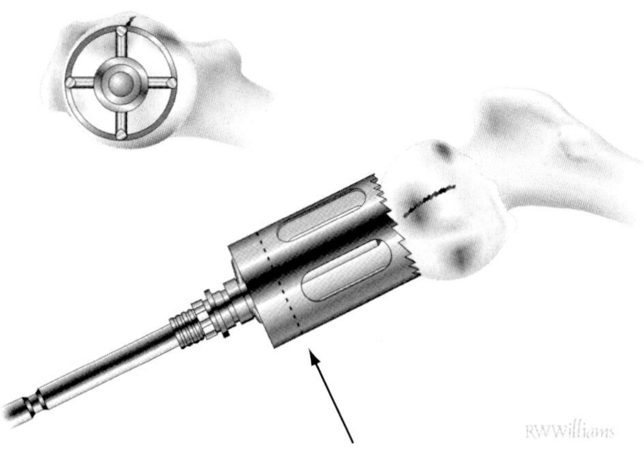

Figure 7-14 Cylindric reaming should be performed very carefully to avoid notching the neck. The spigot-guided reamers have an anthropometric designed stop to prevent reaming into the base of the neck.

Cylindrical Reaming

Reaming commences with an oversized reamer generally two to three sizes larger than the final anticipated size, irrigating copiously to avoid seizing. For the new style reamers (5803) place a spigot over the pin to improve the stability of the reamer (Fig. 7-13). The teeth of the reamer engage the femoral head asymmetrically, so if you are reaming over the pin alone, it is important to start the reaming with intermittent repetitive pressure directed parallel to the axis of the pin so as not to bend it (Fig. 7-14). The spigot technique provides for more stable reaming so the pin rarely bends.

In patients with advanced osteoarthritis, large osteophytes may encircle the entire neck, totally occluding any neck vessel that enters the head-neck junction in the normal hip (Fig. 7-15). If a large amount of bone and osteophyte are removed or if there is any concern about reaming too close to the neck or if there is a relatively short neck and there is concern about reaming into the base of the neck, then stop reaming and complete the bone cut with a curved osteotome. With the new reamers, which are used in conjunction with the spigot, there is a stop in the reamer which prevents reaming into the base of the neck. After each reamer pass it is recommended that the

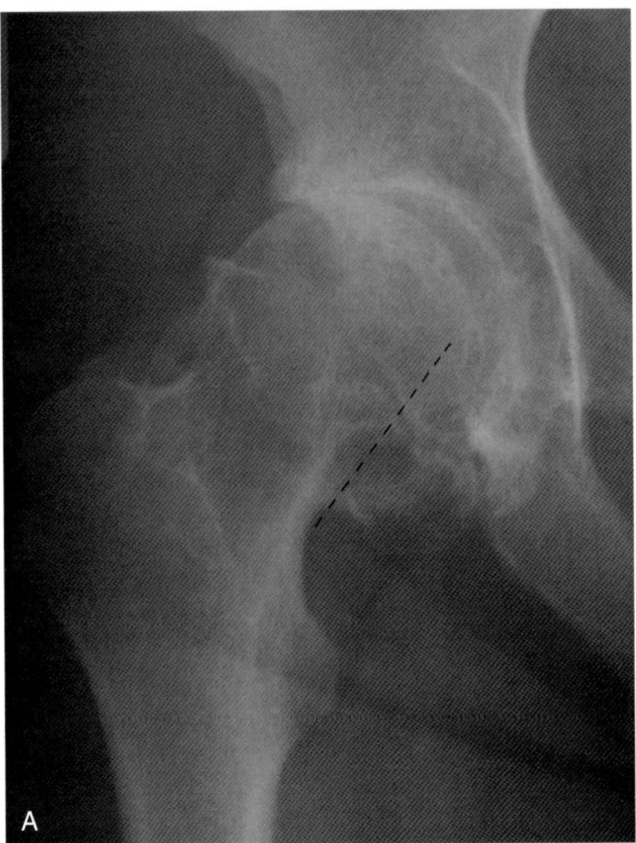

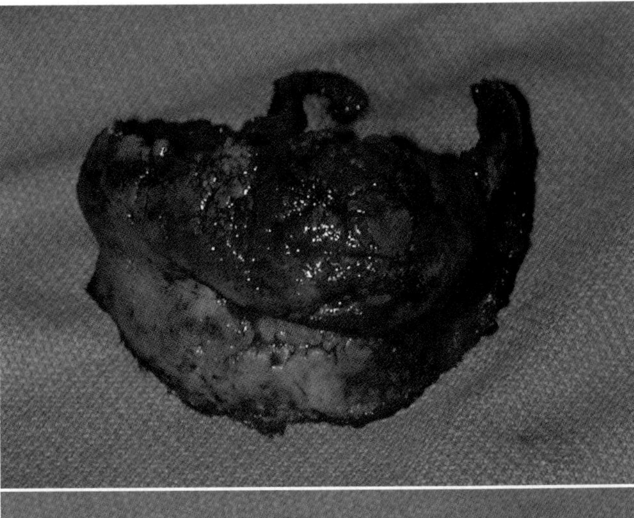

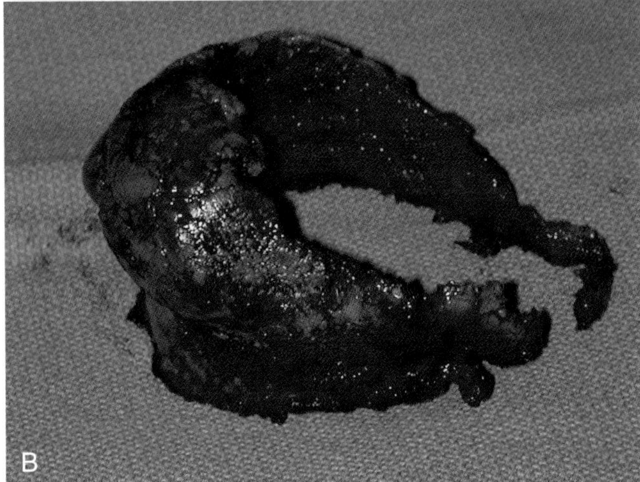

Figure 7-15 **A,** Anteroposterior (AP)-pelvis view of a patient with a very large anterior-inferior and posterior osteophyte. Note that the hip is externally rotated with external rotation contracture. The approximate line of resection is shown. **B,** Gross photo of the very large osteophyte resected with a cylindric reamer. Note the typical osteophyte obliteration of vascular foramina at the head-neck junction.

head-neck junction be carefully assessed by palpation of the remaining offset around the neck. Look for the recesses that may be located superiorly or inferiorly containing soft tissue. In that situation, the pin may be relocated to take advantage of reaming closer to the neck in the location of the recess (Fig. 7-16). Then, a reappraisal of the pin orientation is made with the protractor and the the cylindrical reamer gauge. The pin should be relocated if not optimally positioned based on a careful assessment of the head pathology and the notch checker. Smaller reamers are then used similarly down to approximately one or two sizes greater than the final anticipated size based on templating and intraoperative assessment. If the bone is soft, the head may be dented by the rim of the acetabulum when it is placed under the abductors during acetabular reaming. To avoid this problem, or the consequences of a depression in the head, ream a minimal amount of bone during debulking so some of the stronger even sclerotic bone remains or if head indentation occurs, the final reaming will remove it so that a more uniform circumferential cylindrical reamed area remains. Be careful and stop reaming at the head-neck junction to avoid notching the superior neck.

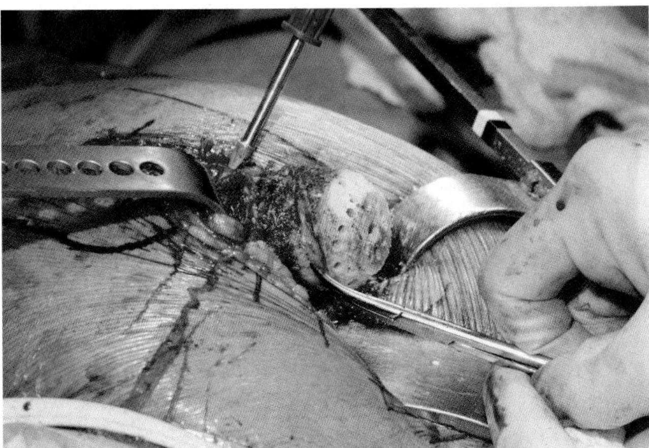

Figure 7-16 Nearly prepared femoral head with a superior recess (hemostat pointer), which is recessed from the adjacent cylindrically reamed head. In this case, it was not necessary to ream closer to the neck.

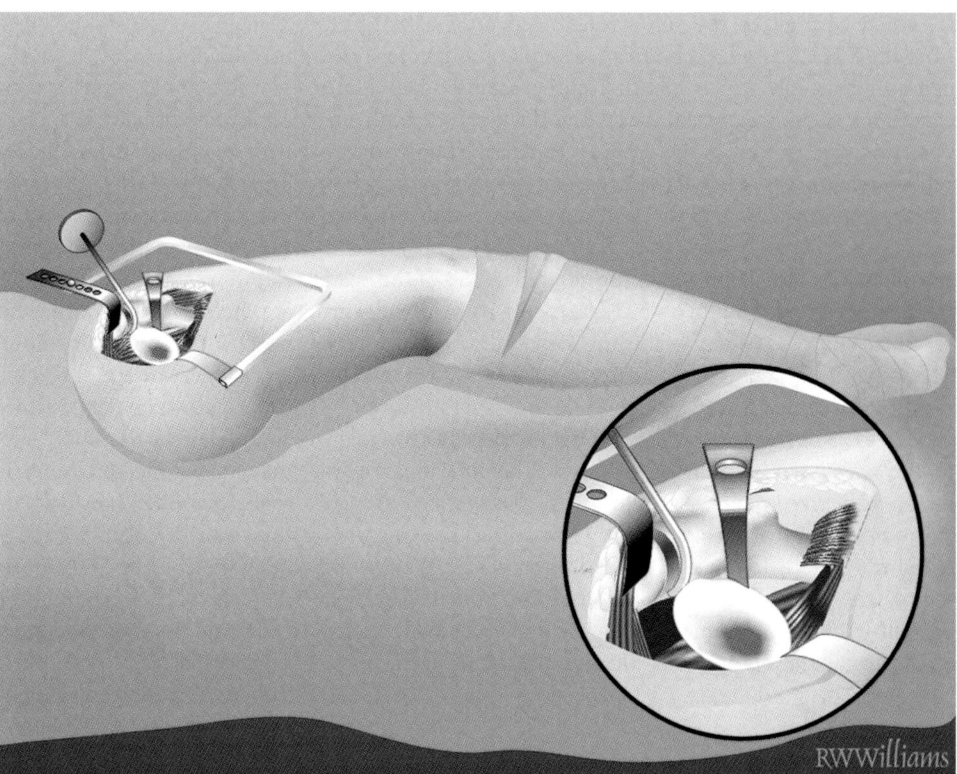

Figure 7-17 Placing the head under the abductor muscles to access the acetabulum.

This is essential because reaming at 140 degrees is generally greater than the neck-shaft angle. This initial reaming is performed to debulk the head and then by further flexion, adduction and internal rotation, the interval between the anterior femoral neck and the acetabulum is increased so that the remaining anterior capsule can be more easily incised or excised. A towel pack is held between the thigh of the assistant surgeon and the leg to assist in internal rotation up to 120° (see Fig. 7-7). A final check is made to remove residual capsule from the acetabulum and occasionally some rim acetabular osteophytes if they are prominent or irregular. Release the reflected head of the rectus femoris and use an elevator to clear gluteus minimus off the ilium to create space for the head. In order to position the femoral head under the abductor muscles pocket superiorly and anteriorly, an assistant with the aid of a dislocator hook placed around the neck pulls the proximal femur superiorly and laterally while the leg is brought into extension and then neutral. The surgeon and assistant working in tandem force the head anteriorly and superiorly (Fig. 7-17). The right-angle Hohman device (Innomed Inc., Savannah, GA) is placed over the anterior wall of the acetabulum to retract the femur anteriorly (Fig. 7-18). The leg may be slightly internally rotated to provide wide access to the acetabulum. The inferior capsule is carefully resected using a malleable retractor to assist in disecting and retracting the soft tissue, which contains blood vessels, just inferiorly. The interval between the capsule and the underlying fat and muscle is used to protect underlying vessels. A double-pointed, inferior acetabular retractor (Innomed Inc., Savannah, GA) is inserted to visualize the entire acetabulum.

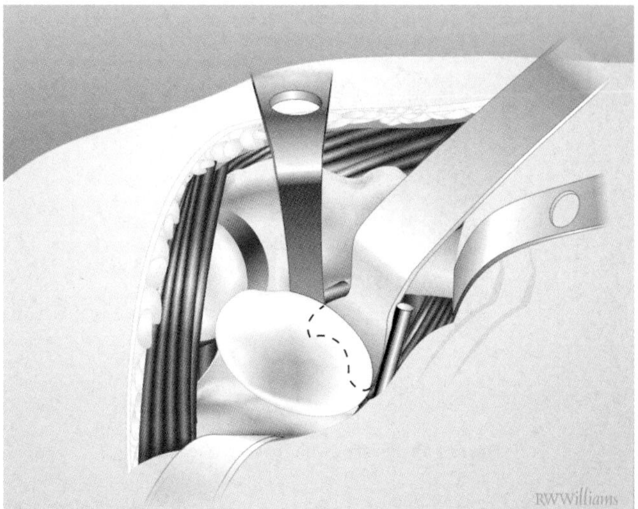

Figure 7-18 The right-angle Hohman device (Innomed Inc., Savannah, GA) is placed over the anterior wall of the acetabulum to retract the femur anteriorly. The Charnley pin holds the posterior capsule. The double-pointed retractor (Innomed Inc., Savannah, GA) is placed inferiorly and helps to visualize the entire acetabulum.

Acetabular Preparation

Acetabular preparation starts with a careful assessment of the thickness of the anterior and posterior walls and the orientation of the acetabulum. Prominent soft tissues and cartilage lying on the floor of the cotyloid foramen are removed. Anatomic reaming is preferred if the acetabulum is normal, in which case all of the soft tissues need not be removed from the fossa. Reaming is performed similar to that of a THR using increasingly larger hemispherical reamers until some cancellous bone is exposed. Assess the thickness of both the posterior wall as well as the anterior wall. For young and/or active patients with hard dense bone, I prefer to ream most of the acetabulum with a "bear claw" aggressive reamer (rather than with "cheese grater" style reamers) (Fig. 7-19). Ream starting with a size that matches the outer diameter of the head so there will good stability of the reamer and avoid jarring and eccentric cutting. When these reamers are sharp, they are very aggressive, but when used with care, they are very efficient. The reaming is directed at a 42-degree angle and generally directed with 20 to 25 degrees of anteversion. It is not necessary to ream to the acetabular floor in most cases. The final bear claw reamer (one size under the line-to-line size) is inserted in such a way as to remove any overhanging rim posteriorly. The final reaming ("line-to-line") is performed with a cheese grater with the size the same as the listed size of the component. This will be approximately 1.5 mm less than the final outside diameter of the acetabular component. The appearance of each of the available sockets is shown in Figure 7-20 and the dimensions in Table 7-2.

Acetabular cysts are curetted and additional soft tissue removed with a high-speed burr, jet lavaged, and then grafted with reamings from the femoral head. These grafts can be impacted with the translucent gauges and a sponge stick but the graft material should not be interposed between the anterior and posterior columns of the acetabulum. The final size, roundness, and especially the depth of the reamed acetabulum are checked using translucent acetabular gauges (Fig. 7-21). The posterior rim of the component may protrude a few millimeters to increase the anteversion of the socket about 10 degrees up to approximately 20 to 30 degrees and to avoid reaming completely to the floor. A final check in three planes is then made using metallic rigid ring gauges (Fig. 7-22). For the thin shells, reaming is performed "line-to-line" (e.g., 58 for a 58-mm thin-walled 3.5-mm thick socket, which is actually 59.3 mm in diameter). The 58-mm ring gauge should completely seat to the floor of the acetabulum in all planes. If the gauge does not reach the floor or is difficult to insert, this is probably due a ridge rim of bone at the acetabular entrance posterioly or possibly anteriorly created because the cutting teeth of reamers are less than a hemisphere. The 59-mm gauge should not go to the floor to provide a press-fit of about 1.3 mm. The press-fit is essentially achieved in the anterior to posterior direction between the anterior and posterior columns of the acetabulum.

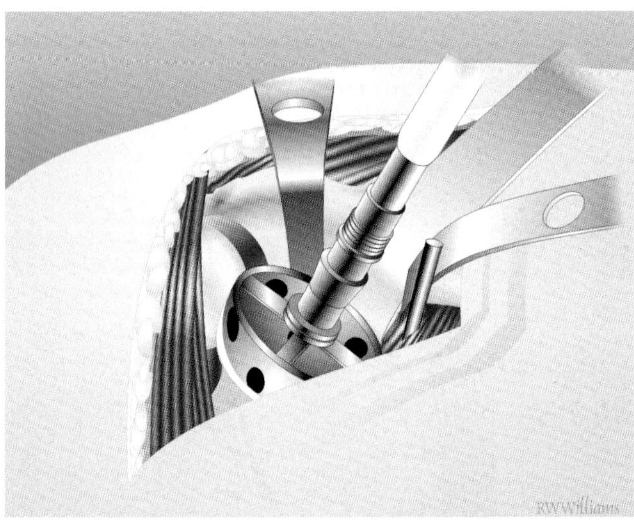

Figure 7-19 Reaming with "bear claw reamer."

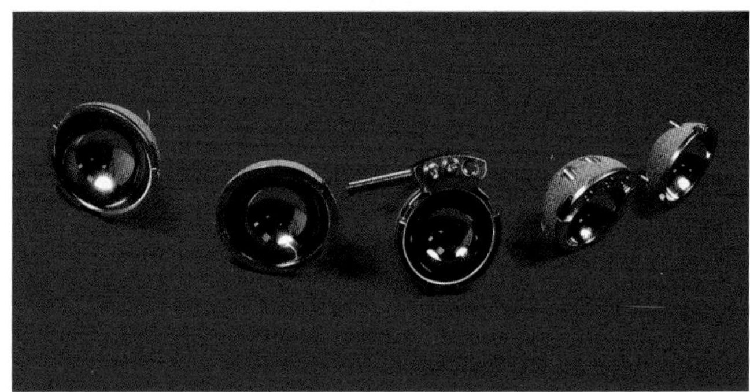

Figure 7-20 The five socket types available for resurfacing with Conserve®Plus. From left to right, thin shell (3.5 mm), thick shell (5.5 mm), quadra-fix shell, super-fix shell, and spiked shell.

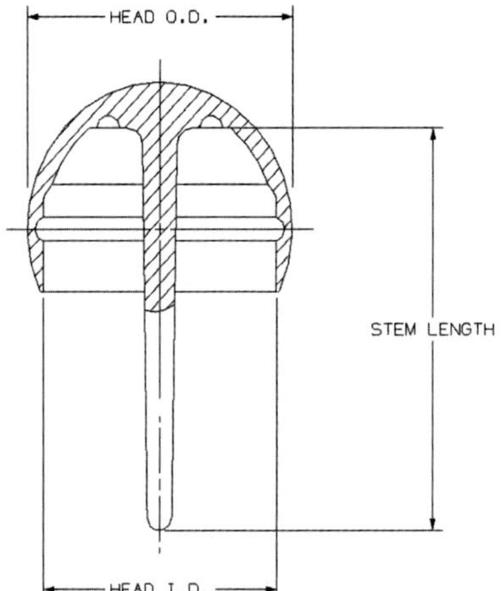

Table 7-2 Wright Medical Acetabular Components available to mate with Conserve®Plus Resurfacing Head or the Big Femoral Head (BFH)

Cup	Differential Between OD and ID*	Sizing Example†	Optional Screws
Conserve Plus Standard	7.5 mm	56 mm OD mates with 50 mmfemoral	No
Conserve Plus Thick Shell*	11.5 mm	60 mm OD mates with 50 mm femoral	No
Conserve Plus Spiked Shell	7.5 mm	56 mm OD mates with 50 mm femoral	No
Quadrafix	8.5 mm	58 OD mates with 50 mm femoral	Yes
Super Fix	14.5 mm	64 mm OD mates with 50 mm femoral	Yes

OD, outer diameter; ID, inner diameter.
**It is recommended to under ream by 1 to 1.5 mm with these sockets.*
†Sizing as reported on the manufacturer's labels.

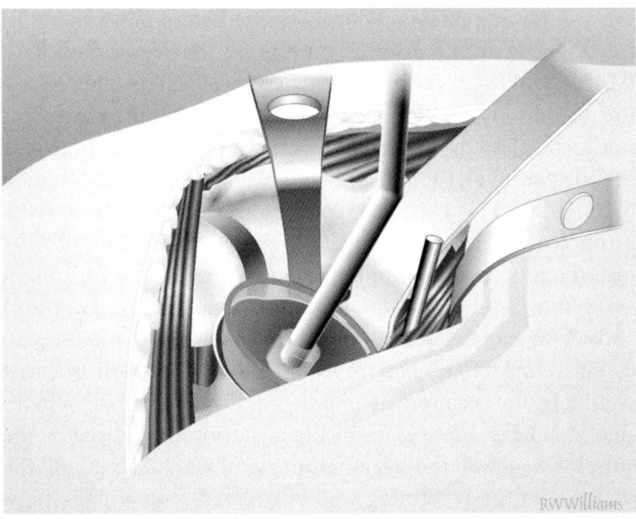

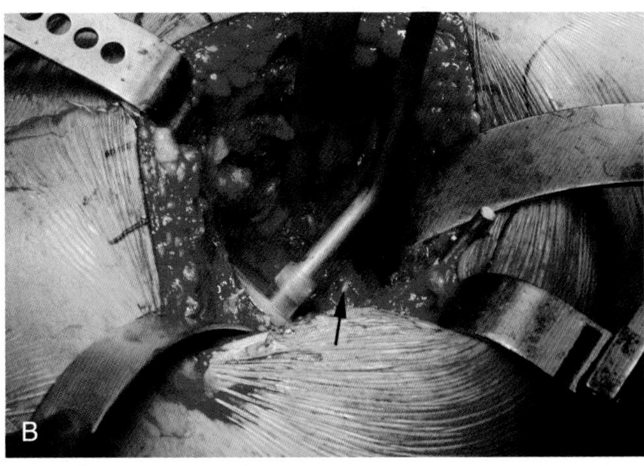

Figure 7-21 **A,** The translucent acetabular gauge is used to assess size, depth, and sphericity of the reamed acetabulum. **B,** The gauge is fully seated and in the correct orientation with more anteversion than normal. The handle is straight up to ascertain lateral coverage. The posterior rim in this case will be a few millimeters proud. Note the protruding anterior wall with osteophyte (*arrow*), which will be osteotomized.

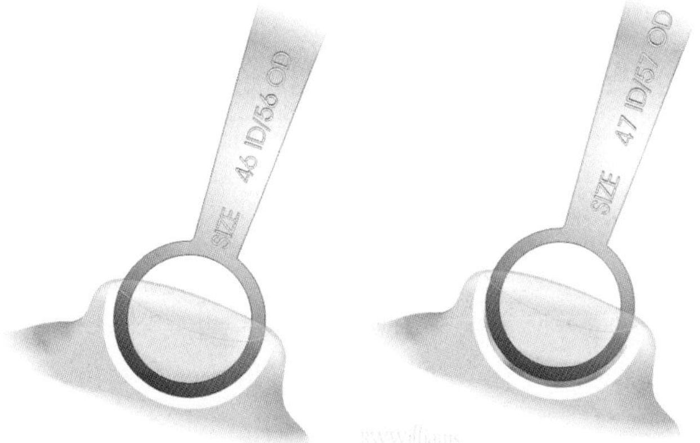

Figure 7-22 A final check of size and roundness of the acetabulum is made with the ring gauges. The 56-mm outside diameter (OD) gauge seats against the bone. The 57-mm gauge does not quite seat.

In some hips with softer bone, it may be possible to push the 59-mm ring gauge to the floor which is satisfactory because, in fact, only a half-millimeter interference fit is sufficient for initial stability with the Conserve®Plus porous-beaded socket. If blood oozes from cancellous bone, a paste graft may be impacted into the interstices of the bone with the clear plastic gauge (see Fig. 7-21). Remove any graft material between the anterior and posterior columns with a sponge stick; otherwise initial stability may be compromised.

Acetabular Implantation

The acetabular component is inserted after a final jet lavage and antibiotic irrigation. The outriggers on the handle of the inserter should be set on 42 degrees of lateral opening (the guide rod will be perpendicular with the patient in the lateral decubitus position) and 15 degrees of anteversion[3] (Fig. 7-23). Our recommendation is to increase the anteversion to 20 to

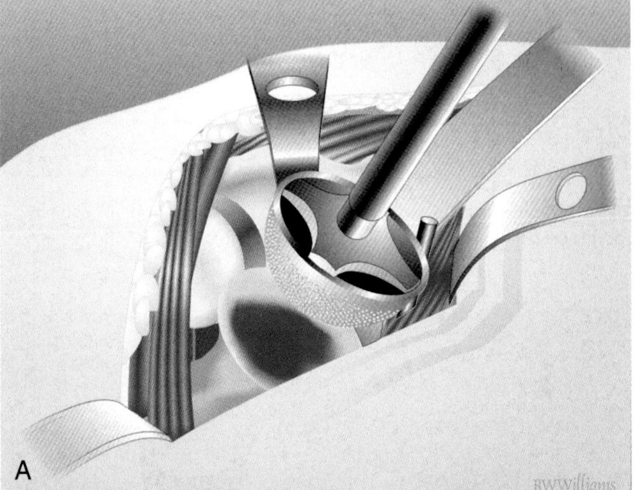

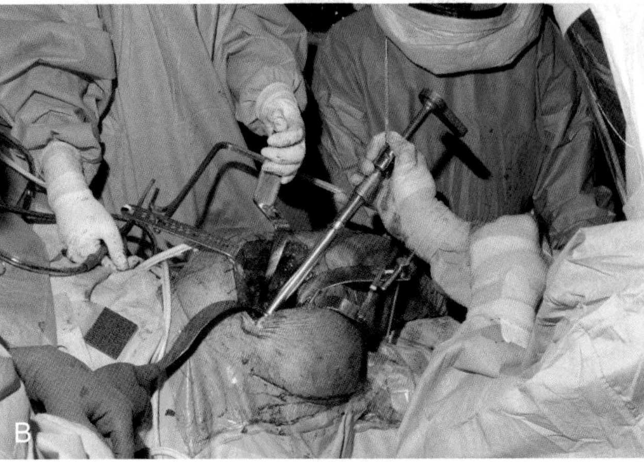

Figure 7-23 **A,** Component insertion with the inserter-extractor attached. **B,** The acetabular component inserter is held by the surgeon at 42 degrees of lateral opening (the "guide rod" is perpendicular to the patient on the table). An assistant impacts the socket.

25 degrees. The surgeon holds the inserter in the optimal position, and the technician or assistant impacts it with a very heavy 10-lb mallet until it is seated. The orientation of the socket should be carefully checked. After the socket is impacted, check the initial stability of the implant at this point by rocking the pelvis, with the inserter still engaged in the socket (Fig. 7-24). If the fixation is insufficient and the pelvic rocking produces any movement, the component should be removed and the acetabular cavity reamed deeper. Repeat the steps to ensure the precision of cavity preparation. The component should be cleaned thoroughly with a jet stream system and any remaining soft tissue removed with a sponge before reinsertion. To free the low profile inserter, pull up on the release and have the assistant rotate counterclockwise a few degrees and remove the inserter by bringing the handle cephalad. If the position is not correct and only a slight correction is needed, an impactor may be placed on the rim and with mallet taps reorient slightly then reimpact (Fig. 7-25). If correction is not possible and the position is not satisfactory, then remove the socket with the inserter, thoroughly clean the socket with a jet stream system and remove soft tissue with a sponge. Again, minor degrees of correction can be accomplished by mallet taps on the rim using an impactor. A ball impactor is then used to insure final seating of the component (Fig. 7-26). Protruding osteophytes (Fig. 7-27) are removed from the posterior and especially the anterior walls of the acetabulum within 1 to 2 mm of the socket, and the remaining wall chamfered with a high-speed burr or sebatome. The technique for inserting other available sockets is similar using appropriately matched translucent gauges, ring gauges, and inserter for the size selected (see Fig. 7-20).

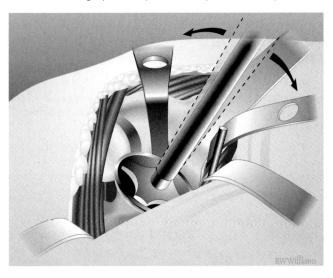

Figure 7-24 It is important to check the fixation of the implant at this point by rocking the pelvis, with the inserter still engaged into the socket.

Final Femoral Head Preparation

The femoral head is delivered again and internal rotation is aided by the towel pack held between the thigh of the assistant surgeon and the leg (see Fig. 7-7). The neck elevator is repositioned and the pin reinserted through the last cylindrical reamer used. A final check is made for pin orientation and a correction is made, if necessary, with the relocator guide

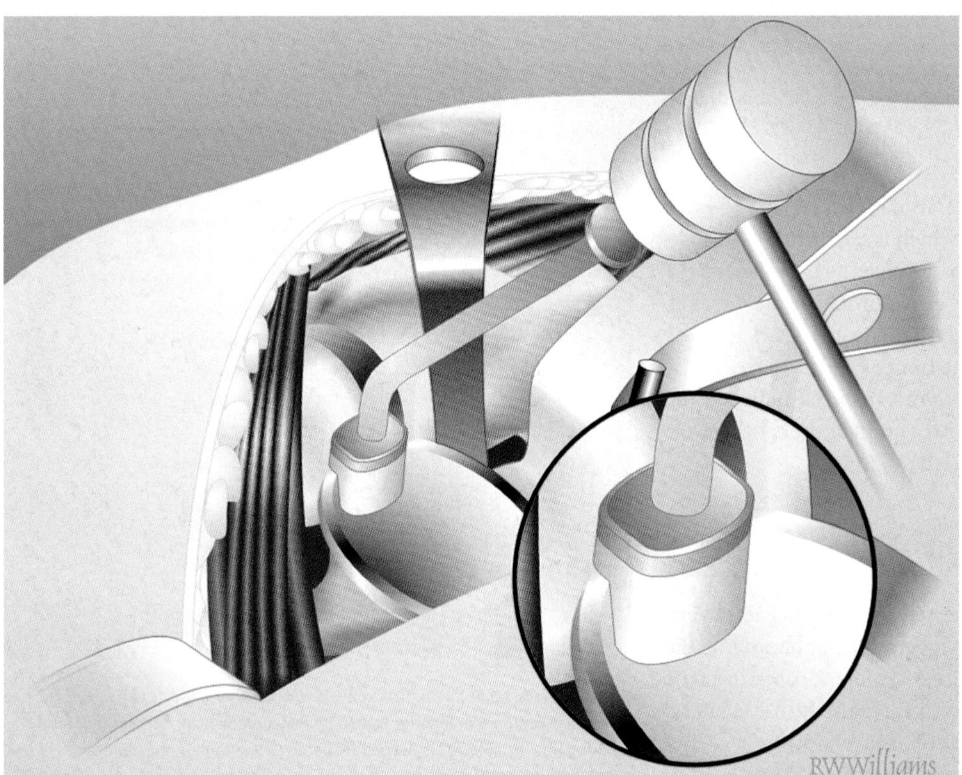

Figure 7-25 Minor degrees of correction may be accomplished by mallet taps on the rim using an impactor.

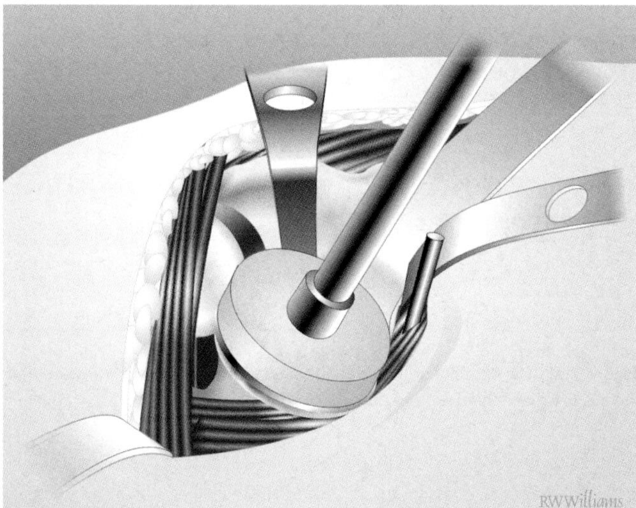

Figure 7-26 The ball impactor is used to ensure full seating of the acetabular component.

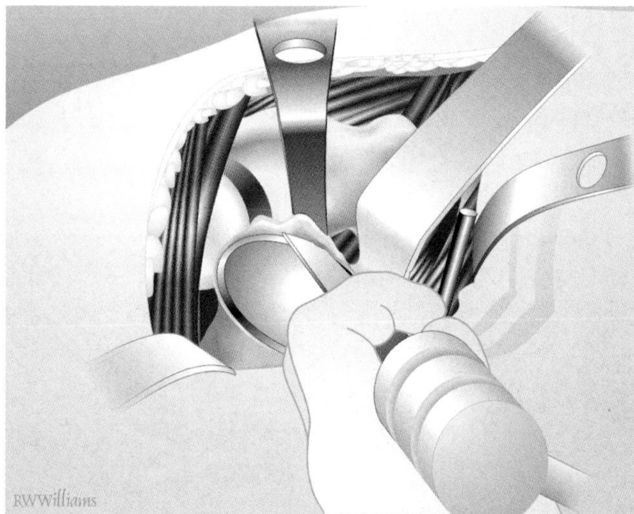

Figure 7-27 Removal of the protruding osteophytes around the acetabulum.

before reaming to the final size. Before the final cylindrical reaming, locate any recessed area from an optimal 360-degree uniform cylindrical reamed surface. It is common to have a recess superior or inferior to the area or occasionally in both locations (see Fig. 7-16). The soft tissue can be removed in order to determine the final contour of the head and neck and to assist in fine tuning the pin by relocation if necessary and before making the final ream. It is imperative that the final ream be made with precision by a single advance of the reamer to ensure a snug fit of the saw cut-off guide. The saw cut-off guide is applied with the tower alignment guide (Fig. 7-28). The tower should be removed in order to be certain that the inferior margin of the guide covers all the reamed bone at the head-neck junction If not. the guide should be tapped downward with a mallet. Two or three (if there is any movement of the guide) short pins are inserted in the guide holes to maintain the cut-off guide position (Fig. 7-29) during the resection of the dome with a saber or oscillating saw (Fig. 7-30). The

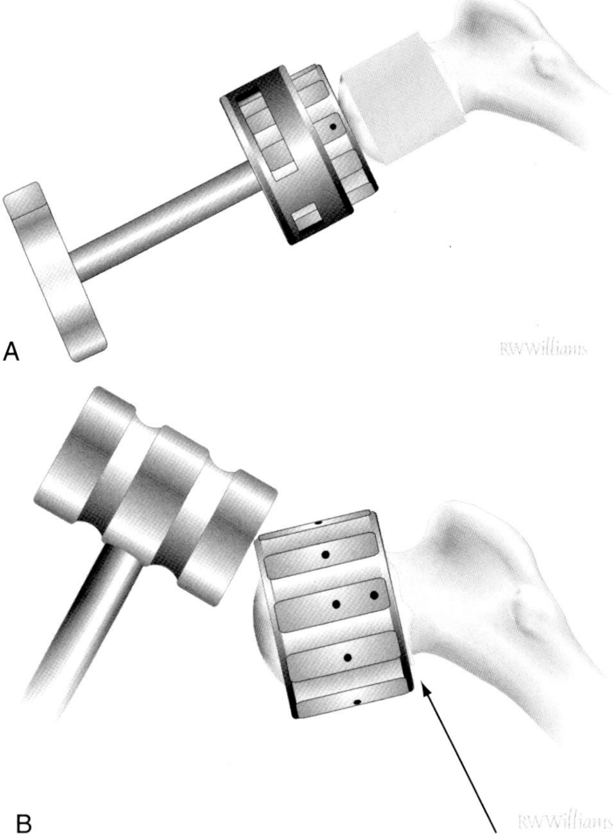

Figure 7-28 **A,** The saw cut-off guide is positioned. **B,** Remove the tower alignment guide and, if necessary, impact with mallet to cover all the reamed bone inferiorly.

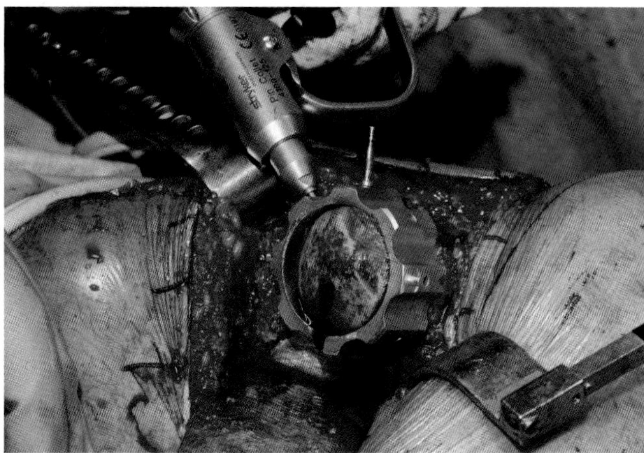

Figure 7-29 Two or three (if there is any movement of the guide) short pins are inserted in the guide holes to ensure stability of the cut-off guide position during the resection of the dome.

dome must be cut absolutely flush and all debris removed or the tower alignment will not seat and cannot be locked snugly by rotation. The starter drill is used to center the tapered metaphyseal stem reamer and for making a hole in the lessor trochanter for the tapered intraosseous suction tip (Fig. 7-31),

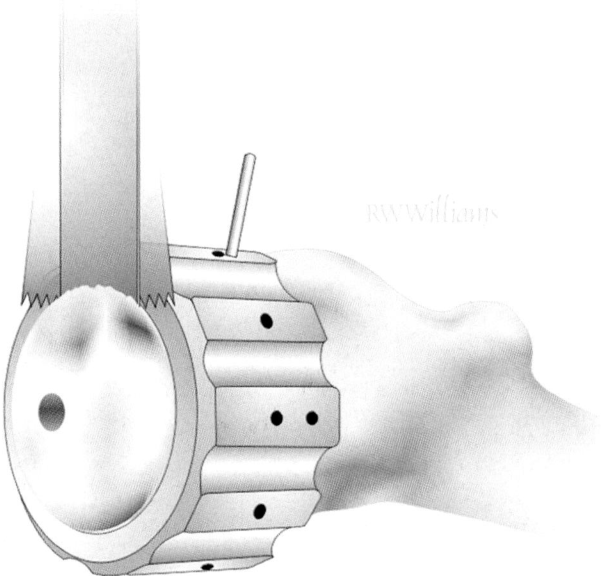

Figure 7-30 Saber oscillating saw. To remove the dome bone.

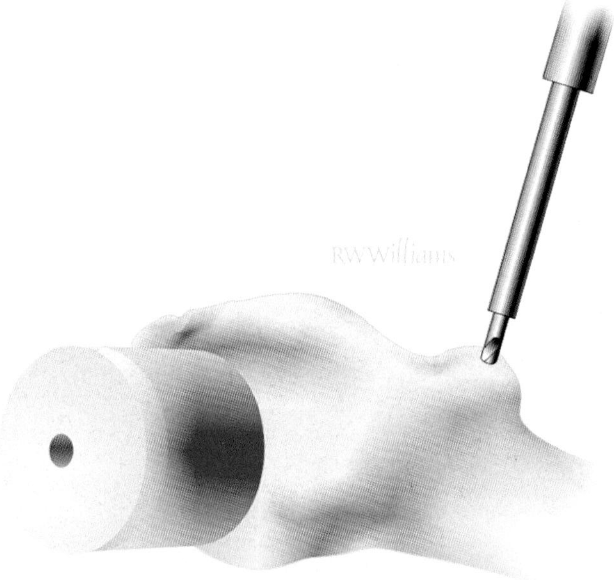

Figure 7-31 The starter drill is used to shape the tapered central hole for the metaphyseal stem reamer and to make a hole in the lessor trochanter for the suction canula.

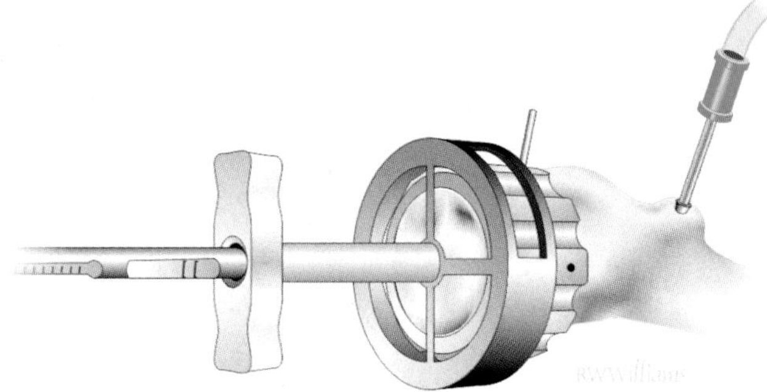

Figure 7-32 The depth of drilling with the stem reamer will depend whether the stem is to be cemented or press-fit.

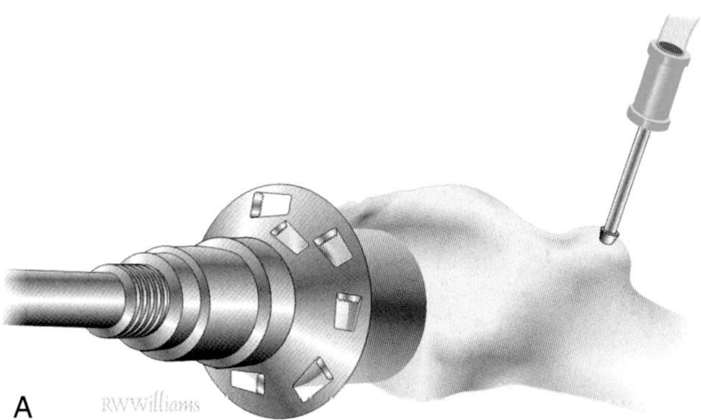

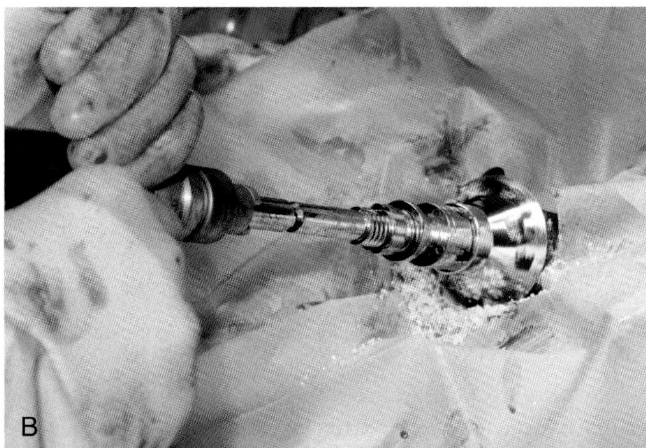

Figure 7-33 **A,** Chamfer reaming is the last step in the shaping of the femoral head. **B,** Use of the vidrape sheet to collect bone chips.

which is connected to wall suction. The depth of drilling with the stem reamer will depend on the chosen method of stem fixation: one or two sizes deeper than indicated if the stem is to be cemented and one size under if it is to be press fitted (Fig. 7-32). I recommend cementing the stem if there are cysts greater than 1 cm or if the component size is less than 48 mm. The appropriate chamfer guide is inserted into the drilled hole after removal of the tower alignment and cut-off guides. The final shape of the femoral head is obtained with the chamfer reamer over the spigot (Fig. 7-33). It is recommended that superior sclerotic bone be removed with the chamfer reamer. If this bone is not removed, then use smaller chamfers down to the corresponding size of the femoral reamer or use a high speed burr to roughen the surface. With the old style 160-degree chamfer reamers, more bone may be removed than necessary and this is especially true when the bone stock is good. In those situations, it is possible to ream with a larger size chamfer (up to three sizes greater than the cylindrical reamer size) to remove less bone and still be able to seat the component. With new style 170-degree chamfer reamers, ream over the spigot. A more bone conserving ream is obtained and, if sclerotic bone remains, this sclerotic bone may be reamed using the next smaller reamer. This enables the surgeon to remove less bone when it is of good quality. Place an "ophthal-

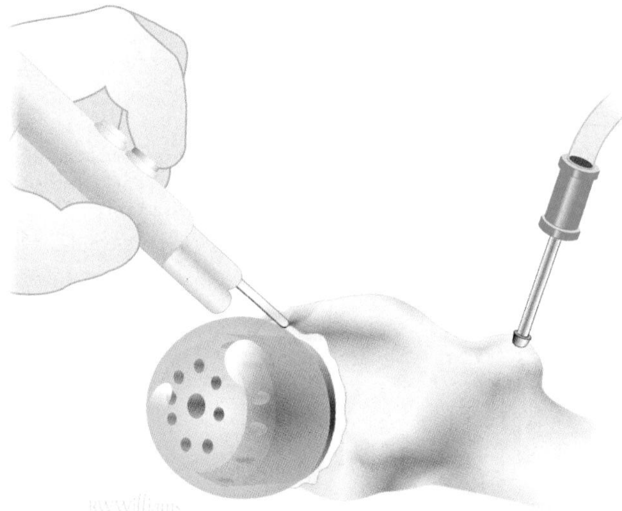

Figure 7-34 A final check of the shaping of the femoral head is done by using the plastic trial. When seated, the trial gives a reference point that should be marked with the electrocautery to ensure seating of the final femoral component after cementation. With the 3803 instruments, rotate the femoral trial about the axis of the central hole, checking for peripheral impingement.

mic vidrape sheet" with a small hole in the center over the head before chamfer reaming to collect bone debris. The plastic trial provides a final check of the prepared surfaces and a cautery mark is made at the head-neck junction to ensure full seating (Fig. 7-34). A trial reduction may be performed if desired to check motion and possible impingement.

With the old style open metallic trial (3803 set) the final check of the femoral head shape is made by rotating the femoral head trial to ensure a cement mantle of about 1 mm all around the femoral head. All cystic material and soft tissue should be removed from the prepared femoral head with a sharp curette and especially a high-speed burr (Fig. 7-35). Additional fixation holes should be made in both the dome and the nonporous chamfered areas using a 1/8 inch or 3.2-mm drill bit (see Fig. 7-35). The hole size is based on maximizing surface area with smaller holes as opposed to larger ones, which are sufficiently durable based on retrieval analysis. Generally 8 to 10 holes are made in the dome and 12 to 20 are made in the chamfered area. Holes are especially important when the bone is dense or sclerotic.[6]

Femoral Head Cementation

Before cementation, the femoral head is cleared of any fat or debris with a jet lavage system and irrigated with duo-biotic. A suction tip is then inserted through the stem hole and connected to wall suction. An additional tapered suction cannula is inserted into a 3.2 mm hole drilled with the starter drill in the lesser trochanter. The tapered suction cannula is tapped in for a tight fit (2 functioning suctions are needed). It is important to clean and dry the surfaces. A carbon blow-dry carbo-jet (Kinamed Inc., Camarillo, CA) is very useful in drying the the bone externally as well as the stem hole internally and to identify any soft or hard tissue that would prevent intimate contact of the cement to the bone[7] (Fig. 7-36). Regard the head as if it were a tooth cavity and prepare it as a dentist would before implantation with an acrylic filling. It must be absolutely clean and dry.

I recommend using regular Surgical Simplex P (Howmedica Inc., Rutherford, NJ) because of the optimal handling characteristics. One package of bone cement is then mixed and poured into the femoral component at about 2 minutes and smoothed with a finger over all the surfaces (Fig. 7-37). At about 4 minutes, when the acrylic reaches the early doughy stage, it is hand-pressurized into the cylindrically reamed portion of the head (Fig. 7-38). If the stem is to be cemented, cement is also hand-pressurized down the central hole after the cleaning and drying and removing the dome suction (Fig. 7-39). The femoral component is then inserted with the acrylic, and hand-pressurized on with the impactor making sure that the component is fully seated[8] (if needed, use the impactor and light repetitive taps with the mallet). Pressure is maintained until the cement has cured. In order to shorten the working and set time to about 10 minutes, the monomer may be heated to above body temperature in a blanket warmer but there must be sufficient time before setting to ensure that the excess cement can be extruded and that the component is fully seated. All excess cement should be trimmed carefully posteriorly, inferiorly, and superiorly with a scalpel, cutting at a right angle to the cup face so that acrylic is not pulled out from the interface. A dental tool is very useful to remove excess cement from the anterior cup-bone margin, using a reflective mirror to visualize and remove excess cement (Fig. 7-40). Next, clean the surfaces with a moist lap pad. Generally, several thousand milliliters of irrigant are used to clean the hip area and keep the maximum temperature low during acrylic setting. Please note this acrylic technique is designed to provide maximum surface area for fixation in the cylindrical reamed bone and to avoid overpenetration of cement. Other cementing techniques must be used for other devices with less than 1-mm clearance using low-viscosity cement, which will pressurize more cement superiorly and potentially less in the cylindrical reamed bone because the forces are in shear. It is our objective to have a nearly circumferential 1-mm cement mantle with penetration of no more than 2 to 3 mm.

Hip Reduction and Closure

After careful removal of all visible or palpable loose pieces of cement and bone debris, the hip is reduced and a complete range of motion performed. It is desirable to stretch the hip in flexion up to as much as 120 degrees, especially in those hips that were very stiff preoperatively. This procedure aids in beginning the rehabilitation. A check for anterior impingement is made by internal rotation of the hip with 90 degrees of flexion. It is desirable to have at least 40 degrees of internal rotation. If this is not possible, then consider removing the anterior osteophyte if that is the cause of the impingement. There should also be 40 degrees of external rotation in extension. With the hip

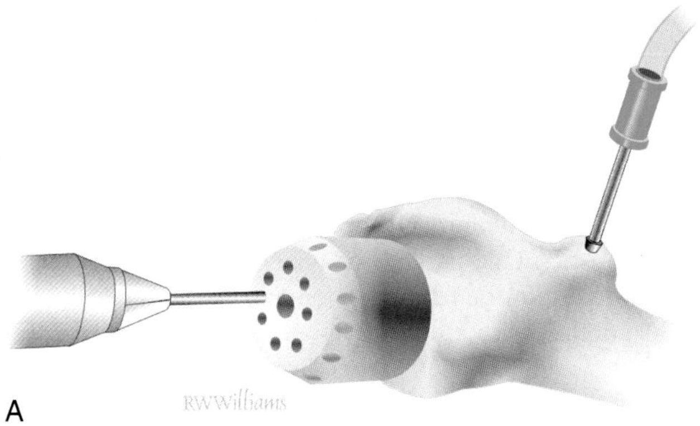

Figure 7-35 **A,** All cystic material and soft tissue should be removed from the prepared femoral head first with a sharp curette and then with a high-speed burr. **B,** Extra fixation holes are drilled in the dome and chamfered area of the prepared femoral head.

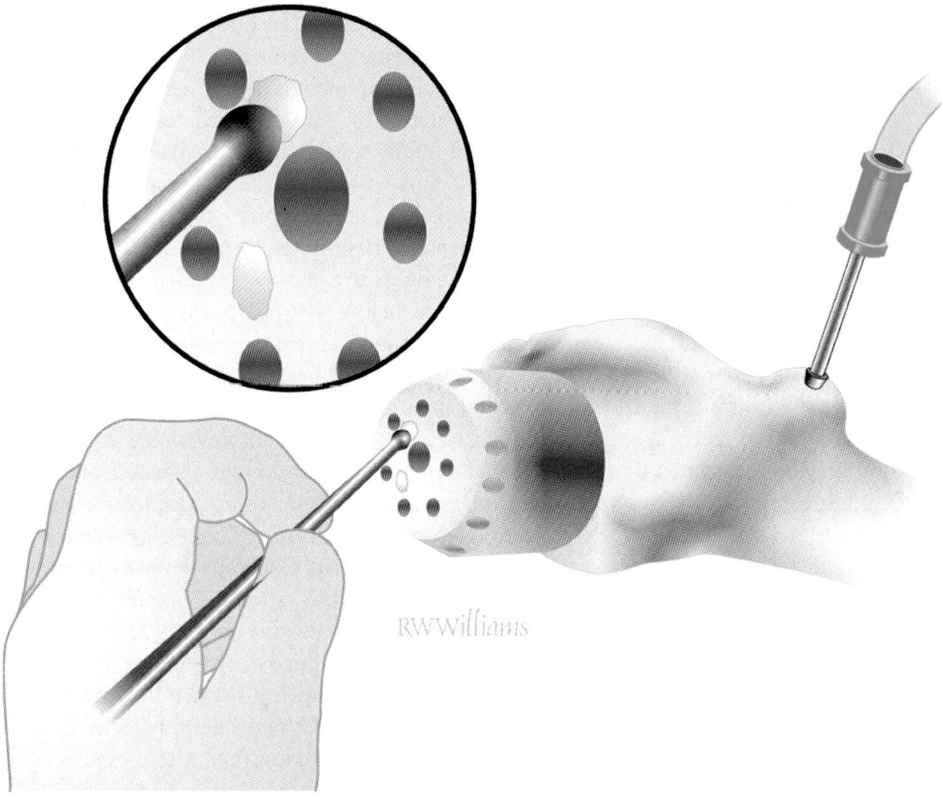

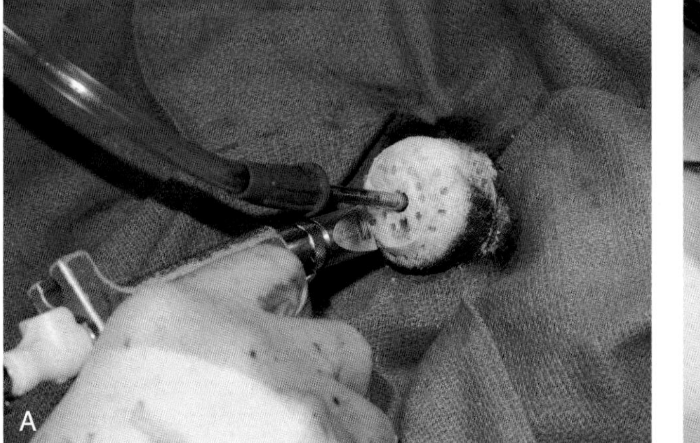

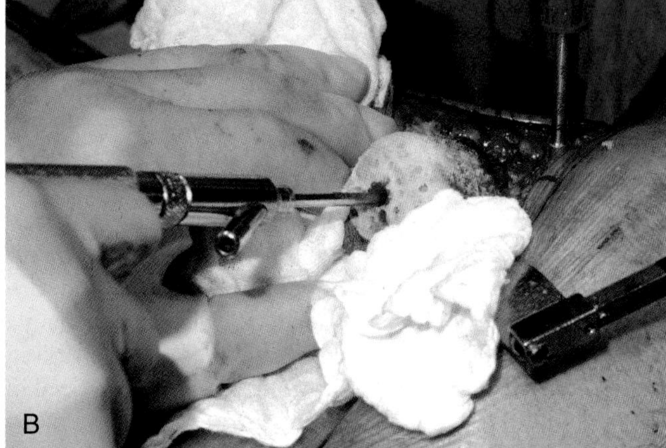

Figure 7-36 The CO_2 blow-dry (Carbo Jet, Kinamed Inc., Camarillo, CA) is useful to dry. **A,** The femoral head before cementation. **B,** The stem hole.

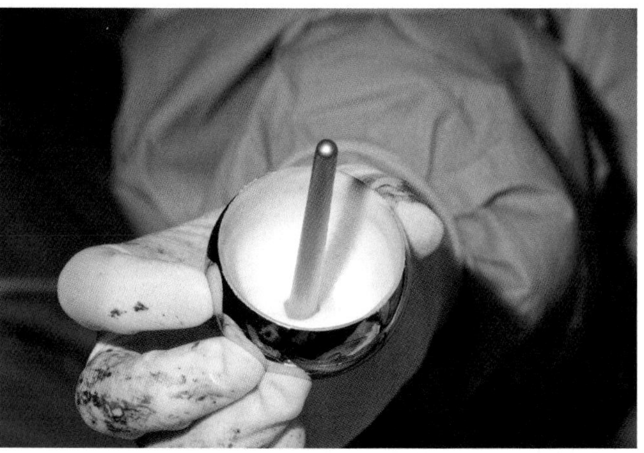

Figure 7-37 The cement is poured into the femoral component and then spread over the entire surface with a finger to provide a thin layer of cement on the metallic surface.

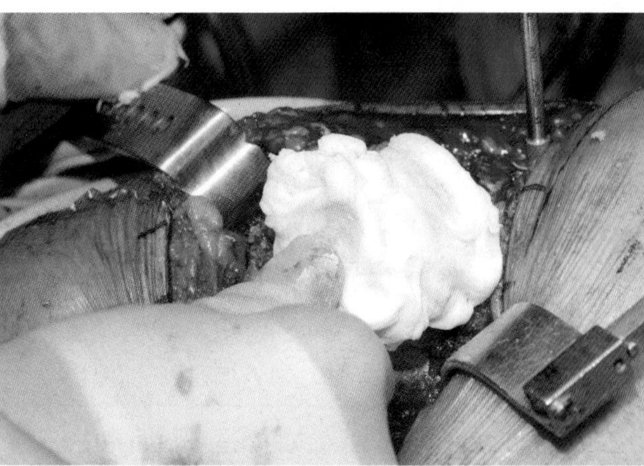

Figure 7-39 Additional cement is pressurized into the head's central hole when the stem is cemented in.

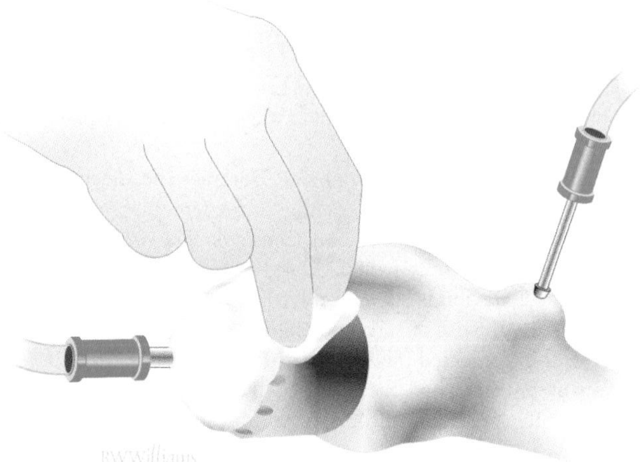

Figure 7-38 The cement is applied and pressurized with the fingers into the bone, especially into the cylindrically reamed surface.

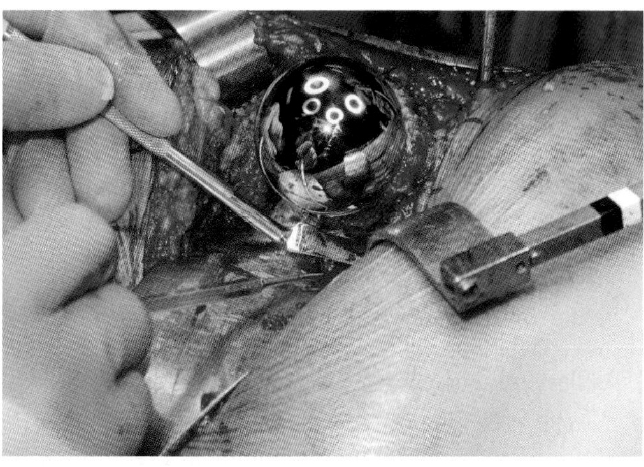

Figure 7-40 A dental tool and special metallic mirror (Innomed Inc. Savannah, GA) are used to visualize the excess cement inferiorly and facilitate its trimming.

and knee extended, push the hip anteriorly to make sure it is stable. If it is unstable, there may be too much socket anteversion and repositioning is indicated. Because the capsule has been released and at least partially resected, one can easily pull the hip out of the socket (so-called Shuck test) but this is anticipated and has not been a problem if proper precautions are carried out (see postoperative management). A final irrigation is done with the remains of 2000 or 3000 mL of saline and 1000 mL of antibiotic solution. The short rotators, and if necessary, the gluteus maximus tendon fascia are repaired with #1 Vicryl, and the wound is closed with one small size 1/8 inch Hemovac drain. Most wounds can be secured with subcuticular closure and Dermabond (Ethicon, Somerville, NJ).

Postoperative Management

Once the anesthesia has worn off, the hip will be stable and special abduction pillow is not necessary. However, it is important to keep pressure on the reduced hip so that dislocation does not occur until the patient is safely in the recovery room and a radiograph is obtained with the feet taped into internal rotation. On several occasions, when this was not doned, a dislocation occurred generally in external rotation. In those cases, with simple traction and internal rotation, the reduction has been successful without recurrence.

All patients are managed with prophylactic antibiotics for 2 days and generally adjusted, low-dose warfarin for three weeks, and then aspirin for an additional 3 weeks. Indomethacin 50 mg is given preoperatively and postoperatively. Twenty five milligrams of indomethacin three times a day or indomethicin XR 75 mg are given for 5 days. All male patients undergoing simultaneous bilateral surgery are given 700 rads of single-dose radiation preoperatively and the indomethacin. Walking begins on the first postoperative day with weight-bearing of at least 50% with crutches or as tolerated. The patients are sometimes discharged on day 2 or by day 3. One more day is generally needed if a one stage bilateral surgery was performed. Crutches are used for 3 to 4 weeks to allow for soft tissue healing and restoration of more normal lubrication, and a cane is occasionally used for an additional 1 to 2 weeks. Patients return to driving when they have control of their leg, and most return to work 2 to 4 weeks after surgery. Low-impact sports are generally permitted at 4 to 5 months postoperatively.[3] Contact or impact sports should be restricted for 10 to 12 months. For hips that have cysts greater than 1 cm, contact sports are not recommended.

Pitfalls

The main pitfalls possibly associated with the described technique are the following:

1. Notching the superior femoral neck cortex during cylindrical reaming, which could weaken the femoral neck and lead to femoral neck fracture. The guiding pin should be as accurately positioned as possible before reaming commences. The pin should be relocated at any time up until the final ream to ensure optimal positioning of the component.
2. Reaming into the anterior osteophyte when there is no structural cortex underneath. This can weaken the femoral neck because these osteophytes often become a structural part of the neck. We suggest a slight anterior translation of the femoral component associated with a slight posterior to anterior positioning of the component to preserve the osteophyte, if possible, as long as sufficient internal rotation in flexion is possible.
3. Leaving debris on the femoral head and failure to properly dry the head during cement application. This is a critical moment in the surgical procedure that determines the quality of the initial fixation of the femoral component and ultimately the long term durability. Remember the fixation area is markedly reduced when compared with a stem of a THR.

References

1. Amstutz H, Beaulé P, Dorey F, Le Duff M, Campbell P, Gruen T: Metal-on-metal hybrid surface arthroplasty—surgical technique. J Bone Joint Surg 2006;88A:234-249.
2. Amstutz H, Beaulé P, Dorey F, Le Duff M, Campbell P, Gruen T: Metal-on-metal hybrid surface arthroplasty: two to six year follow-up. J Bone Joint Surg 2004;86A:28-39.
3. Amstutz H, Beaulé P, Le Duff M: Hybrid metal-on-metal surface arthroplasty of the hip. Operative Techniques in Orthopedics 2001;11:1-10.
4. Beaulé P, Amstutz H: Surface arthroplasty of the hip revisited: current indications and surgical technique. In Singha, R (ed): Hip Replacement: Current Trends and Controversies. New York, Marcel Dekker, 2002, pp 261-297.
5. Freeman M: Some anatomical and mechanical considerations relevant to the surface replacement of the femoral head. Clin Orthop Rel Res 1978;134:19-24.
6. Amstutz H, Le Duff M, Campbell P, Dorey F: The effects of technique changes on aseptic loosening of the femoral component in hip resurfacing. Results of 600 Conserve Plus with a 3-9 year follow-up. J Arthroplasty 2007;22:481-489.
7. McTighe T, Reynolds H, Matsen F, Murray W, Skinner H, Guevara J, Roche K: The use of carbon dioxide gas for preparation of bony surfaces in cemented total joint arthroplasty. ISTA, 1995.
8. Amstutz H, Campbell P, Le Duff M: Fracture of the neck of the femur after surface arthroplasty of the hip. J Bone Joint Surg 2004;86A:1874-1877.

CHAPTER 8

Indications for Metal-on-Metal Hybrid Hip Resurfacing

Harlan C. Amstutz

Introduction

Although metal-on-metal (MM) surface arthroplasty can be selected for most patients who need a prosthetic solution for end-stage osteoarthritis (OA) of the hip, either primary or secondary, it is particularly indicated for young patients when conventional total hip replacement (THR) may not last a lifetime and the patient may likely require revision surgery. The results in those patients who had good bone quality traditionally were better even with early designs, materials, and techniques. Those patients were predominantly male, and men have a greater surface area for femoral fixation. The ideal case also has a high head-neck ratio (greater than 1.2).

When we initiated hip resurfacing in the 1970s, THR complication rates were high and survivorships low in young patients. Although durability improved in the early 1990s, a high percentage required revision before 10 years, and revision procedures were less satisfactory. There clearly was a need for improved THRs, and because of the inherent advantages, a more reliable resurfacing. When we started our clinical trials, there was no access to MM, alumina-alumina, or improved cross-linked polyethylene (PE) for THRs the United States. Although from our earlier experience with the THARIES and porous surface replacements (PSR), we knew that survivorships were likely to be better in patients with good bone quality than in patients with a deficient bone stock. Therefore, we set out to define the indications by operating on patients with bone stock deficiencies, even if they were severe, if the patient was young enough and was destined to require a second replacement in his or her lifetime based on survivorship data then available. Our early experience, perhaps not surprisingly, validated this hypothesis, with lower survivorships in those patients. Our ideal patient became a man younger than 65 years of age with OA, good bone quality, and a head-neck ratio of less than 1.2 (Fig. 8-1). However, having photographed the femoral heads before cementing the femoral component and then correlating the clinical and pathologic results obtained by retrieval analysis with our initial bone quality, we were able to define the risk factors for failure among our initial cohort of hips. We identified both bone quality and especially bone preparation issues, which had not been optimally identified with our previous hip resurfacing experience. From this analysis, the Surface Arthroplasty Risk Index (SARI)[1] was developed, which remains helpful for defining indications and technical issues, especially for surgeons initiating their experience. The items involved in the computation of the SARI are listed in Table 8-1.

Even more importantly, this analysis enabled us to improve the quality of bone preparation and cementing techniques with a second-generation and, subsequently, a third-generation technique. The current technique includes cementing in the stem in hips with risk factors. However, the improvement even with second-generation techniques has resulted in marked improvement in survivorships[2] to the extent that the SARI is less relevant as a predictor of early or midterm failure when these techniques are used. Figure 8-2 illustrates the various categories under which femoral head defects were listed. This has broadened the indications for my patients to the extent that short- and medium-term loosening have been essentially eliminated, even for those with large defects or other risk factors (Fig. 8-3). For these patients with risk factors, our general recommendation is to restrict impact activities to ensure durability, although for those who need very high activitiy levels in their profession or choose to participate in sports, the results have been surprisingly good so far, but more follow-up is needed.

Today's THRs are better than ever with anticipated long-term durability if the right design and materials are implanted by an experienced surgeon and the patient takes reasonable care not to abuse the device. However, the minimally bone invasive, anatomically accurate, and easily revisable hip resurfacings have the same appeal for older patients that younger patients recognize, even though it is hoped that one implant should get them through their lifetime. For surgeons with considerable experience who have eliminated the sources of short-term failures, almost every patient may be a candidate for resurfacing, irrespective of age. Figure 8-4 shows the equity

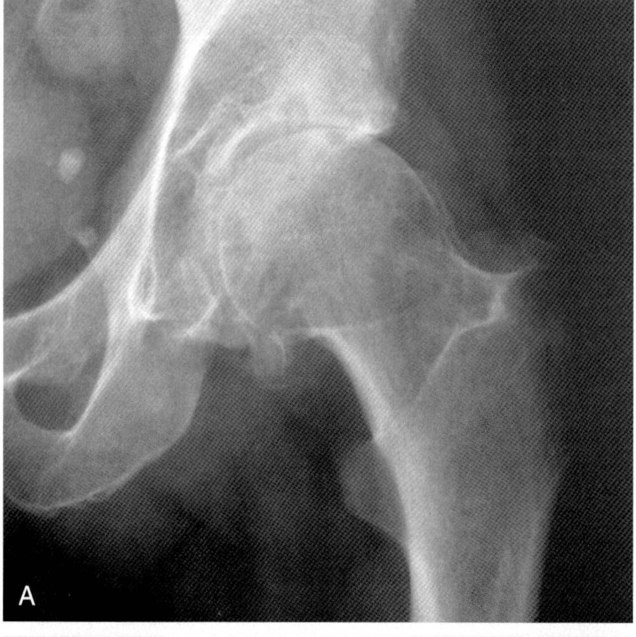

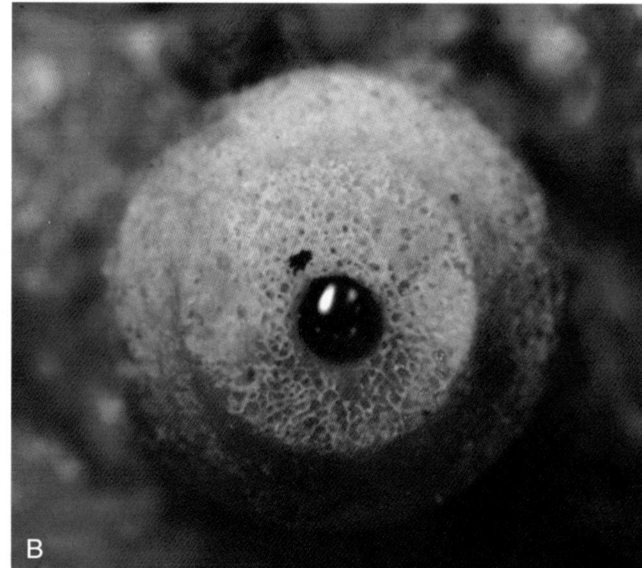

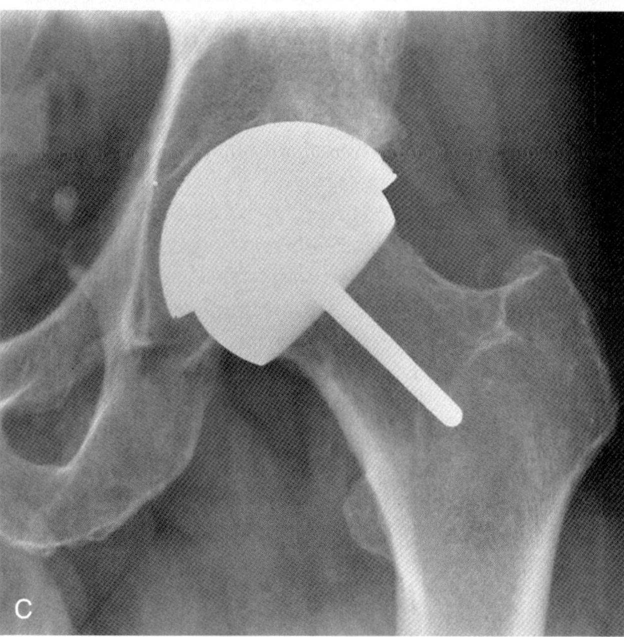

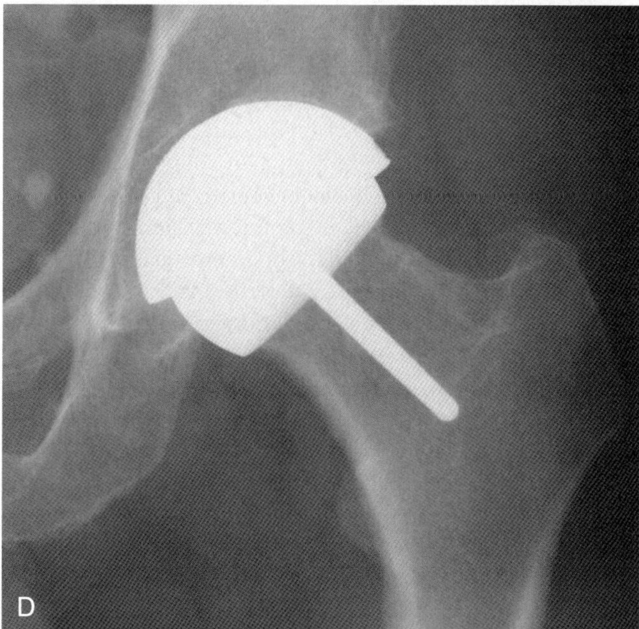

Figure 8-1 A, Preoperative anteroposterior radiograph of a 60-year-old man with primary osteoarthritis of the left hip (hip # 7 in our overall series). The head-neck ratio is 1.34. **B,** Intraoperative photograph of the femoral head after preparation for cementing. Note the excellent bone quality of the cancellous bone in this case, which is sufficient for proper bone-cement interlocking. **C,** Immediate postoperative radiograph showing the neutral positioning of the femoral component (130-degree stem-shaft angle). **D,** Ten years after surgery, the components show impeccable fixation and minimal femoral neck remodeling changes. The patient stopped playing tennis but remains very active and is an avid golfer. His University of California-Los Angeles (UCLA) scores are 9, 10, 10, and 8 for pain, walking, function, and activity, respectively.

Table 8-1 Items Involved in Computation of the SARI

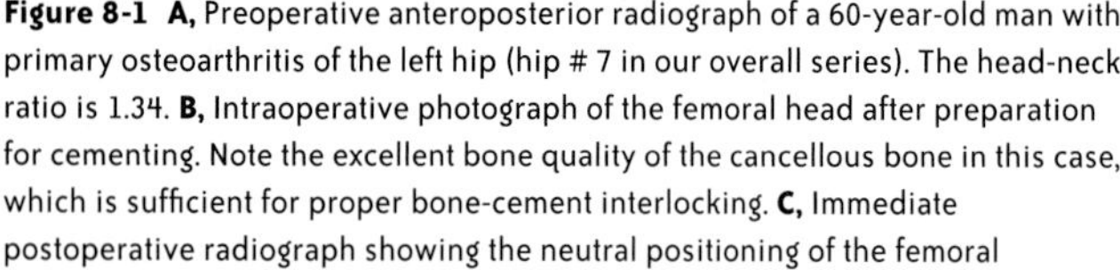

Item	Points
Weight <82 kg	2
Femoral cysts >1 cm	2
Activity >6 (UCLA score)	1
Previous surgery on the operated hip	1

SARI, Surface Arthroplasty Risk Index; UCLA, University of California-Los Angeles.

of the results in our patient population stratified in groups of 10 years. At the present time, our experience in the patients older than 70 years of age is not extensive, with only 20 hips (2% of our study group). Although we regularly include men and women younger than 65 years of age, we recommend that surgeons who do not have extensive experience with resurfacing initiate their trials after a solid educational background with male patients younger than 55 years with a large head size and good bone quality. It is important to explain alternatives, risk factors, and potential complications to each

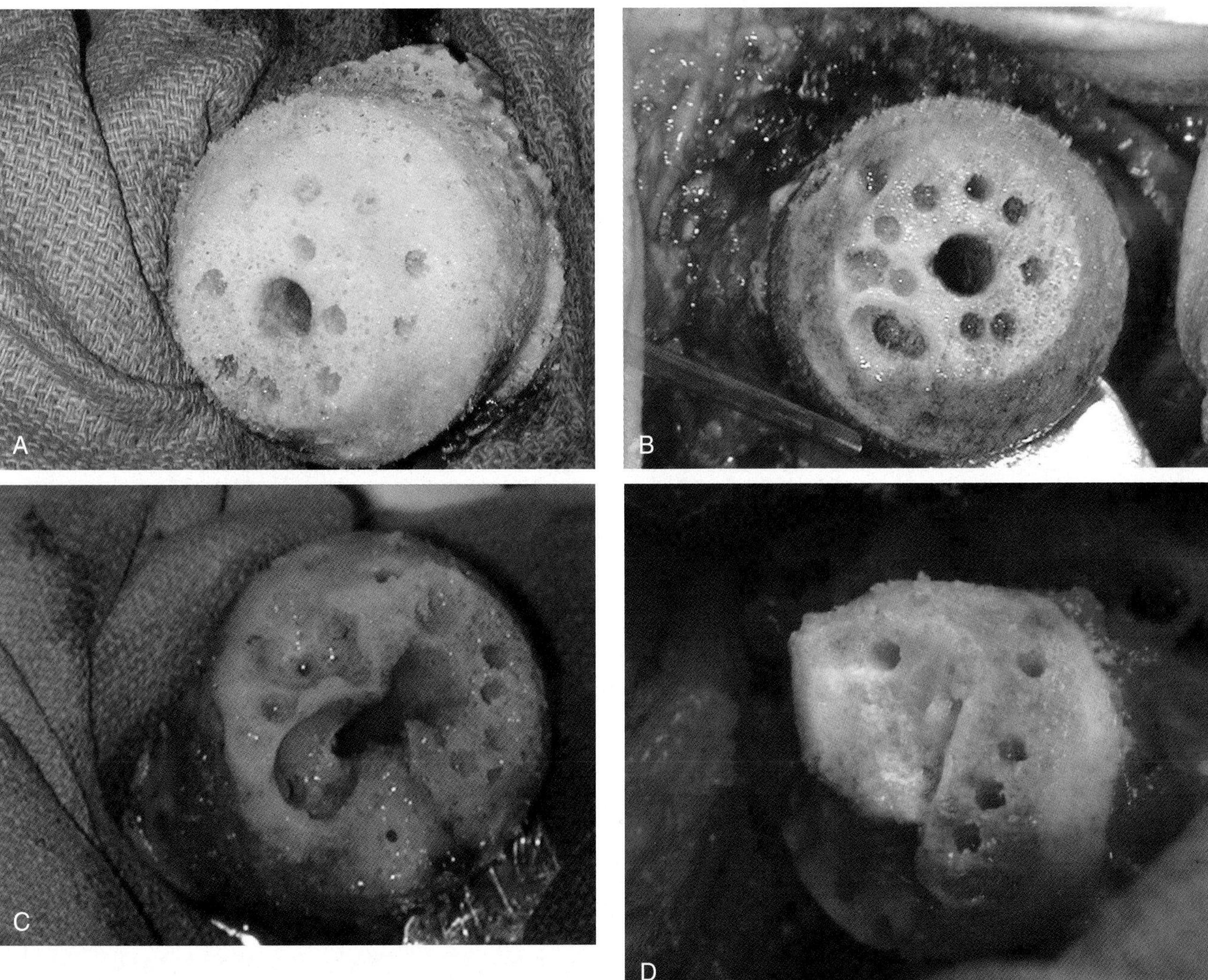

Figure 8-2 The four categories under which femoral heads were rated in terms of the extent of the defects measurable after femoral head preparation. **A,** Category 0: no defect is visible. **B,** Category 1: one or several defects less than 1 cm in size. **C,** Category 2: one or several defects, the largest being 1 to 2 cm in size. **D,** Category 3: one or several defects, the largest being greater than 2 cm in size.

patient. When we initiated MM resurfacing, the stability and range of motion (ROM) achieved were distinct advantages compared with THRs at that time. Today, if a surgeon uses a Big Femoral Head (Wright Medical Technology, Arlington, TN) with a THR (a construct we began using on most THR patients in 1998), that advantage goes away and the prime advantages of resurfacing are preservation of femoral bone, maintenance of leg length because it is an anatomic replacement, and the ability to convert easily to a THR.

Timing of the Procedure

The quality of the bone in the femoral head is more important for hip resurfacing than for conventional THR, in which the femoral head is resected before stem insertion. Therefore, for a THR, the patient may delay surgery with minimal penalty if he so chooses, even though the head becomes more eroded and cystic degeneration occurs.

However, for hip resurfacing, a patient should consider surgery as soon as his or her symptoms and disability warrant consideration of a THR, before the bone quality deteriorates, because the better the bone quality (if all other factors such as technique or subsequent patient activity are equal), the more likely a long-term durable result will be achieved.

Conservative treatment options include reducing the stress on the hip, physical therapy, and medications. Physical therapy and exercises are directed at preserving muscle strength and ROM within the limits of pain, but it is not recommended to stretch the hip, especially in cases of impingement. Recommended medications include anti-inflammatory agents. Weight reduction is highly desirable, because 1 pound weight loss equals 3 pounds in stress reduction on the hip while walking! The use of a cane or walking stick is also a very effective means of reducing the stress on the hip.

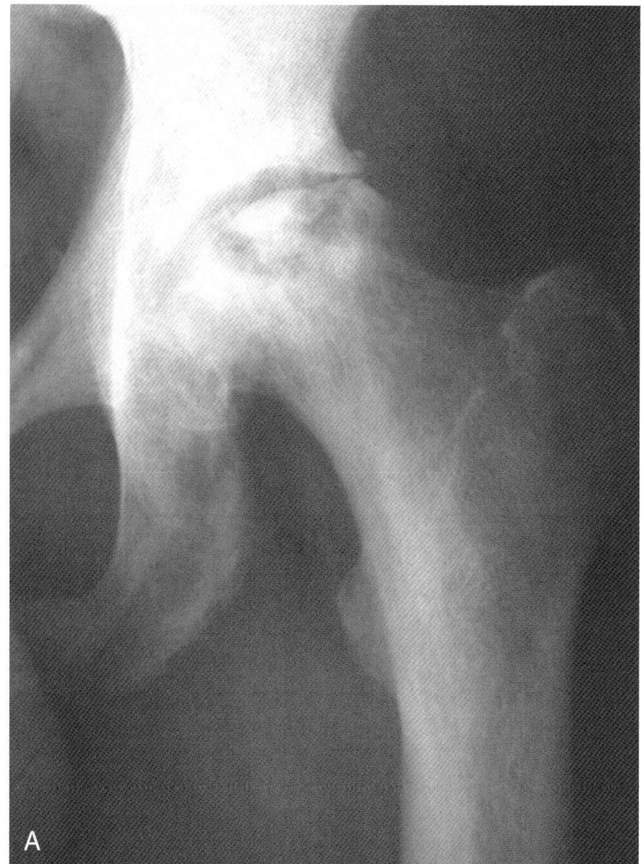

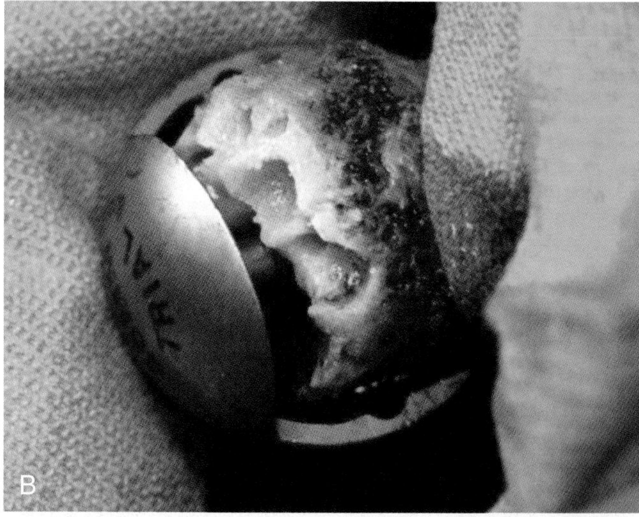

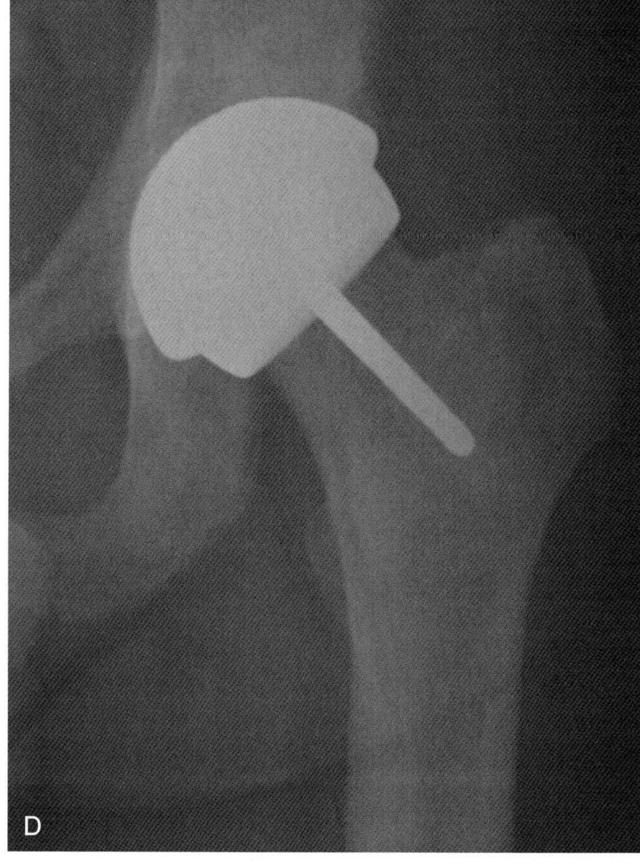

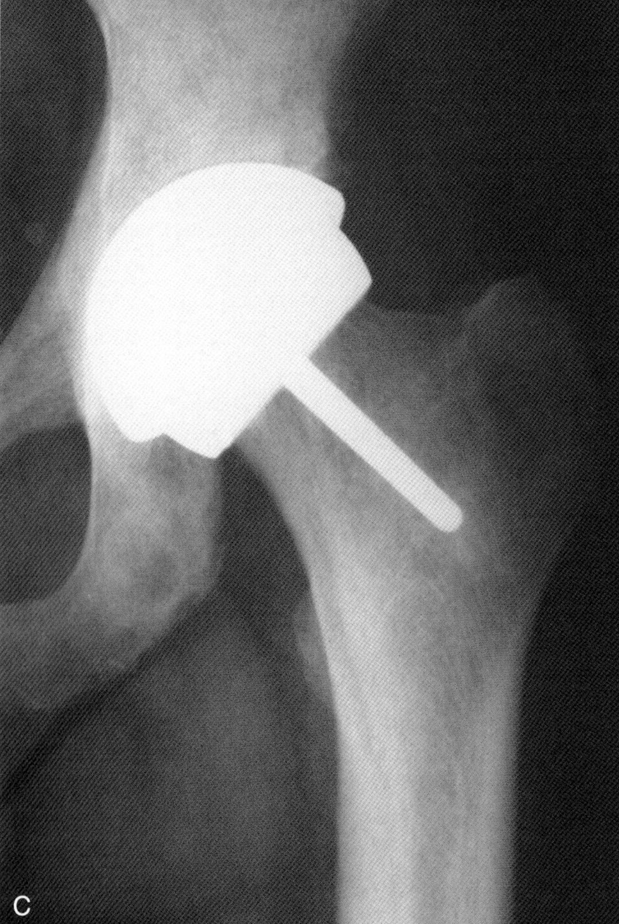

Figure 8-3 **A,** Preoperative anteroposterior radiograph of a 46-year-old man (hip # 328 in our overall series) with osteonecrosis of the left hip, Ficat stage IV. The patient has sickle cell disease. **B,** Intraoperative photograph of the femoral head after preparation for cementing. The application of the femoral template allows an estimation of the magnitude of the bone defects left after removal of all the necrotic bone. Additional holes were drilled, especially in the sclerotic bone, to increase the size of the bone-cement interface and ensure proper initial fixation. **C,** Immediate post-operative radiograph showing a slight varus positioning of the femoral component (136-degree stem-shaft angle). The short metaphyseal stem was cemented to further increase the area of fixation between bone and cement. **D,** Seven years after surgery, there are no signs of loosening and the femoral neck shows a slight remodeling change superiorly, although there is no neck narrowing. His University of California-Los Angeles (UCLA) scores are 10, 10, 10, and 7 for pain, walking, function, and activity, respectively.

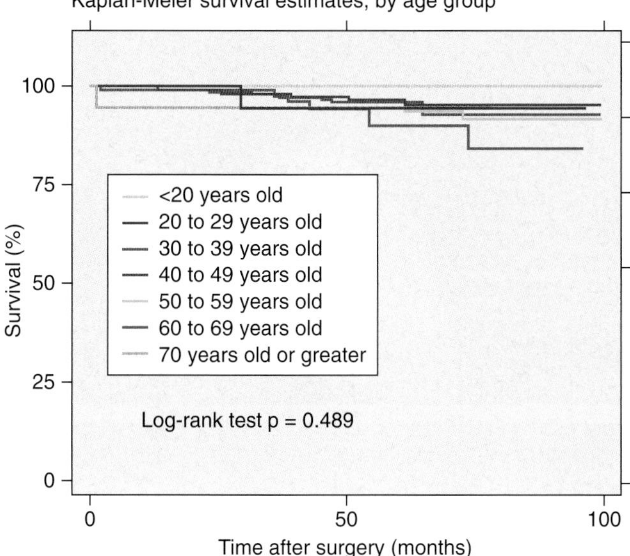

Figure 8-4 Kaplan-Meier survivorship curves of seven age groups constituted on the basis of 10-year intervals. The time to conversion to a total hip replacement was used as endpoint.

Selection of the optimal treatment plan should be consistent with the degree of pain, the amount of hip disability, and the nonsurgical and surgical alternatives. The individual's anticipated life span will also influence the selection of treatment.

Are There Special Considerations for Patients Who Have a High Body Mass Index?

In our experience, heavy patients present for evaluation and treatment earlier than other patients because of symptoms from the heavy loading compared with those who are normal or light weight, but there was no difference in femoral cyst size between the group with a body mass index (BMI) of 30 or greater and those with a BMI of less than 30 (P = 0.400). However, from a survivorship standpoint with all hips included from the beginning of our experience, we found that a 5-point increase in BMI was associated with a twofold decrease of the risk of revision and, therefore, a high BMI does not constitute a contraindication for hip resurfacing.[3]

However, technically, resurfacing is more challenging in patients with increased girth either due to fat, muscle, or a combination of both because a greater degree of exposure is needed, not only to deliver the head for preparation but also to translate the head out of the way to completely visualize and access the acetabulum for reaming and socket implantation. Because of surgical difficulties, I emphasize weight reduction. However, if the patient cannot or will not lose weight and is having increased disability, then either THR or resurfacing should be considered.

An ample incision length and full gluteal release from the linea aspera are mandatory. We strongly recommend debulking the head, especially with large femoral head sizes (>48 mm), to facilitate access to the acetabulum.

The deep wound makes pin centering and head preparation more difficult, and it is important to check the accuracy of each preparation step.

Indications for Bilateral Simultaneous Hip Resurfacing

Those patients who present with bilateral symptomatic arthritic hips should be considered for simultaneous procedures if the pain and severity of disease dictate the need for bilateral surgery, the patient is generally healthy (less than 65 years of age), and the surgeon is experienced (proficient) with the procedure. If the patient has just become symptomatic or has a pain rating of 6 or more with early arthritic radiographic changes and it is estimated that the other hip would not need surgery for 2 or more years, then my preference would be to operate only on one hip. Unfortunately, there are no studies available that describe and quantify the natural history of OA, and allow one to make a scientific prediction. However, complete joint obliteration and reduced contact area, either due to anatomic dysplasia or dysplasia secondary to lateral head extrusion related to the presence of medial osteophytes, often leads to early cyst formation. The surgeon and the patient also need to consider age, rehabilitation time, and the economics.

For bilateral resurfacing, we suggest operating on the worst hip first and making certain that extra care is given to preventing complications. The hips are radiated with 800 rads within 24 hours of surgery (the closer the better) to minimize the risk of heterotopic ossification (HO) in addition to the usual indomethacin preoperatively and for 5 days postoperatively. Generally, 1 g of antibiotic are given throughout the procedure for both hips.

Special Indications for Metal-on-Metal Hip Resurfacing

Special indications include cases in which a conventional THR cannot be inserted, or inserted with considerable difficulty, and or with risk factors for failure, such as the following:

1. Abnormal proximal femur in the intertrochanteric or subtrochanteric region, where insertion of a conventional stem would be impossible or require an osteotomy to realign the femur before an arthroplasty (see Fig. 17-6).
2. Abnormal bone, where arthroplasty would be almost impossible to perform because of the absence of a femoral canal, such as melorrheostosis (Fig. 17-1) and osteopetrosis (i.e., marble bone disease, Fig. 17-2).
3. Patients who have had previous septic arthritis, sepsis in the subtrochanteric region such as from a prior trauma, or who have a high risk for sepsis. Resurfacing in these situations poses less risk because the intramediary canal is not

violated. If a recurrence or infection develops, it can be more easily dealt with.

4. Patients who have a high risk for postoperative dislocations following conventional hip arthroplasty with conventional ball sizes, that is, patients with dysplasia, Erhlos-Danlos syndrome, postpoliomyelitis, or other patients who demonstrate severe joint laxity with or without neuromuscular deficiencies. (The stability objective can also be met with THR using a BFH.)
5. Young patients who would be at risk for requiring multiple revisions in their lifetime. A revision, should it be required after resurfacing, can be performed with a comparable outcome to primary THR because the socket fixation has proven reliable and a stem can be easily inserted into the virgin femoral canal. There are many patients who require high levels of activity in their profession. Although any arthroplasty may be at risk of failure with these patients, the long-term morbidity risk is minimized with resurfacing because of the relatively easy conversion to a THR with BFH, as opposed to revising a stem-type conventional replacement.
6. Patients who require excessive ROM for their profession preferentially would have freedom for doing their occupation without the fear of dislocation. (This objective can also be met with THR using a BFH.)
7. Providing a normally functioning hip with a bone-saving device allows the patient to delay surgery and can substantially minimize morbidity and maintain optimal outcomes. We now know the functional results are at least as good and, in some cases, better than a THR.
8. Delaying surgery is important because new technology in improving fixation and reduction of wear and any adverse consequences by modification of existing or by development of new bearing materials is likely. For example, there are new technologies to reduce wear and potential adverse toxicity by a type A HM (hardened metal now introduced with the wrought femoral component), which has already been introduced with the Conserve®Plus or possibly in the future with an alumina femoral component.
9. Patients who have unusual anatomy and biomechanics, which would be difficult to replicate with a THR, such as an extremely long or valgus neck (Fig. 8-5).

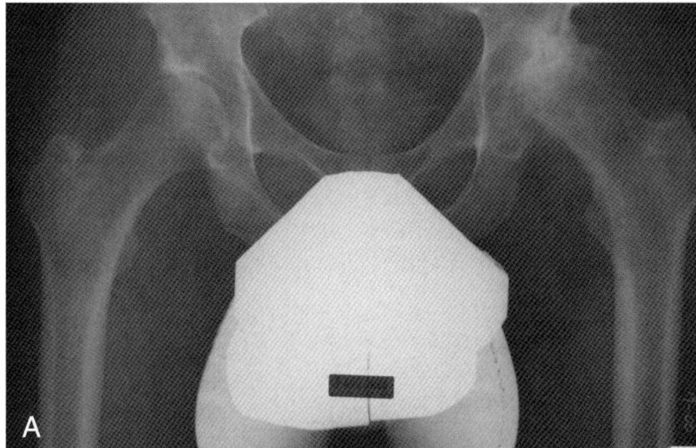

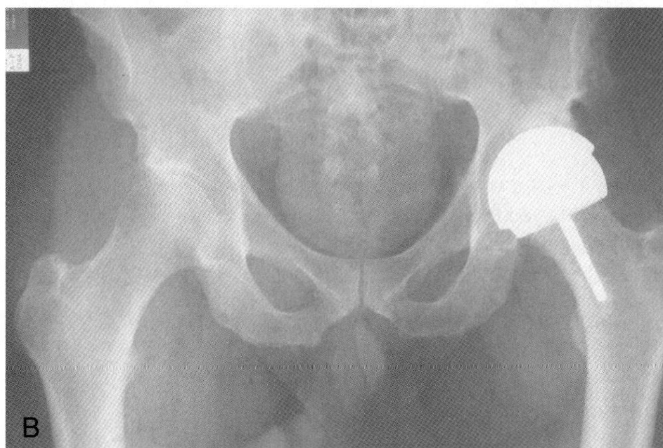

Figure 8-5 **A,** Preoperative anteroposterior radiograph of a 59-year-old man with posttraumatic osteoarthritis of the left hip. Note the unusually long femoral neck and the high neck-shaft angle (140 degrees). **B,** Four months after surgery. Leg length was preserved, and the component was placed in valgus (stem-shaft angle of 149 degrees). His University of California-Los Angeles (UCLA) scores at 4 months were 8, 8, 6, and 4 for pain, walking, function, and activity, respectively.

Contraindications to Metal-on-Metal Hip Resurfacing

1. Patients with severe cystic degeneration or in whom the cyst extends into the cylindrically reamed portion, so that fixation is not circumferential with a uniform cement mantle in this important area (Fig. 8-6).
2. Patients with severe or potentially severe renal dysfunction. Although the Conserve®Plus MM bearing of the prosthesis has extremely low wear, especially with newly introduced type A (HM) femoral component, metal wear particles are released and metal ions that are normally excreted by the kidneys may accumulate to a greater degree in a patient with renal dysfunction. With potential toxicity yet to be identified, how much renal function is essential or desirable is unknown. The only report in the literature[4] indicates that ion levels were 100 times higher in two patients with renal failure with an MM THR than other patients with the same THR, and that these levels did not decrease with the patients on dialysis. However, these levels did decrease when the patients subsequently had a renal transplant (cobalt levels decreased to 7.3 and 7.4 μg/L, and chromium levels decreased to 10.2 and 12.2 μg/L, respectively).

We have observed one 37-year-old patient who had steroid-induced avascular necrosis (AVN) and underwent resurfacing with a McMinn device who subsequently underwent renal transplant 4 years postoperatively and is now 11 years postoperative. His ion levels are similar to those of other patients with the same device (cobalt serum 2.128 ppb, cromium serum 1.8668 ppb, cromium urine

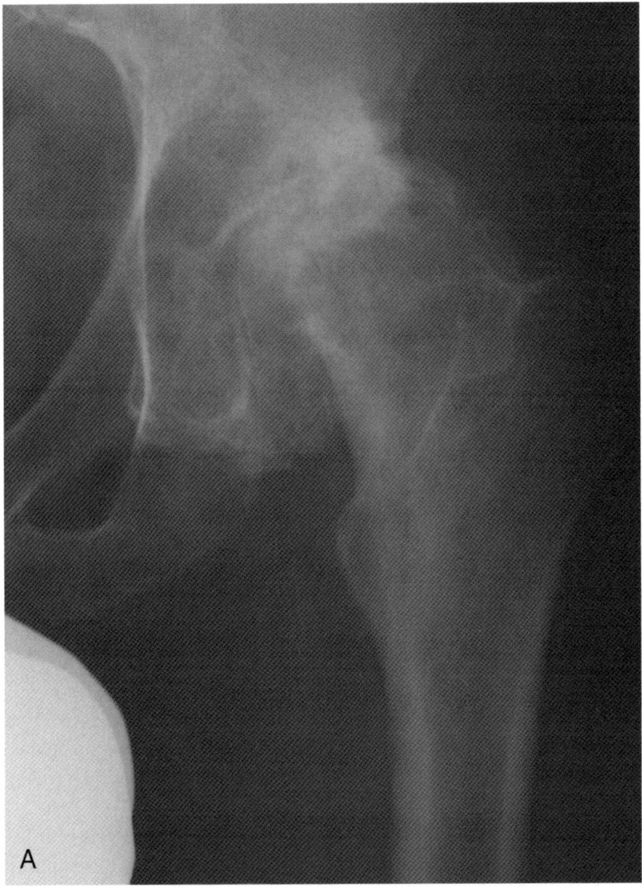

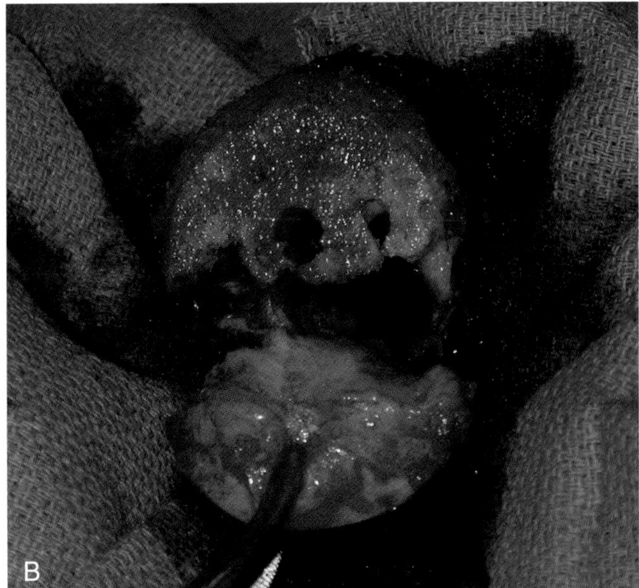

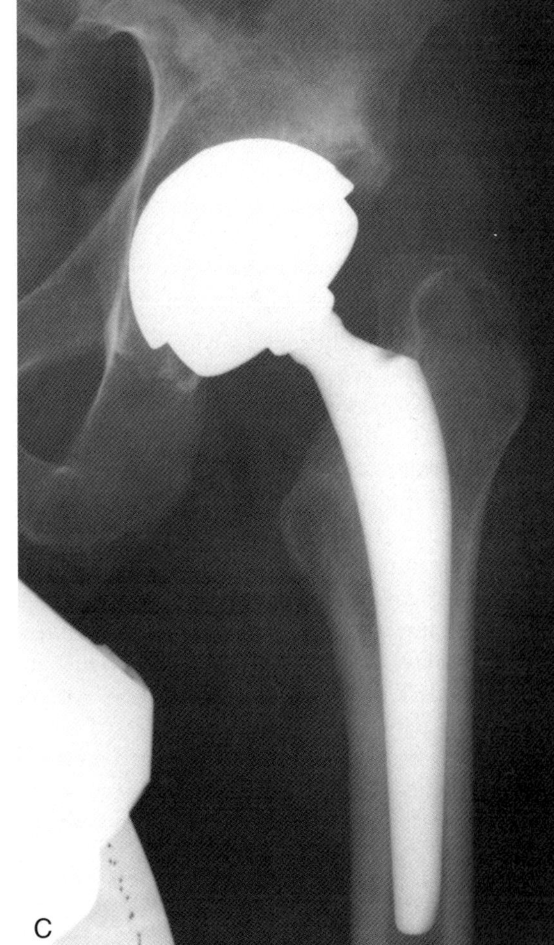

Figure 8-6 **A,** Preoperative anteroposterior radiograph of a 44-year-old man with osteoarthritis. Note the extensive cystic formation on the superior aspect of the femoral neck. The patient was advised to have a total hip replacement but implored us to evaluate at surgery if there was any opportunity to perform a resurfacing procedure. **B,** After reaming of the femoral head, the femoral neck revealed the anticipated large cavitary defect, and a large portion of the head fractured due to the torque of chamfering, confirming our initial impression that resurfacing was contraindicated. **C,** The hip was treated with an anthropometric total hip (ATH) standard-sized grit-blasted femoral stem and Big Femoral Head (Wright Medical Technology, Arlington, TN). One year after surgery, his University of California-Los Angeles (UCLA) scores are 10, 10, 10, and 10 for pain, walking, function, and activity, respectively.

2.511 ppb), and his serum creatinine was 1.7 at his last follow-up visit. It is recommended that surgeons discuss potential ion toxicity with patients who have had impaired renal function and learn what is the risk of subsequent impairment.

3. Patients with active sepsis. However, if a patient has a septic hip, it is recommended to débride the hip to consider hip resurfacing, which may be performed subsequently with more safety than if it were a stem-type device because the intramedullary canal is not violated (entered). If there was

a recurrence, then the surgical treatment would be simpler because it would more likely be local and not extend into the intramedullary canal.

4. Patients with severe osteoporosis (the degree has not yet been identified). Certainly, hips with higher degrees of osteoporosis would be more vulnerable to fracture if errors in technique produced a notch or there were other imperfections in technique such as incomplete seating of the femoral component.

Relative Contraindications

1. Patients with extensive femoral head cystic degeneration (single or multiple cysts greater than 1 cm) or a small femoral component size (<48 mm) when resurfacing is performed with inadequate technique or by an inexperienced surgeon. Older patients with both characteristics might be better served with a conventional stem-type THR. Our statistical analysis pointed out that these variables are important factors in the survivorship of the prosthesis, especially with our early technique.[1] Although our follow-up with the improved technique is shorter than with the initial technique (4 to 6 years compared with 6 to 10 years), the loosening and radiographic signs of loosening have been significantly reduced from 9% to 1%.[2] The younger the patient, the larger the cystic degeneration that may be acceptable because there is no optimal alternative. However, meticulous bone preparation is necessary and the patient must be advised to restrict high-impact physical activities.
2. Age limits are not well defined. Older male patients with good bone quality are acceptable candidates. Our experience to date is that resurfacing is a good alternative to stem-type THA and, in time, may be preferable. Longer term results will be necessary from both modern types of devices. There is no doubt that resurfacing is less forgiving than THA, but in experienced surgical hands, the complication rates are similar. The case of older women is more controversial because of existing or anticipated osteopenia. There is literature which supports that fact that women who develop OA rarely have osteoporosis and subsequent fractures of the neck of the femur, whereas those with osteoporosis rarely develop OA.[5-8] However, there are exceptions and a paucity of data to make a strong recommendation regarding bone quantity and resurfacing at this time. Clearly, the risks must be considered and thoroughly discussed with the prospective patient.
3. Women of childbearing age. At this time, there is no clinical evidence of toxicity in women who have borne children or in their off-spring.[9] Furthermore, Sierra et al[10] have shown that childbirth is not affected by the presence of a conventional THA, and pregnancy after THA is not associated with decreased survival of the prosthesis. In my series, 83 women of childbearing age (>45 years old) have undergone hip implantation surgery, and five have delivered nine healthy children now ranging from 6 months to 7 years old. In addition, at least 15 other normal births after MM resurfacing have been reported in recent international meetings. In a recent article, Ziaee et al[11] reported on the ion levels of 10 pregnant patients and concluded that the placenta has a modulatory effect on the rate of metal ion transfer. At the present time, there is no known contraindication to using MM hip resurfacing, although the numbers of progeny are small and further experience and follow-up is needed. However, it is important for the surgeon to thoroughly discuss risks and potential hazards as well as the benefits with any potential candidates in the child-bearing age.
4. Patients with severe dysplasia of the hip (Crowe class III to IV) and a leg-length discrepancy of more than 2.5 cm. The possibility of equalizing a leg-length discrepancy greater than 1.5 cm is limited and almost entirely derived from moving the socket distal to the anatomic location. Large discrepancies are more effectively equalized with a stem-type THR.

References

1. Beaulé P, Dorey F, Le Duff M, Gruen T, Amstutz H: Risk factors affecting early outcome of metal on metal surface arthroplasty of the hip in patients 40 years old and younger. Clin Orthop 2004;418:87-93.
2. Amstutz H, Le Duff M, Campbell P, Dorey F: The effects of technique changes on aseptic loosening of the femoral component in hip resurfacing. Results of 600 Conserve Plus with a 3-9 year follow-up. J Arthroplasty 2007;22:481-489.
3. Le Duff M, Amstutz H, Dorey F: Metal-on-metal hip resurfacing for obese patients. J Bone Joint Surg Am 2007;89;2705-2711.
4. Brodner W, Grohs J, Bitzan P, Meisinger V, Kovarik J, Kotz R: Serum cobalt and serum chromium level in 2 patients with chronic renal failure after total hip prosthesis implantation with metal-metal gliding contact. Z Orthop Ihre Grenzgeb 2000; 138:425-429.
5. Arden NK, Griffiths GO, Hart DJ, Doyle DV, Spector TD: The association between osteoarthritis and osteoporotic fracture: the Chingford Study. Br J Rheumatol 1996;35:1299-1304.
6. Cumming R, Klineberg R: Epidemiological study of the relation between arthritis of the hip and hip fractures. Ann Rheum Dis 1993;52:707-710.
7. Dequeker J, Johnell O: Osteoarthritis protects against femoral neck fracture: the MEDOS study experience. Bone 1993;14 Suppl 1:S51-S56.
8. Foss M, Byers P: Bone density, osteoarthrosis of the hip, and fracture of the upper end of the femur. Ann Rheum Dis 1972; 31:259-264.
9. Brodner W, Grohs J, Bancher-Todesca D, Dorotka R, Meisinger V, Gottsauner-Wolf F, Kotz R: Does the placenta inhibit the passage of chromium and cobalt after metal-on-metal total hip arthroplasty? J Arthroplasty 2004;19:102-106.
10. Sierra R, Trousdale R, Cabanela M: Pregnancy and childbirth after total hip arthroplasty. J Bone Joint Surg Br 2005;87:21-24.
11. Ziaee H, Daniel J, Datta A, Blunt S, McMinn D: Transplacental transfer of cobalt and chromium in patients with metal-on-metal hip arthroplasty: a controlled study. J Bone Joint Surg Br 2007; 89:301-305.

CHAPTER 9

Results of Conserve® Plus Hip Resurfacing

Harlan C. Amstutz

Michel J. Le Duff

Introduction

The series of patients resurfaced with Conserve®Plus we examined in this section started in November of 1996 with the first hip ever implanted with this design. The indications for the procedure at the time were very wide. There were no exclusion criteria either for bone quality (cysts) or quantity (osteoporosis) unless the procedure became technically infeasible. Patients were included if they were young enough and thought to require more than one replacement in their lifetime, or slightly older but had high anticipated activity levels related to their occupation or desired recreation. The surgery was performed even though these patients were thought to present possible risk factors for shortened durability. All etiologies were included, and there were no restrictions related to gender, anticipated patient activity, or body characteristics (e.g., body mass index [BMI]). The series was initiated before cross-linked polyethylene or ceramic-on-ceramic for total hip replacements was available in the United States, and metal-on-metal devices were in clinical trial. The patients were presented with alternative treatments (total hip replacement [THR] or other types), performance data, and potential complications that were revelant to the time period of their initial consultation.

In a group of more than 1100 patients, 1000 Conserve®Plus were implanted in 838 patients by the senior author (HCA) between this date and September of 2006, and this cohort will represent our study group. During this period, HCA also performed 439 other hip procedures in 375 patients, including 21 other total hip resurfacing procedures, 207 revisions of previous arthroplasties, 32 hemisurface arthroplasties, 175 primary conventional total hip replacements, and four other surgeries.

The series started with custom components, and from 11/26/96 to 3/10/00, 293 hips were implanted before the U.S. Food and Drug Administration requested that official clinical trials be implemented by Wright Medical Technology Inc. After this period, a Single-Center Investigational Device Exemption (IDE) was started, and from 3/23/00 to 8/3/00, 63 hips were implanted (including three hips implanted under compassionate use because the patients did not meet one of the U.S. Food and Drug Administration (FDA) exclusion criteria, which excluded patients less than 18 years of age and initially inflammatory joint disease). After this period, the multicenter IDE started with an initial cohort, and from 8/22/00 to 10/2/01, 112 hips were implanted, including

- Six compassionate use
- Forty training arm cases, in which surgeons from other sites participated in the operative procedure
- One inflammatory arm

Following the initial cohort, the clinical trials went to a continued access phase, and from 10/30/01 to 6/30/05, 348 hips were implanted (including two compassionate use). The remaining devices of this series (184 hips) were implanted between 8/18/05 and 9/5/06 under a physician-directed application. From the geographic point of view, our series was also unique because a large number of our patients came from long distances across the United States or beyond. Only 28% came from Southern California, and 54% came from a different state or country. This was related to Dr. Amstutz being the only surgeon in the country to perform this procedure regularly until the multicenter IDE started and, later, from the patients' desire to have their surgery done by the surgeon who developed and had the most experience with the procedure. Figure 9-1 shows the spread of our Conserve®Plus patients over the United States. The regular follow-up of these out-of-state patients was made possible essentially by the senior author traveling across the country and setting up satellite clinics in more than 20 different locations. The patients who could not attend these clinics or visit our center in Los Angeles were instructed to follow-up with a local orthopaedist, who would forward to us clinical and radiographic data, so a phone interview could subsequently be set up with the patient to discuss the findings.

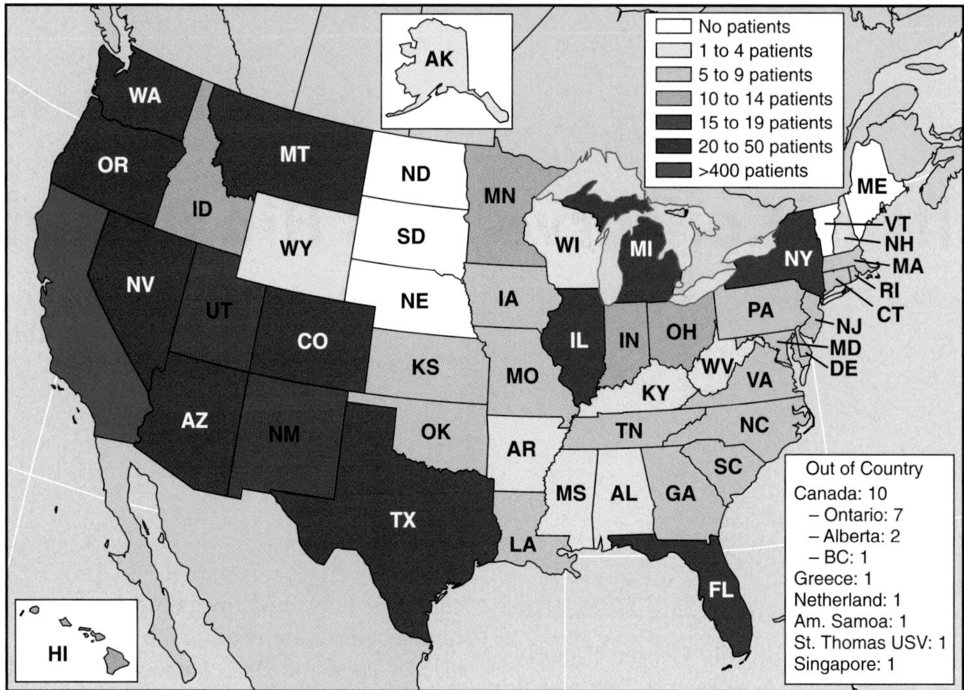

Figure 9-1 Concentration of patients per state over the U.S. territory.

From the initiation of the series, a documentation of the bone quality of the femoral head was made by taking intraoperative photographs of the femoral head after completion of the preparation, before the cement is applied. The size of the largest bone defect visible on the intraoperative photograph was assessed by a measurement of its largest dimension, normalized to the known dimension of the cylindrically reamed femoral head.[1,2] These data were instrumental in the process of identification of the risk factors for failure of metal-on-metal hip resurfacing during our early experience[1,3] and used as control variables in the subsequent statistical analyses that led to the development of the most recent and more effective surgical techniques.[4]

Demographics of the Study Group

A summary of the overall demographics of the study group is presented in Table 9-1.

In the following sections, we investigate the possible changes in patient characteristics over the course of the series.

Age at Surgery

The age of the patients in this series varied considerably (range, 14 to 78 years) because the senior author did not use this criteria for exclusion. However, the average of 50 years illustrates that a majority of patients seeking the resurfacing procedure were young compared with the usual age of patients undergoing conventional THR. The distribution of patient age at surgery is shown in Figure 9-2. An evolution could be observed in this field, and patient age became slightly higher after the first half of the series (48.6 years for the first 500 hips versus 51.5 years for the last 500, $P = .00002$). A possible explanation for this is the shift in etiology from 62.8% to 76.4% of idiopathic or "primary" osteoarthritis cases between the first and the second 500 procedures. Idiopathic osteoarthritis tends to develop later in life than osteoarthritis secondary to other etiologies.

This shift does not represent a deliberate selection from the senior author who continued to include all resurfaceable cases in the series but is probably a reflection of the new awareness of the patients and referring physicians that resurfacing is a viable solution for most osteoarthritis cases, not just cases of end-stage arthritis happening before the usually acceptable age for a conventional THR.

Male/Female Ratio

The male/female ratio remained constant during the whole series with a higher proportion of men (74.7%) than women (25.3%). This result is typical of most modern generation metal-on-metal resurfacing series.[5-9]

Patient Height, Weight, and Body Mass Index

The average patient body characteristics (height, weight, and BMI) did not change throughout the series. However, patients with a BMI equal or greater to 35 were excluded from the study between 5/18/01 and 6/30/05 at the request of the FDA, who insisted that this modification of the IDE protocol be

Table 9-1 Demographics of the Study Group

	Average	Range
Age at surgery (years)	50.0	14 to 78
Height, Males (cm)	179.1	155 to 203
Height, Females (cm)	164.9	140 to 183
Weight, Males (kg)	88.8	57 to 164
Weight, Females (kg)	67.1	42 to 119
BMI Males	27.6	18.4 to 46.4
BMI Females	24.6	17.5 to 42.3
Gender (n = 838 Patients)	**Count**	**%**
Males	626	74.7
Females	212	25.3
Charnley Class (n = 838 Patients)	**Count**	**%**
A	511	61.0
B	280	33.4
C	47	5.6
Etiology (n = 1000 Hips)	**Count**	**%**
Idiopathic OA	696	69.6
ON	83	8.3
DDH	103	10.3
Epiphyseal dysplasia	4	0.4
Post-traumatic OA	43	4.3
Inflammatory OA	11	1.1
SCFE	17	1.7
LCP	21	2.1
Rheumatoid	12	1.2
Ankylosing spondylitis	5	0.5
Pigmented villonodular synovitis	2	0.2
Melorheostosis	1	0.1
Arthrokatadysis	1	0.1
Osteopetrosis	1	0.1
Femoral Defect Size (n = 1000 Hips)	**Count**	**%**
No defect	361	36.1
<1 cm	292	29.2
1-2 cm	247	24.7
>2 cm	100	10.0
Previous Surgeries (n = 1000 Hips)	**Count**	**%**
Hemiresurfacing	2	0.2
Osteotomy	13	1.3
Coring	12	1.2
Pinning	17	1.7
Judet graft	1	0.1
Acetabular reconstruction	2	0.2
ORIF	3	0.3
Free vascularized fibular graft	2	0.2
Other	1	0.1
Total	53	5.3

BMI, body mass index; DDH, developmental dysplasia of the hip; LCP, Legg-Calve-Perthes disease; OA, osteoarthritis; ON, osteonecrosis; ORIF, open reduction internal fixation; SCFE, slipped capital femoral epiphysis.

made to the section that defined the indications, because of the belief that those patients might be at higher risk for femoral neck fracture. Thus far, our data have shown opposite results.[10]

Charnley Class

The distribution of the patients between the three classes of the Charnley classification remained constant throughout the series. The occurrence of bilateral disease is high (only 51% of the hips operated on overall did not show contralateral affection) and 162 patients have had bilateral Conserve®Plus resurfacing performed either in one or two separate operations. This figure most likely will increase in the years to come as patients who are classified as Charnley class B develop further symptoms in their contralateral hip, or for many others, who have some anatomic defect with signs of either femoroacetabular impingement (FAI) or dysplasia, become Charnley class B when they become symptomatic.

Etiology

As mentioned in the section devoted to patient age, the prevalence of patients who underwent surgery for idiopathic osteoarthritis increased significantly over the course of implantation of these 1000 hips. On the other hand, the overall number of hips operated for secondary arthritis decreased: Osteonecrosis cases represented 11% in the first 500 hips and only 5.6% in the second half of the series. Similarly, but to a lesser extent, the number of hips operated on for developmental dysplasia of the hip decreased from 11.4% to 9.2%, and the number of hips operated on for post-traumatic osteoarthritis decreased from 5.4% to 3.2%. Rheumatoid disease, inflammatory arthritis, and other unusual etiologies combined to account for an additional 3.8% decrease in prevalence between the first and second halves of the series.

Femoral Head Defects

There was an evolution between the beginning of the series and its second half in the proportion of femoral heads with cystic defects (Table 9-2). The second half of the series presented more femoral heads without defects and fewer femoral heads with defects (Mann-Whitney U test, $P = .0001$). This

Table 9-2 Changes in Proportion of Femoral Heads with Important Cystic Defects

	First 500 Hips (%)	Second 500 Hips (%)
No defect	31.9	40.1
<1 cm	19.0	39.5
1 cm to 2 cm	34.9	14.6
>2 cm	14.2	5.8

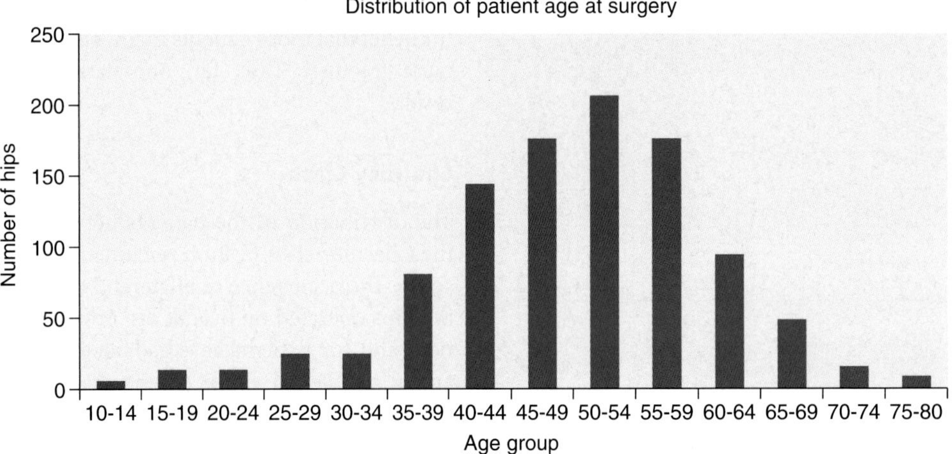

Figure 9-2 Distribution of patient age at surgery, in increments of 5 years.

evolution is consistent with the increase in idiopathic osteoarthritis cases and more young patients seeking treatment earlier.

Previous Surgeries

The prevalence of previous surgeries performed on the hips prior resurfacing dropped from 37 (7.4%) in the first 500 hips to 15 (3.0%) in the second half of the cohort. This result is also consistent with the modification in incidence of the etiologies over time of implantation.

Component Sizes

Although the femoral component of the Conserve®Plus prosthesis remained the same during the entire series, a second thinner acetabular component (3.5-mm wall thickness) was introduced and used at our center, beginning on 10/30/03. All of the early cases were implanted with the original 5-mm wall thickness cup.

Six hundred and fifty-one hips were implanted with the 5-mm shell, 347 with the thin shell, and two hips (one patient) with the Superfix cup, an asymmetric cup used to restore the normal biomechanics of the hip and leg lengths in case of superolateral acetabular defect of one hip and loss of femoral head height on the contralateral hip. Two hips were implanted with a double socket with the Conserve®Plus 5-mm shell cemented into a porous-coated surface replacement socket before the introduction of the SuperFix, which in each instance would have been used today to fill the acetabular defects. The thinner acetabular component enables the surgeon to preserve more bone on either the acetabular side or the femoral side, or both. In our series, we compared component sizes between the hips implanted with the 5-mm shells and those implanted with the thin shell. The two groups were comparable in height (175.8 cm for the thin shells versus 175.3 cm for the 5-mm shell group, $P = .438$), weight (83.3 kg for the thin shells versus 83.2 kg for the 5-mm shell group, $P = .942$), and BMI (26.8 for the thin shells versus 26.9 for the 5-mm shell group, $P = .586$). The gain was 2.2 mm ($P = .0001$) on the femoral side and –0.8 mm ($P = .0001$) on the acetabular side, showing that the 5-mm shell was already allowing a minimal amount of acetabular bone to be removed and that the main advantage of the thin shells resides in the ability to increase the size of the femoral component in order to maximize the fixation area and accommodate proximal femoral geometries characterized by a low head/neck ratio without the risk of notching the neck with the cylindrical reamer.

Femoral Bone Grafting

Twenty-five hips were grafted on the femoral side before the femoral component was cemented into place. In 17 cases, autologous grafting was performed using the paste from the reamings, and in eight cases, bone chips from allograft were used, often in combination with paste. The indications for grafting were the presence of a major bone defect after preparation of the femoral head, in particular in cases where a previous surgery (pinning, coring, and so on) left a defect considered too deep to fill with cement only. The average age of this group of patients was 41.2 years, and the average defect size was 21.7 mm. The average follow-up for this group is 6.5 years (range, 1.3 to 8.5 years)

Out of 25 hips, one was revised for loosening of the femoral component at 31 months (Fig. 9-3). Two hips present a radiolucency around the femoral metaphyseal stem. These two hips have been implanted for more than 7 years, they have now shown these lucencies for more than 6 years, and the patients are still asymptomatic. Our results do not either support or refute the use of bone graft, but our feeling at this time is not to graft because of the loss of valuable surface area for acrylic fixation except in those cases in which a very large defect was present in the neck and intertrochanteric area from

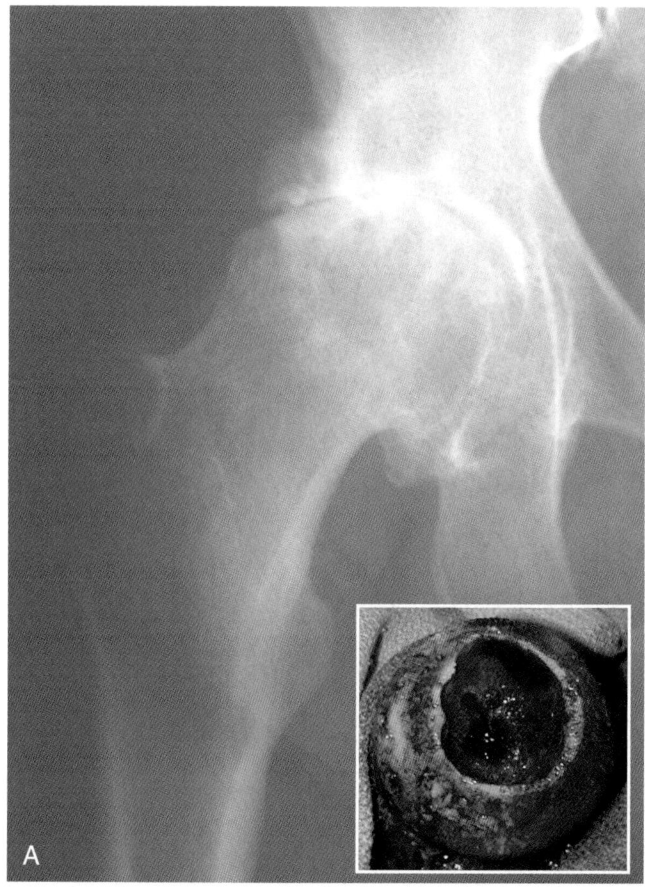

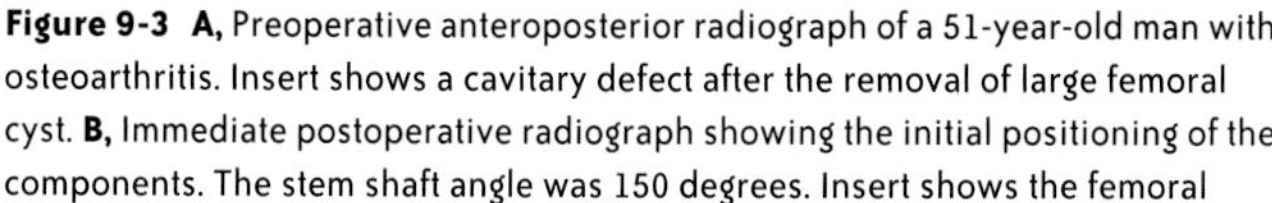

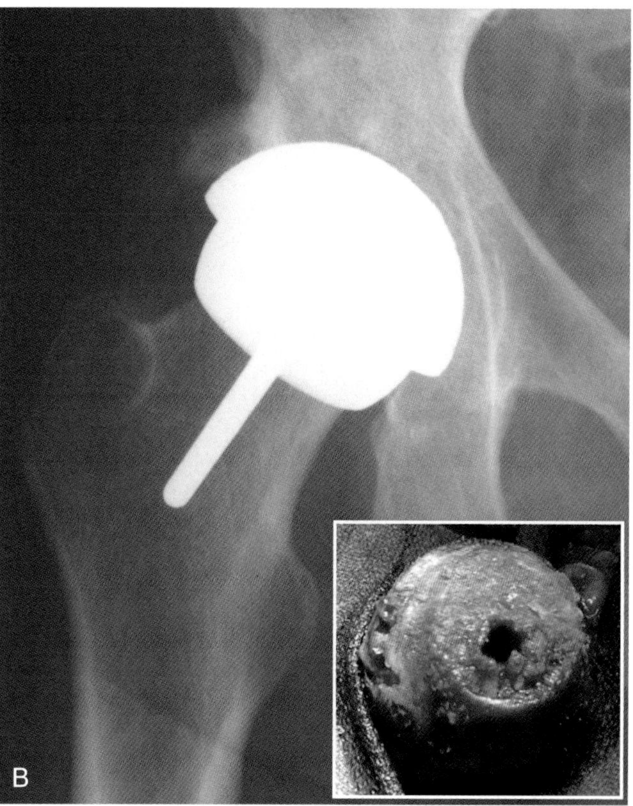

Figure 9-3 **A,** Preoperative anteroposterior radiograph of a 51-year-old man with osteoarthritis. Insert shows a cavitary defect after the removal of large femoral cyst. **B,** Immediate postoperative radiograph showing the initial positioning of the components. The stem shaft angle was 150 degrees. Insert shows the femoral head after grafting of the defect, just before cementation of the femoral component. Note the complete absence of any fixation holes in the chamfered area because the bone was thin.

previous coring, fibular grafting, or residual after removal of an intertrochanteric nail. In those situations, the graft is inserted distal to the head-neck junction.

Results

The average follow-up for the whole series of 1000 hips was 5.4 years (range, 1.0 to 10.8 years).

Clinical Scores

The average preoperative University of California-Los Angeles (UCLA) hip scores for the whole cohort were 3.6 ± 1.2 (standard deviation [SD]) for pain, 6.4 ± 1.4 for walking, 5.8 ± 1.6 for function, and 4.7 ± 1.5 for activity. The postoperative UCLA hip scores at last follow-up were 9.4 ± 0.9 for pain, 9.6 ± 0.9 for walking, 9.5 ± 1.2 for function, and 7.5 ± 1.6 for activity. All postoperative UCLA scores marked a significant improvement over the preoperative scores ($P < .0001$).

The average preoperative Short Form-12 (SF-12) scores were 32.97 ± 8.43 for the physical component and 48.04 ± 12.61 for the mental component. The average postoperative SF-12 scores were 50.90 ± 8.72 and 53.67 ± 8.97, and these improvements were also significant ($P < .0001$). In comparison, the average physical and mental components for the general U.S. population are 50.12 ± 9.45 and 50.04 ± 9.59.[11]

Specific data for the computation of the Harris Hip Score (HHS) were collected after hip #292 (with the beginning of the Conserve®Plus IDE), so an average preoperative score for the whole cohort is not available. However, the average postoperative HHS was 93.3 ± 8.9.

Conversions to Total Hip Replacement

There have been 32 successful conversions to total hip arthroplasty in this series. Eight were consecutive to a fracture of the femoral neck and occurred at an average of 11.1 months (range, 1 to 50 months). There were 20 conversions performed for aseptic loosening of the femoral component at an average time of 53.6 months (range, 23 to 103 months). Among these

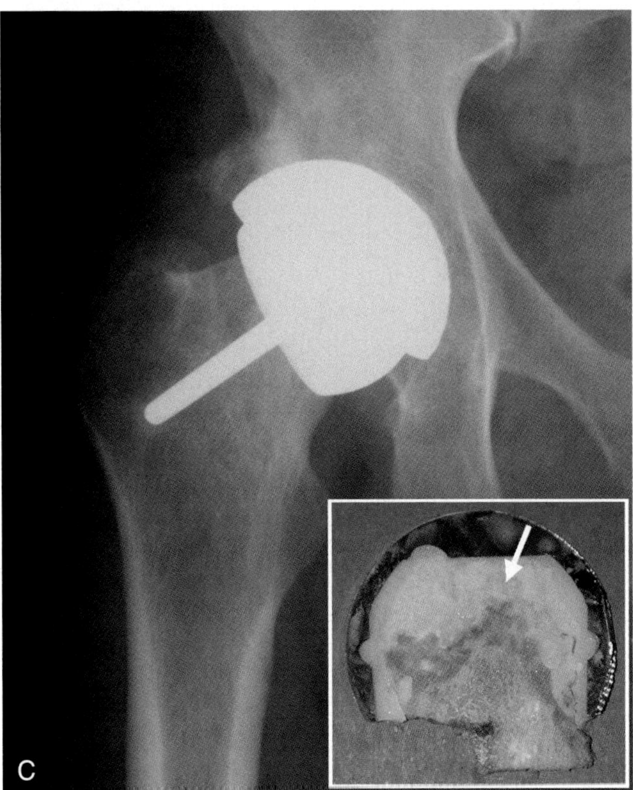

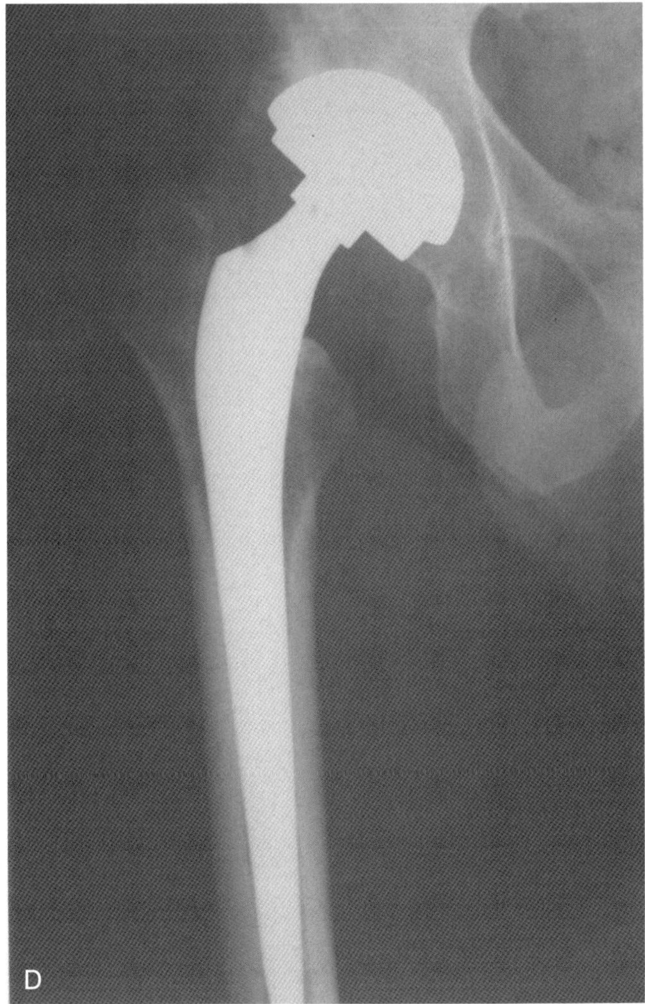

Figure 9-3, cont'd C, Thirty-one months after surgery, the femoral component tipped into varus. Insert shows a cut section of the retrieved femoral component. The bone graft material was necrotic bone with no evidence of new vascularity or repair. **D,** Four and a half years after conversion to total hip replacement. The femoral component was revised to an anthropometric total hip (ATH) long-stem grit-blasted size 9 and a 44 mm unipolar Big Femoral Head (Wright Medical Technology, Arlington, TN) matching the dimensions of the original acetabular component that was left in situ.

28 conversions secondary to aseptic failure of the femoral component, 21 were performed by the senior author and the well-fixed acetabular component was left in situ in 18. The remaining three underwent a revision of both components because a unipolar femoral head matching the inner diameter of the acetabular shell was not available at the time of surgery.[12]

There was one more conversion for aseptic femoral failure that could not be properly identified because the revision was performed at an outside institution and we were not provided with the retrieved implant or sufficient information to classify the failure.

Two hips were converted to THR for late hematogenous sepsis, one 13 months after resurfacing in a two-stage procedure and the other 36 months after resurfacing with a direct exchange. Both acetabular and femoral components were revised in either operation.

One hip was converted to THR 50 months after surgery because of recurrent subluxation secondary to impingement of the lesser trochanter against the ischium in an unusual case of developmental dysplasia of the hip with a prior valgus femoral osteotomy in which the neck/shaft angle was increased and the offset markedly reduced.

There were no conversions to THR consecutive to a loosening of the acetabular component in this series. This result is of great importance because it justifies the concept of resurfacing in young and active patients, who are likely to undergo more than one procedure during their lifetime: the durability of well-fixed porous-coated acetabular components retained at revision surgery has been demonstrated,[13] and the availability of unipolar femoral heads matching the socket dimensions potentially provides lifetime prosthetic solutions to the young patient with end-stage osteoarthritis.

Femoral Neck Fracture

Of eight femoral neck fractures, six occurred in femoral components that had been implanted with a 1-mm cement mantle (n = 926) for a prevalence of 0.6%. The other two occurred in femoral components that had been implanted with a tight fit, in which the cylindrical reaming diameter is identical to the inner diameter of the femoral component (n = 74), for a prevalence of 2.7%.

For the six fractures with a 1-mm cement mantle, the following risk factors have been identified[14]:

- Incomplete seating of the femoral component (component left proud)
- Uncovered reamed bone below the limit between the neck and the component, creating a 360-degree stress riser.
- Large cysts and osteopenia
- Overpenetration of cement
- Trauma (fall or extreme range of motion on a given movement)

Most cases did not present just one but a combination of these factors, highlighting the multifactorial nature of this mode of failure (Fig. 9-4).

Femoral Component Loosening

Femoral component aseptic loosening has been the dominant mode of failure in this series. However, modifications of the surgical technique (described in Chapter 7 and summarized at the end of the present chapter) have considerably reduced the prevalence of femoral loosening and the rate of appearance of metaphyseal stem radiolucencies. Table 9-3 shows the prevalence of radiolucencies and femoral loosenings sorted by generation of femoral fixation technique.

A rigorous comparison between generations of surgical technique can be made only through a time-dependent analysis to make a fair assessment of the progress, if any. This was made in a recent publication[4] demonstrating the improvement between first- and second-generation technique, using the time to appearance of a metaphyseal stem radiolucency as an endpoint. Figure 9-5 shows a case illustration of femoral component loosening in a hip treated with the first generation of femoral fixation technique.

Our initial publications identified the risk factors for femoral loosening, which are essentially related to the size of the area of fixation between bone and cement, and quality of the bone (size of femoral defects).[1,3] The immediate application of the progress made in the quality of the initial fixation is an advantage for the patients presenting the previously highlighted risk factors, as illustrated in Figure 9-6, which shows the difference in survivorship between first- and second-generation technique in patients with poor bone quality (femoral defects >1 cm).

Table 9-3 Prevalence of Radiolucencies and Femoral Loosenings Sorted by Generation of Femoral Fixation Technique

	Femoral Loosening	Stem Radiolucencies	Total	Follow-up (Months)
First generation (n = 300)	17 (5.7%)	11 (3.7%)	28 (9.3%)	97 (84-124)
Second generation (n = 371)	2 (0.5%)	2 (0.5%)	4 (1.1%)	64 (36-84)
Third generation (n = 329)	0 (0%)	0 (0%)	0 (0%)	20 (7-36)

Complications

There were a total of 55 complications in this series for an overall complication rate of 5.5%. Twenty of these events required a surgical intervention of some sort. The breakdown by according adverse event is presented in the following sections.

Dislocations

There were nine dislocations in this series, all but one occurring within the first month postoperatively. Two necessitated reoperation, one of them being converted to THR, as mentioned in the previous section, and one undergoing cup reorientation 3 days after initial surgery, when it was deemed a potential for recurrent dislocation or increased wear was present. All of the others were treated with closed reduction and have been stable since. Three of these dislocations were explained by a malposition of the acetabular component (either excessive abduction angle or excessive anteversion of the cup), four by a traumatic event, one by a proximal femoral geometry deemed unsuitable for resurfacing, and one by an extensive dissection of the soft tissues surrounding the joint to retrieve a scalpel blade fractured during surgery.[15]

Sepsis

There were six instances of sepsis in the series occurring at an average of 10.8 months after surgery (range, 0.3 to 35). Two of these patients underwent conversion to THR, as mentioned earlier. The other four were treated with débridement of the infected tissues surrounding the prosthesis and antibiotics. There has been no recurrence of the infection in any of them since the treatment.

Heterotopic Ossification

The incidence of heterotopic ossification (HO) Brooker grade III or IV was 7% in the first 400 hips using the protocol outlined in Chapter 7, with 1% having reduction of motion. Three hips in two patients required removal of heterotopic bone because of a significant limitation of range of motion, at an average of 15.4 months (range, 8 to 27 months). Preoperatively, 700 rads of radiation therapy was given before the surgical débridement and there was no reccurrence. One other patient has significant reduction of motion but has not undergone heterotopic bone removal 5.5 years postoperatively. The prevalence of HO that did not affect the patients' quality of life will be discussed later in the radiographic analysis section.

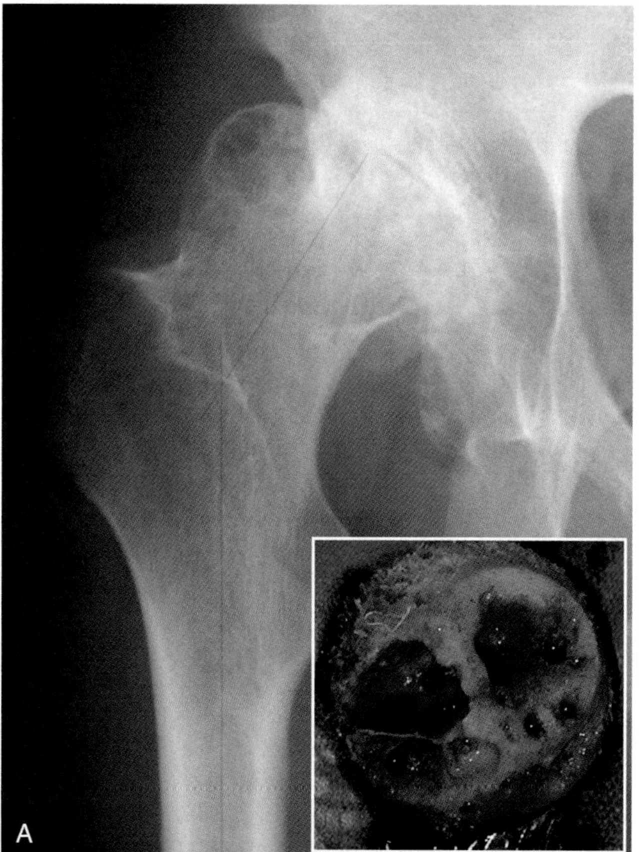

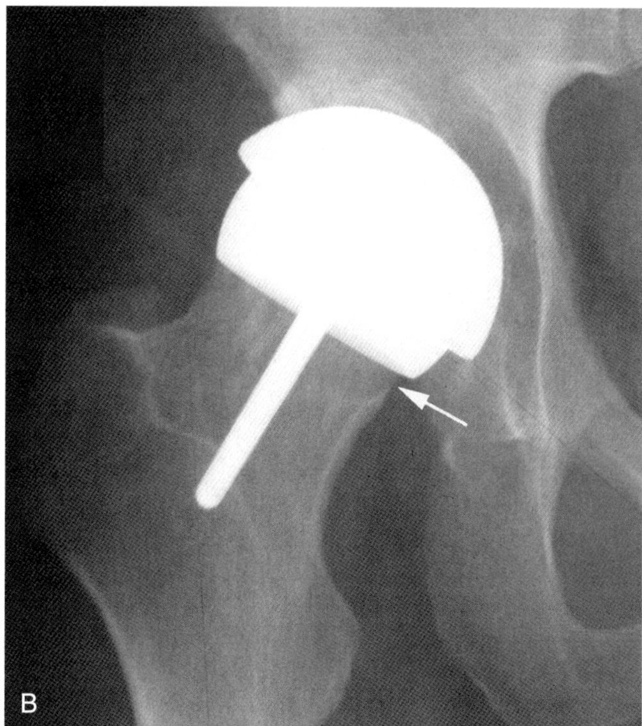

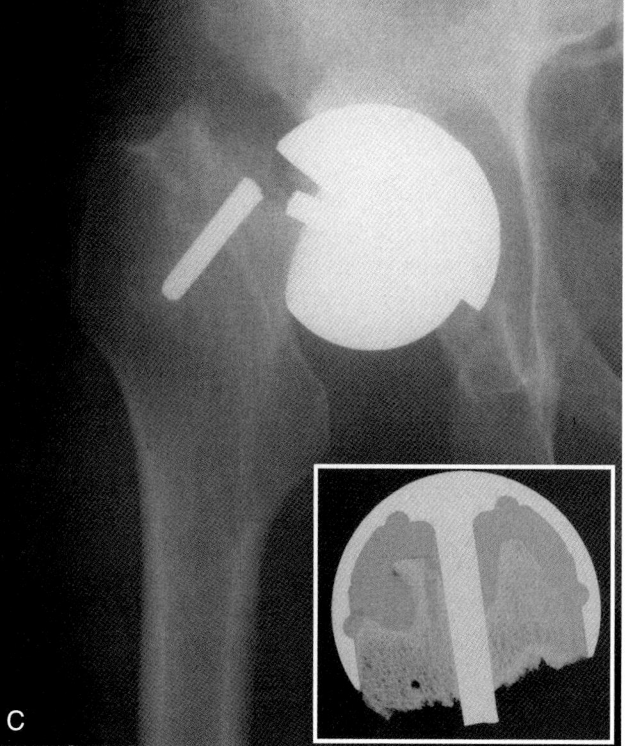

Figure 9-4 A, Preoperative anteroposterior radiograph of a 57-year-old man with developmental dysplasia of the hip. Insert shows the femoral head after preparation and reveals two large cystic defects. **B,** Immediate postoperative radiograph. An area of uncovered reamed bone is visible at the junction of the component and the medial aspect of the femoral neck *(arrow)*. **C,** Five months after surgery, the patient slipped and fell on icy ground and sustained a femoral neck fracture. Insert shows a microradiograph of the retrieved component. Note that the component was incompletely seated (proud), leaving a thick layer of cement in the dome area.

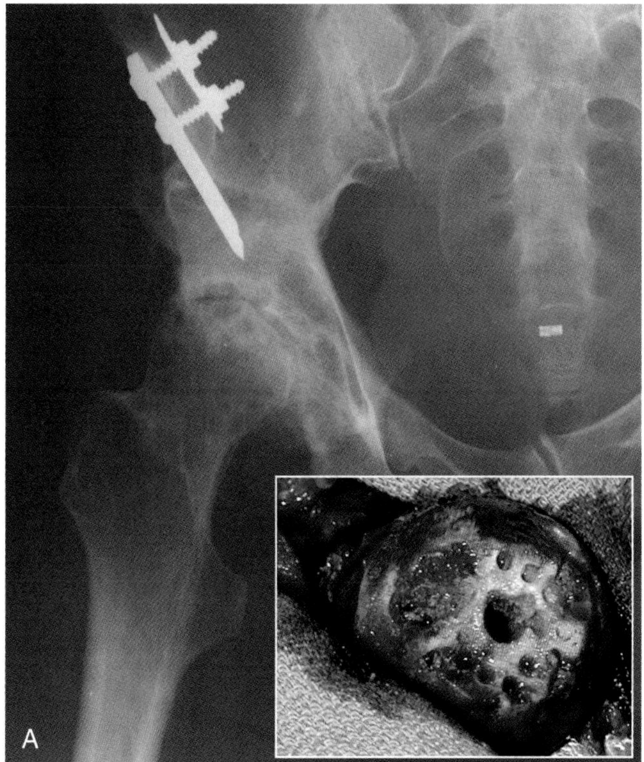

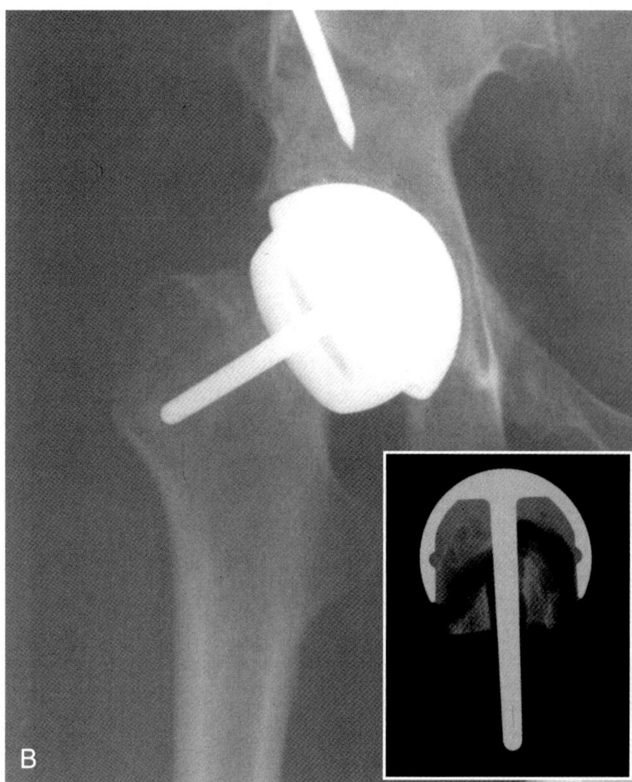

Figure 9-5 **A,** Preoperative anteroposterior radiograph of a 43-year-old woman with developmental dysplasia of the hip. Insert shows the femoral head after preparation, an example of the first generation of cementing technique. Very few drilled holes (to secure the bone-cement interface), and residual cystic material are visible. **B,** Thirty-nine months after surgery, the femoral component is loose (tipped into varus with a large metaphyseal stem radiolucency). Insert shows a microradiograph of a cut section of the retrieved head. There was a nonunion within the viable bone, with histologic evidence of ongoing bone repair at this site.

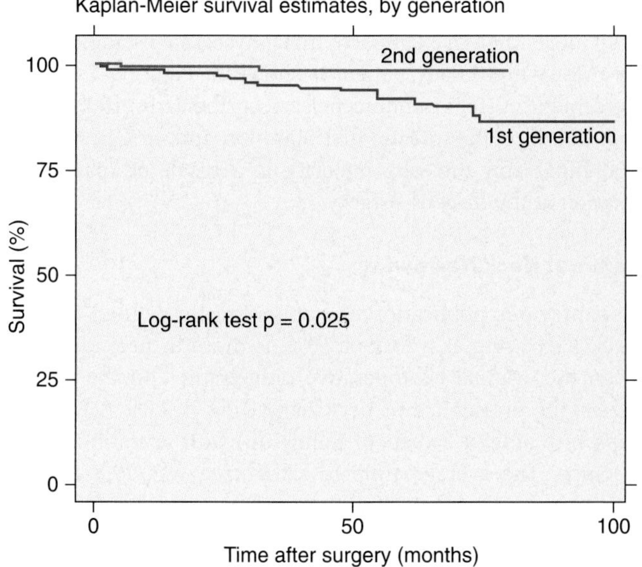

Figure 9-6 Kaplan and Meier survival estimates of the Conserve®Plus implanted by the senior author grouped by generation of femoral fixation technique, for patients with poor bone quality (femoral head defects >1 cm). Any conversion to total hip replacement was used as the endpoint.

Nerve Palsy

There were a total of 17 femoral nerve palsies in the series, and two of these cases presented pre-existing neural dysfunctions. All but one (a long thoracic nerve palsy, which had no relationship with the surgery and started 2 months after surgery) were identified in the recovery room. Of these 16, there were 15 femoral nerve palsies, which all resolved completely within a few months without treatment, and one peroneal nerve palsy associated with a common femoral artery thrombus and compartment syndrome. In this isolated case, the recovery was incomplete with permanent sequalae. The overall rate of femoral nerve palsy (1.5%) was relatively high but primarily attributed to an unsatisfactory anterior pelvic stabilizer in use from September of 2000 until May 2003, which provided good pelvic stability but, during the procedure, may have pressed on the femoral triangle and was likely primarily responsible for 12 of these 16 cases. After the use of this positioner was discontinued, the rate dropped to 0.4% and there has not been a single case of nerve palsy for the last 220 hips. The facility with which the procedure is now performed is probably also a factor with less femoral head pressure on the juxtapositioned femoral nerve during acetabulum preparation and socket implantation.

Blood-Related Complications

There were a total of 14 blood-related adverse events: four thrombophlebitis, one common femoral artery thrombus, six hematomas, and three bleeds. The thromboembolic phenomena were treated with warfarin sodium (Coumadin; four cases) or heparin (one case). Four hematomas resolved spontaneously, one was evacuated, and one resolved after holding Coumadin for 2 days.

Two bleedings resolved after holding prophylactic treatment, and the third one required re-exploration to repair a traumatized branch of the profunda. All of these events resolved without sequelae, except that the artery thrombus required thrombectomy of vessel and surgical release of the associated compartment syndrome.

Clicking

A small percent of patients report clicking, metallic sensations, or noises in the postoperative period, which are thought to be due to separation of the metallic surfaces before the capsule has healed. Rarely do the clicks persist. A grinding metallic sensation may occur when a patient stands, before initiating walking. However, with hip motion, this sensation disappears. This is due to the metal surfaces contacting one another without lubricant, and when walking is initiated, lubrication is entrained in between the surfaces and the sensation disappears. Finally, the patient may feel a click, or it may be audible if the components impinge such as in a patient with extreme degrees of motion or laxity. We have not observed any cases of squeaking or evidence of iliopsoas bursitis with the Conserve Plus but we have always been inserting this low-profile socket below the anterior pelvic wall. None of the noises or sensations described earlier are painful or thought to be pathologic.

Other Complications

There were six other adverse events recorded in this series:

In two hips, a re-exploration was required immediately postoperatively because debris (bone in one case and cement in the other) were trapped inside the joint space, revealed by an unusual appearance of the prosthesis on the anteroposterior postoperative radiograph. One of the five hips operated with a transtrochanteric approach had a non-union of the greater trochanter associated with trochanteric bursitis and necessitated wire removal. One hip was reoperated immediately after surgery to modify the abduction angle of the acetabular component, without any dislocation, when it was identified on the postoperative radiograph that this angle was too high. One hip had to be reoperated and a cup exchange performed because of a mismatch of components during the initial surgery. The inside diameter of the socket was 44 mm, but a 42-mm outside diameter head was implanted by mistake. The difference was small enough so that the range of motion check routinely performed did not reveal any malfunction of the joint. High ion levels after 1 year indicated the need for revision of the cup, which was exchanged for a custom-made Conserve®Plus shell with an outside diameter of 55 mm and an inside diameter of 42 mm. Finally, one hip needed acetabular reconstruction after the acetabular shell protruded through the acetabular wall. The patient was heavy, had poor bone quality, and had undergone simultaneous bilateral resurfacing (the event occurred on the first hip operated). In addition, the wall had presumably been further weakened by over-reaming.

Radiographic Analysis

Metaphyseal Stem Radiolucencies

Metaphyseal stem radiolucencies have been associated with impending aseptic loosening of the femoral component in modern-generation metal-on-metal resurfacing.[1] In the present series, 13 hips in 12 patients presented metaphyseal stem radiolucencies at the last radiographic follow-up. However, only one was associated with clinical symptoms of component loosening in a patient who was deported and lost to follow-up before a revision of the component could be performed. The other 12 hips have now shown these radiolucencies for an average of 67.4 months (range 31 to 90 months) with no clinical sign of loosening. The average activity level is less than the overall group with only 6.9 (range 4 to 10) whereas three patients maintained a high level of physical activity. These data suggest that the presence of a metaphyseal stem radiolucency, although certainly revealing a degree of micromotion at the bone-component interface, is not a reliable predictor for the onset of symptoms due to a femoral component loosening. Nonetheless we consider hips showing a metaphyseal stem radiolucency at risk for femoral component loosening. An example of metaphyseal stem radiolucency in a nonsymptomatic patient is shown in Figure 9-7. A high percentage of stem radiolucencies occurred early (100% in the first 500 hips, 85% in the first 300 hips, and 46% in the first 100 hips) and the vast majority is a result of inadequate fixation at the time of surgery.

Femoral Neck Narrowing

In a previous publication, we operationally defined femoral neck narrowing as a loss of 10% or more in neck diameter from the original postoperative radiograph.[16] In the present series, the prevalence of neck narrowing is 2.8% (21 of 753 hips with at least 2 years of follow-up) with seven in the first 70 hips. The average time to narrowing was 29.8 months (range, 9 to 47 months). Fifty percent stopped progressing. Two underwent revision for femoral component loosening. The average cup angle was 44.4 degrees (range, 22 to 64 degrees). Sixty-five percent had femoral head defects larger than 1 cm observed during surgery. Four had a cemented metaphyseal stem, but there was no difference in incidence with the rest of the group (P = .753) and the functional outcome was not affected (average HHS 93.0, range 81 to 100).

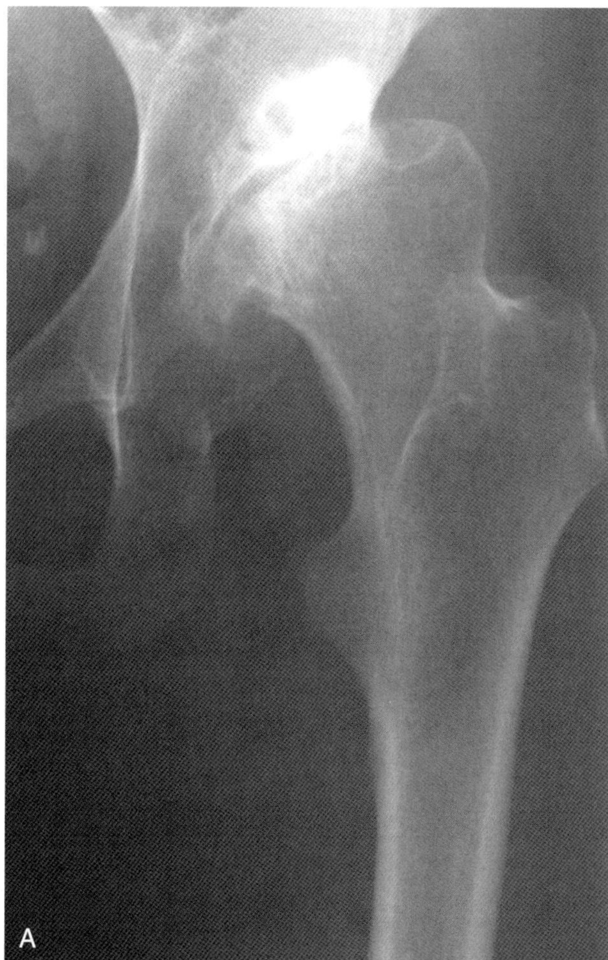

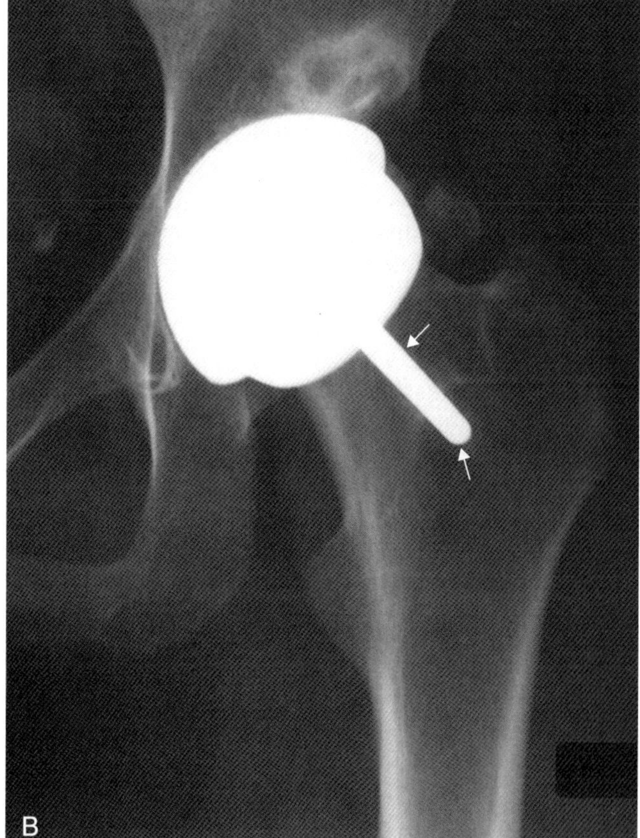

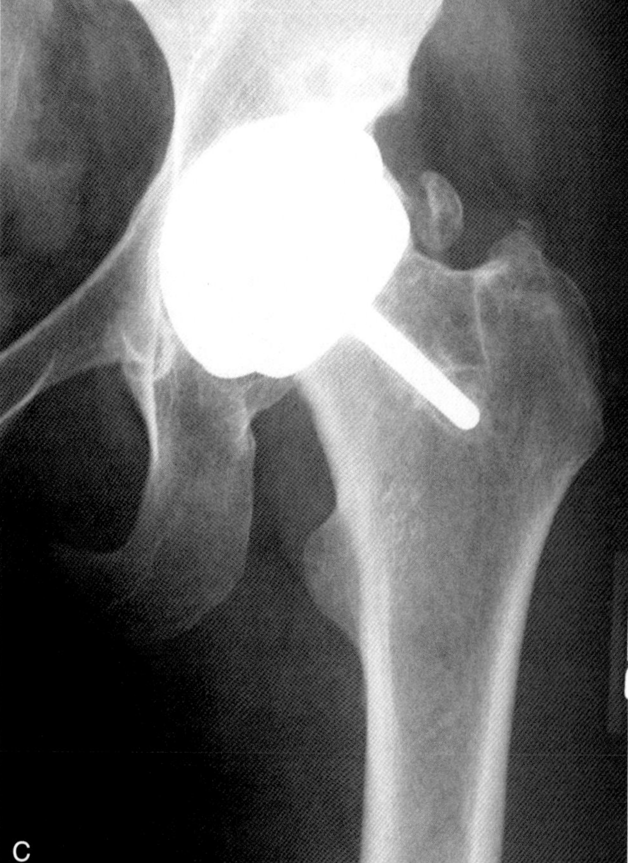

Figure 9-7 **A,** Anteroposterior radiograph of a 40-year-old woman with developmental dysplasia of the hip. **B,** Ten months after surgery, a metaphyseal stem radiolucency appeared on the follow-up radiograph. **C,** Eight and a half years after surgery, the radiolucency is still present and the patient is completely asymptomatic (University of California-Los Angeles [UCLA] scores of 10, 10, 10, and 7 for pain, walking, function, and activity, respectively). The radiolucency has now been visible for 90 months without clinical signs of loosening. She has avoided impact activities.

Although the etiology and significance are unknown, possible causes include stress shielding (due to reduction of femoral head diameter in hips resurfaced with the thick shells) or external pressure due to synovitis or pseudotumors. With the introduction of the thin socket shell, the reamed femoral bone diameter and component size, on average, are now 2 mm larger than they were with the 5-mm shells, thus adding area for fixation but the impact on neck narrowing is as yet unknown. Osteolysis, defined as bone resorption related to metal particulate debris, might be an additional possible etiology. The prevalence of neck narrowing in the current series seems to be less than with other currently used metal-on-metal resurfacing designs. Lilikakis[17] and Hing[18] reported 27% and 27.6% of neck narrowing for the Cementless Cormet 2000 (Corin Medical, Cirencester, UK) and the Birmingham Hip Resurfacing (Smith and Nephew, Finsbury Orthopedics Ltd, Surrey, UK), respectively.

Heterotopic Ossification

The cause of HO is unknown, most likely multifactorial, and probably related to muscle trauma and bone debris. It is also related to gender and ethnicity, which makes comparisons between procedures and prophylactic treatments difficult. The incidence might be higher after metal-on-metal resurfacing than with total hip replacement both because of muscle and soft tissue stretching during the reaming and implantation of the socket and because of the increased amount of bone debris generated during the preparation of the femoral head. However, there are currently no data to support this statement.

In the current series, we recorded the presence of HO according to the Brooker scale[19] on the first 700 hips implanted to ensure a minimum radiographic follow-up of 2 years. The overall incidence of HO was 23.6%, with 13.9% of grade I, 4.6% of grade II, 4.5% of grade III, and 0.6% of grade IV. As expected, women were less affected than the men, with 10.5% overall, only grade I (7.6%) or grade II (2.9%). There was an evolution over time in the overall incidence of HO, and the first 300 hips showed a higher overall prevalence than the next 400 (30.6% versus 18.4%, Mann-Whitney U test, $P = .0002$). When examining the HO grades with clinical significance (Brooker III and IV), the prevalence decreased from 7% to 3.5% between the first 300 and the next 400 hips. This difference was significant (Chi-square, $P = .0404$). It is probable that a change in technique by using a so-called eye sheet to catch the debris before it could get into the tissues during chamfer reaming and increasing the irrigation to 4000 mL coupled with the facility of the operation were factors in the reduction of the incidence.

Survivorship Analysis

Implant survival techniques have been used on a regular basis over the course of the last 10 years of experience with Conserve®Plus

1. As a means to compare the overall results of the prosthesis to previous designs
2. To establish the efficacy of modifications in the surgical technique[4]
3. To compare the results of subgroups within the population of patients implanted with Conserve®Plus and to identify risk factors for the procedure[3]

For the entire study group, the current Kaplan and Meier survival estimates of the prosthesis, using any conversion to total hip replacement as endpoint are 98.0% at 3 years (95% confidence interval [CI], 96.6% to 98.9%), 96.3% at 4 years (95% CI, 94.3% to 97.7%), 94.6% at 5 years (95% CI, 91.9% to 96.4%), and 91.3% at 8 years (95% CI, 86.9% to 94.3%). These numbers represent conservative estimates of the performance of the device and are likely to improve as the follow-up of the recent cases increases because most of the early failures happened in the first 100 hips that were operated on, during the phase of development of the device and the procedure. As an example, we reported a survival rate of 94.4% at 4 years in January of 2004,[1] a rate that is now 2% better with the addition of 3 years of follow-up and a total of 550 patients at this level of follow-up.

In comparison with early resurfacing designs, these results are already far better and indicate the superiority of the Conserve®Plus with a metal-on-metal bearing over the metal-on-polyethylene ones, which showed 70% survival at 5 years and 40% and 8 years with the Wagner design,[20] for example. In Figure 9-8, we plotted the survivorship curves of the Conserve®Plus study group and the THARIES devices implanted by the senior author at UCLA in the 1970s and 1980s.

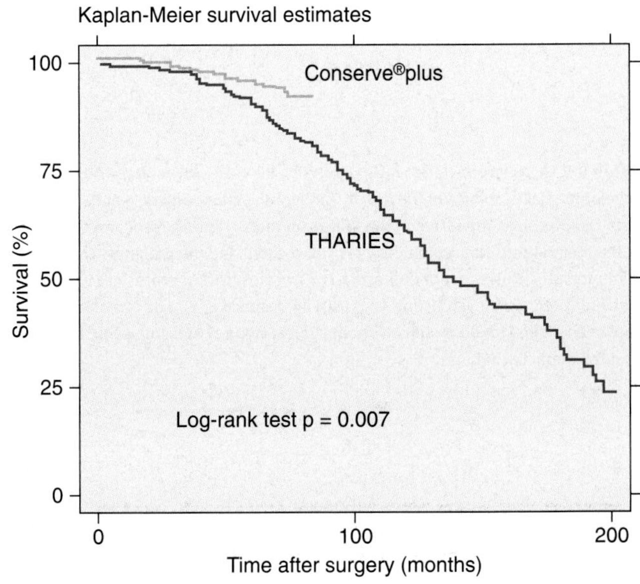

Figure 9-8 Comparative Kaplan and Meier survival estimates of the Conserve®Plus and the THARIES implanted by the senior author, using any conversion to total hip replacement as the endpoint.

In a previous publication,[4] we showed the efficacy of surgical technique implemented gradually between hip #100 and hip #300 on the prevention of femoral component loosening. There was a significant improvement ($P = .016$) of the second 300 hips over the first 300 in a time-dependent analysis using as an endpoint the time to appearance of a metaphyseal stem radiolucency, suggesting potential femoral component loosening. The combination of changes affecting the initial component fixation (adding fixation holes in the dome and chamfered areas) and cleansing and drying using a suction tip in the dome hole, were significantly related to the improvement of the results. In this analysis, the Cox proportional hazard ratio was used, allowing a control for possible covariates like the surface arthroplasty risk index (SARI), an indicator of the overall risk for failure that we calculated for each hip in the series. The SARI had been previously developed from a series of 94 hips in patients 40 years old or younger,[3] in which independent variables influencing the results had been identified and weighted to yield the following scoring system:

- Weight less than 82 kg = 2 points
- Femoral head defects greater than 1 cm in size = 2 points
- Previous surgery on the operated hip = 1 point
- Activity level (UCLA scoring system) of 7 or more = 1 point

The SARI was subsequently validated when applied to the first 400 hip implants,[1] and a significant increase ($P = .004$) in the risk of early failure found in patients with a SARI greater than 3. However, the adverse effect of a high SARI score has been mitigated in our later cases by the very significant improvement in initial fixation due to improved technique, which has resulted in the absence of stem radiolucencies and loosening despite risk factors.

One of the main results of survivorship analyses in the first generation of metal-on-polyethylene resurfacing devices were the differences between etiologies, with the advantage to primary (idiopathic) osteoarthritis over the other etiologies ($P = .011$).[21] In the present series, this effect has not been observed with up to 10 years of follow-up, and the survivorship curves of the various etiologies are not statistically different ($P = .437$, log rank test) as illustrated in Figure 9-9.

The age of the patient at surgery has been considered so far a factor influencing the long-term survivorship of the prostheses, whether resurfacing or conventional stem type design.[22] As a matter of fact, age is considered an inversely proportional surrogate variable for patient activity level, which is much more difficult to quantify.[23] In the present series, we compared the survivorship results of the older patients (50 years of age and older) with those of patients younger than 50 years. We found no difference in prosthetic survivorship between the two patient groups, even after adjustment for SARI scores (Cox ratio 0.837, 95% CI, 0.403 to 1.738, $P = .634$). This result is in contrast with the literature related to conventional THA. It could be somewhat attributed to the prosthetic design but certainly reflects the very high activity level of all the patients

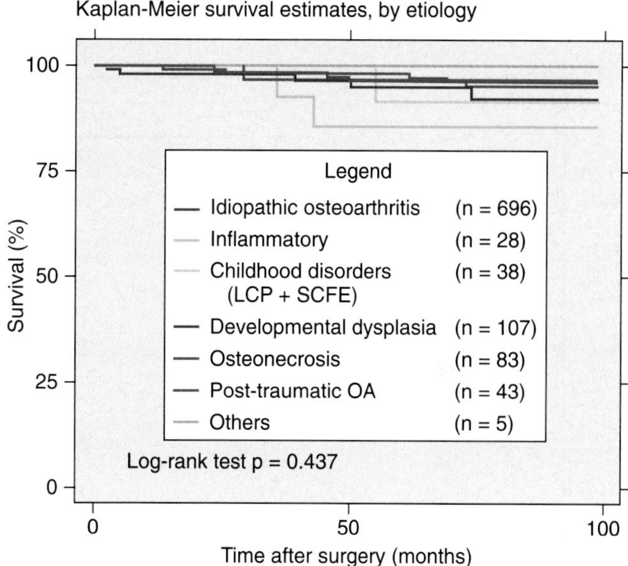

Figure 9-9 Kaplan and Meier survival estimates of the Conserve®Plus implanted by the senior author, sorted by etiology, and using any conversion to total hip replacement as the endpoint.

in this series, both younger and older. The average UCLA activity score for either group was 7.6 ± 1.6 (SD) ($P = .487$, Mann-Whitney U test).

The affect of obesity on the outcome of THA remains a controversial topic. A review of the literature by Stukenborg-Colsman et al[24] concluded that obesity appears to have a negative impact on the results of total hip and knee arthroplasty. However, a recent publication from McLaughlin and Lee[25] showed no difference in revision rate of uncemented THR at a mean follow-up of 14.5 years. In light of these indecisive data, many physicians take a conservative approach and are reluctant to refer patients for surgery or operate when their BMI is high.[26] In the present series, we found that the 5-year survivorship results of the patients with a BMI equal or greater than 30 (the official definition for obesity) were 98.6% at 5 years (95% CI, 94.5% to 99.7%), using any revision as endpoint. Looking at the entire cohort, the effect of BMI on survivorship was more linear than dichotomous, and creating 3 groups (BMI less than 25, BMI 25 to less than 30, and BMI 30 or more) gave a significant linear trend, even after adjusting for femoral defect size ($P = .013$) as illustrated in Figure 9-10. This is consistent with the positive association between weight and medium-term prosthetic survival in resurfacing that we had suggested in previous publications.[1,3] There are certainly several possible explanations for this result, among which the increased average size of the femoral component needed to resurface the patients from the study group, a difference of 1.5 mm ($P < .0001$) associated with the greater proportion of men in the study group. Also a greater BMI is correlated with a greater bone mineral density of the proximal femur,[27] so the study group benefited from a better bone quality (independently from cyst formation) for implantation of the femoral component. Finally, the study group had a lower postoperative

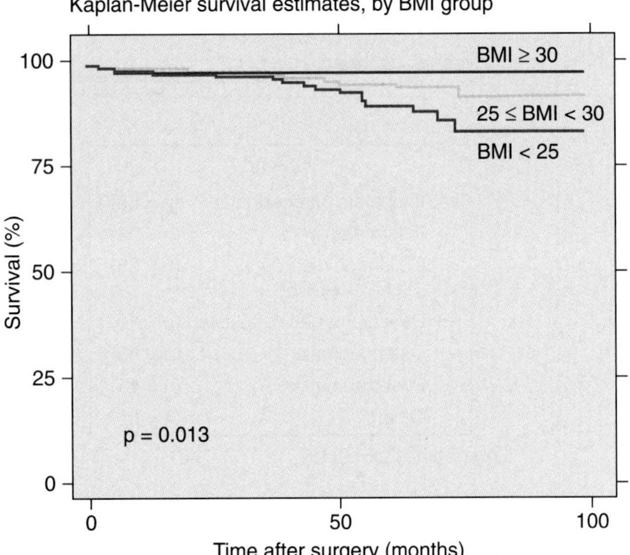

Figure 9-10 Kaplan and Meier survival estimates of the Conserve®Plus implanted by the senior author, sorted by body mass index group, and using any conversion to total hip replacement as the endpoint.

activity score (even though 62% still engage regularly in some sort of sporting activity), and this factor may have contributed to reduce the amount of aseptic loosening in comparison with the rest of the cohort.

Summary of Design and Technique Changes to Reduce Complications and Improve Durability

Femoral Neck Fractures

1. Avoidance of technical errors. Special care should be taken to precisely ream the head and fully seat the component.
2. Development of the thin Conserve®Plus acetabular shells for a greater preservation of the acetabular bone without notching the femoral neck.
3. Improved instrumentation with dome stops to prevent reaming into the femoral neck.

Femoral Loosening

1. Markedly improved bone preparation and cleaning (facilitated by the use of Carbo-Jet).
2. Added stem cementation in hips with risk factors.

Dislocation

1. Experience with insertion and assessment of component orientation. A conscious effort is needed to avoid verticalization of the socket.
2. Introduction of low-profile socket inserter to better visualize the acetabulum during insertion.
3. Check stability, with range of motion performed in both flexion and extension, and make appropriate adjustments to avoid impingement. Remove the socket, if necessary; clean of all soft tissue; and reinsert. This can be performed with relative ease with the Conserve®Plus. The facility to do this varies with other systems.

Nerve Palsy

1. Avoid any potential pressure on the femoral triangle area and the femoral nerve by secure pelvic stabilization on the symphysis area, sacrum and trunk.
2. Debulk the femoral head especially posteriorly and inferiorly to facilitate the exposure for acetabular preparation.

Heterotopic Bone

1. Shorten operating time.
2. More irrigation (increase to 4000 mL).
3. Protection of tissues from bone debris while reaming, especially with the chamfer reamer.
4. Position the femoral head during reaming of the acetabulum to minimize trauma to the abductor muscles.

Comparison to Other Published Results in the Literature

The survivorship after hip resurfacing with good bone quality is apparent, although none of the other reports have as long and detailed a follow-up, including serial anteroposterior and cross-table lateral radiographs as reported in our review. McMinn reported on 446 hips resurfaced with the McMinn and BHR with a 3-year mean follow-up with 99.8% survivorship with good bone quality. However, this was not a consecutive series and did not include personal follow-up and complete x-ray analysis.[7] Treacy reported on 144 BHR with a 98% 5-year survivorship with good bone quality.[8] Two further studies report good short-term results with the BHR with good bone quality.[5,6] Schmalzried published the results of a series of 91 hips that had good bone quality with a 2-year follow-up with the Conserve®Plus.[28] There were no neck fractures or other short-term failures. In contrast to these reports, Cutts reported results of 65 hips resurfaced by five surgeons with a 21% failure rate with the Cormet prosthesis.[29] Failures included six neck fractures, four socket loosenings, one osteonecrosis (ON), one case of sepsis, and two cases of increased pain.

There are no published results in the literature of a comparable series to that reported in this chapter, in which challenging hips with significant risk factors have been resurfaced. The fact that we have demonstrated a significant improvement in survivorship in these challenging hips emphasizes the importance of surgical technique. Other studies with thorough clinical and x-ray analysis are needed to establish long-term efficacy of those resurfaced with comparable risk factors.

References

1. Amstutz H, Beaulé P, Dorey F, Le Duff M, Campbell P, Gruen T: Metal-on-metal hybrid surface arthroplasty: two to six year follow-up. J Bone Joint Surg 2004;86A:28-39.
2. Amstutz H, Ball S, Le Duff M, Dorey F: Hip resurfacing for patients under 50 years of age. Results of 350 Conserve Plus with a 2-9 year follow-up. Clin Orthop 2007;460:159-164.
3. Beaulé P, Dorey F, Le Duff M, Gruen T, Amstutz H: Risk factors affecting early outcome of metal on metal surface arthroplasty of the hip in patients 40 years old and younger. Clin Orthop 2004;418:87-93.
4. Amstutz H, Le Duff M, Campbell P, Dorey F: The effects of technique changes on aseptic loosening of the femoral component in hip resurfacing. Results of 600 Conserve Plus with a 3-9 year follow-up. J Arthroplasty 2007;22:481-489.
5. De Smet K: Belgium experience with metal-on-metal surface arthroplasty. Orthop Clin North Am 2005;36:203-213.
6. Back D, Dalziel R, Young D, Shimmin A: Early results of primary Birmingham hip resurfacings. An independent prospective study of the first 230 hips. J Bone Joint Surg 2005;87B:324-329.
7. Daniel J, Pynsent PB, McMinn D: Metal-on-metal resurfacing of the hip in patients under the age of 55 years with osteoarthritis. J Bone Joint Surg 2004;86 B:177-188.
8. Treacy R, McBryde C, Pynsent P: Birmingham hip resurfacing arthroplasty. A minimum follow-up of five years. J Bone Joint Surg Br 2005;87:167-170.
9. Vendittoli P, Lavigne M, Roy A, Lusignan D: A prospective randomized clinical trial comparing metal-on-metal total hip arthroplasty and metal-on-metal total hip resurfacing in patients less than 65 years old. Hip International 2006;16:873-881.
10. Le Duff M, Amstutz H, Dorey F: Metal-on-metal hip resurfacing for obese patients. J Bone Joint Surg Am 2007;89: 2705-2711.
11. Ware J, Kosinski M, Keller S: SF-12: How to Xcore the SF-12 Physical and Mental Health Summary Scales. Lincoln, RI, Quality Metric Inc., 1998.
12. Ball S, Le Duff M, Amstutz H: Early results of conversion of a failed femoral component in hip resurfacing arthroplasty. J Bone Joint Surg Am 2007;89:735-741.
13. Beaulé P, Dorey F, Le Duff M: Fate of cementless acetabular components retained during revision of a femoral component of a total hip arthroplsty. J Bone Joint Surg 2003;85-A:2288-2293.
14. Amstutz H, Campbell P, Le Duff M: Fracture of the neck of the femur after surface arthroplasty of the hip. J Bone Joint Surg 2004;86 A:1874-1877.
15. Prasad R, Amstutz HC, Sparling EA: Use of a magnet to retrieve a broken scalpel blade. J Arthroplasty 2000;15:806-808.
16. Beaulé P, Le Duff M, Campbell P, Dorey F, Park S, Amstutz H: Metal-on-metal surface arthroplasty with a cemented femoral component: A 7-10 year follow-up study. J Arthroplasty 2004; 19:17-22.
17. Lilikakis A, Vowler S, Villar R: Hydroxyapatite-coated femoral implant in metal-on-metal resurfacing hip arthroplasty: minimum of two years follow-up. Orthop Clin North Am 2005; 36:215-222.
18. Hing C, Young D, Dalziel R, Bailey M, Back D, Shimmin A: Narrowing of the neck in resurfacing of the hip—a radiological study. J Bone Joint Surg Br 2007;89:1019-1024.
19. Brooker A, Bowerman J, Robinson R, Riley L: Ectopic ossification following total hip replacement. Incidence and a method of classification. J Bone Joint Surg 1973;55A:1629-1632.
20. Howie DW, Campbell D, McGee M, Cornish BL: Wagner resurfacing hip arthroplasty. The results of one hundred consecutive arthroplasties after eight to ten years. J Bone Joint Surg Am 1990;72:708-714.
21. Amstutz H, Grigoris P, Dorey F: Evolution and future of surface replacement of the hip. J Orthop Sci 1998;3:169-186.
22. Kim WC, Grogan T, Amstutz HC, Dorey F: Survivorship comparison of THARIES and conventional hip arthroplasty in patients younger than 40 years old. Clin Orthop 1987;214: 269-277.
23. Dorey FJ, Amstutz HC: The need to account for patient activity when evaluating the results of total hip arthroplasty with survivorship analysis. J Bone Joint Surg Am 2002;84-A:709-710.
24. Stukenborg-Colsman C, Ostermeier S, Windhagen H: What effect does obesity have on the outcome of total hip and knee arthroplasty. Review of the literature. Orthopade 2005;34: 664-667.
25. McLaughlin J, Lee K: The outcome of total hip replacement in obese and non-obese patients at 10- to 18-years. J Bone Joint Surg Br 2006;88:1286-1292.
26. Sturmer T, Dreinhofer K, Grober-Gratz D, Brenner H, Dieppe P, Puhl W, Gunther K: Differences in the views of orthopaedic surgeons and referring practitioners on the determinants of outcome after total hip replacement. J Bone Joint Surg Br 2005;87:1416-1419.
27. Pocock N, Eisman J, Gwinn T, Sambrook P, Kelly P, Freund J, Yeates M: Muscle strength, physical fitness, and weight but not age predict femoral neck bone mass. J Bone Miner Res 1989;4:441-448.
28. Schmalzried T, Silva M, de la Rosa M, Choi E, Fowble V: Optimizing patient selection and outcomes with total hip resurfacing. Clin Orthop Relat Res 2005;441:200-204.
29. Cutts S, Datta A, Ayoub K, Rahman H, Lawrence T: Early failure modalities in hip resurfacing. Hip International 2005;15: 155-158.

CHAPTER 10

Modes of Failures: Fractures and Loosening

Patricia A. Campbell
William Lundergan

Introduction

In the early 1970s, several centers in Europe, Japan, and the United States adopted surface replacement arthroplasty as a means of treating young patients with a variety of degenerative hip diseases.[1,2] Over the following years, those centers reported their early results and detailed the complications that were common to stem-type hip replacement (such as component loosening) as well as those that were unique to the resurfacing operation (such as neck fracture) (Table 10-1). Almost without exception, the analysis of early failures led to changes in prosthetic design, patient selection criteria, and surgical technique. For example, the earliest Imperial College London Hospital (ICLH) resurfacing design employed a polymeric femoral component and a metal acetabular component. Retrieval analysis showed that this was associated with loosening, so the two component materials were switched. In addition, the large trochanteric osteotomy and invasive screw fixation were associated with neck fracture, so the surgical technique was modified, reducing the incidence of neck fractures.[3]

Despite progress from these and other improvements, surface arthroplasty was largely abandoned in the 1980s because of poor mid- and late-term survivorship, but Amstutz et al[4,5] pursued the technique and emphasized the continuing need for evolution and optimization of the technique, materials, instrumentation. and implant design. This included the analysis of failures performed at a specialized laboratory at the University of California-Los Angeles (UCLA). Concurrent with the analysis of stem-type hip replacement failures, it was eventually shown that the majority of hip replacement failures were the result of inadequate materials, especially ultra-high-molecular-weight polyethylene (UHMWPE).[6-8] Although this situation has now been overcome by the introduction of metal-on-metal resurfacings, the study of first-generation failures provides a basis for understanding modern resurfacing failures, particularly when long-term retrievals are included. This retrospective introduction also highlights the advances that modern generation resurfacings provide the contemporary orthopaedic surgeon.

First-Generation Failure Modes

Amstutz et al[9] described four main failure modes in first-generation resurfacings (Box 10-1 Resurfacing Modes of Failure), and the first three are discussed further later.

Aseptic Loosening

Aseptic loosening is one failure mode that resurfacing components have in common with conventional hip replacements. Aseptic loosening, particularly on the acetabular side, was the most common cause for failure among 163 failures of 586 Total Hip Articular Replacement Arthroplasty (THARIES, DePuy, Warsaw, IN) resurfacings performed by the author.[10,11] Implant retrieval analysis and wear measurements of the retrieved PE liners determined that aseptic loosening was the result of PE wear debris–induced interfacial bone resorption.[12] The larger size of the resurfacing bearings compared with the small ball size (22-32 mm) used in conventional total hip replacement was found to be disadvantageous in terms of a higher PE wear rate[13,14] such that there was a clear wear penalty for the larger bearings. The close proximity of the interfaces to the source of the debris was also thought to make resurfacings more vulnerable to wear-induced osteolysis.[15]

Femoral Loosening

The observation of bone erosion at the margins of the femoral component and the neck by an invasive membrane communicating with the joint and containing abundant polyethylene debris supported this contention.[16-18] In 1990, Howie et al[19] detailed the histopathologic findings of 72 Wagner resurfacings that were revised from 8 to 70 months postoperatively and devised a classification of loosening based on the integrity of

Table 10-1 Complications Common to Stem-type Hip Replacement and Unique to Resurfacing Arthroplasty

Authors	Implant Types	# Retrievals Incidence of Failure (%)	Predominant Failure Mode	Authors' Reason for Failure	Comments
Howie et al[18]	Wagner	72 (n/a)	Aseptic loosening both	Polyethylene wear-induced bone loss	Four grades of loosening
Sedel et al[52]	Spherocylindric (Luck)	38 (18%)	Variable	1 sepsis, 3 unsatisfactory technique, 1 unexplained, 2 due to predisposed factors	
Cotella et al[20]	ICLH Double-Cup	92 (23%)	Aseptic loosening both	Erosive cellular response to polyethylene debris	No difference in cemented and uncemented
Schreiber et al[29]	ICLH Double-Cup	43 (24%)	Aseptic loosening femoral	Adverse biomechanical stresses disrupts cement-bone interface	
Morberg et al[23]	8 Wagner, 11 ICLH and 6 KMI	25 (n/a)	Aseptic loosening both	Excessive joint forces disturbed interface, Negative long-term effects of the cement	AVN not seen
Bell et al[17]	Wagner	18 (9%)	Aseptic loosening acetabular	Combination of mechanical and biologic factors	AVN not seen
Bogoch et al[16]	Indiana	6 (n/a)	Femoral neck fracture	Fracture through viable/ nonviable bone junction	3 of 6 had AVN
Amstutz et al[9]	THARIES	n/a (12%)	Aseptic loosening acetabular	Osteolysis by wear-induced histiocytic tissue	AVN not seen
Milgram and Rana[53]	Cementless double-cup arthroplasty	31 (n/a)	Aseptic loosening femoral	Continuation of degenerative arthritic processes	AVN, fibrous replacement of bone common
Morberg et al[54]	ICLH double cup	11 (n/a)	Aseptic loosening acetabular	Gradual deterioration of bone at the cement interface	AVN not seen
Duijsens et al[55]	Gerard (cementless)	61 (41%)	Aseptic loosening femoral	Resorption of femoral head & neck	Femoral head resorption in 33

AVN, avascular necrosis; ICLH, Imperial College London Hospital; KMI, Kinetics Medical Incorporated; THARIES, Total Hospital Articular Replacement with Internal Eccentric Shells.

BOX 10-1 Resurfacing Modes of Failure

Mode I Aseptic loosening
Mode II Femoral neck fracture
Mode III Wear-induced osteolysis
Mode IV Sepsis

the femoral cement–bone interface. Four grades were defined: 0 = bone-cement contact ;1 = connective tissue–cement contact; 2 = slightly loose; 3 = markedly loose. In the grade 3 cases, there was marked loss of femoral head shape and replacement of the proximal bone by a thick fibrous tissue. Macrophages and wear particles, predominantly of polyethylene, were identified in all four grades, including those that were solidly fixed. Although polymethyl methacrylate bone cement particles were acknowledged to be a possible contributing factor to the histiocytic response at the interface, particularly in loose cases, PE particles were thought to be more important in the initiation of bone resorption at the bone-cement interface and the progression of the loosening process.

The key role of UHMWPE was supported by a comparison of cemented and cementless femoral ICLH components in which the failure rates were comparable.[20] Similarly, a detailed analysis of failed noncemented surface arthroplasties showed PE particles to be abundant in the osteolytic lesions well within the femoral head (Fig. 10-1).[21] Loosened components were characterized by the presence of an interfacial fibrous membrane, bone resorption of the adjacent bone (often with bone formation on the bone surface away from the membrane), invasion of marrow by macrophages with wear debris and often by the atrophy of cancellous bone. Generally, femoral heads remained viable.[18,22,23]

Acetabular Loosening

In Amstutz' series, 90% of the acetabular failures occurred from bone-cement loosening, with 10% from dissociation, that is, when the liner came out of the acrylic bed. The former occurred by the same wear-induced bone resorption process that was described around conventional hip replacement failures.[24] The rate at which wear-induced osteolysis undermined the fixation of cemented implants was found to be greater in smaller components.[12]

Cement-Related Loosening

The majority of first-generation hip resurfacings used cement fixation, and the biological response to bone cement has been

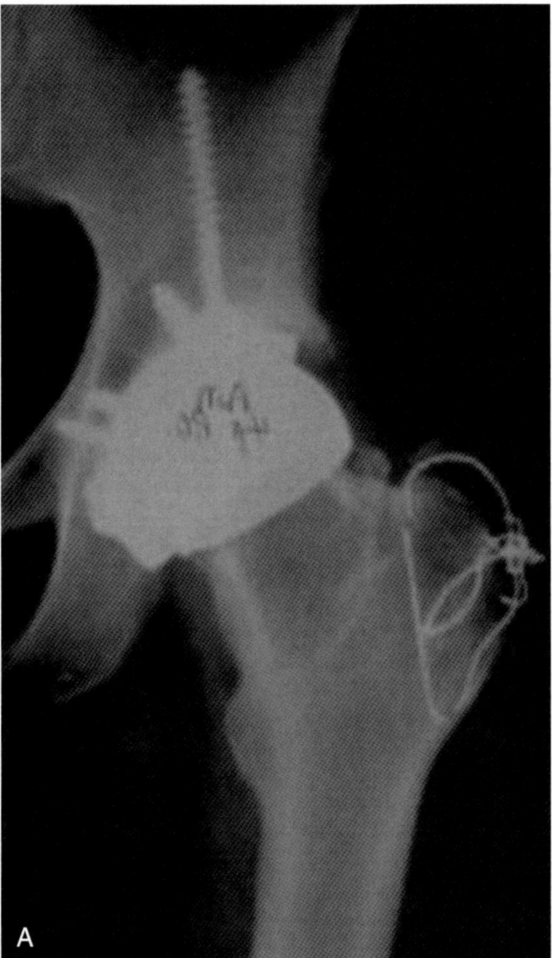

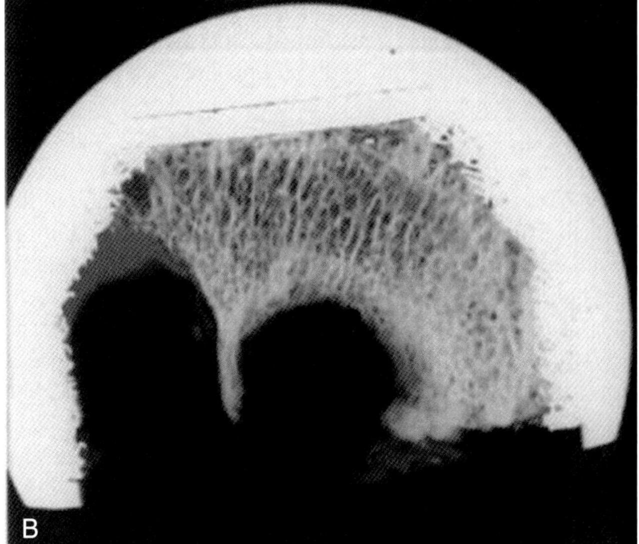

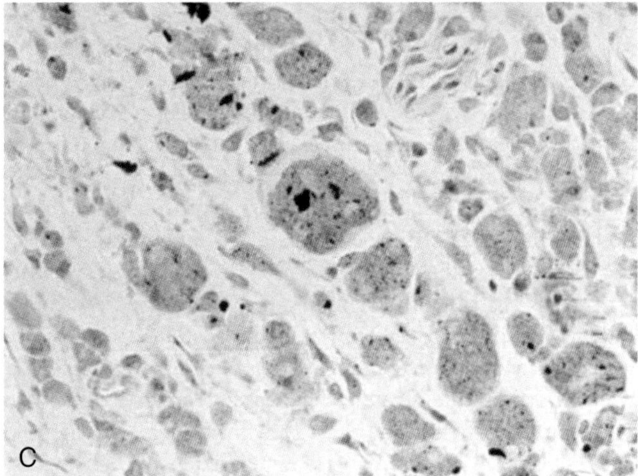

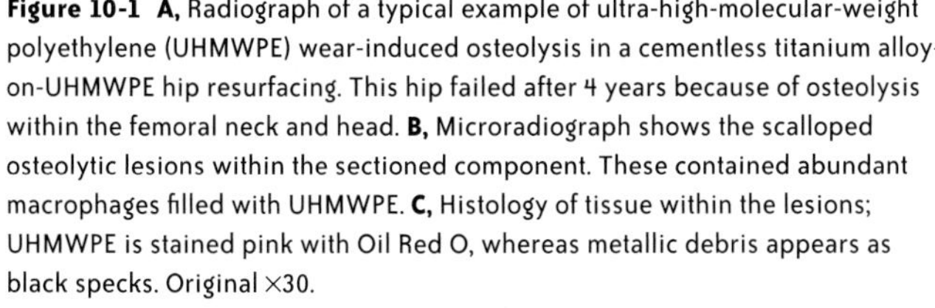

Figure 10-1 **A,** Radiograph of a typical example of ultra-high-molecular-weight polyethylene (UHMWPE) wear-induced osteolysis in a cementless titanium alloy-on-UHMWPE hip resurfacing. This hip failed after 4 years because of osteolysis within the femoral neck and head. **B,** Microradiograph shows the scalloped osteolytic lesions within the sectioned component. These contained abundant macrophages filled with UHMWPE. **C,** Histology of tissue within the lesions; UHMWPE is stained pink with Oil Red O, whereas metallic debris appears as black specks. Original ×30.

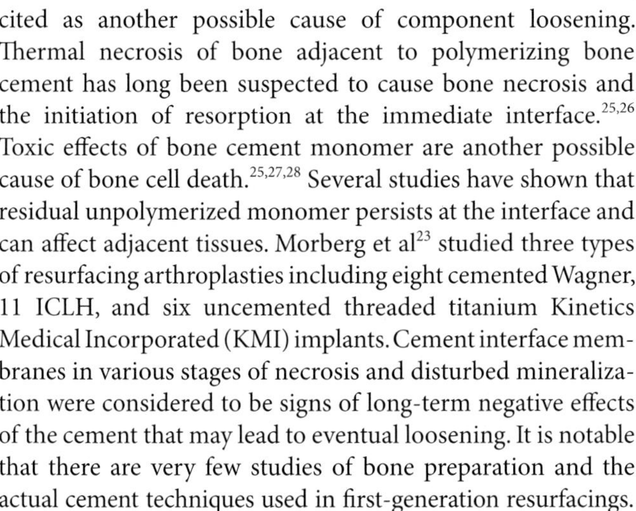

cited as another possible cause of component loosening. Thermal necrosis of bone adjacent to polymerizing bone cement has long been suspected to cause bone necrosis and the initiation of resorption at the immediate interface.[25,26] Toxic effects of bone cement monomer are another possible cause of bone cell death.[25,27,28] Several studies have shown that residual unpolymerized monomer persists at the interface and can affect adjacent tissues. Morberg et al[23] studied three types of resurfacing arthroplasties including eight cemented Wagner, 11 ICLH, and six uncemented threaded titanium Kinetics Medical Incorporated (KMI) implants. Cement interface membranes in various stages of necrosis and disturbed mineralization were considered to be signs of long-term negative effects of the cement that may lead to eventual loosening. It is notable that there are very few studies of bone preparation and the actual cement techniques used in first-generation resurfacings.

Mechanical Causes of Loosening

In contrast to the biologic basis of femoral loosening, biomechanical theories have been proposed to explain loosening failures. Theoretical finite element models of hip resurfacing have predicted failure because of the altered stresses on the bone. Schreiber et al[29] created a finite element model patterned after the cemented ICLH femoral component with two different conditions; one attached cement to the cortical bone of the femoral neck, whereas the other attachment was only between cancellous bone and the component. The model was statically loaded with 1680 N to correspond to the one-legged stance of an individual of about 600 N weight with the component in a valgus position (15 degrees to the vertical). In the cortical bone–fixed model, tolerable stress concentrations occurred at the margins of the shell and the femoral neck, whereas the cancellous bone under the component was largely stress shielded. The authors questioned whether the interlock between the cortical bone and the cement can be maintained sufficiently to handle the tensile and shear forces their model predicts. In the cancellous bone–fixed model, the cancellous bone at the rim of the component is loaded in excess of the normal physiologic loads, whereas the cancellous bone in the medial corner of the component is stress shielded. The authors postulate that the microfracturing of the overloaded cancellous bone could initiate a progressive breakdown of the cement interface because fibrous tissue fills the gap created when the trabeculae fail to heal and re-establish fixation. At the same time, the stress-shielded cancellous bone will atrophy and be unable to support the component, which will then migrate in a varus direction. These models have known limitations and did not include important features such as variable bone density. Nor do they account for the different cementing techniques (such as filling cysts or adding fixation key holes). Although there are a small number of cases of long-term retrievals of cemented resurfacings that show the features predicted by models such as these (Fig. 10-2), there are more cases that do not match the predictions of the FEA models, highlighting once again the complex and multifaceted nature of bone remodeling in response to implants.

Mjoberg[30] postulated that migration of resurfacing components measured with roentgen stereophotogrammetry was the result of the instability from the fibrous tissue layer that formed as a result of heat injury to bone following cement polymerization. Alternatively, one can postulate that lack of initial cement fixation could have the same outcome. The presence of cement interface membranes was noted in cases with poor cement penetration of relatively thin layers of cement in failed Conserve®Plus implants, whereas extensive penetration of cement did not necessarily cause membrane formation.[31] The affect of cement on bone and survivorship of hip resurfacing components is discussed further later.

Femoral Neck Fracture

This unique failure mechanism has been attributed to surgical technique errors, poor patient selection, and biologic and mechanical causes. The incidence of neck fractures in first-generation resurfacing failures was variable; although some clinicians reported high rates,[16] in the 586 THARIES series of Amstutz et al,[9] only eight of 163 failures were caused by neck fracture. These eight THARIES fractures were attributed to fatigue failure of the bone as judged histologically by the presence of microfractures and healing fracture callus. The role of avascular necrosis (AVN) of the femoral head in femoral neck fractures was a controversial issue, with several authors reporting a high incidence of AVN,[16] but the total number of cases examined was low, exaggerating the apparently high percentage of AVN failures (for example, three of six fractures reported[16]). In larger series, the incidence of AVN was much lower.[10,18,32] It is worth noting that during that early era of resurfacing, some surgeons recommended using a surgical approach to the hip, which may have left more of the extraosseous blood supply to the femoral head intact (such as the transtrochanteric approach by Amstutz,[9] and the anterior approach by Wagner[33]) as opposed to the posterior approach commonly used in modern metal-on-metal hip resurfacings.

Wear Debris–Induced Osteolysis

Amstutz et al[9] included a separate classification of failure specifically for wear debris–induced osteolysis. This was in response to a high incidence of revisions for enigmatic pain in their series of titanium-on-UHMWPE porous-coated resurfacings. Radiographs of these cases typically showed cavitary, osteolytic defects within the femoral neck, extending under the femoral component (see Fig. 10-1). Sections through the revised femoral components typically showed good ingrowth fixation and the presence of osteolysis caused by an invasive histiocytic pseudogranulomatous tissue. The implants were not yet loose because bone ingrowth was typically present, and revisions were carried out after fracture of the osteolysis-weakened femoral necks or to prevent fracture. The cells making up the invasive tissue were laden with titanium and UHMWPE debris.

Although the titanium implants were replaced by cobalt chromium components, the osteolysis caused by UHMWPE-laden cells continued to be a major cause of failure. Interestingly, hemiresurfacing components revised after a longer in vivo service life lacked the invasive granulomatous tissue and the femoral head bone was generally well preserved in both cemented and cementless designs (Fig. 10-3). This observation motivated the change away from PE in resurfacing components.

Key Findings from the First-Generation Failures

There is general agreement that the histiocytic reaction to UHMWPE wear debris was the major cause of aseptic loosening, and this was the motivation for the reintroduction of metal-on-metal bearings. Although there are similarities between the first- and second-generation resurfacings, as can be seen from Table 10-2, there have been significant design and technique changes. The impact of these changes on failure modes in contemporary metal-on-metal hip resurfacings is discussed in the following section.

Implant Retrieval Analysis of Contemporary Metal-On-Metal Hip Resurfacings

Approximately 40,000 metal-on-metal hip resurfacings have been implanted over the past decade and short- to mid-term clinical results have been encouraging, as discussed in other chapters of this book. It was anticipated that the change to wear-resistant metal-on-metal bearings would remove the most onerous cause of failure of the previous generation, that

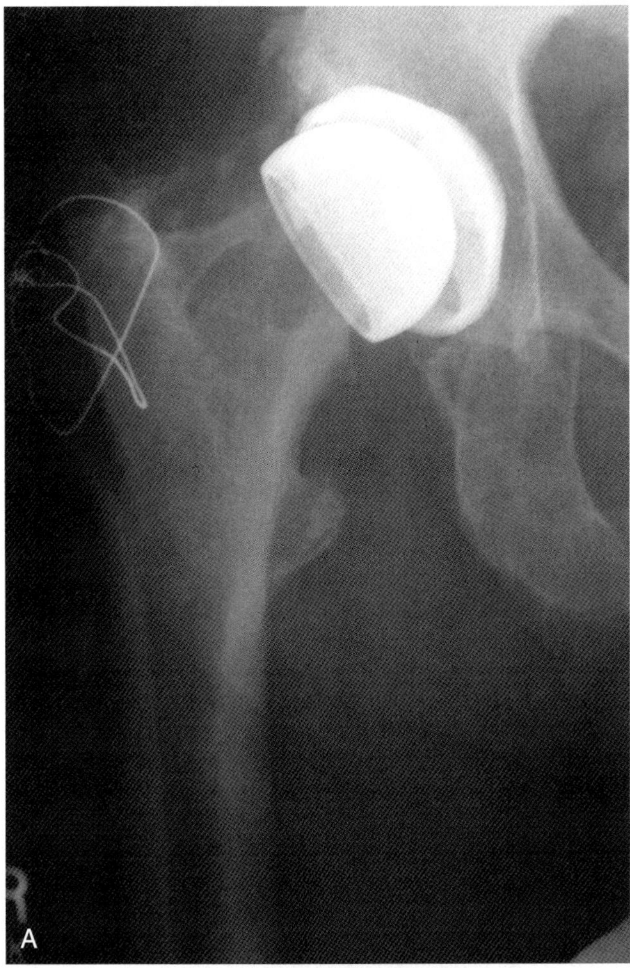

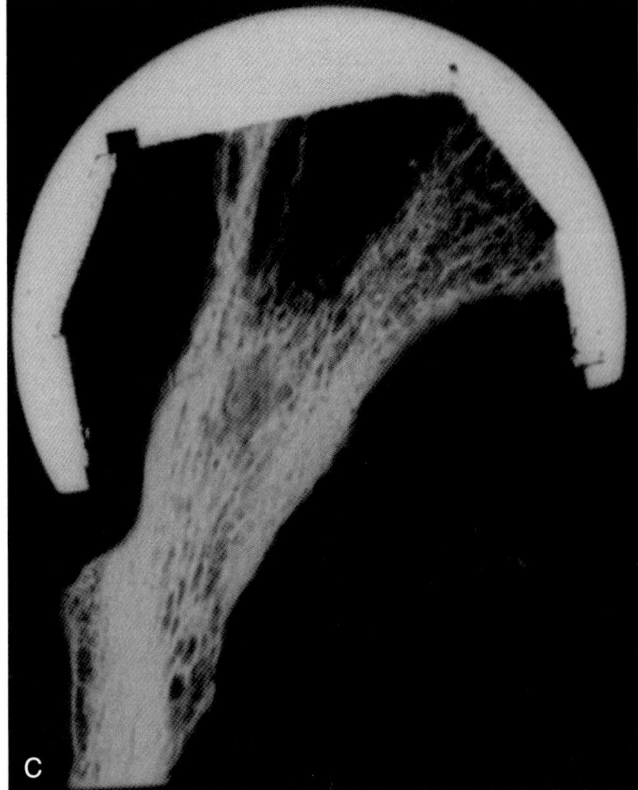

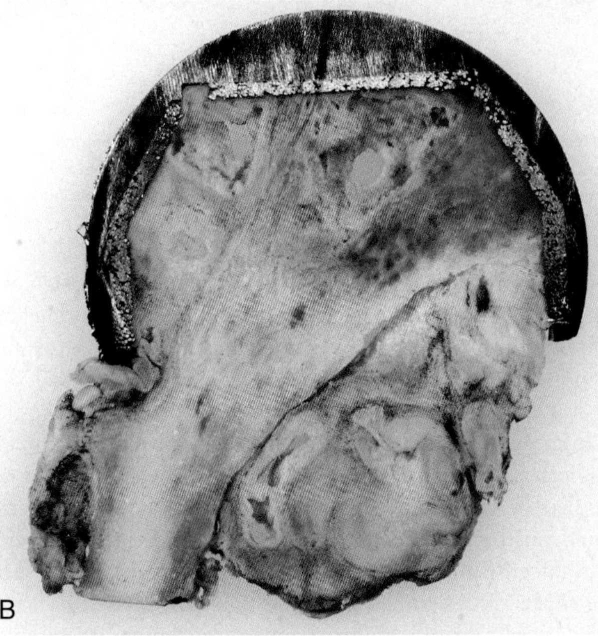

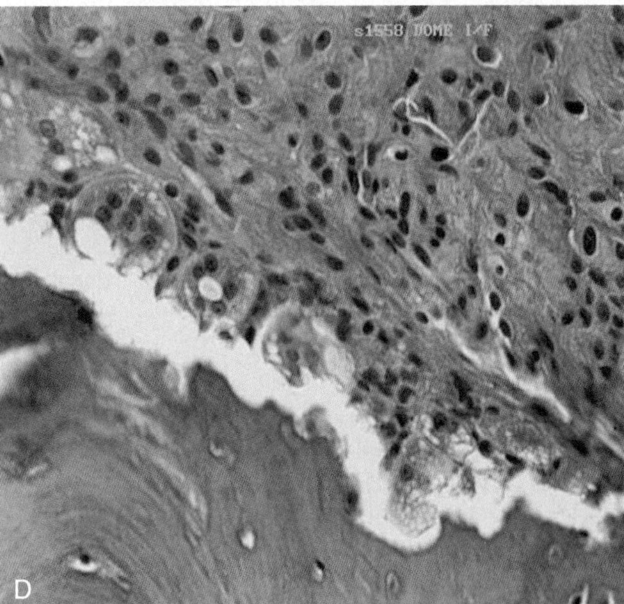

Figure 10-2 **A,** Radiograph of a 12-year retrieval of a porous-coated titanium–on–ultra-high-molecular-weight polyethylene hip resurfacing that failed because of wear-induced osteolysis. **B,** Section through the femoral head showing remodeling of the bone into a strong supportive column, reminiscent of the predictions in finite element models. **C,** Microradiograph of the section. **D,** Histology of the soft tissue showing histiocytic tissue. H&E, original ×20.

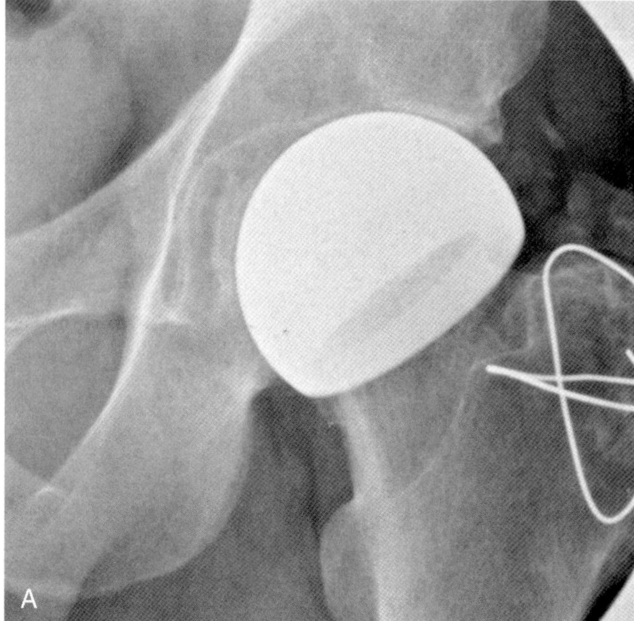

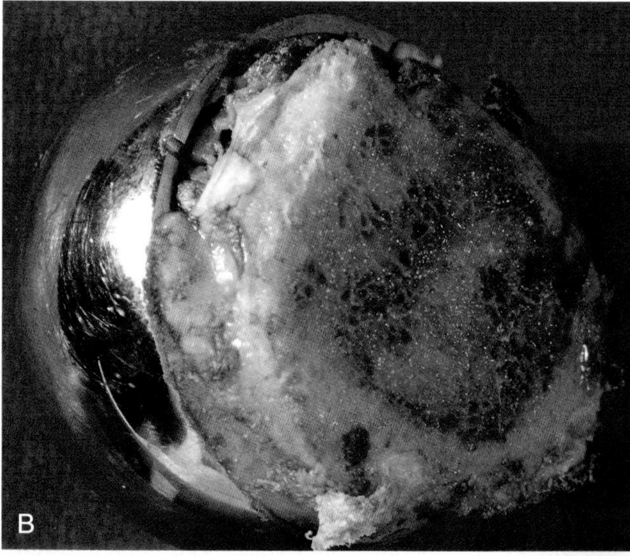

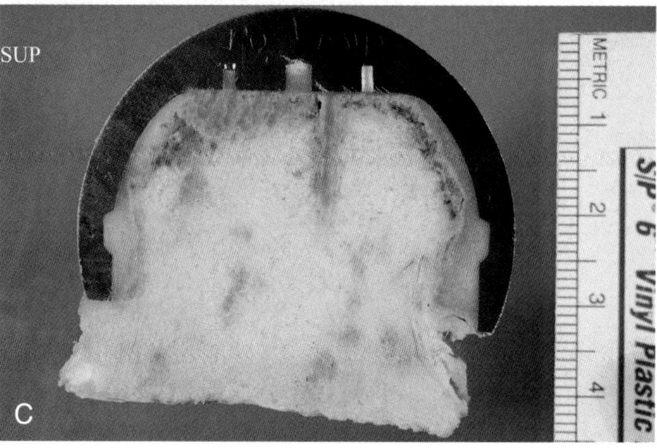

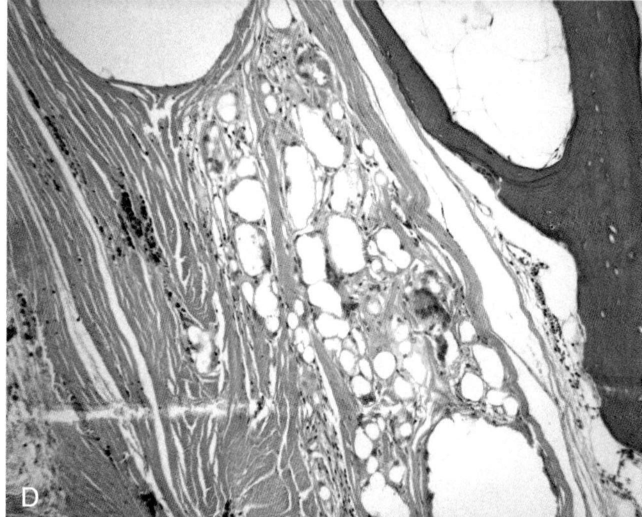

Figure 10-3 **A,** Radiograph of a hemiresurfacing component that was revised for acetabular erosion after 23 years. **B,** The retrieved femoral head showing good preservation of the femoral neck. **C,** Section through the femoral head. Despite limited cement penetration, there is minimal interface membrane formation and no osteolysis. **D,** Histology of the cement interface showing a thin fibrous membrane containing occasional titanium-filled macrophages. H&E, original ×10.

is, wear-induced osteolysis, but this would also place more emphasis on surgical technique and adequate fixation.[31] This appears to be an accurate prediction. Two failure modes predominate—femoral neck fracture and femoral loosening.[34,35] The number of reported implant retrieval analyses of modern hip resurfacing is small, but valuable insights have been gained into factors associated with these two important causes of failure.[31,36] These thin or non-existent cement mantles are the focus of this chapter.

Femoral Neck Fracture

The reported incidence of neck fracture in modern resurfacings is approximately 2%, although it is variable among the different centers and with the various designs currently in clinical use (Table 10-3). Whether this variability reflects the influence of surgeon experience and criteria for patient selection or more fundamental aspects of component design and surgical technique remains to be determined. Shimmin et al[34] reviewed the resurfacing experience within the Australian National Registry of joint replacements and reported that fractures of the femoral neck were twice as likely in women than men, and were more prevalent when the femoral implant was placed in varus. The 50 fractures in the study were not studied histologically, so the role of cement or vascularity could not be commented upon. As more designs are being introduced, future data from the Australian registry may show the effects of design and cement philosophy.

Campbell et al have carried out extensive studies of failed hip resurfacings.[31] These included mostly the Conserve®Plus design (Wright Medical Technologies, Arlington, TN), which was undergoing a clinical trial within the United States, and the Birmingham Hip Resurfacing (BHR, Smith and Nephew, Memphis, TN) which is the predominant design in Europe

Table 10-2 Similarities and Differences between First- and Second-generation Hip Resurfacings

Feature	Variables	First Generation (THARIES)	Metal-on-metal Generation
Acetabular component	Design	Eccentric (–3 mm)	Hemispherical
	Fixation	Cemented	Cementless
	Coverage	165-170° (depending on size)	160-180°
Femoral component	Design	No stem	Metaphyseal stem
	Fixation	Cemented	Cemented
	Placement	Variable	More precise
Surgery	Approach	Anterior, or transtrochanteric	Posterior
	Retinacular vessel sparing or sacrificing	Vessel sparing	Vessel sacrificing
	Capsule sparing or sacrificing	Sacrificing	Variable
Head preparation	Reaming	Anatomic (matching neck/shaft angle)	140 degrees
	Cleaning and drying	Variable	Meticulous cleaning recommended
	Fixation holes	Variable	Multiple recommended
Cementing technique	Mantle thickness	Variable	0 to 1 mm by design
	Application	Circumferential (Hand)	Circumferential (Hand or applied within the component)
		Suction not used	Transtrochanteric suction
	Viscosity	Doughy	Low-viscosity or doughy
	Volume used	Variable	Typically half volume of femoral shell

Table 10-3 The Reported Incidence of Neck Fracture in Modern Hip Resurfacings

Authors	Implant Type	Incidence (number) of Revisions (All Causes)	Incidence (number) of Fractures (per Total Number of Hips)	Total Number of Hips	Follow-Up	AVN related
Treacy et al, 2005 (UK)[56]	BHR	2% (3)	<1% (1)	144		1
De Smet, 2005 (Belg)[57]	BHR	1% (3)	<1% (1)	252		0
Daniel et al, 2004 (UK)[58]	BHR	<1% (1) ave 3.3 yrs	<1% (1)	446 (excluding 1996 group)	3.3 years average	1
Back et al, 2005 (Aus)[59]	BHR	<1% (1) ave 3 yrs	0	230	3 years average	n/a
Shimmin & Back, 2005 (Aus)[34]	BHR	2% (69)	1.46% (50)	3497 (89 surgeons)		Histology was not reported
Little et al, 2005 (UK)[37]	BHR	4% (13)	2.1% (8)	377		12/13 patchy necrosis
Nishii et al, 2007 (Japan)[60]	BHR	4% (2)	2% (1)	48	5 years minimum	not stated
Amstutz current (USA)	Conserve Plus	3.1% (26)	1% (8)	800		4 (2 with 1-mm PMMA)
Amstutz et al, 2004 (USA)[44]	Conserve Plus	3.1% (19)	<1% (5) 4-80 wk	600		1
Lilikakis et al, 2005 (Eur)[61]	Cormet	4% (3)	0	70		n/a
Grigoris et al, 2006 (UK)[2]	Durom	0	0	100	2 years minimum	n/a
Howie et al, 2005 (Aus)[62]	McMinn	73% (8)	18% (2)	11		not stated
Pollard et al, 2006 (UK)[63]	BHR	6% (4)	4.7% (3)	63	5 years average	1

ave, average; AVN, avascular necrosis; BHR, Birmingham Hip Replacement; PMMA, polymethyl methacrylate.

and Australia. Failures ranged from 1 week to several years postoperatively. Of the 98 failures submitted for analysis, the most common cause of failure was femoral neck fracture (32%). The majority of these occurred within 2 months of surgery, but in seven cases, the average time to fracture was 15 months. Histologic analysis of the short-term fractures showed that the break occurred through areas of healing cancellous and cortical bone at the component/neck region (Fig. 10-4). Many of these fracture failures were also found to be incorrectly or improperly seated, resulting in uncovered reamed

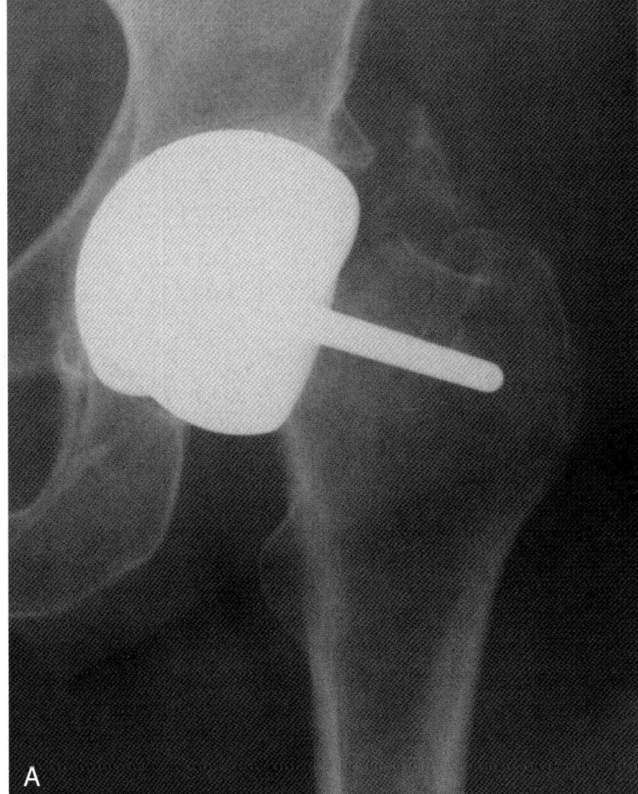

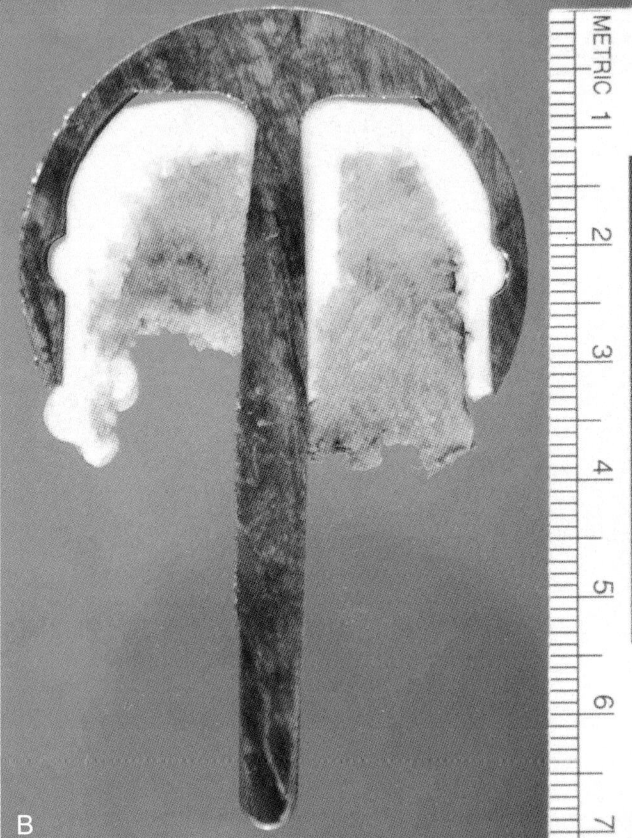

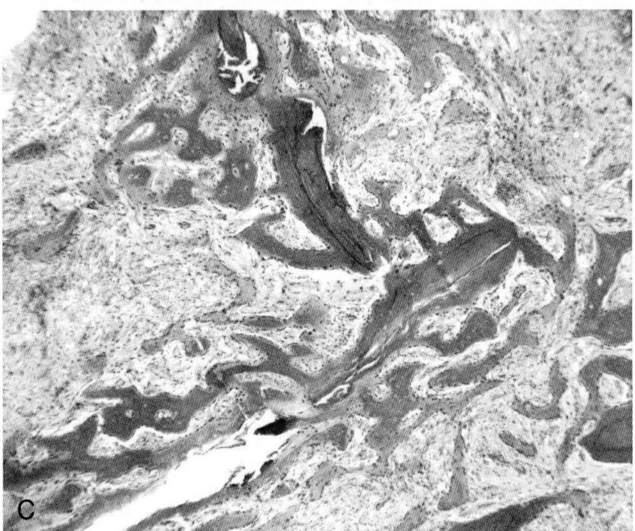

Figure 10-4 **A,** Radiograph showing a typical example of a short-term resurfacing fracture associated with a technical error that weakened the femoral neck. **B,** Cut section showing that the implant was not properly seated. **C,** When examined histologically, the break can be seen to occur through an area of weak, healing new bone.

bone in the femoral neck, which could act as a stress riser. Additionally, the damage may have occurred if the surgeon applied excessive force to seat the component, especially with components that have thin or non-existent mantles, and compounded if there was weak bone or component misalignment. Notching has been found both in fractured and successful resurfacings.[34,37] Although stress fractures occurring under MMSA components have been reported to heal if noted early and the hip is protected by a period of non–weight bearing,[38] bone undergoing repair following stress fracture is a site of weakness for eventual fatigue failure. Thus, many of these failures can be considered to have a dual-phase failure mode; the original trauma to the bone occurs at surgery, but the actual failure process takes place several weeks or months later. Several subcapital fractures were found after retrieval in components that were revised for pain or femoral migration. Again, it is postulated that these represent dual-phase events, with the original event possibly occurring at surgery, but the healing process provides weeks or months of durability.

Similar findings were reported by Morlock et al[36] following the analysis of fracture patterns and histology among 55 femoral resurfacing failures. Early fractures were associated with uncovered reamed bone and microfractures, with associated healing. The authors speculated that failure occurred when forces and moments on the bone exceeded the strength of the weakened bone. Pseudoarthrosis features were commonly found within the components and were attributed to a "two-time" fracture time line. The cause of the initial injury was suggested to be either trauma or surgically induced damage, such as excessively high implantation forces.

The Role of Vascularity in Fracture

In contrast, Little et al[37] proposed that fractures occurred because femoral head bone was devascularized and weakened during the surgery, specifically because resurfacing was performed through the posterior approach, which destroys the extraosseous blood supply to the femoral head. This proposition was based on the histologic observation of extensive background necrosis (where necrotic bone is surrounded by newly formed bone) among 12 of 13 failed resurfacings from a cohort of 377, mostly BHR, implants from the authors' institution. However determinations were made on a single section, which may not be representative of the entire femoral head. A study of the oxygen tension changes during the resurfacing surgery was performed by the same research group to support the histologic findings of necrosis. These studies showed that tissue dissection and dislocation during the posterior approach led to a marked reduction in oxygen supply to the sampled areas of the femoral head.[39] Because the volume of bone sampled by the probe was not disclosed, it is not clear if the measurements reflect a similar loss of blood supply throughout the femoral head. Khan et al,[40] using cefuroxime, a cephalosporin routinely given for antibiotic prophylaxis during hip surgery as an indicator of the blood supply to the femoral head, reported that the posterolateral approach was associated with a significant reduction in the blood supply compared with the transgluteal approach. Recent studies on resurfaced femoral heads with PET scans reported good bone viability levels, but it is not clear if this is due to preservation of the original supply or re-establishment of temporarily compromised vascularity.[41,42]

Extensive background necrosis was less commonly observed by Campbell et al.[31] A modification of the scheme used by Howie et al[43] (Fig. 10-5A) was applied to look specifically at bone viability in 25 failed hip resurfacings. The bone in the dome region, the middle of the head, and the cup/neck edges were assessed at the light microscopic level using image analysis software (Image One, West Chester, PA). Bone viability was judged by the presence of osteocyte nuclei in the majority of lacunae of the bone trabeculae. Typically, several millimeters of partially necrotic bone (i.e., showing background necrosis) were present below the cement, whereas bone within the head, away from the cement, appeared to be more consistently viable (Fig. 10-5B and C). Further study is needed to better understand the factors influencing the vascularity of the resurfaced femoral head, particularly if cement is abandoned in favor of porous ingrowth fixation.

Avascular Necrosis and Fractures

In contrast to the short-term fractures, longer term fractures tend to be associated with extensive or complete avascular necrosis of the femoral head.[31,36] These occur after a year or more and often are associated with a clinical history of pain but without radiographic indication of loosening. Histologic analysis typically shows no evidence of repair to the original cut surfaces, indicating that the devascularization occurred at the time of surgery (Fig. 10-6). This can occur in various ways (Box 10-2). The interface between the dead bone in the proximal part of the component and the viable bone of the femoral neck is comparable to the healing zone of a primary femoral head undergoing avascular necrosis, that is, active bone resorption and formation occurring within a vascularized fibrotic or fibrocartilaginous stroma. There is incomplete removal of the dead bone, but often extensive new bone formation resulting in a sclerotic bone margin demarcating the two zones. The interface is a site of mechanical weakness, and fatigue failure eventually occurs at this location, although it may take several years.

Femoral Loosening

Resurfacing femoral loosening failures can be divided into those in which the femoral component was grossly loose or completely detached at the time of revision and those that were still connected to the bone but showed radiographic changes and were associated with pain. This mode of failure is currently less common in modern generation hip resurfacings because of the higher rate of early failure from fracture and the relatively short follow-up time but it can be anticipated to become more common with time. Amstutz et al reported that seven of 12 hips from a group of 400 Conserve®Plus resurfacings with average 3.5 years follow-up were revised for femoral loosening.[44] The demographics of the patients who had loosening failures were not different from the remainder of the group, but the sectioned femoral heads showed that these cases had large areas of cystic degeneration, and the implants were incompletely seated in three of them. All of these femoral heads were viable, but failure occurred at the cement-bone interface. Membranes were typically present between the cement and bone, and in three cases that were completely dissociated from the component, fibrous tissue had replaced large portions of the proximal femoral bone,

BOX 10-2 Forms of Devascularization

- Disruption of blood vessels with dislocation
- Dissection
- Mechanical trauma
- Chemical trauma
- Heat trauma
- Microembolism
- Arterial and venous outflow blockage

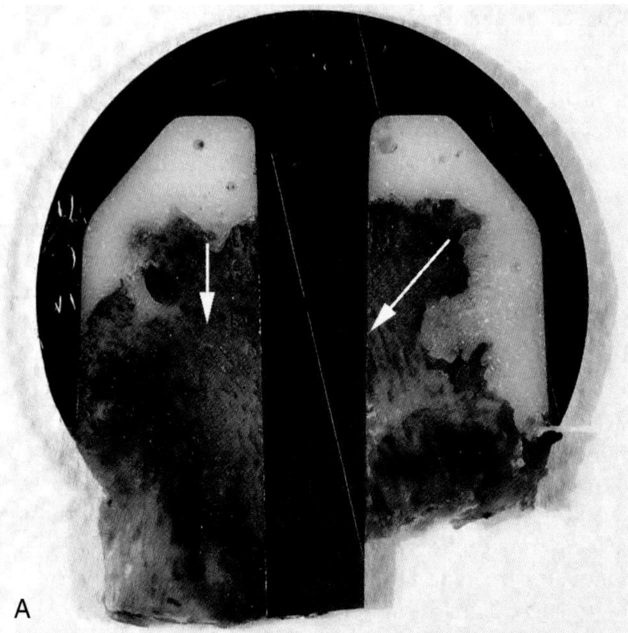

Dome depth vs. percentage live bone

Percent live bone: 100.0, 90.0, 80.0, 70.0, 60.0, 50.0, 40.0, 30.0, 20.0, 10.0, 0

Depth (mm): 1, 2, 3, 4, 5, 6, 7

B

Chamfer depth vs. percentage live bone

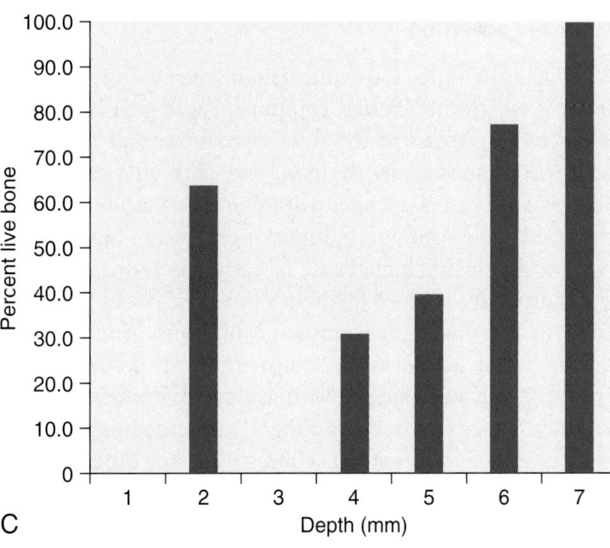

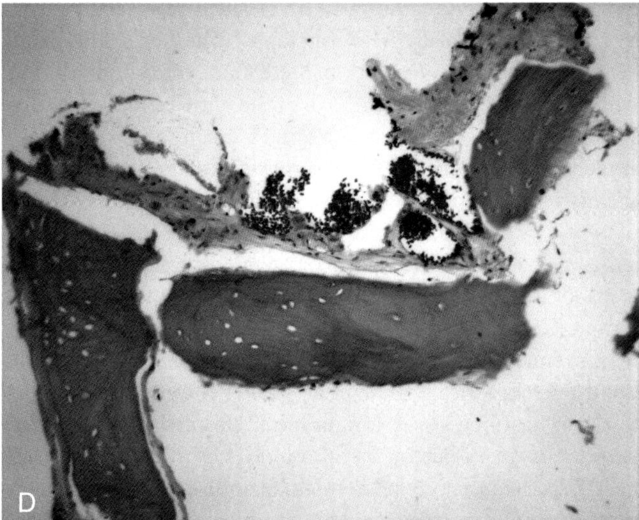

Figure 10-5 **A,** This is a middle section from a BHR that was revised after 1 month for femoral neck fracture. The thick but poorly penetrated cement layer is likely to have thermally damaged the underlying bone. The viability of the bone was assessed histologically along the lines shown in the figure. **B,** Graph showing that the percentage of viable bone is increasing away from the cement interface measured at the dome. **C,** Graph showing that the percentage of viable bone is increasing away from the cement interface measured from the chamfer. **D,** Histology of the cement interface showing empty osteocyte lacunae, which is indicative of dead bone. H&E, original ×4.

reminiscent of failed Wagner components in first-generation resurfacings.[18]

Role of Cement in Femoral Loosening

The return to cement fixation in modern resurfacing has again raised questions about the best cement technique—how much is needed for fixation without putting the femoral head bone at risk of thermal necrosis or excessive penetration? Accompanying the various resurfacing designs are differing philosophies regarding the optimal amount, timing, and distribution of cement.[31] In vitro studies have generally recommended restraint in the amount of cement used for the fixation of resurfacing components, but the most widely used type of resurfacing to date, the BHR, typically uses large amounts of low-viscosity cement for femoral fixation.

Retrieval analyses of both failed and nonfailed femoral resurfacing components have noted the wide variety in amount and distribution of cement, even considering the different cement philosophies among the main resurfacing designs. Campbell et al[31,36,45] studied the relationship between the amount and distribution of cement and femoral fracture and

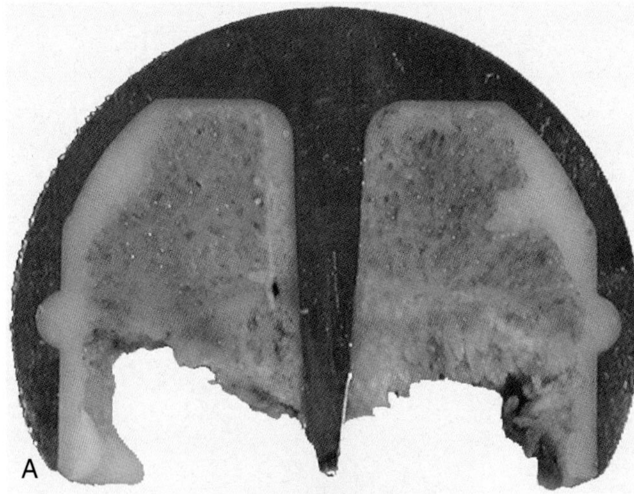

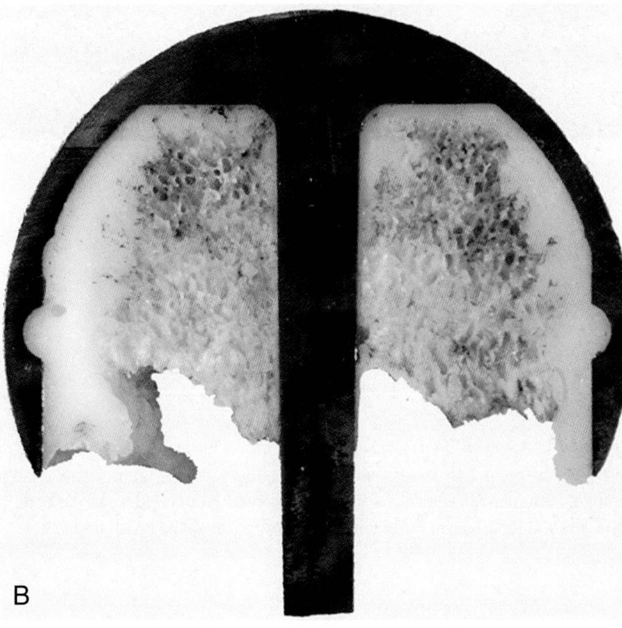

Figure 10-6 These Conserve®Plus resurfacing components fractured as the result of avascular necrosis that was apparently induced at the time of implantation surgery. Note the similar fracture pattern. **A,** Revised after 7 months. **B,** Revised after 14 months.

loosening. The most obvious cause of loosening is the inadequacy of cement fixation due to a combination of poor preparation of the bone and reduced surface area due to cystic degeneration, particularly when this is amplified by small component size. Cases in which the implant lifts easily from the femoral head remnant leaving cement attached to the component are consistent with insufficient cement, loss of initial fixation by necrosis of the interdigitated bone with subsequent membrane formation, or insufficient initial interdigitation to provide fixation (Fig. 10-7).

A less obvious cause of loosening failure is overcementing. As noted earlier, cement thermal necrosis of bone does occur and the resulting bone removal and replacement by fibrous membranes can undermine fixation and contribute to loosening.[26] Campbell et al[31] studied this association in a group of 48 resurfacings that failed for neck fracture, femoral loosening, and nonfemoral reasons. The thickness of the cement mantle, and the degree of cement penetration into cancellous bone were measured in a blinded manner in each of the three sections (anterior, middle, and posterior). The overall amount of cement within the bone was also measured. The cases that failed from femoral loosening contained a statistically significantly higher amount of cement than those that fractured or failed from nonfemoral causes. It is suspected that the practice of filling cystic defects with cement contributed to the negative effects without contributing to the fixation, because the cysts are often lined with soft tissue or sclerotic bone, both of which are an impediment to cement penetration if the surgeon does not remove all of this material. These large volumes of cement may contribute to thermal necrosis. However the effects of cement can apparently be reduced by adequate lavage, intertrochanteric suction, and early hip reduction.[46]

Campbell et al[31] also found that membranes were not always present at the cement interface, even when cementing had been extensive. The interface between cement and bone varied considerably from a thin lining of giant cells to thick fibrous tissue containing histiocytes and blood vessels. Bone healing occurred around necrotic trabeculae when present and often grew to within a few microns of bone cement with little intervening tissue.

Intuitively, this would seem to be the most advantageous situation for the transfer of stresses through the implant, cement, and to the bone, whereas by contrast, the intervention of interfacial membranes would likely reduce the direct transfer of stresses transmitted to the bone and potentially lead to increasing thickness of the membrane. However, the resurfacing finite element analysis model of Ong et al[47] based on the BHR prosthesis found that the nonphysiologic stresses that occurred following the application of the implant to the bone were partly restored when the bone was fully debonded from the implant. Their model predicted that there would be bone resorption from the proximal femoral head and bone apposition around the distal stem.

Watanabe et al[48] modeled a well-fixed, BHR-type cemented resurfacing in which the load was directed through the center of the head during the first peak (1320 N), valley (1200 N) and second peak (1600 N) of the gait cycle of an individual using crutches. Regardless of loading condition, cortical bone stress concentrations occurred adjacent to the rim of the prosthesis and were highest in the posteroinferior region. The peak compressive cortical bone stress values were close to the ultimate strength of femoral bone, and the authors cautioned against using resurfacing components in patients with osteopenia. Stress shielding of the cancellous bone under the rim of the component was noted during the valley phase of the gait cycle but was not predicted for the femoral neck. The cancellous bone of the femoral head under the component was not studied in this model, but other models predicted cancellous bone stress shielding under the component.[49,50] The failure of cancellous bone to withstand the altered loading following

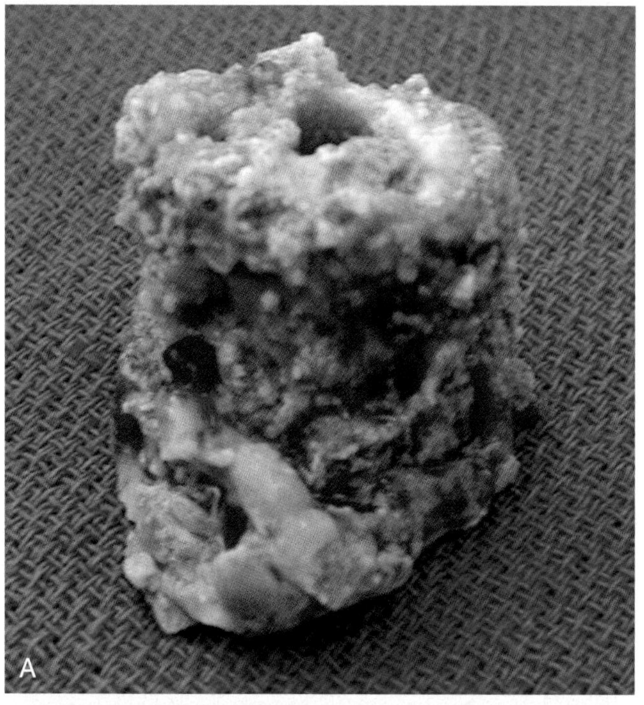

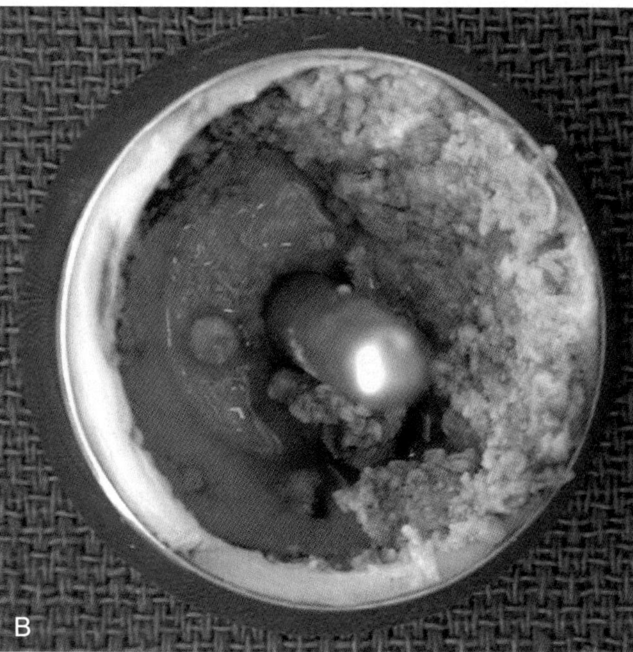

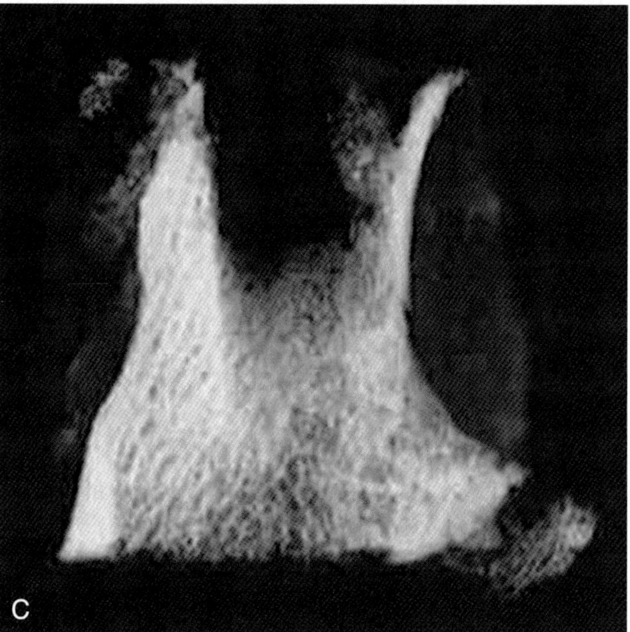

Figure 10-7 **A,** This is the typical appearance of a femoral failure in which there has been complete dissociation between the cement and the bone. **B,** The remnant femoral head is partially transformed into fibrous tissue, and the bone is generally viable. **C,** Microradiograph of a section through the head remnant.

resurfacing may lead to microfractures,[51] whereas other areas of the head may undergo stress shielding with subsequent bone resorption,[29] but only follow-up retrieval studies will confirm or refute these predictions.

If remodeling takes place, the bone can be strengthened to withstand the increased stresses. During remodeling, however, movement between the bone and the cement cannot be tolerated[29] if a fibrous interface is to be avoided. This healing process may be difficult to achieve when patients are encouraged to begin early post-operative activity. The role of an early return to high activity or impact sports in the breakdown of the cement-bone interface has not been determined. Retrieval analyses of long-term resurfacings show variable amounts of bone remodeling and cases with proximal bone thinning are seen. However, the loss of proximal bone is often accompanied by solidification of the bone elsewhere, and this can provide remarkable durability despite major bone loss (see Fig. 10-2). This highlights the remarkable adaptive capability of the human femoral head to withstand the damage induced by resurfacing.

References

1. Amstutz HC, Le Duff MJ: Background of metal-on-metal resurfacing. Proc Inst Mech Eng [H] 2006;220:85-94.
2. Grigoris P, Roberts P, Panousis K, Jin Z: Hip resurfacing arthroplasty: the evolution of contemporary designs. Proc Inst Mech Eng [H] 2006;220:95-105.
3. Freeman MA: Some anatomical and mechanical considerations relevant to the surface replacement of the femoral head. Clin Orthop Relat Res 1978;134:19-24.
4. Amstutz HC, Thomas BJ, Jinnah R, Kim W, Grogan T, Yale C: Treatment of primary osteoarthritis of the hip. A comparison of total joint and surface replacement arthroplasty. J Bone Joint Surg 1984;66A:228-241.
5. Amstutz HC, Grigoris P, Dorey FJ: Evolution and future of surface replacement of the hip. J Orthop Sci 1998;3:169-186.
6. Galante JO, Lemons J, Spector M, Wilson PDJ, Wright TM: The biologic effects of implant materials. J Orthop Relat Res 1991;9:760-775.
7. Amstutz HC, Campbell P, Clarke IC, Kossovsky N: Mechanism and clinical significance of wear debris-induced osteolysis. Clin Orthop Relat Res 1992;276:7-18.
8. Schmalzried TP, Jasty M, Harris WH: Periprosthetic bone loss in total hip arthroplasty. Polyethylene wear debris and the concept of the effective joint space. J Bone Joint Surg 1992;74A: 849-863.
9. Amstutz HC, Campbell P, Nasser S, Kossovsky N: Modes of failure of surface replacements. In Amstutz HC (ed): Hip Arthroplasty. New York, Churchill Livingstone, 1991, pp 507-534.
10. Amstutz HC, Dorey F, O'Carroll PF: THARIES resurfacing arthroplasty. Evolution and long-term results. Clin Orthop Relat Res 1986;213:92-113.
11. Amstutz HC: Assessment of the failed hip replacement. In Amstutz HC (ed): Hip Arthroplasty. New York, Churchill Livingstone, 1991, pp 469-472.
12. Mai MT, Schmalzried TP, Dorey FJ, Campbell PA, Amstutz HC: The contribution of frictional torque to loosening at the cement-bone interface in Tharies hip replacements. J Bone Joint Surg 1996;78A:505-511.
13. Kabo JM, Gebhard JS, Loren G, Amstutz HC: In vivo wear of polyethylene acetabular compenents. J Bone Joint Surg 1993;75B:254-258.
14. Clarke IC, Gustafson A, Jung H, Fujisawa A: Hip simulator ranking of polyethylene wear—comparisons between ceramic heads of different sizes. Acta Orthop Scand 1996;67:128-132.
15. Schmalzried TP, Guttmann D, Grecula M, Amstutz HC: The relationship between the design, position, and articular wear of acetabular components inserted without cement and the development of pelvic osteolysis. J Bone Joint Surg 1994; 76A:677-688.
16. Bogoch ER, Fornasier VL, Capello WN: The femoral head remnant in resurfacing arthroplasty. Clin Orthop Relat Res 1982;167:92-105.
17. Bell RS, Schatzker J, Fornasier VL, Goodman SB: A study of implant failure in the Wagner resurfacing arthroplasty. J Bone Joint Surg 1985;67A:1165-1175.
18. Howie DW, Campbell D, McGee M, Cornish BL: Wagner resurfacing hip arthroplasty. The results of one hundred consecutive arthroplasties after eight to ten years. J Bone Joint Surg 1990; 72:708-714.
19. Howie DW, Cornish BL, Vernon-Roberts B: Resurfacing hip arthroplasty: Classification of loosening and the role of prosthetic wear particles. Clin Orthop Relat Res 1990;255:144-159.
20. Cotella L, Railton GT, Nunn D, Freeman MA, Revell PA: ICLH double-cup arthroplasty, 1980-1987. J Arthroplasty 1990;5: 349-357.
21. Nasser S, Campbell PA, Kilgus D, Kossovsky N, Amstutz HC: Cementless total joint arthroplasty prostheses with titanium-alloy articular surfaces. A human retrieval analysis. Clin Orthop Relat Res 1990;261:171-185.
22. Campbell P, Mirra J, Amstutz HC: Viability of femoral heads treated with resurfacing arthroplasty. J Arthroplasty 2000;15: 120-122.
23. Morberg P, Albrektsson T, Reigstad A, Rokkum M, Lindgren U, Svensson O, Romanus B: A qualitative and quantitative study of retrieved femoral heads in three different types of resurface hip arthroplasties. J Arthroplasty 1993;8:617-624.
24. Schmalzried TP, Kwong LM, Jasty M, Sedlacek RC, Haire TC, O'Connor DO, Bragdon CR, Kabo JM, Malcolm AJ, Harris WH: The mechanism of loosening of cemented acetabular components in total hip arthroplasty. Clin Orthop Relat Res 1992;274:60-78.
25. Albrektsson T, Linder L: Bone injury caused by curing bone cement. A vital microscopic study in the rabbit tibia. Clin Orthop Relat Res 1984;183:280-287.
26. Mjoberg B, Pettersson H, Rosenqvist R, Rydholm A: Bone cement, thermal injury and the radiolucent zone. Acta Orthop Scand 1984;55:597-600.
27. Willert HG: Tissue reactions around joint implants and bone cement. In Chapchal G (ed): Arthroplasty of the Hip. Stuttgart, Germany, Georg Thieme, 1973, pp 11-21.
28. Jefferiss CD, Lee AJ, Ling RS: Thermal aspects of self-curing polymethylmethacrylate. J Bone Joint Surg Br 1975;57:511-518.
29. Schreiber A, Jacob HAC, Stalder M, Cserhati MD, Züllig R: Loosening of the femoral component of the ICLH double cup hip prosthesis. A biomechanical investigation with reference to clinical results. Acta Orthop Scand 1984;55(suppl):207.
30. Mjoberg B: Fixation and loosening of hip prostheses. A review. Acta Orthop Scand 1991;2:500-508.
31. Campbell P, Beaule P, Ebramzadeh E, Le Duff M, De Smet K, Lu Z, Amstutz H: A study of implant failure in metal-on-metal surface arthroplasties. Clin Orthop Relat Res 2006;453:35-46.
32. Bradley GW, Freeman MA, Revell PA: Resurfacing arthroplasty. Femoral head viability. Clin Orthop Relat Res 1987;220: 137-141.
33. Wagner H: Surface replacement arthroplasty of the hip. Clin Orthop Relat Res 1978;134:102-130.
34. Shimmin AJ, Back D: Femoral neck fractures following Birmingham hip resurfacing: A national review of 50 cases. J Bone Joint Surg 2005;87B:463-464.
35. Amstutz HC, Beaule PE, Dorey FJ, Le Duff MJ, Campbell PA, Gruen TA: Metal-on-metal hybrid surface arthroplasty: two to six-year follow-up study. J Bone Joint Surg 2004;86A:28-39.
36. Morlock MM, Bishop N, Ruther W, Delling G, Hahn M: Biomechanical, morphological, and histological analysis of early failures in hip resurfacing arthroplasty. Proc Inst Mech Eng [H] 2006;220:333-344.
37. Little CP, Ruiz AL, Harding IJ, McLardy-Smith P, Gundle R, Murray DW, Athanasou NA: Osteonecrosis in retrieved femoral heads after failed resurfacing arthroplasty of the hip. J Bone Joint Surg 2005;87B:320-323.

38. Cossey AJ, Back DL, Shimmin A, Young D, Spriggins AJ: The nonoperative management of periprosthetic fractures associated with the Birmingham hip resurfacing procedure. J Arthroplasty 2005;20:358-361.
39. Steffen RT, Smith SR, Urban JP, McLardy-Smith P, Beard DJ, Gill HS, Murray DW: The effect of hip resurfacing on oxygen concentration in the femoral head. J Bone Joint Surg 2005;87B: 1468-1474.
40. Khan A, Yates P, Lovering A, Bannister GC, Spencer RF: The effect of surgical approach on blood flow to the femoral head during resurfacing. J Bone Joint Surg Br 2007;89:21-25.
41. Forrest N, Welch A, Murray AD, Schweiger L, Hutchison J, Ashcroft GP: Femoral head viability after Birmingham resurfacing hip arthroplasty: assessment with use of [18f] fluoride positron emission tomography. J Bone Joint Surg 2006;88(suppl 3):84-89.
42. McMahon SJ, Young D, Ballok Z, Badaruddin BS, Larbpaiboonpong V, Hawdon G: Vascularity of the femoral head after Birmingham hip resurfacing. A technetium Tc 99m bone scan/single photon emission computed tomography study. J Arthroplasty 2006;21:514-521.
43. Howie DW, Cornish BL, Vernon-Roberts B: The viability of the femoral head after resurfacing hip arthroplasty in humans. Clin Orthop Relat Res 1993;291:171-184.
44. Amstutz HC, Campbell PA, LeDuff MJ: Fracture of the neck of the femur after surface arthroplasty of the hip. J Bone Joint Surg 2004;86A:1874-1877.
45. Howald R, Kesteris U, Klabunde R, Krevolin J: Factors affecting the cement penetration of a hip resurfacing implant: An in vitro study. Hip International 2006;16:S82-S89.
46. Gill H, Campbell P, Murray D, DeSmet K: Pulse-lavage and early joint relocation reduce thermal damage potential during hip resurfacing. J Bone Joint Surg 2007;89B:16-20.
47. Ong KL, Kurtz SM, Manley MT, Rushton N, Mohammed NA, Field RE: Biomechanics of the Birmingham hip resurfacing arthroplasty. J Bone Joint Surg 2006;88B:1110-1115.
48. Watanabe Y, Shiba N, Matsuo S, Higuchi F, Tagawa Y, Inoue A: Biomechanical study of the resurfacing hip arthroplasty: finite element analysis of the femoral component. J Arthroplasty 2000;15:505-511.
49. Huiskes R, Strens PHGE, van Heck J, Slooff TJJ: Interface stresses in the resurfaced hip. Finite element analysis of load transmission in the femoral head. Acta Orthop Scand 1985;56:474-478.
50. de Waal Malefijt MC, Huiskes R: A clinical, radiological and biomechanical study of the TARA hip prosthesis. Arch Orthop Trauma Surg 1993;112:220-225.
51. Huiskes R, Strens P, Vroemen W, Slooff TJ: Post-loosening mechanical behavior of femoral resurfacing prostheses. Clin Mater 1990;6:37-55.
52. Sedel L, Travers V, Witvoet J: Spherocylindric (Luck) cup arthroplasty for osteonecrosis of the hip. Clin Orthop Relat Res 1987; 219:127-135.
53. Milgram JW, Rana NA: Pathologic evaluation of the failed cup arthroplasty: a review of 32 cases. Clin Orthop Relat Res 1981;158:158-179.
54. Morberg PH, Johansson CB, Reigstad A, Rokkum M: Vital staining of bone in stable, retrieved femoral surface replacement prostheses: A microscopic study of undecalcified ground sections. J Arthroplasty 2001;16:1004-1009.
55. Duijsens AW, Keizer S, Vliet-Vlieland T, Nelissen RG: Resurfacing hip prostheses revisited: Failure analysis during a 16-year follow-up. Int Orthop 2005;29:224-228.
56. Treacy RB, McBryde CW, Pynsent PB: Birmingham hip resurfacing arthroplasty. A minimum follow-up of five years. J Bone Joint Surg 2005;87B:167-170.
57. De Smet KA: Belgium experience with metal-on-metal surface arthroplasty. Orthop Clin North Am 2005;36:203-213.
58. Daniel J, Pynsent PB, McMinn DJ: Metal-on-metal resurfacing of the hip in patients under the age of 55 years with osteoarthritis. J Bone Joint Surg 2004;86B:177-184.
59. Back DL, Dalziel R, Young D, Shimmin A: Early results of primary Birmingham hip resurfacings. An independent prospective study of the first 230 hips. J Bone Joint Surg 2005;87B:324-329.
60. Nishii T, Sugano N, Miki H, Takao M, Koyama T, Yoshikawa H: Five-year results of metal-on-metal resurfacing arthroplasty in Asian patients. J Arthroplasty 2007;22:176-183.
61. Lilikakis AK, Vowler SL, Villar RN: Hydroxyapatite-coated femoral implant in metal-on-metal resurfacing hip arthroplasty: minimum of two years follow-up. Orthop Clin North Am 2005;36:215-222.
62. Howie DW, McGee MA, Costi K, Graves SE: Metal-on-metal resurfacing versus total hip replacement-the value of a randomized clinical trial. Orthop Clin North Am 2005;36:195-201.
63. Pollard TCB, Baker RP, Eastaugh-Waring SJ, Bannister GC: Treatment of the young active patient with osteoarthritis of the hip. J Bone Joint Surg 2006;88B:592-600.

CHAPTER 11

Reaction to Wear Products

Patricia A. Campbell
Karren Midori Takamura

Introduction

Despite the greatly improved wear resistance provided by metal-on-metal bearings, articulation inevitably produces wear particles. Some of the larger (phagocytosable submicron to several microns) particles interact with cells such as macrophages and trigger cellular reactions leading to the production of inflammatory cytokines. The majority of wear particles from metal-on-metal implants are nanometer-sized, that is, an order of magnitude smaller than phagocytosable particles and these probably enter the cell differently, avoiding many of the cytokine pathways associated with inflammatory cytokines. This would be consistent with the lesser degree of histiocytic inflammation around metal-on-metal joints.[1-3]

Much has been learned about the cellular processes involved in wear particle–induced reactions, including osteolysis, and the reader is referred to several excellent review articles on this topic.[4-6] Metal wear particles, particularly the nanometer-sized ones, can rapidly corrode and become detectable in the blood and urine as metal ions. The chemical and biologic processes involved in the corrosion of wear particles are beyond the scope of this chapter. In this chapter, we review what is known about cobalt and chromium corrosion products in the context of patients with metal-on-metal hip replacements. In particular, the important factors influencing the measurement of metal ions and the effects of large amounts of wear products are discussed. For perspective, it is useful to review the role of cobalt and chromium in normal bodily processes and to establish the typical background exposure patients have to these metals in their daily lives.

Cobalt is a beneficial trace element that forms part of vitamin B_{12}. Although there is no set recommended daily allowance for cobalt, the Food and Agricultural Organization of the United Nations and the World Health Organization recommend 2.4 μg of vitamin B_{12} per day, which is equivalent to 0.1 μg of cobalt/day,[7] and it is found in fish, nuts, green leafy vegetables, and cereals. In healthy people, high levels of cobalt (50-100 mg cobalt/day)[7] increase red blood cell production, and in the past, it was used to treat anemia. In the 1960s, a Canadian brewery used a cobalt-based substance to stabilize beer foam, and some individuals who ingested large amounts of beer also ingested relatively large amounts of the cobalt (0.04-0.14 mg cobalt per kg body weight/day).[8] This resulted in edema from cardiac failure, and liver injury from hepatic ischemia and polycythemia; several deaths were reported. It is not conclusive whether these effects were a direct result of the amount of cobalt or from excessive drinking that caused these problems, because the symptoms were similar to alcoholic cardiomyopathy.

Excessive levels of exposure to inhaled cobalt can also be harmful: serious effects on the lungs have been observed in some industrial workers who were exposed to high levels of cobalt particulates in combination with tungsten carbides, forming so-called hard metal lung diseases.[9,10] Because hard metal lung disease develops only in a small proportion of exposed workers, it has been suggested that individual sensitivity plays an important role in the response to the material. Cobalt particulates alone are thought to be much less harmful.[11]

Cobalt has not been shown to cause cancer in humans by inhalation, oral, or dermal exposure, but it is classed as a possible carcinogen by the International Agency for Research on Cancer (IARC).[12]

Chromium compounds exist with two valencies (trivalent [III] and hexavalent [VI]), and it is mostly the latter form that is associated with adverse health effects, particularly in industrial settings involving activities such as stainless steel welding, chrome plating, or chromite mining. Occupational or environmental exposure to chromium VI can cause upper respiratory problems including lung cancer or perforations of the nasal mucosa.[13] In small amounts, the ingestion of hexavalent chromium poses a minimal health risk because it is quickly oxidized in the gut to the less dangerous and less bioavailable trivalent form.[14-16]

Trivalent chromium is an essential nutrient that participates in sugar, protein, and fat metabolism. It is present in meat, whole-grain products, fruits, vegetables, and spices, but most foods only have less than 2 μg per serving. There is no set recommended daily allowance for chromium, but 50 to 200 μg of chromium (III) per day is recommended for adults.[8] Recently, chromium supplementation has become popular to enhance metabolism for dieting and to increase sports performance,[17] and chromium is prevalent in many sports drinks, food bars and vitamins. Chromium VI is classed as a known carcinogen by the IARC, but metallic chromium and chromium III are unclassifiable with current knowledge.[12]

Production of Cobalt and Chromium Ions from Hip Replacements

Overview of Wear Mechanisms, Particle Production, and Corrosion

The tribologic mechanisms involved in metal-on-metal hip replacements are reviewed in Chapter 4. Briefly, depending on factors such as diameter, clearance, surface roughness, and lubricant efficiency, wear particles are presumably generated during articulation.[18] In the clean, controlled conditions of a hip simulator, well-functioning metal-on-metal bearings produce nanometer-sized particles[19]; in vivo–generated particles have a larger size range,[20,21] possibly because of the more variable wear processes including third-body wear, and the more irregular pattern of use, for example the diurnal start-stop of a human joint.

The particles are both globular and needle-shaped and are composed of the alloy material and oxides from the articulating surface, including chromium-rich oxides,[20] as well as organometallic phosphates.[22] Recently, structural studies have suggested that globular wear particles result from torn-off nanocrystals, whereas the needle-shaped particles are generated by fractured epsilon-martensite.[23]

The particles are released into the joint fluid, where they may come into contact with phagocytic cells, primarily of the macrophage lineage, and become internalized. Although some cells may be distributed away from the joint through the vascular and lymphatic systems,[24,25] many of them remain in the local tissues.[26] This results in the accumulation of particles within synovial phagocytic cells and tissue histiocytes in the joint-lining tissues. Particles can also be stored freely in the interstitial fluids, synovial fluid, and the fluids that can accumulate within tissue bursas. Additionally, particles can be bound up in fibrin lining bursas, joint tissues, or within bone cysts.

In all scenarios, the particles are likely to begin chemically transforming as soon as they interact with the joint and cellular fluids. In an interesting study by Haynes et al,[27] the treatment of macrophages with a compound that prevented a drop in pH within phagosomes around ingested cobalt chromium particles significantly reduced the toxicity of those particles, supporting the importance of intracellular corrosion to ion production. Other studies with elemental analysis by transmission electron microscopy of ultrathin sections of macrophages from aseptically loosened total hips and knees showed that the chemical composition of phagocytosed particles was different from that of the implanted alloys: cobalt and titanium were reduced, often down to zero, whereas chromium and aluminum persisted.[28] These results were interpreted to mean that enhanced corrosion of wear particles by phagocytic cells may contribute significantly to the adverse biologic effects including cell and tissue necrosis.

The small size of the particles presents an enormous collective surface area for corrosion and the complex chemical dynamics of the process are likely to vary as the particle moves from the implant surface to the synovial fluid, intracellular cytoplasm or the bloodstream. Metal alloys corroding in an aqueous environment do not release metal ions in proportion to the element's abundance in the alloy because of the complex electrochemical processes occurring in vivo and the corrosion resistance effect of the stable passivation layer that results in preferential chromium oxide formation on the outer surface.[29,30] Similarly, metal-binding proteins can be expected to have relative affinity for cobalt and chromium that differs from the amounts in the alloy.[31] Other substances that the particles encounter can enhance or inhibit corrosion; for example, transferrin is thought to enhance chromium dissolution, whereas calcium phosphates, which deposit onto the surface of implanted metals, are thought to reduce the dissolution of cobalt and chromium.[22]

Depending on the chemistry of the periparticle fluid,[22] various corrosion products can be produced, including soluble and insoluble forms of various salts and metal-protein complexes, free radicals, and reactive oxygen species.[32,33] These will vary in size, stability, solubility, and consequently, in their bioavailability.[34-36] In one study of the bioaccessibility of various cobalt compounds in human serum and simulated body fluids, the species of cobalt compound, as well as the properties of the surrogate fluids, especially pH, had a major impact on cobalt solubility. It was noted that the cobalt in the form used in implantable devices was less likely to dissolve than other forms.[37] It is thought that synovial fluid contains a ligand (a molecule that binds to another to form a more complex biomolecule) that is highly reactive with chromium, resulting in increased dissolution of chromium compared with serum.[22]

The binding of the various cobalt and chromium products affects the storage and excretion dynamics in vivo. In vitro studies on the binding capacity of blood cells and serum for cobalt and chromium chloride solutions showed that chromium binding to both cells and serum was increased 20-fold over cobalt.[34] Chromium in its hexavalent form can enter cells much more readily than the trivalent form. It is thought to bind mostly to nucleoproteins.[29] In serum, chromium binds selectively to the serum protein siderphilin (transferrin). The intracellular process of reduction of hexavalent chromium to trivalent form is thought to be harmful to chromosomes and other intracellular organelles,[38] and DNA damage has been documented secondary to exposure of cells to soluble forms of cobalt and chromium.[39-41]

In a series of elegant studies comparing the intracellular effects of particulate cobalt and chromium generated in either nanometer or micron sizes by a pin-on-plate tribometer, Papageourgiou et al[33] reported that nanometer-sized particles rapidly corroded inside cells and produced different forms of DNA damage and more extensive damage than microparticles of the same dose. Direct in vivo effects of such DNA changes, however, have not been reported. Ingestion/excretion studies have indicated that chromium VI is reduced to chromium III before entering the bloodstream, which is why the U.S. Environmental Protection Agency allows up to 0.10 mg/L (100 parts per billion) of chromium VI in the water supply.[14,15]

Overview of Measuring Metal Ions

In addition to the complexities involved in dissolution and binding kinetics of wear products from metal-on-metal implants, the complex inter-relationships between ion levels with wear rate, implant, and clinical factors are also poorly understood. The following section reviews the current literature and highlights some of the known and unknown areas relevant to the ion levels that are reported in metal-on-metal implants.

Measurement Methods

It should be noted that the analytic tools needed to measure ions in the blood or urine are operated at close to the qualitative and quantitative detection limits of the equipment. The choice of equipment and the need for strict anticontamination procedures, rigorous calibration, and therefore, operator expertise to avoid measurement errors are important factors in the production of sound data. It is thought that the considerable differences in the literature values, often several orders of magnitude in range, for normal levels of trace elements in human tissues and body fluids reflect methodologic differences and contamination effects.[30,42] For this reason, these types of measurements are usually performed in specialty laboratories where strict quality control methods are followed.

Inductively coupled plasma mass spectroscopy (ICP-MS) and graphite furnace atomic absorption spectrophotometry (GF-AAS) are the most commonly used methods to measure ion levels in blood and urine of patients with implants. The former uses a plasma source to dissociate the metal sample into atoms and ions, which are then separated based on atomic mass-to-charge ratio. The ICP-MS has excellent detection limits and can detect more than one element at once, reducing the sample size and time needed,[43] but it has a high initial capital cost and requires skill to use because some elements create polyatomic interferences, giving inaccurate results.[44] For example, the carbon from the organic compounds in the serum and the argon from the ICP source may interact to give the same atomic mass as the main isotope of chromium. However, this problem can be circumvented by using high-resolution ICP-MS (HR-ICP-MS).[45] This instrument is used in several research centers involved in the study of patient ion levels and has already been noted to have improved the detection of low levels of ions.[46]

Graphite furnace atomic absorption spectrophotometry uses a graphite tube electrically heated to 3000° C to turn the sample into a cloud of atomic gas. Light from the cathode lamp passes through the sample, and atoms of interest absorb the light, which is then measured by the detector. In the flame atomic absorption spectrometry (FAAS), either an air/acetylene or a nitrous oxide/acetylene flame is used instead of the electrically heated graphite tube. GF-AAS is desirable because it has very good detection limits and moderate pricing, and there are few spectral interferences.[43] However, it has a longer analysis time because only single elements are detected and there can be chemical interferences. Some laboratories preferentially measure cobalt using ICP-MS and chromium using GF-AAS.[47]

Regardless of the method used, it is important that the instrument is calibrated against standardized control samples provided by a recognized authority such as the National Institute for Standards and Technology and that the calibration be provided with the data. Furthermore, because of intra- and intersample variation, the results of individual samples tested in triplicate should preferably be presented as a mean with standard deviation.

The large degree of variability in patient ion levels makes it important to present the group data in such a way that the outliers can be shown without skewing that data; the box plot and the median value are suitable for this purpose.[44] Indeed, when the data are presented as a box plot, it also becomes apparent that some patient ion levels may be only minimally changed from preoperative levels over time. The reasons for these low levels are unclear, but again, it is likely to be multifactorial.

Last, it must be emphasized that, although these tools can provide data on the concentrations of cobalt and chromium in patient-derived samples, they cannot provide information about their chemical form (for example trivalent versus hexavalent chromium) or biologic activity.[48]

Choice of Test Matrix

Ions can potentially be measured in all bodily fluids, but the main dispute currently among researchers is whether serum or whole blood is the optimal matrix. Each has advantages and disadvantages (Table 11-1). In an attempt to standardize methods, a consensus document recommended that serum be used because it is relatively easy to test.[44] In contrast, proponents of whole blood testing argue that including the red cells in the analysis allows a more accurate assessment of the total chromium levels because, although hexavalent chromium and cobalt can both bind strongly to blood cells, only hexavalent chromium is capable of passing through cell membranes. It has been postulated that the increases in the chromium level of the cell fraction of blood may indicate that chromium VI is being pooled in the red cells.[49] Studies to date have not been conclusive in determining if the chromium released from implants is trivalent or hexavalent, and further studies are needed.

Table 11-1 Advantages and Disadvantages of the Various Ion Measurement Instruments

	FAAS	GF AAS	ICP-AES	ICP-MS
Detection limits	Very good for some elements	Excellent for some elements	Very good for most elements	Excellent for most elements
Sample throughput	10-15 sec/element	3-4 min/element	1-60 elements/min	All elements in <1 min
Interferences				
Spectral	Very few	Very few	Many	Few
Chemical (matrix)	Many	A lot	Very few	Some
Physical (matrix)	Some	Very few	Very few	Some
Sample volumes required	Large	Very small	Medium	Very small—medium
Semiquantitative analysis	No	No	Yes	Yes
Capital costs	Low	Medium-high	High	Very high
Running costs	Low	Medium	High	High
Relative system costs	1×	2×	4-7×	10-20×

FAAS, flame atomic absorption spectrometry; GFAAS, graphite furnace atomic absorption spectrophotometry; ICP-AES, inductively coupled plasma-atomic emission spectrophotometry; ICP-MS, inductively coupled plasma mass spectroscopy.

Urine analysis for ions can be informative, although it is prone to high variations because of fluctuations in concentration and may be more prone to accidental contamination. Twenty-four–hour collections are recommended,[44] and presenting the results in terms of creatinine levels can overcome the dilution/concentration effects.[50] One major research center using AAS does not routinely test for cobalt in urine.[51] Elimination by the gastrointestinal tract may also be important but this route is not usually measured.

A small number of studies have measured both serum and whole blood to measure the validity of serum as an accurate measurement of systemic exposure to metal ions. Daniel et al[52] compared the serum and whole blood ion levels of 262 concurrent specimens using HR-ICP-MS. This was a heterogenous group of patients up to 10 years postoperatively and included bilateral resurfacings. The average differences between serum and whole blood levels were 0.84 µg/L and 2.1 µg/L for cobalt and chromium, respectively, which were statistically significant. The differences were not even over the range of concentrations, being higher with lower values. This led to the conclusion that serum and whole blood metal ion levels should not be used interchangeably or interconvertibly.

Vendittoli et al[53] compared metal ion concentrations in whole blood, serum, and erythrocytes in patients with metal-on-metal resurfacings between 1 and 2 years postoperatively. They found significant differences between whole blood and serum concentrations of cobalt and chromium and whole blood and erythrocyte concentrations of cobalt, but not chromium. This study indicated an overestimation of serum-derived values. Khan et al[54] looked at relationships between blood, plasma, and serum cobalt levels in patients with metal-on-metal hip resurfacings. Those results indicated that serum and plasma cobalt levels were higher compared with whole blood, and they concluded that whole blood does not give accurate intracellular levels because it contains both blood cells and the fluid part. It should be noted that in all of these studies, the samples would have to be carefully handled to avoid the lysing of red cells, which would then contaminate the serum fraction and reduce the accuracy of the results.[52] Using ICP-MS, Kim et al[55] prospectively assessed ions in serum, erythrocytes, and urine of 60 patients who underwent resurfacing. They reported a strong correlation between serum and erythrocyte cobalt levels but a poor correlation between serum and erythrocyte chromium levels (Box 11-1).

Cobalt and Chromium Levels in Total Hip Replacement

Metal-Polyethylene Total Hip Replacements

It is important to note that even with a standard metal-on-polyethylene (M-PE) total hip replacement, small amounts of metal ions are produced, although in the absence of third-body wear or impingement, these are more likely to come from the Morse taper than the well-functioning M-PE bearing. Jacobs et al[56] have published the results of serum levels for cobalt and chromium measured prospectively by GF-AAS in 75 patients with various types of total hip replacements including porous-coated cobalt-chromium alloy stems and titanium stems that had cobalt-chromium femoral balls articulating against polyethylene. Most patients had levels of cobalt below the detection limit of 0.3 ppb, whereas chromium in the serum and urine were increased up to 7.5-fold over preoperative values or around 0.2 ppb.[38] Ions can be detected in blood from patients with other types of implanted devices such as total knee and spinal replacement hardware. For example, cobalt in serum of patients with the Maverick Total Disk Arthroplasty (Medtronic Sofamor Danek, USA, Inc., Memphis, TN) at an average of 14.8 months was mean 4.75 ppb with standard deviation of 2.71 ppb.[57] Cobalt median serum levels in patients with unilateral cobalt-chromium Foundation total knee

BOX 11-1 Choice of Test Matrix

Whole Blood	Serum
More difficult to test due to complexity of matrix components, requires digestion	Relatively easy to test, few confounding matrix variables
Easy to collect, minimal contamination	Requires anticontamination facilities to promptly separate serum fraction from clot
Includes the metal bound in red cells	Does not include red cell metal

BOX 11-2 Trends Seen with Hip Resurfacing Ion Levels

Run-in then steady state	Wear is higher in the run-in period, the run-in period varies
Large diameters	Minimal wear penalty for large diameters
Variability of results	Multifactorial causes of ion levels
Outliers	High levels probably reflect malfunctioning implants
Comparison with total hip replacement	Steady state levels can be comparable to total hip replacement levels

arthroplasty (Plus Orthopedics, Marl, Germany) was 3.28 ppb at 66 months.[58] These levels are likely to increase if the implants become loose or are damaged by third-body wear.[59]

Metal-on-Metal Total Hip Replacement Ion Levels

Early-generation metal-on-metal bearings often suffered early failure in association with high wear because of poor implant tolerance, manufacturing quality, and design limitations.[60] Metallosis and high systemic levels of ions were noted in such early failures.[61,62] Even when these problems were not in affect, ion levels in patients with first-generation metal-on-metal implants were possibly marred by nonstandard methods of specimen collection and analysis[38]; refinements in technique now allow the detection of levels of only a few parts per billion.

Several longitudinal studies of contemporary metal-on-metal total hip replacements have been published, and a general trend is beginning to emerge, namely that well-functioning high-carbon-cobalt-chromium alloy bearings produce about a 5- to 10-fold increase over preoperative values, resulting in median postoperative values for cobalt of 1 ppb.[63] At a minimum follow-up of 10 years, the median serum cobalt and chromium levels of 72 patients with a high carbon metal-on-metal total hip where the bearing was the only cobalt-chromium in the system were reported as 0.75 ppb (range 0.3-50.1 ppb) and 0.95 (range 0.3-58.6 ppb), respectively.[46] Two patients had markedly elevated levels as seen in the upper range values—one was revised after 10 years, and there was acetabular osteolysis but there was no obvious cause for the elevation; the other was found to have an elevated rim liner in combination with a skirted femoral head, which may have caused impingement. The latter problem has been reported previously.[64]

Surface Arthroplasty Ion Levels

The earliest studies of ion levels in patients with an early-generation surface arthroplasty design noted higher levels than in patients with long-term first-generation metal-on-metal total hip replacements; mean serum cobalt at average 295 months in 8 patients with McKee-Farrar hips was 0.9 ppb, whereas the mean serum cobalt at average 12 months in 6 patients with McMinn resurfacings was 3.77 ppb.[38] Implant retrieval analysis of some failed early-generation metal-on-metal hip resurfacings found that implant manufacturing problems resulted in a small but important amount of out-of-roundness that may have increased wear and ion levels.[65] Improvements in manufacturing have led to reductions in wear, and Campbell et al[66] noted that wear was undetectable in some short-term retrievals of modern resurfacing designs. However, other reports have noted variable levels of wear and ions in hip resurfacings. Table 11-2 summarizes some of the current literature and shows that ion levels in various designs of hip resurfacing can be comparable to total hip replacement levels.

Despite the shortage of longitudinal prospective ion studies in patients who have undergone hip resurfacing, some early conclusions can be made, however, regarding the ion levels in patients with metal-on-metal hip resurfacing (Box 11-2). The early run-in period can be discerned from most published longitudinal studies and appears to last up to a year. Back et al,[47] who studied 16 patients with the Birmingham Hip Resurfacing (BHR) (Smith & Nephew, Memphis, TN) prostheses, noted a 6-month peak in serum cobalt, whereas chromium peaked at 9 months. At 2 years, both levels were below these high peaks but remained above preoperative levels. A study of 25 patients with Conserve®Plus (Wright Medical Technology, Arlington, TN) noted that cobalt peaked at 3 months, whereas chromium peaked at 6 months in serum and 12 months in urine, although a marked degree of variability was measured in all time periods.[51] When compared with serum ion levels in 27 patients with 28-mm total hips, the average 12-month serum cobalt level in 25 metal-on-metal hip resurfacing implants was slightly lower (2.24 ppb vs. 1.07 ppb). This was possibly due to the monoblock, nonmodular design wherein the predominant source of wear products is the bearing, whereas the modular junctions and screw threads present in the total hip replacement added to the bearing-derived wear products.

Table 11-2 Reported Metal Ion Levels in Hip Resurfacing Patients

Author	Reference	Implant	Analytic Technique	Blood Sample	No. of Implants	Mean Time in vivo (mo)	Median Cobalt Level (ppb)	Median Chromium Level (ppb)	Notes
Back et al 2005	47	BHR	ICP-MS (serum cobalt), GFAAS (serum chromium)	Serum	n = 20 enrolled	Preoperatively	0.34	0.31	
		BHR		Serum		3	2.95	3.93	
		BHR		Serum		6	3.33	4.42	
		BHR		Serum		12	2.37	4	
		BHR		Serum		24	1.86	3.53	
Daniel et al 2007	82	BHR	HR-ICP-MS	Whole blood	n = 26	12	1.3 (0.43-3.77), mean	2.4 (0.7-3.82), mean	
Witzleb et al 2007	76	BHR	GF-AAS	Serum	n = 56	3	2.17	1.96	
		BHR		Serum	n = 50	12		4.2	
		BHR		Serum	n = 23	24	4.28	5.12	
Skipor et al 2002	83	Conserve Plus	GF-AAS	Serum	n = 17	3	1.26 ± 0.37	1.88 ± 0.48	Mean +/− 95% C.I.
		Conserve Plus		Serum	n = 10	6	1.2 ± 0.77	2.02 ± 0.98	
		Conserve Plus		Serum	n = 21	12	1.07 ± 0.26	1.80 ± 0.45	
Kim et al 2006	55	Conserve Plus	ICP-MS	Erythrocyte	n = 60	12	0.8	1.2	
		Conserve Plus		Serum		12	1.1	1.9	
		Conserve Plus		Erythrocyte		24	1.1	1.2	
		Conserve Plus		Serum		24	1.6	3.3	
Allan et al 2007	74	Cormet 2000	HR-ICP-MS	Serum	n = 37	6	3.7	4.52	
		Cormet 2000		Serum		12	4.31	5.12	
		Cormet 2000		Serum		24	2.75	3.75	
		Cormet 2000		Serum		36	2.6	4.28	
Vendittoli et al 2007	53	Durom	HR-ICP-MS	Whole blood	n = 64	Preoperatively	0.15 (0.15)	0.92 (0.54)	Mean (S.Dev)
		Durom		Whole blood	n = 50	3	0.90 (0.42)	2.01 (1.12)	
		Durom		Whole blood	n = 51	6	0.80 (0.32)	1.89 (0.96)	
		Durom		Whole blood	n = 53	12	0.67 (0.35)	1.61 (1.04)	
		Durom		Whole blood	n = 27	24	0.59 (0.26)	1.37 (0.65)	
		Durom		Serum	n = 34	12-24	0.83 (0.33-1.45)	1.59 (0.61-3.23)	
		Durom		Erythrocyte	n = 22	12-24	0.46 (0.2-0.88)	0.92 (0.3-2.6)	
		Durom		Whole blood	n = 41	12-24	0.63 (0.25-1.52)	1.33 (0.4-4.5)	
Jacobs et al 1996	38	McMinn and Wagner SA	GF-AAS	Serum	McMinn (n = 4) Wagner SA (n = 2)	12.4	3.77	3.86	First-generation resurfacings

BHR, Birmingham Hip Resurfacing; GFAAS, graphite furnace atomic absorption spectrophotometry; HR-ICP-MS, high-resolution ICP-MS; ICP-MS, inductively coupled plasma mass spectroscopy

Factors Possibly Affecting Ion Levels In Vivo

Metallurgy

Issues such as different choices of test matrix (whole blood, serum, erythrocytes, urine) and the measurement instrumentation continue to confound the comparison of data between different centers studying different implant types. This problem, in turn, makes it difficult to draw conclusions regarding the relationship between implant and clinical variables that are suspected to have a contributory effect. For example, the question of the role played by metallurgy on wear resistance and ion load is still controversial. Of the more than a dozen designs of hip resurfacings available, about half are manufactured using an as-cast material, whereas the remainder undergo some type of heat treatment following casting. Proponents of the as-cast metallurgy maintain that this will provide superior wear resistance, whereas proponents of heat treating argue that the effect of other factors such as clearance and roundness are more important. The relationship between in vivo ion levels and component metallurgy will be difficult to demonstrate because of the multifactorial nature of in vivo wear.[67] The longitudinal monitoring of large patient cohorts may be required before such questions can be answered. Atypically high ion levels have been reported for implants using a low carbon alloy,[67-69] which is consistent with higher wear rates demonstrated by these alloys in hip simulator tests and in retrievals. Low carbon alloys are no longer used in metal-on-metal pairings.

Implant Position

Component position has been found to influence wear,[66] and hence, ions.[70] Hip simulator wear tests have shown that cup angle adversely affects wear[71] because the focal contact involved with edge leading created a deep wear stripe of atypically high wear and prevented the bearing reaching steady-state wear. When the serum ion levels of 60 total hip replacement patients with a titanium alloy stem and 28-mm Metasul (Zimmer, Warsaw, IN) bearings were studied by AAS and correlated with acetabular inclination (which ranged from 23 to 63 degrees), there was no statistically significant effect of inclination angle except for the three patients with the steepest acetabular components (58, 61, and 63 degrees).[70] Those levels were markedly elevated compared with the overall group median values, and it was recommended that sockets of metal-on-metal pairings not exceed 50 degrees.

In another study of 28-mm metal-on-metal bearings by the same authors,[72] the effect of cup angle greater than 50 degrees was mixed; two patients with cups inserted at 58 degrees had normal cobalt ion levels (1 to 2 ppb), whereas one with a cup angle of 62 degrees had 35 ppb. Such observations highlight the complex interrelationship between the many factors influencing wear and ion levels in patients with metal-on-metal bearings.

Large-diameter bearings such as resurfacings may be sensitive to the effects of component position. Buddhdeve et al[73] measured whole blood levels of chromium and cobalt using IC-PMS and found a positive correlation between ion levels and inclination angle (which ranged from 28 to 55 degrees). The authors recommended that an inclination angle of 40 degrees should be used. Allan et al[74] and De Smet et al[75] reported similar findings regarding cup inclination, but the latter also emphasized the role of cup version angle in high serum ion levels. Femoral component position is also likely to influence wear and ion levels,[66] highlighting the importance of surgical technique in obtaining optimal lubrication and low wear in large metal-on-metal bearings.

When a group of 111 patients who had undergone hip resurfacing were compared with a group of 74 patients who had undergone total hip replacement with a comparable range of cup inclination angles (ranging from 42 to 50 degrees and 34 to 48 degrees respectively), no statistically significant correlation between angle and ion level was found in either group in part due to high variability in both.[76] However, none of the cups exceeded 50 degrees, which is the level thought to be associated with high wear. The authors noted, however, that a patient with outlier values (up to 10-fold higher than the larger group median) who was not included in the longitudinal study, had a cup inclination angle of 61 degrees.

Patient Activity

The role of patient activity in metal-on-metal implant wear and ion levels is controversial. Several prospective large cohort studies of metal-on-metal total hip replacement patients have failed to find any correlation between ion levels and activity scores.[72,77] Several small studies have tried to measure ions before and after exercise. Heisel et al[78] studied the effects of exercise on ion levels by measuring serum and urine by GFAAS in seven patients (three with a 36-mm total hip replacement bearing and four with a 49-mm resurfacing bearing), and reported that no rise occurred after sixty minutes of strenuous treadmill exercise. Khan et al[79] used ICP-MS to measure metal ion levels before and after exercise in five patients with small-diameter (28-mm Metasul) and 10 patients with large-diameter implants (38-mm to 54-mm Cormet or Birmingham resurfacings). The study participants walked or jogged at their own pace for 1 hour, and metal ion levels were higher after exercise in both groups. In contrast, the serum ion levels in an Ironman triathlete with a Birmingham resurfacing remained stable during a 4-week period, which covered prerace training and the Ironman event (11 hours of swimming, biking, and marathon running); only a small rise in urine chromium was detected after the race, but this reverted to prerace levels within 48 hours.[50]

Component Diameter

Theoretically, the large-diameter metal-on-metal hip resurfacing bearings are tribologically advantaged compared with the smaller diameter of stem-type hip replacements and this has been shown in the clean, controlled environment of the hip simulator.[80,81] In patients where multiple factors affect ion levels, the effect can be more difficult to detect and the large-diameter advantage has been disputed. Clarke et al[67] reviewed the current literature and presented numerous examples where the ion levels were higher in several different types of resurfacing components compared with 28-mm total hip replacements. The authors concluded that large-diameter metal-on-metal bearings experience higher run-in wear for a longer period and hypothesized that this may be due to higher radial mismatch (clearance) in resurfacings, although allowing that a number of other factors from metallurgy to implant position could be contributing factors. Daniel et al[82] compared the urine and whole blood ion levels of 26 patients with 50- and 54-mm BHR implants at 2 years postoperatively, and 58 patients with 5 years of BHR use, with 28 patients with a 28-mm Metasul total hip replacement at 1 to 3 years and 23 with 4 to 6 years Metasul use. There was no statistically significant differences in urinary or whole blood cobalt and chromium levels at either time period, and the authors concluded that diameter did not affect whole blood levels of ions. Skipor et al[83] also reported no significant differences between total hip replacement patient levels compared with a hip resurfacing made by the same manufacturer.

Bilateral Implants

There is limited information about the ion levels of patients who have bilateral resurfacings. Studies of these patients is complicated by the variable timing of the second hip surgery which can range from simultaneous to several years. Several studies have noted that bilateral patients often have the highest ion levels.[38,76] One study of six bilateral total hip replacements and seven Conserve®Plus hip resurfacings was performed using serum cobalt and chromium and urine chromium levels measured by GFAAS.[84] The second surgery was performed from 3 to 20 months in the total hip replacement group and from 5 to 46 months in the resurfacing group. All patients demonstrated increased values following implantation of the second implant and some were more than double the unilateral values.

Preliminary data from a larger series of patients who underwent bilateral resurfacing including five simultaneous and 10 staged from 4 to 48 months after the first hip were compared with a group of 39 patients with unilateral resurfacing components implanted by the same surgeon (Harlan C. Amstutz, unpublished data, 2007). Again, all patients demonstrated elevations after the second hip, but the staged bilaterals had lower ion levels compared with simultaneous bilaterals at the same postoperative period. These observations highlight the complex, multifactorial nature of ion production, storage, and clearance.[85]

Areas of Concern

Effect on the Fetus

Women of childbearing age are recipients of metal-on-metal surface arthroplasty implants, and there is concern over the effects of ions on the fetus. Some surgeons refuse to implant metal-on-metal hips in women of childbearing age; others recommended that women have the baby before the resurfacing, or postpone pregnancy until at least a year after the resurfacing. Data have now been reported to show that cobalt and chromium do indeed cross the placenta. Ten women with BHR implants consented to provide their blood and blood from the umbilical cords of their newborns. The women in the study had low levels of ions, but cobalt and chromium were detected in cord blood, although there was a barrier effect with 29% of maternal chromium levels and 60% of maternal cobalt levels passing into the umbilical cord blood.[86] Similar findings have been noted in two women who underwent hip resurfacing with the Conserve®Plus, which was developed by this book's editor (Harlan C. Amstutz, MD, unpublished data) (Table 11-3). Children born to those mothers have been apparently normal, as were the seven others from three mothers, but the levels of ions in both the studied mothers and babies were within the normal range (see Table 11-2, serum cobalt range 1.1-2.1 ppb). Further studies are needed to provide data on the effects on the fetus, where much higher levels of ions are detected.

Chromosome and DNA Damage

One group in Bristol, England has spearheaded research into the effects of metal ions on DNA and chromosomes. Chromosomal changes have been demonstrated in patients with various types of joint replacements including metal-on-polyethylene and metal-on-metal devices.[40,87] There was a statistically significant increase of both chromosome translocations (relocation of a chromosomal segment in a different position in the genome) and aneuploidy (chromosome loss and gain) detected by fluorescent in situ hybridization in peripheral blood lymphocytes of 95 patients with the Metasul metal-on-metal total hips at 6, 12, and 24 months after surgery.[41] The cause for the increased aberrations was not known, and several possible confounding factors were recognized (such as age and smoking) but were not thought to be responsible. There were no statistically significant correlations between chromosome translocation indices and cobalt or chromium concentrations, but they did correlate with molybdenum levels despite their low levels. Similar aberrations have been shown to occur with titanium, and the clinical implications from this and other studies by the Bristol group are as yet unclear because there is no confirmed case of an implant-induced cancer to date.[88,89] The multifactorial nature of DNA damage makes linking the results of these studies to a clinical problem very difficult.[90]

Kidney Disease and Ion Clearance

Both cobalt and chromium can be excreted through the kidneys. Cobalt is quickly cleared by the kidneys. However, chromium tends to be more slowly excreted because it occurs in a biphasic manner with the rapid excretion of small dialyzable molecules, followed by a slower excretion of the larger and more prevalent molecules (such as the siderophilin-chromium complex).[29] Kidney disease may interfere with this clearance, leading to systemic accumulation. Brodner et al[91] reported that markedly elevated serum cobalt and serum

Table 11-3 Levels of Ions Reported in Two Mothers and Their Offspring

Sample	Cobalt ppb	Chromium ppb
Mother #1 Maternal serum	1.13	2.23
Maternal red cells	1.4	1.5
Baby (cord blood serum)	0.6	0.7
Baby (cord blood red cells)	1.0	0.1
Breast milk 3 wk post-partum	0.4 (a second sample was nondetectable)	0.5 in two samples
Maternal urine 3 wks post-partum	1.45	2.1
Mother #2 serum prenatal	1.19	2.52
Mother 2 urine prenatal		4.77
Mother 2 urine 16 mo postnatal		3.98
Baby 2 (cord blood serum)	1.11	0.48
Baby 2 urine at 16 months		0.085*

Mother #1 59 months postoperative unilateral Conserve Plus surface arthroplasty.
Mother #2 51 months postoperative unilateral Conserve Plus surface arthroplasty.
**Consistent with laboratory data of children from mothers who did not undergo implant surgery. Note that all of the maternal values are within the typical range for this implant.*

chromium levels (for example, 105 ppb cobalt and 60 ppb chromium in one patient, 119 Co and 75 ppb Cr in the other) were measured in two patients with endstage chronic renal disease but the levels returned to normal after renal transplantation. Chronic renal disease is usually considered to be a contraindication for the use of a metal-on-metal articulation. One patient of this book's editor has a metal-on-metal surface arthroplasty that was implanted 4 years before renal transplantation; at his last follow-up at 11 years, the ion levels are normal (serum cobalt 2.06 ppb, serum chromium 0.83 ppb).

Outliers

One concern with the use of metal-on-metal bearings is risk of long-term exposure of joint tissues to accumulating wear products, both particulate and nonparticulate in nature. Nearly all ion studies report one or more high level outlier (a case that exceeds 3 times the standard deviation of the group). For example, the case shown in Figure 11-1 has been one of two outliers within a prospective study of patients who have undergone metal-on-metal surface arthroplasty. Compared with the group (n = 20) median cobalt at 2 years of 1.13 ppb, this patient had a level of 59.6 ppb. The patient is asymptomatic and presents a clinical quandary: Should these implants be revised under the assumption that they are malfunctioning even if the problem is not clear from the radiographs? There is a known level of risk from revision surgery that must be balanced against the unknown risk of the local and systemic effects of high ion levels. More data are needed to help surgeons make this important treatment decision.

Metal Allergy/Sensitivity

According to most immunology textbooks, the term "allergy" refers to one of the four specific types of hypersensitivity (Box 11-3), but differs from the delayed-type hypersensitivity (DTH, type 4) which is the form describing a patient reacting to a metal implant.[35] Occasional reports of implant failure because of an apparent metal allergy have appeared in the orthopaedic literature since metal implants were used.[92-94] It is now recognized that a small number of patients will suffer from a form of allergy or hypersensitivity to constituents of the metal-on-metal bearings even in the absence of high wear.[35,95,96] The histologic features of the reaction characterizing the joint tissues from these hypersensitive patients are different from the classic textbook form of type 4 DTH.[97] For this reason, the term aseptic lymphocytic vasculitis–associated lesions

BOX 11-3 Hypersensitivity Definitions

Type	Description
Type I (allergy)	Involves a soluble antigen reacting with immunoglobulin E (IgE), leading to mast-cell activation (e.g., asthma)
Type II	Cell or matrix antigens are bound by immunoglobulin G (IgG), leading to activation of phagocytic cells (e.g., penicillin reaction)
Type III	Cellular antigens bound by immunoglobulin G (IgG), leading to activation of phagocytic cells or the complement cascade (e.g., serum sickness)
Type IV (delayed-type hypersensitivity)	Soluble antigens bind to T cells, leading to macrophage or eosinophil activation (e.g., contact dermatitis)
Aseptic lymphocytic vasculitis–associated lesions	Infiltrates of T and B cells, often with plasma cells, arranged perivascularly or diffuse, often forming a tidemark around an area of necrosis. Fibrin build-up is common along the capsule or bursa surface

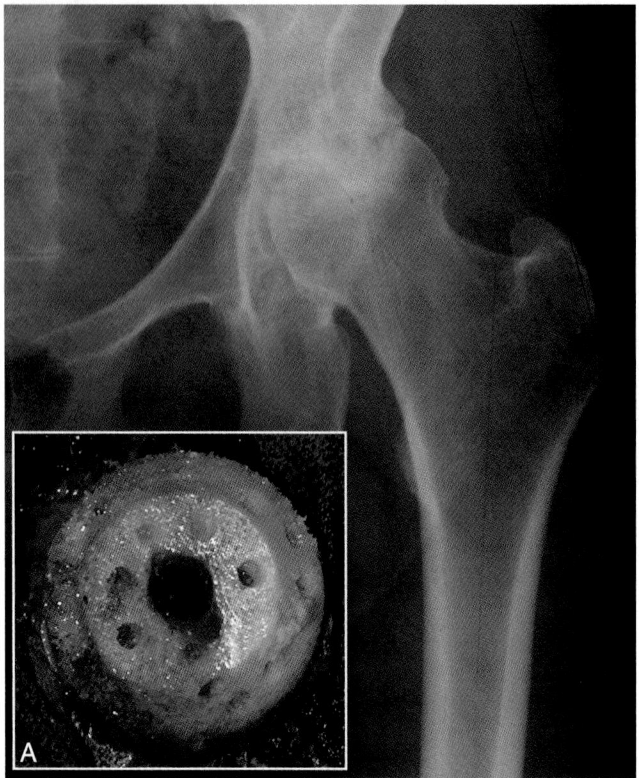

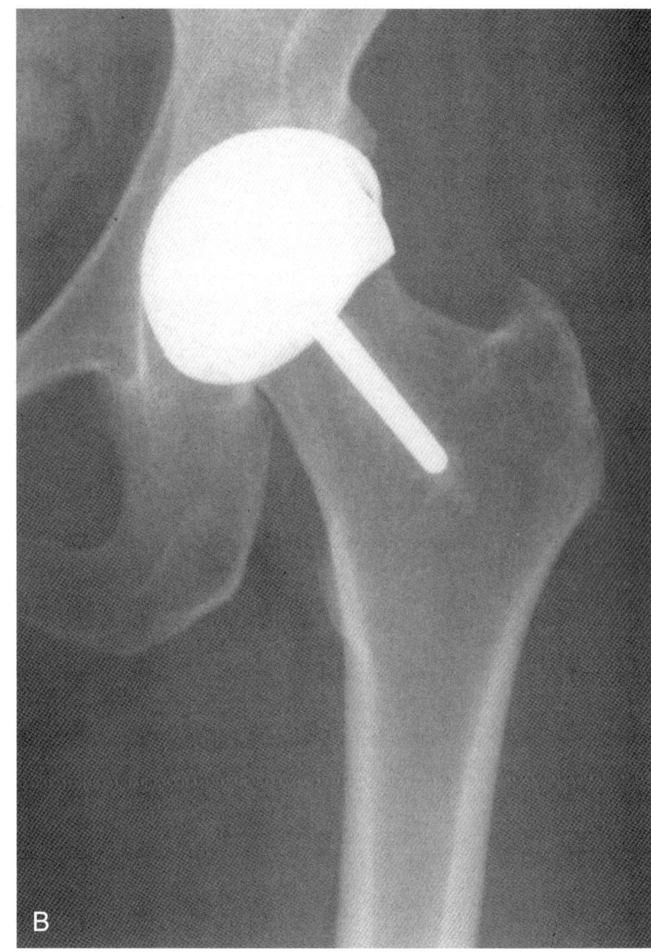

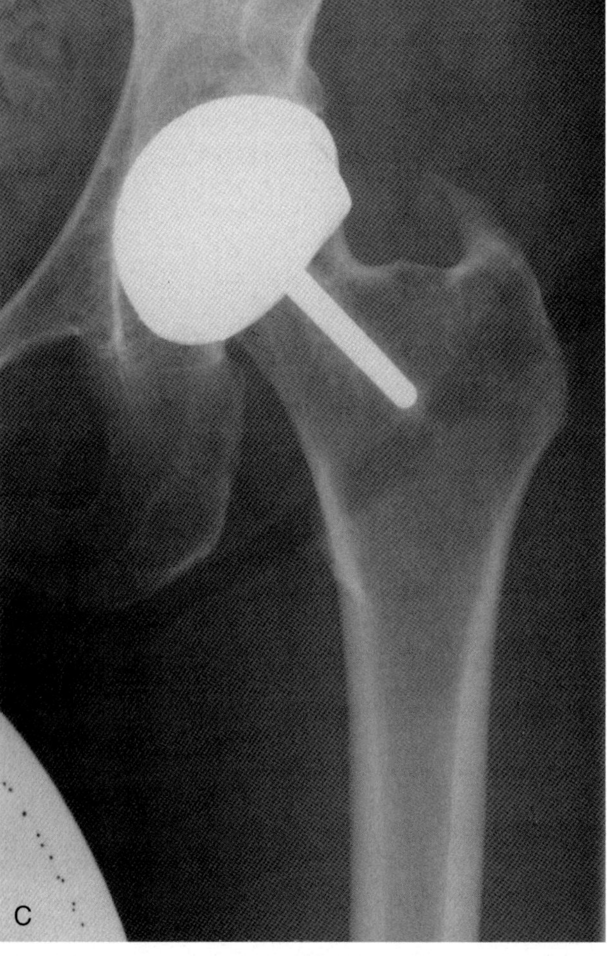

Figure 11-1 **A,** Anteroposterior x-ray of a 68-year-old woman who had extreme generalized ligamentous laxity–associated and primary osteoarthritis of the left hip. The insert shows the good bone quality of the femoral head after preparation for cementation. **B,** Anteroposterior radiograph taken 3 months after metal-on-metal resurfacing. The acetabular component appears to be open laterally 47 degrees and anteverted approximately 30 degrees. **C,** Anteroposterior view 6 years after surgery. The patient is asymptomatic with University of California-Los Angeles (UCLA) scores of 10 for pain walking and function and 7 for activity. Flex, 150 degrees; AB-add, 100 degrees; and rotation arc, 120 degrees. Note the normally observed remodeling change laterally, presumably from neck-socket impingement during Yoga stretches. Her ion levels are very high (cobalt in serum 56.9 ppb at 2 years, 36.7 at 6 years).

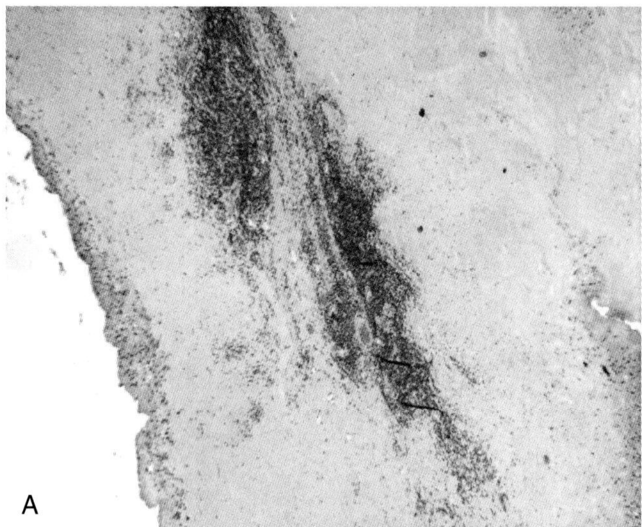

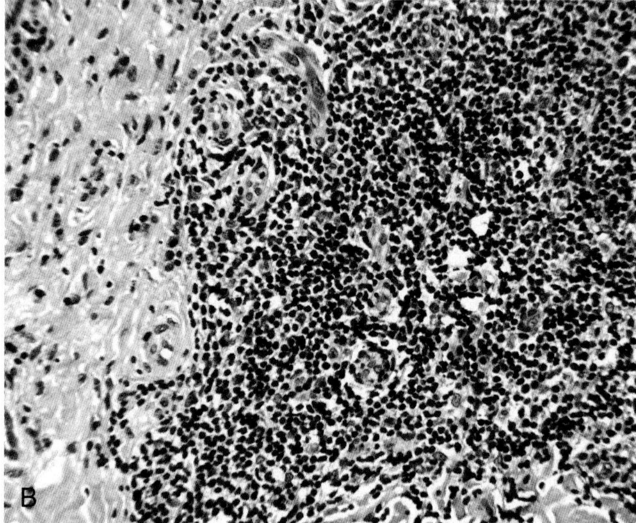

Figure 11-2 **A,** Histology of tissues around the metal-on-metal surface arthroplasty of a patient revised for unexplained pain after 20 months (s2206). **B,** Higher power micrograph showing the characteristic lymphocytic infiltrates of aseptic lymphocytic vasculitis–associated lesions.

(ALVAL) has been coined to describe the histological features associated with an allergy-like reaction in the joint tissues.[98] An example is given in Figure 11-2; the characteristics are infiltrates of lymphocytes, often with plasma cells and frequently these are arranged perivascularly. These infiltrates appear to be denser and more extensive in patients with clinical signs of metal allergy (ongoing pain, typically in the groin; effusion often forming an enlarged bursa or groin mass) in the absence of infection or mechanical causes. Lesser numbers of lymphocytes are commonly found in tissues of patients with failed metal-on-metal implants in the absence of such clinical features and the reason for their presence in the tissues is unclear.[1,66]

Diagnosing metal sensitivity can be difficult: If all possible causes for the patient's pain can be eliminated by imaging or hematologic testing, a diagnosis of metal sensitivity should be entertained and if confirmed, the cobalt chromium bearings should be removed.

Skin Sensitivity and Hip Sensitivity

It has been estimated that 10% to 15% of the general population has a dermal sensitivity to metal; nickel is the most common sensitizer in humans, followed by cobalt and chromium.[35] For this reason, there is concern that patients with a dermal sensitivity will also have an adverse reaction to a cobalt-chromium hip replacement. Several excellent review articles address this issue, and each generally agrees that there is little evidence to support this concern.[35] A retrospective survey of patients with a metal-on-metal hip resurfacing was carried out among this book editor's patient cohort. They were asked about reactivity to jewelry (type of jewelry involved, the metal involved, and the nature of the reaction). One hundred seventy-eight patients responded (142 male 36 female) and 21 (5.6%) reported they had a dermal problem, mostly to steel or "cheap" jewelry in the form of rashes, redness and itching. Of those 21, 11 were male and 10 were female, but because most of the overall patient cohort was male, the proportion of women with skin reactions was higher. However, none of these patients had any problems with their hip replacement. An example is provided in Figure 11-3.

Metal-Induced Toxicity

Some of the component metals of the alloys used for total joint prostheses can be toxic (inducing cell death) when a certain threshold level accumulates in the cells, tissues, or joint fluids. Numerous in vitro studies have attempted to establish which material and form (particle or corrosion products) of the alloys could be toxic in patients. The studies typically involved exposure of various types of cells to variable doses of particles or to fluids in which particles had been incubated, releasing soluble corrosion products. For example, Rae et al[99] incubated primary monolayer cultures of human synovial fibroblasts with various preparations of alloy metals for up to 18 days. The cultures exposed to particulate pure metals were poisoned by cobalt and vanadium but were not affected by nickel, chromium, molybdenum, titanium, or aluminum. Some of the early studies have been criticized for using excessively high doses of particles,[100] but similar results have been found by other groups using more clinically relevant particles in doses closer to the expected implant-related level.[101,102] Interestingly, the toxicity of cobalt particles is enhanced when they are freshly produced compared with particles that have "aged," presumably because the latter are coated with a passivation film that reduces the corrosion product exchange with the cells.[103,104] The age of the cells was also found to influence the cellular response, with "older" cells (allowed to reproduce in vitro for 15 generations) showing a greater loss of viability and more complex aneuploidy than younger cells (allowed to reproduce for five generations).

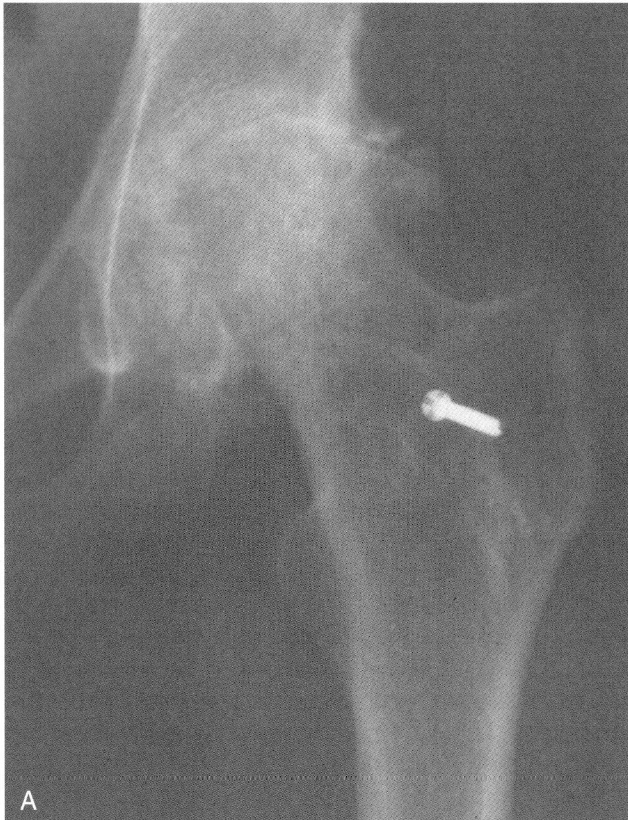

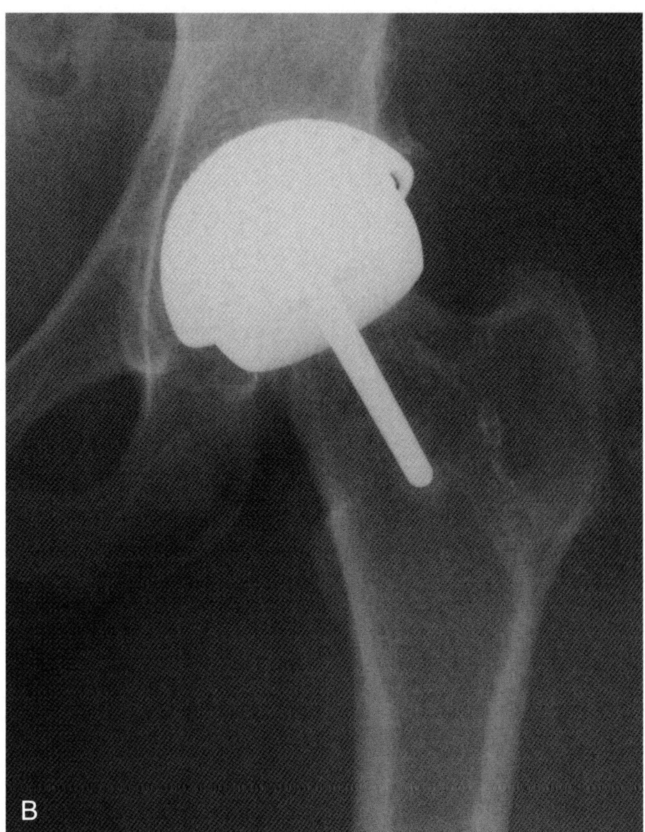

Figure 11-3 **A,** Preoperative radiograph of a 53-year-old woman with successful Conserve®Plus metal-on-metal surface arthroplasty, despite a known dermal reactivity to metal jewelry. **B,** Radiograph at 5.5 years.

Hallab et al,[105] who have extensive experience in these types of studies, have studied the proliferation response and viability of osteoblasts, fibroblasts and lymphocytes after exposure in culture to aluminum, cobalt, trivalent chromium, iron, molybdenum, nickel, vanadium, and sodium solutions at different concentrations. Only cobalt and vanadium were found to be toxic in the concentrations likely to be found in synovial fluid, whereas chromium was less toxic. The relative prevalence of soluble cobalt indicates that it would be the more important determinant of local tissue toxicity around metal-on-metal surface arthroplasties, and reports of extensive necrosis in cases with high wear support that local toxic reactions do occur.[23,65]

Retrieval specimens submitted for analysis to the Implant Retrieval Lab of Orthopaedic Hospital have provided a clear demonstration of the risks to the local tissues when there is excessive wear from a failed metal-on-metal bearing. Extensive tissue necrosis of periprosthetic tissues and surrounding muscle or enlarged, partly necrotic bursae filled with fibrin have all been encountered in cases with high wear and metallosis. Reports are beginning to appear describing masses in the hip, fluid hernias, and similar pathologic entities, and some of these have their origin in a local tissue reaction to metal-induced toxicity (some may be related to metal sensitivity).

Reactions further from the joint have also been reported; Case et al[24] compared the extent and effects of dissemination of wear debris in 13 patients with metal implants with grossly variable degrees of wear and damage. Metal was found in local and distant lymph nodes, bone marrow, liver, and spleen only in those cases with gross wear or damage. The amount of metal as measured from ICP-MS of periprosthetic tissues was highest in four cases with loose prostheses (two stainless steel total hips at 7.5 and 8.5 years, one cobalt-chrome Thomson hemiarthroplasty at 9 years, and a steel and titanium knee at 14 years). Histologically, there was a higher concentration of metal in the iliac lymph nodes closest to the joints, and more metal was present in cases that were loose. Particles were concentrated in sinus macrophages, causing mild inflammation, but around the loose total knee, the accumulation of the metal-laden cells resulted in large numbers of granulomas and extensive necrosis of the lymphoid tissue. At the transmission electron level, changes in the nuclei of macrophages with ingested metal particles suggested an apoptotic (cellular self-destruction) response. In vitro studies have confirmed that cobalt and chromium exposure can induce both necrosis and apoptosis depending on dose and exposure time.[106]

Summary

This chapter focused on nonparticulate wear products; little is known about these products, but it is likely that individual differences in local and systemic reaction will present a clinical and histologic spectrum. Much is yet to be learned about their long-term effects, particularly at the genetic level, but the wider interest in monitoring metal-on-metal bearings with ion measurements, and the continued provision of retrieval specimens for analysis should provide further information in the future. Metal sensitivity reactions, although seemingly rare, will remain a clinical problem until a screening test is developed. It is hoped that a better understanding about the potential consequences of high wear will encourage surgeons to carefully monitor their patients and to revise hip problems quickly to avoid possible metal-induced problems.

References

1. Campbell P, Mirra J, Doorn P, Mills B, Alim R, Catelas I: Histopathology of metal-on-metal hip joint tissues. In Rieker C, Oberholzer S, Wyss U (eds): World Tribology Forum in Arthroplasty. Göttingen, Germany, Hans Huber, 2000, pp 167-180.
2. Doorn PF, Mirra JM, Campbell PA, Amstutz HC: Tissue reaction to metal on metal total hip prostheses. Clin Orthop Rel Res 1996;329(suppl):S187-S205.
3. Willert H-G, Buchhorn GH, Semlitsch M: Particle disease due to wear of metal alloys. Findings from retrieval studies. In Morrey BF (ed): Biological, Material, and Mechanical Considerations of Joint Replacement. New York, Raven Press, Ltd, 1993, pp 129-146.
4. Archibeck MJ, Jacobs JJ, Roebuck KA, Glant TT: The basic science of periprosthetic osteolysis. Instructr Course Lect 2001;50:185-195.
5. Ingham E, Fisher J: Biological reactions to wear debris in total joint replacement. Proc Inst Mech Eng [H] 2000;214:21-37.
6. Revell PA, al-Saffar N, Kobayashi A: Biological reaction to debris in relation to joint prostheses. Proc Inst Mech Eng [H] 1997;211:187-197.
7. World Health Organization website. Accessed July 20, 2007. http://www.who.int/ipcs/publications/cicad/cicad69%20.pdf
8. Agency for Toxic Substances and Disease Registry. http://www.atsdr.cdc.gov/toxprofiles/tp33-c3.pdf
9. Huaux F, Lasfargues G, Lauwerys R, Lison D: Lung toxicity of hard metal particles and production of interleukin-1, tumor necrosis factor-alpha, fibronectin, and cystatin-c by lung phagocytes. Toxicol Appl Pharmacol 1995;132:53-62.
10. Lison D, De Boeck M, Verougstraete V, Kirsch-Volders M: Update on the genotoxicity and carcinogenicity of cobalt compounds. Occup Environ Med 2001;58:619-625.
11. De Boeck M, Lardau S, Buchet JP, Kirsch-Volders M, Lison D: Absence of significant genotoxicity in lymphocytes and urine from workers exposed to moderate levels of cobalt-containing dust: a cross-sectional study. Environ Mol Mutagen 2000;36:151-160.
12. McGregor DB, Baan RA, Partensky C, Rice JM, Wilbourn JD: Evaluation of the carcinogenic risks to humans associated with surgical implants and other foreign bodies—a report of an IARC Monographs Programme Meeting. International Agency for Research on Cancer. Eur J Cancer 2000;36:307-313.
13. Baruthio F: Toxic effects of chromium and its compounds. Biol Trace Elem Res 1992;32:145-153.
14. Paustenbach DJ, Finley BL, Mowat FS, Kerger BD: Human health risk and exposure assessment of chromium (VI) in tap water. J Toxicol Environ Health A 2003;66:1295-1339.
15. Finley BL, Scott PK, Norton RL, Gargas ML, Paustenbach DJ: Urinary chromium concentrations in humans following ingestion of safe doses of hexavalent and trivalent chromium: implications for biomonitoring. J Toxicol Environ Health 1996;48: 479-499.
16. Losi ME, Amrhein C, Frankenberger WT, Jr: Environmental biochemistry of chromium. Rev Environ Contam Toxicol 1994;136:91-121.
17. Anderson RA: Chromium metabolism and its role in disease processes in man. Clin Physiol Biochem 1986;4:31-41.
18. Liu F, Jin Z, Roberts P, Grigoris P: Importance of head diameter, clearance, and cup wall thickness in elastohydrodynamic lubrication analysis of metal-on-metal hip resurfacing prostheses. Proc Inst Mech Eng [H] 2006;220:695-704.
19. Firkins PJ, Tipper JL, Saadatzadeh MR, Ingham E, Stone MH, Farrar R, Fisher J: Quantitative analysis of wear and wear debris from metal-on-metal hip prostheses tested in a physiological hip joint simulator. Biomed Mater Eng 2001;11: 143-157.
20. Catelas I, Medley JB, Campbell PA, Huk OL, Bobyn JD: Comparison of in vitro with in vivo characteristics of wear particles from metal-metal hip implants. J Biomed Mater Res 2004; 70B:167-178.
21. Doorn PF, Campbell PA, Amstutz HC: Metal versus polyethylene wear particles in total hip replacements. A review. Clin Orthop Rel Res 1996;329(suppl):S206-S216.
22. Lewis AC, Kilburn MR, Heard PJ, Scott TB, Hallam KR, Allen GC, Learmonth ID: The entrapment of corrosion products from CoCr implant alloys in the deposits of calcium phosphate: a comparison of serum, synovial fluid, albumin, EDTA, and water. J Orthop Rel Res 2006;24:1587-1596.
23. Buscher R, Tager G, Dudzinski W, Gleising B, Wimmer MA, Fischer A: Subsurface microstructure of metal-on-metal hip joints and its relationship to wear particle generation. J Biomed Mater Res B Appl Biomater 2005;72:206-214.
24. Case CP, Langkamer VG, James C, Palmer MR, Kemp AJ, Heap PF, Solomon L: Widespread dissemination of metal debris from implants. J Bone Joint Surg 1994;76:701-712.
25. Urban RM, Jacobs JJ, Tomlinson MJ, Gavrilovic J, Black J, Peoc'h M: Dissemination of wear particles to the liver, spleen, and abdominal lymph nodes of patients with hip or knee replacement. J Bone Joint Surg 2000;82:457-476.
26. Lewis CG, Belniak RM, Hopfer SM, Sunderman J, William F: Cobalt in periprosthetic soft tissue. Acta Orthop Scand 1991;62:447-450.
27. Haynes DR, Rogers SD, Howie DW, Pearcy MJ, Vernon-Roberts B: Drug inhibition of the macrophage response to metal wear particles in vitro. Clin Orthop 1996;323:316-326.
28. Shahgaldi BF, Heatley FW, Dewar A, Corrin B, Hennig FF, Raithel HJ, Schaller KH, Dohler JR: In vivo corrosion of cobalt-chromium and titanium wear particles. Nickel-, chrom- and cobalt-concentrations in human tissue and body fluids of hip prosthesis patients. J Bone Joint Surg 1995;77B:962-966.
29. Yang J, Black J: Competitive binding of chromium, cobalt and nickel to serum proteins. Biomaterials 1994;15:262-268.
30. Michel R, Hofmann J, Loer F, Zilkens J: Trace element burdening of human tissues due to the corrosion of hip-joint prostheses made of cobalt-chromium alloys. Arch Orthop Trauma Surg 1984;103:85-95.
31. Betts F, Wright T, Salvati EA, Boskey A, Bansal M: Cobalt-alloy metal debris in periarticular tissues from total hip revision

arthroplasties. Metal contents and associated histologic findings. Clin Orthop Rel Res 1992;276:75-82.
32. Hallab NJ, Jacobs JJ, Skipor A, Black J, Mikecz K, Galante JO: Systemic metal-protein binding associated with total joint replacement arthroplasty. J Biomed Mater Res 2000;49:353-361.
33. Papageorgiou I, Brown C, Schins R, Singh S, Newson R, Davis S, Fisher J, Ingham E, Case CP: The effect of nano- and micron-sized particles of cobalt-chromium alloy on human fibroblasts in vitro. Biomaterials 2007;28:2946-2958. Epub 2007 Mar 2941.
34. Venezia C, Karol MH: Comparison of cobalt and chromium binding to blood elements. Toxicology 1984;30:125-133.
35. Hallab N, Merritt K, Jacobs JJ: Metal sensitivity in patients with orthopaedic implants. J Bone Joint Surg 2001;83A:428-436.
36. Beyersmann D: Interactions in metal carcinogenicity. Toxicol Lett 1994;72:333-338.
37. Stopford W, Turner J, Cappellini D, Brock T: Bioaccessibility testing of cobalt compounds. J Environ Monit 2003;5:675-680.
38. Jacobs JJ, Skipor AK, Doorn PF, Campbell P, Schmalzried TP, Black J, Amstutz HC: Cobalt and chromium concentrations in patients with metal on metal total hip replacements. Clin Orthop Rel Res 1996;329(suppl):S256-S263.
39. Case CP, Langkamer VG, Howell RT, Webb J, Standen G, Palmer M, Kemp A, Learmonth ID: Preliminary observations on possible premalignant changes in bone marrow adjacent to worn total hip arthroplasty implants. Clin Orthop Rel Res 1996;329(suppl):S269-S279.
40. Doherty AT, Howell RT, Ellis LA, Bisbinas I, Learmonth ID, Newson R, Case CP: Increased chromosome translocations and aneuploidy in peripheral blood lymphocytes of patients having revision arthroplasty of the hip. J Bone Joint Surg 2001; 83:1075-1081.
41. Ladon D, Doherty A, Newson R, Turner J, Bhamra M, Case CP: Changes in metal levels and chromosome aberrations in the peripheral blood of patients after metal-on-metal hip arthroplasty. J Arthroplasty 2004;19:78-83.
42. Michel R, Nolte M, Reich M, Löer F: Systemic effects of implanted prostheses made of cobalt chromium alloys. Arch Orthop Traumatic Surg 1991;110:61-74.
43. Thermo Scientific: AAS, GFAAS, ICP or ICP-MS? Which technique should I use? http://www.thermo.com/eThermo/CMA/PDFs/Articles/articlesFile_18407.pdf
44. MacDonald SJ, Brodner W, Jacobs JJ: A consensus paper on metal ions in metal-on-metal hip arthroplasties. J Arthroplasty 2004;19:12-16.
45. Case CP, Ellis L, Turner JC, Fairman B: Development of a routine method for the determination of trace metals in whole blood by magnetic sector inductively coupled plasma mass spectrometry with particular relevance to patients with total hip and knee arthroplasty. Clin Chem 2001;47:275-280.
46. Grubl A, Marker M, Brodner W, Giurea A, Heinze G, Meisinger V, Zehetgruber H, Kotz R: Long-term follow-up of metal-on-metal total hip replacement. J Orthop Rel Res 2007;25: 841-848.
47. Back DL, Young DA, Shimmin AJ: How do serum cobalt and chromium levels change after metal-on-metal hip resurfacing? Clin Orthop Rel Res 2005;438:177-181.
48. Jacobs JJ, Gilbert JL, Urban RM: Corrosion of metal orthopaedic implants. J Bone Joint Surg 1998;80:268-282.
49. Bartolozzi A, Black J: Chromium concentrations in serum, blood clot and urine from patients following total hip arthroplasty. Biomaterials 1985;6:2-8.
50. De Haan R, Campbell P, Reid S, Skipor AK, De Smet K: Metal ion levels in a triathlete with a metal-on-metal resurfacing arthroplasty of the hip. J Bone Joint Surg Br 2007;89:538-541.
51. Skipor A, Campbell P, Paterson L, Amstutz H, Schmalzried T, Jacobs J: Serum and urine metal levels in patients with metal on metal surface arthroplasty. J Mater Sci Mater Med 2002;13:1227-1234.
52. Daniel J, Ziaee H, Pynsent PB, McMinn DJ: The validity of serum levels as a surrogate measure of systemic exposure to metal ions in hip replacement. J Bone Joint Surg Br 2007;89:736-741.
53. Vendittoli PA, Mottard S, Roy AG, Dupont C, Lavigne M: Chromium and cobalt ion release following the Durom high carbon content, forged metal-on-metal surface replacement of the hip. J Bone Joint Surg Br 2007;89:441-448.
54. Khan M, Kuiper J, Richardson J: Relationship between blood, plasma and serum cobalt levels in patients with metal on metal hip replacement. Orthopaedic Research Society (ORS); 2007 San Diego Convention Center. San Diego, CA, Poster no. 1657.
55. Kim P: Cobalt and chromium levels in patients with metal on metal hip resurfacing prostheses. Toronto, Canada, Canadian Orthopaedic Association, 2006.
56. Jacobs JJ, Skipor AK, Patterson LM, Hallab NJ, Paprosky WG, Black J, Galante JO: Metal release in patients who have had a primary total hip arthroplasty. A prospective, controlled, longitudinal study. J Bone Joint Surg 1998;80:1447-1458.
57. Zeh A, Planert M, Siegert G, Lattke P, Held A, Hein W: Release of cobalt and chromium ions into the serum following implantation of the metal-on-metal Maverick-type artificial lumbar disc (Medtronic Sofamor Danek). Spine 2007;32:348-352.
58. Luetzner J, Krummenauer F, Lengel AM, Ziegler J, Witzleb WC: Serum metal ion exposure after total knee arthroplasty. Clin Orthop Relat Res 2007;461:136-142.
59. Tager K: Aspects of loosening in McKee-Farrar endoprostheses. In Buchorn GH, Willert HG (eds): Technical Principles, Design and Safety of Joint Implants. Seattle, Hogrefe Huber, 1994, pp 72-81.
60. McKellop H, Park S-H, Chiesa R, Doorn P, Lu B, Normand P, Grigoris P, Amstutz H: In vivo wear of three types of metal on metal hip prostheses during two decades of use. Clin Orthop Rel Res 1996;329(suppl):S128-S140.
61. Dielert E, Milachowski K, Schramel P: [The role of the alloy-specific elements iron, cobalt, chromium and nickel in aseptic loosening of total hip joint prosthesis]. Z Orthop Ihre Grenzgeb 1983;121:58-63.
62. Jones DA, Lucas HK, O'Driscoll M, Price CHG, Wibberley B: Cobalt toxicity after McKee hip arthroplasty. J Bone Joint Surg 1975;57B:289-296.
63. MacDonald SJ: Can a safe level for metal ions in patients with metal-on-metal total hip arthroplasties be determined? J Arthroplasty 2004;19:71-77.
64. Delaunay CP: Metal-on-metal bearings in cementless primary total hip arthroplasty. J Arthroplasty 2004;19:35-40.
65. Campbell P, McKellop H, Alim R, Mirra J, Nutt S, Dorr L, Amstutz HC: Metal-on-metal hip replacements: wear performance and cellular response to wear particles. In Disegi JA, Kennedy RL, Pilliar R: Cobalt-Base Alloys for Biomedical Applications, ASTM STP 1365. West Conshohocken, PA, American Society for Testing and Materials; 1999, pp 193-209.
66. Campbell P, Beaule P, Ebramzadeh E, Le Duff M, De Smet K, Lu Z, Amstutz H: A study of implant failure in metal-on-metal surface arthroplasties. Clin Orthop 2006;453:35-46.

67. Clarke IC, Donaldson T, Bowsher JG, Nasser S, Takahashi T: Current concepts of metal-on-metal hip resurfacing. Orthop Clin North Am 2005;36:143-162, viii.
68. Lhotka C, Szekeres T, Steffan I, Zhuber K, Zweymuller K: Four-year study of cobalt and chromium blood levels in patients managed with two different metal-on-metal total hip replacements. J Orthop Res 2003;21:189-195.
69. Milosev I, Pisot V, Campbell P: Serum levels of cobalt and chromium in patients with Sikomet metal-metal total hip replacements. J Orthop Res 2005;23:526-535.
70. Brodner W, Grubl A, Jankovsky R, Meisinger V, Lehr S, Gottsauner-Wolf F: Cup inclination and serum concentration of cobalt and chromium after metal-on-metal total hip arthroplasty. J Arthroplasty 2004;19:66-70.
71. Wang A: Future bearing technologies. Presented at Tribos; 2007 Queensland, Australia.
72. Brodner W, Bitzan P, Meisinger V, Kaider A, Gottsauner-Wolf F, Kotz R: Serum cobalt levels after metal-on-metal total hip arthroplasty. J Bone Joint Surg 2003;85-A:2168-2173.
73. Buddhdev P, Tarassoli P, Powell J, Skinner J, Hart A: Cup inclination angle and whole blood levels of cobalt and chromium ions after hip resurfacing. In American Association of Orthopaedic Surgeons, 2007. San Diego, American Academy of Orthopaedic Surgeons, 2007.
74. Allan DG, Trammell R, Dyrstad B, Barnhart B, Milbrandt JC: Serum cobalt and chromium elevations following hip resurfacing with the Cormet 2000 device. J Surg Orthop Adv 2007; 16:12-18.
75. De Smet KA, De Haan R, Ebramzadeh E, Campbell P: Blood metal ions and x-ray follow up as a predictor for problems and outcome in hip resurfacing arthroplasty. Presented at International Society for Technology in Arthroplasty (ISTA); 2007, Paris, France.
76. Witzleb WC, Ziegler J, Krummenauer F, Neumeister V, Guenther KP: Exposure to chromium, cobalt and molybdenum from metal-on-metal total hip replacement and hip resurfacing arthroplasty. Acta Orthop 2006;77:697-705.
77. Jacobs JJ, Skipor AK, Doorn PF, Campbell P, Schmalzried TP, Black J, Amstutz HC: Wear in metal-on-metal THR: serum and urine chromium concentrations. J Bone Joint Surg 1996-1997;20:733-734.
78. Heisel C, Silva M, Skipor AK, Jacobs JJ, Schmalzried TP: The relationship between activity and ions in patients with metal-on-metal bearing hip prostheses. J Bone Joint Surg 2005;87:781-787.
79. Khan M, Kuiper J, Takahashi T, Richardson J: Exercise related rise in cobalt serum levels: a method to measure in vivo wear in different designs of metal-on-metal bearings. In 52nd Annual Meeting of the Orthopaedic Research Society, 2006 Chicago IL, 0513.
80. Chan FW, Bobyn JD, Medley JB, Krygier JJ, Tanzer M: The Otto Aufranc Award. Wear and lubrication of metal-on-metal hip implants. Clin Orthop Rel Res 1999;369:10-24.
81. Clarke MT, Lee PT, Arora A, Villar RN: Levels of metal ions after small- and large-diameter metal-on-metal hip arthroplasty. J Bone Joint Surg 2003;85:913-917.
82. Daniel J, Ziaee H, Salama A, Pradhan C, McMinn DJ: The effect of the diameter of metal-on-metal bearings on systemic exposure to cobalt and chromium. J Bone Joint Surg Br 2006; 88:443-448.
83. Skipor AK, Campbell PA, Patterson LM, Gitelis S, Berger RA, Amstutz HA, Jacobs JJ: Metal ion levels in patients with metal-on-metal hip replacements. In Society for Biomaterials 28th Annual Meeting Transactions; 2002 Tampa, FL.
84. Skipor A, Campbell P, Gitelis S, Berger R, Schmalzried T, Amstutz H, Jacobs J: Metal ion levels in patients with metal-on-metal bilateral surface and total hip arthroplasty. In: 51st Annual Meeting of the Orthopaedic Research Societs, 2005.
85. Jakobsen SS, Danscher G, Stoltenberg M, Larsen A, Bruun JM, Mygind T, Kemp K, Soballe K: Cobalt-chromium-molybdenum alloy causes metal accumulation and metallothionein up-regulation in rat liver and kidney. Basic Clin Pharmacol Toxicol 2007;101:441-446.
86. Ziaee H, Daniel J, Datta AK, Blunt S, McMinn DJ: Transplacental transfer of cobalt and chromium in patients with metal-on-metal hip arthroplasty: A controlled study. J Bone Joint Surg Br 2007;89:301-305.
87. Case CP: Chromosomal changes after surgery for joint replacement. J Bone Joint Surg 2001;83:1093-1095.
88. Visuri T: Cancer risk after metal on metal hip prosthesis. In Rieker C, Windler M, Wyss U: METASUL. A Metal-on-Metal Bearing. Bern, Switzerland, Hans Huber; 1998, pp 149-156.
89. Tharani R, Dorey FJ, Schmalzried TP: The risk of cancer following total hip or knee arthroplasty. J Bone Joint Surg 2001; 83-A:774-780.
90. Paustenbach DJ, Finley BL, Kacew S: Biological relevance and consequences of chemical- or metal-induced DNA cross-linking. Proc Soc Exp Biol Med 1996;211:211-217.
91. Brodner W, Grohs JG, Bitzan P, Meisinger V, Kovarik J, Kotz R: [Serum cobalt and serum chromium level in 2 patients with chronic renal failure after total hip prosthesis implantation with metal-metal gliding contact]. Z Orthop Ihre Grenzgeb 2000;138:425-429.
92. Evans EM, Freeman MAR, Miller AJ, Vernon-Roberts B: Metal sensitivity as a cause of bone necrosis and loosening of the prosthesis in total joint replacement. J Bone Joint Surg 1974;56B:626-642.
93. Vernon-Roberts B, Freeman MAR: Morphological and Analytical Studies of the Tissues Adjacent to Joint Prostheses: Investigations Into the Causes of Loosening of Prostheses. In: Schaldach, M., and Hofmann, D. Advances in Hip and Knee Joint Technology. New York: Springer-Verlag; 1976. 148-186.
94. Deutman R, Mulder THJ, Brian R, Nater JP: Metal sensitivity before and after total hip arthroplasty. J Bone Joint Surg 1977;59A:862-865.
95. Gawkrodger DJ: Metal sensitivities and orthopaedic implants revisited: the potential for metal allergy with the new metal-on-metal joint prostheses. Br J Dermatol 2003;148:1089-1093.
96. Willert H, Buchorn G, Fayaayazi A, Lohmann C: Histopathological changes around metal/metal joints indicate delayed type hypersensitivity. Preliminary results of 14 cases. Osteologie 2000;9:2-16.
97. Davies AP, Willert HG, Campbell PA, Learmonth ID, Case CPL: An unusual lymphocytic perivascular infiltration in tissues around contemporary metal-on-metal joint replacements. J Bone Joint Surg 2005;87:18-27.
98. Willert H-G, Buchhorn GH, Dipl-Ing, Fayyazi A, Flury R, Windler M, Koster G, Lohmann CH: Metal-on-metal bearings and hypersensitivity in patients with artificial hip joints. A clinical and histomorphological study. J Bone Joint Surg 2005;87:28-36.

99. Rae T: The toxicity of metals used in orthopaedic prostheses. An experimental study using cultured human synovial fibroblasts. J Bone Joint Surg 1981;63B:435-440.
100. Howie DW, Rogers SD, McGee MA, Haynes DR: Biologic effects of cobalt chrome in cell and animal models. Clin Orthop Rel Res 1996;329(suppl):S217-S232.
101. Haynes DR, Rogers SD, Hay S, Pearcy MJ, Howie DW: The differences in toxicity and release of bone-resorbing mediators induced by titanium and cobalt-chromium-alloy wear particles. J Bone Joint Surg 1993;75A:825-834.
102. Germain MA, Hatton A, Williams S, Matthews JB, Stone MH, Fisher J, Ingham E: Comparison of the cytotoxicity of clinically relevant cobalt-chromium and alumina ceramic wear particles in vitro. Biomaterials 2003;24:469-479.
103. Haynes DR, Crotti TN, Haywood MR: Corrosion of and changes in biological effects of cobalt chrome alloy and 316 L stainless steel prosthetic particles with age. J Biomed Mater Res 2000; 49:167-175.
104. Roesems G, Hoet PH, Dinsdale D, Demedts M, Nemery B: In vitro cytotoxicity of various forms of cobalt for rat alveolar macrophages and type II pneumocytes. Toxicol Appl Pharmacol 2000;162:2-9.
105. Hallab NJ, Anderson S, Caicedo M, Brasher A, Mikecz K, Jacobs JJ: Effects of soluble metals on human peri-implant cells. J Biomed Mater Res A 2005;74:124-140.
106. Huk OL, Catelas I, Mwale F, Antoniou J, Zukor DJ, Petit A: Induction of apoptosis and necrosis by metal ions in vitro. J Arthroplasty 2004;19:84-87.

CHAPTER 12

Primary Osteoarthritis

Harlan C. Amstutz

Michel J. Le Duff

Introduction

In a hip replacement practice, the most common diagnosis justifying surgical intervention is end-stage osteoarthritis. The joint is replaced when the articular cartilage is completely worn, the joint space obliterated, and femoral and acetabular subchondral bone are in contact with one-another. However, the etiologies leading to this stage of degeneration vary greatly.

Etiology

Traditionally, osteoarthritis (OA) has been subdivided into primary and secondary types, with the latter due to childhood disorders, after trauma, or any other known etiologic disease. Primary OA was reserved for a disease entity thought to be idiopathic where the etiology was less well defined or vaguely thought to be due to primary cartilage disease, wear, or overload. Today, most of the patients whose hips become symptomatic due to OA in either the young or in middle age without the obvious secondary etiologic characteristics are nonetheless due to anatomic abnormalities described previously as a pistol grip deformity or a lateral osteochondral bump, which may cause femoral-acetabular impingement depending on the degree of femoral head offset[1] and the degree of dysplasia. With more studies and as our understanding of pathogenesis of arthritis increases, there may ultimately be no idiopathic osteoarthritis remaining. An anatomic deformity was first suggested by Murray, who identified the bumps on anteroposterior (AP) radiographs alone and believed them to be a minor degree of slipped epiphysis.[2] Ganz and colleagues[3,4] have taken this concept further and correlated the abnormality with a symptom complex and physical signs of femoroacetabular impingement. Most of these deformities are located anteriorly, and cause pain and limitation of motion when the hip is flexed, adducted, and internally rotated. There is also a more unusual form of posterior impingement in extension and external rotation. The natural history is unknown, and although it is common in whites, the prevalence is still to be determined. The bump may be more apparent on the Johnson or cross-table lateral view[1] (Fig. 12-1), and it is associated with reduced anterior and lateral offset and a low head-neck ratio (<1.3), which causes a cam-like impingement when the aspherical portion of the head contacts the acetabulum or when a normal femur contacts an abnormal pelvis, leading to a pincer-type impingement.[3] In both situations, as the disease advances, the prominence grows as an osteophyte and there is progressive loss of internal rotation to a greater degree in flexion than in extension. Pathologically, this may result in labral tears, possibly initiating the disease and contributing to its progression. This injury mechanism has since been observed and documented by other groups.[5,6]

The OA progresses with a large osteophyte in the floor of the acetabulum, covering the acetabular fossa, and there is lateral luxation of the femoral head mimicking or adding to a degree of acetabular dysplasia often present. As the joint space is obliterated, high contact stresses generated laterally may be the cause or may be associated with the formation of cystic disease in the head or the acetabulum. There may also be other factors in the pathogenesis of the cystic disease. However, it is my observation that hips that become very stiff have a more concentric narrowing and demonstrate a lesser tendency to cystic degeneration. These observations are important in advising a patient when to have a follow-up radiograph in the early stages of the disease when the patient is not yet in need of a replacement. For example, if a patient has an eccentric joint space with high contact stresses laterally, a radiograph might be indicated in 6 months as opposed to a year or more for the hip that is stiff and has a more uniform femoral to acetabulum contact on the AP radiograph. Other factors, that may play an etiologic role or may be associated with a progression of the disease include the orientation of the acetabulum in either anteversion or retroversion.

Inflammatory OA is a relatively rare type of osteoarthritis. It is characterized by joint concentric space narrowing and bony erosions and a tendency to protrusio with small or absent (at least initially) head-neck junction osteophytic proliferation similar to rheumatoid arthritis but without serologic aberration (i.e., absence of rheumatoid factor and so on) and other manifestations of rheumatoid arthritis. There is usually a variable degree of granulomatous-like synovial proliferation in the acetabular fossa.

Arthrokatadesis is a condition associated with a progressive protrusio beyond the medial wall of the pelvis, and it has an accompanying loss of motion. It has an entirely unknown etiology.

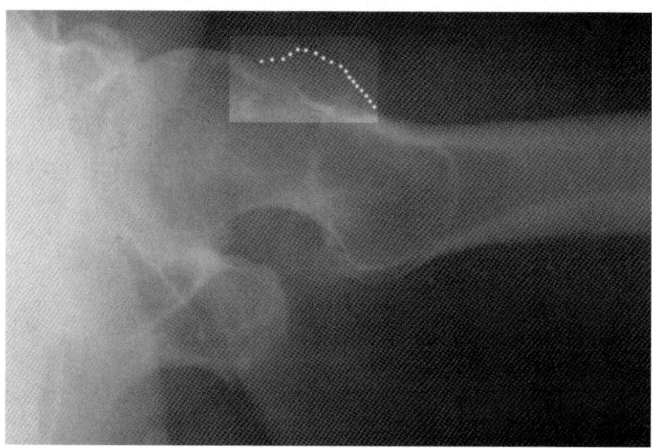

Figure 12-1 Preoperative cross-table (Johnson) lateral x-ray of a 63-year-old man with primary osteoarthritis. The anterior offset ratio was 0.11, as calculated per Eijer et al.[1] Note the absence of concavity on the anterior aspect of the femoral head/neck junction and the presence of an anterior osteophyte (*dotted outline in the enhanced contrast area*).

Finally, there is a rapidly progressive and very destructive type of osteoarthritis in which there is a rapid destruction of the head and occasionally of the acetabulum as well (Fig. 12-2). The condition may or may not be associated with trauma and excessive use of anti-inflammatory or pain killing drugs in association with continued high-activity use.

Idiopathic OA occurs in the absence of any of the abovementioned signs of impingement, inflammatory, arthrokatadesis, or destructive forms of OA.

Medical Management

Weight reduction, eliminating impact activity, acetaminophen (Tylenol), and the judicious use of nonsteroidal anti-inflammatory drugs are the mainstays of medical management. Weight reduction is highly desirable because 1 pound of weight loss equals 3 pounds in stress reduction on the hip while walking. The use of a cane or walking stick is also a very effective means of reducing stress on the hip, but is a hard sell in our society today. Physical therapy and exercises are directed at preserving muscle strength. However, exercises to maintain or increase range of motion, although often prescribed, are not indicated if there is an anatomic impingement because that will only lead to aggravation of the symptoms and progression of osteophytes. Swimming is the best exercise because it is

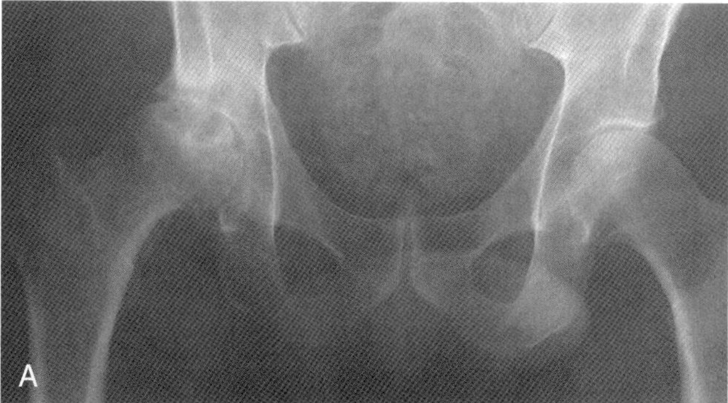

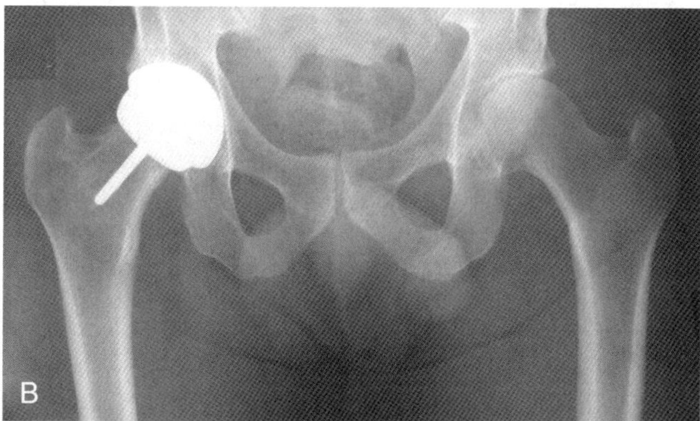

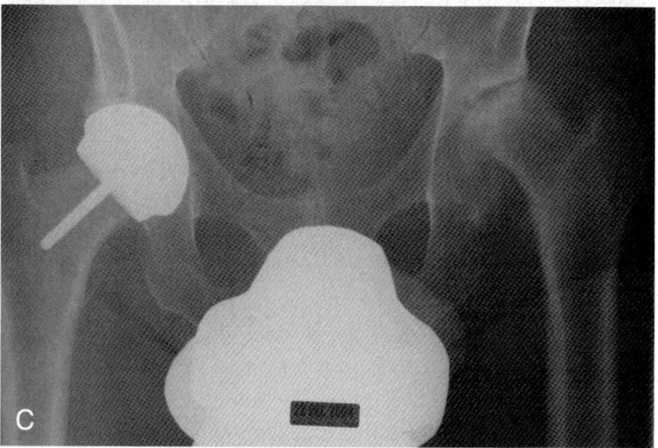

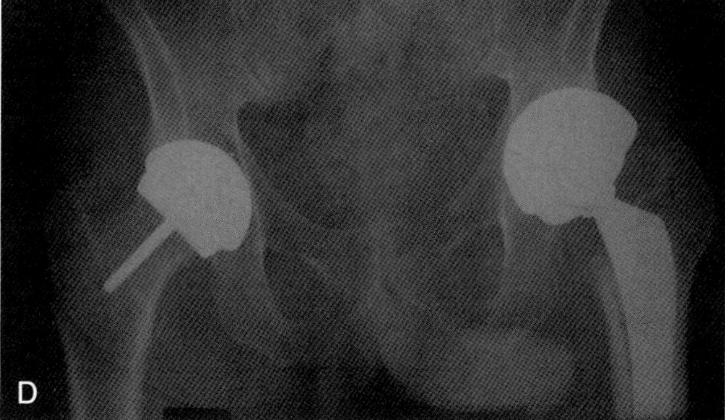

Figure 12-2 **A,** Preoperative anteroposterior radiograph of a 56-year-old man with osteoarthritis and reduced lateral offset of the right hip. The left hip shows no signs of arthritis but presents a similarly reduced offset. **B,** The right hip underwent Conserve®Plus resurfacing and is shown here 3 years after surgery. The left hip is showing a slight joint space narrowing. **C,** One year later, the left hip has undergone a rapid phase of inflammatory type degeneration, both on the femoral and the acetabular sides. **D,** A total hip replacement using Big Femoral Head technology and a Superfix cup was elected to compensate for the large acetabular defect and to equalize the leg lengths.

Table 12-1 Demographics of the Patients Operated for Primary Osteoarthritis

	Men	Women	Combined
Age (years)	52.7 (29-77)	55.2 (30-78)	53.2 (29-78)
Weight (kg)	89.7 (60-164)	68.4 (45-107)	85.5 (45-164)
Height (cm)	179.3 (155-203)	164.9 (147-183)	176.5 (147-203)
BMI	27.9 (18.9-46.4)	25.1 (18.3-42.3)	27.3 (18.3-46.4)
Femoral component size (mm)	49.4 (42-64)	43.3 (38-50)	48.2 (38-64)
Small femoral components (<48 mm)	89 (15.9%)	126 (92.6%)	215 (30.9%)
Cysts >1 cm	147 (26.3%)	44 (32.4%)	191 (27.4%)
Charnley class			
A	264 (57.6%)	72 (62.1%)	336 (58.5%)
B	178 (38.9%)	39 (33.6%)	217 (37.8%)
C	16 (3.5%)	5 (4.3%)	21 (3.7%)

BMI, body mass index.

relieved from gravity, and is not associated with extreme ranges of motion.

Surgical Treatment

With the increasing durability and overall success of total hip replacement (THR) and hip resurfacing, operations such as femoral osteotomy and arthrodesis are no longer satisfactory treatment in societies with advanced medical care. More recently hip arthroscopy and femoral osteoplasty have emerged as possible temporary procedures for femoroacetabular impingement to alleviate symptoms and perhaps forestall progression of advancing OA.[7] Ganz has popularized the trochanteric flip[8] as the preferred approach for chondro-osteoplasty, whereas some surgeons have performed the procedure arthroscopically. Neck fractures have been reported after arthroscopic removal, although Mardones et al[9] have reported that up to 30% of the neck width may be removed safely with contouring, but further determinations on safety and efficacy are needed.

Furthermore, because the natural history of the condition and the long-term results are unknown, the indications and effectiveness for the procedure must be considered preliminary. Indications for the procedure need to be defined because of the variability in the progression of radiographic signs and symptoms of arthritis in patients who have signs of impingement on the contralateral hip after having arthroplasty. We simply do not know enough about various factors (i.e., the morphology [size and shape] of the bump and offset, age and relationship with activity), that might influence the progression. This becomes very important for surgeons and patients in the decision-making process for treatment, in light of the improving results and durability of resurfacing.

Patient Demographics

From our cohort of 1000 Conserve®Plus resurfacing procedures, 696 were performed in 574 patients with a diagnosis of primary osteoarthritis. There were 458 men (79.8%) and 116 women (20.2%). The average age of the group was 53.2 years (range, 29 to 78 years). The demographics of this group of patients are shown in Table 12-1.

Fifty-five patients had bilateral arthroplasty at the same operation, and 67 patients had staged bilateral procedures between 1 and 92 months after the first side (average, 32 months).

Fourteen patients had a contralateral conventional total hip replacement.

In this series, the vast majority were younger than 65 years of age. However, 64 hips have been resurfaced in patients older than 65 (12 bilateral), with three having contralateral THR. In this subgroup, there were 12 women and 40 men (23%/77%), 22 hips (34%) were resurfaced with femoral components smaller than 48 mm, and 23 hips (36%) had femoral head defects greater than 1 cm in size. There were no differences in risk factors with the group of patients who were younger than 65.

Operative Considerations

The optimal orientation of the component is slightly more anterior and superior (lateral), positioned in relation to the central neck axis (to increase the anterior and superior offset), which will permit more flexion and abduction without potential impingement than in a truly neutral position. The lateral position also minimizes any possibility of notching when reaming (Fig. 12-3). The low-profile Conserve®Plus socket is inserted in more than anatomic anteversion (30-35 degrees), with the anterior rim well below the iliopubic rim. The rim of bone is removed to within 1 mm of the socket ideally, and the anterior wall is chamfered away from the socket rim with a high-speed burr. Patients who have impingement-induced or aggravated osteoarthritis invariably present a large anterior neck osteophyte (Fig. 12-4). When these osteophytes increase

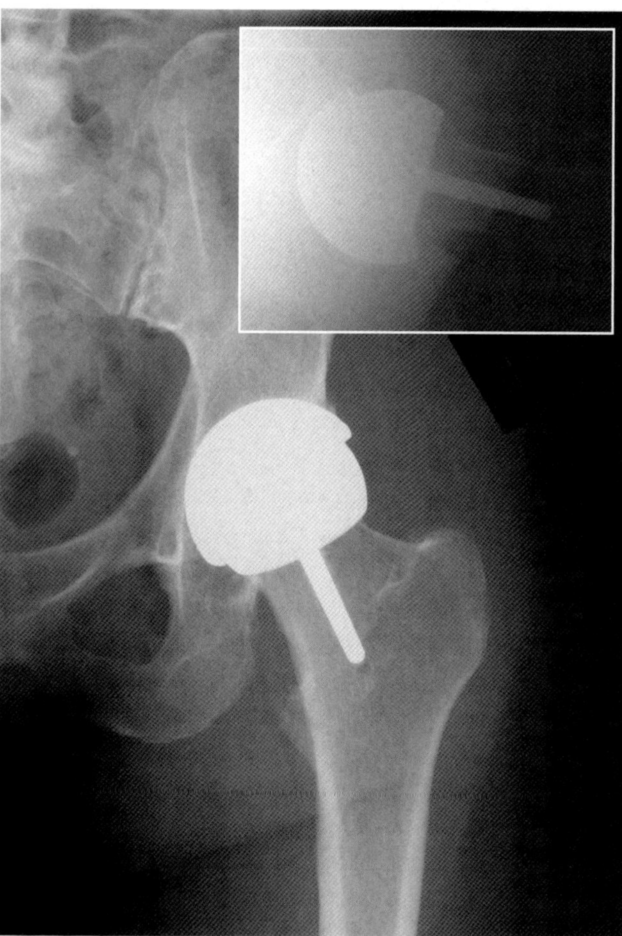

Figure 12-3 Anteroposterior radiograph of a 55-year-old woman immediately after surgery, with the Johnson lateral view in insert. This illustration highlights an optimal femoral component positioning after resurfacing with a slight superior and anterior translation of the component with respect to the central axis of the femoral neck.

in size, the neck cortex underneath may atrophy so that the osteophyte undoubtedly provides some structural support. In our view, they should not be removed unless there is less than 40 to 45 degrees of internal rotation in 90 degrees of flexion after insertion of the components. Our hypothesis that these osteophytes do contain structural bone is supported by our observation that they do not disappear or remodel and generally remain intact for up to 10 years postoperatively. When the osteophytes are small, they are generally soft and probably can be removed, but because they rarely cause an impingement problem, I suggest leaving them because it is impossible to assess their potential role in the neck structural integrity.

In cases in which the osteophytes are large, center the pin initially so as to remove the inferior portion of the head and the osteophyte close to the medial cortex, using oversized reamers. Then serially improve pin centering so that the final reaming axis will be just superior to the central axis of the neck, producing a larger offset superiorly. This will help avoiding any tendency to notch the superior neck (laterally) (see Fig. 12-4).

Results

Clinical Scores

The average University of California-Los Angeles hip scores all improved significantly ($P < .0001$) between preoperative and last follow-up visits. The pain score increased from 3.7 ± 1.2 to 9.5 ± 0.7, the walking score from 6.6 ± 1.4 to 9.7 ± 0.8, the function score from 6.0 ± 1.6 to 9.6 ± 1.1, and the activity score from 4.8 ± 1.6 to 7.7 ± 1.6. These results were significantly ($P < .009$) greater than those of the other etiologies combined with 9.5 versus 9.1 for pain, 9.7 versus 9.4 for walking, 9.6 versus 9.3 for function, and 7.7 versus 7.1 for activity. After 2 years of follow-up, only four patients had pain scores less than 8 and none less than 7. The most active patients in this series are found among the patients operated for primary OA, as illustrated in Figure 12-5.

The Short Form-12 (SF-12) scores also improved significantly ($P < .0001$). The average physical component was 33.5 ± 8.7 preoperatively and 51.0 ± 8.6 at the last follow-up, and the mental component increased from 48.8 ± 12.4 to 54.6 ± 7.8. Compared with the other etiologies, there was no difference in the physical component of the SF-12 ($P = 0.4053$). However, the mental component of the SF-12 was significantly higher for the OA group (54.6 versus 51.5, $P < .0001$). The postoperative Harris hip score (HHS) was 93.6 ± 8.4. We do not report the preoperative HHSs because they were not recorded until hip #293 (March 2000), which corresponds to the beginning of the Investigaional Device Exemption. The postoperative HHS was slightly higher for the OA group compared with the rest of the cohort, without reaching significance though (93.6 versus 92.4, $P = 0.0929$).

Range of Motion

The preoperative and postoperative range of motion measurements are summarized in Table 12-2.

Compared with the other etiologic groups, the patients with primary osteoarthritis differed significantly in postoperative rotation arc. However, the postoperative difference of 2.7 degrees on average may be statistically significant but has no real clinical implication. Preoperatively, the patients with primary OA had slightly reduced adduction and rotation arc compared with the other etiologies, and this is related to the morphology of the impingement type of OA with a larger anterior osteophyte and loss of internal rotation. The loss of internal rotation is invariably greater in flexion than extension, and the patient often presents with an external rotation contracture.

Conversions to Total Hip Replacement

There were 18 conversions to THR in this series. Six were consecutive to fractures of the femoral neck, 10 secondary to loosening of the femoral component, one due to a femoral failure of unknown nature, and one consecutive to a late

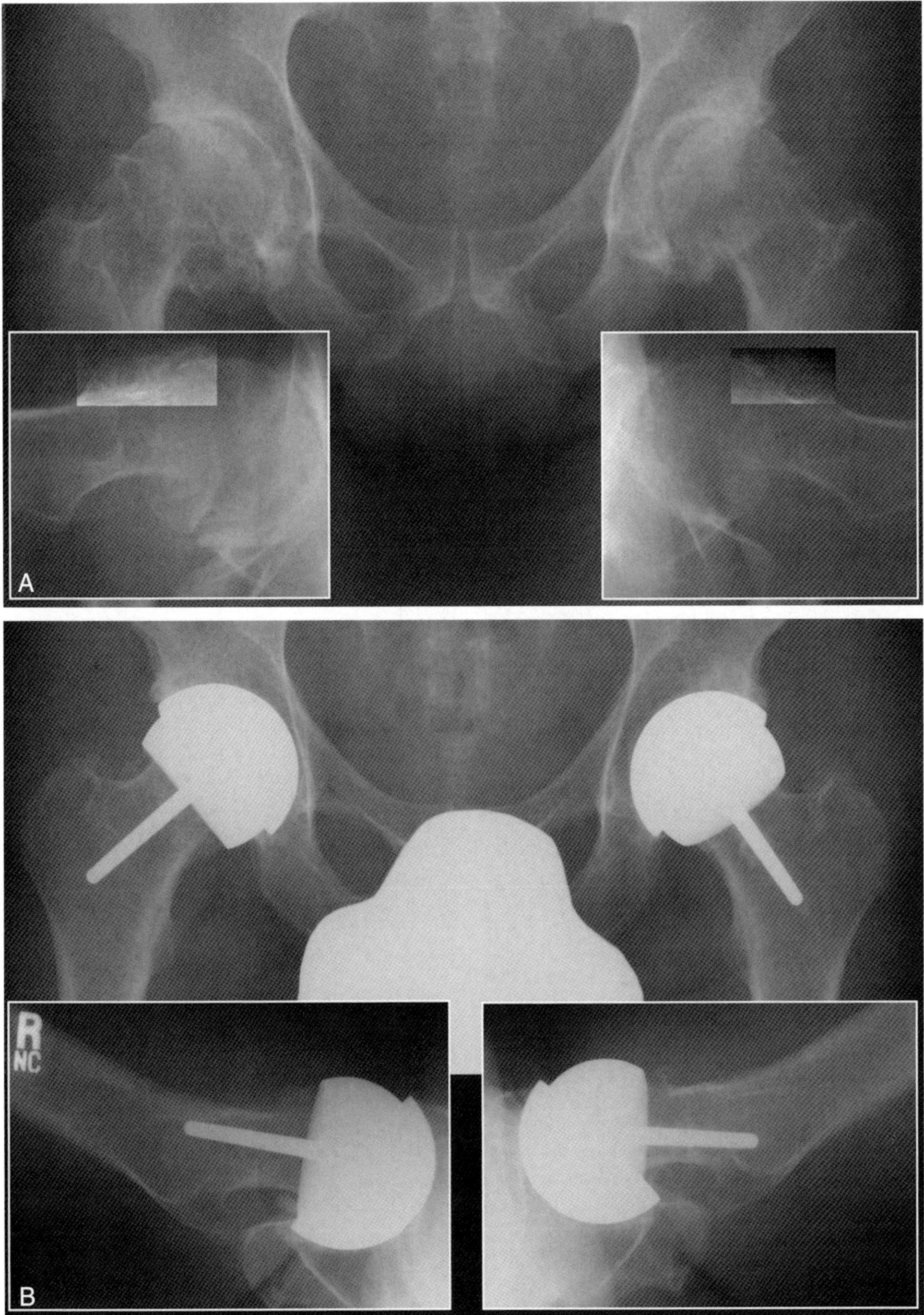

Figure 12-4 **A,** Anteroposterior radiograph of a 48-year-old man with bilateral primary osteoarthritis. Note the large osteophytes on both lateral and medial aspects of the femoral necks. The inserts show the anterior osteophytes (the contrast was enhanced in the regions of interest) on the Johnson lateral radiographs. **B,** Anteroposterior radiograph and Johnson lateral inserts of the same patient 4 months after one-stage bilateral resurfacing. The large anterior osteophyte on the right side was preserved by orienting the femoral component posterior to anterior.

hematogenous sepsis. Figure 12-6 illustrates a case of femoral neck fracture and Figure 12-7 a case of femoral component loosening, which are the two dominant modes of failure observed thus far in thus patient population.

Using any cause for revision as end point, the Kaplan-Meier survivorship results for this group of patients were the following (Fig. 12-8):

3 years: 98.1% (95% confidence interval [CI] 96.2 to 99.0)

4 years: 96.9% (95% CI, 94.5 to 98.3)

5 years: 95.9% (95% CI, 92.9 to 97.7)

8 years: 93.3% (95% CI, 88.5 to 96.2)

In this cohort, we evaluated the difference in survivorship between hips implanted with large (>46 mm) and small size

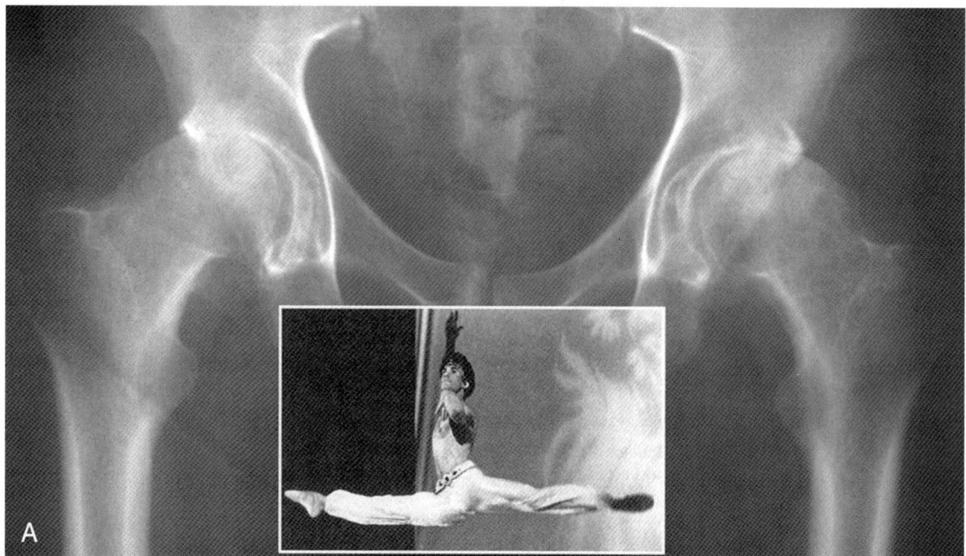

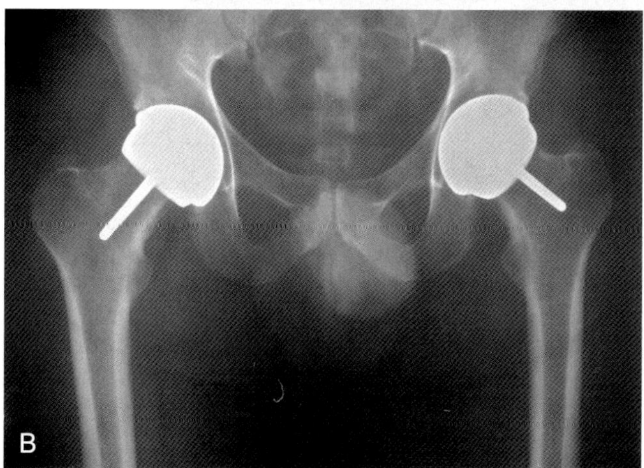

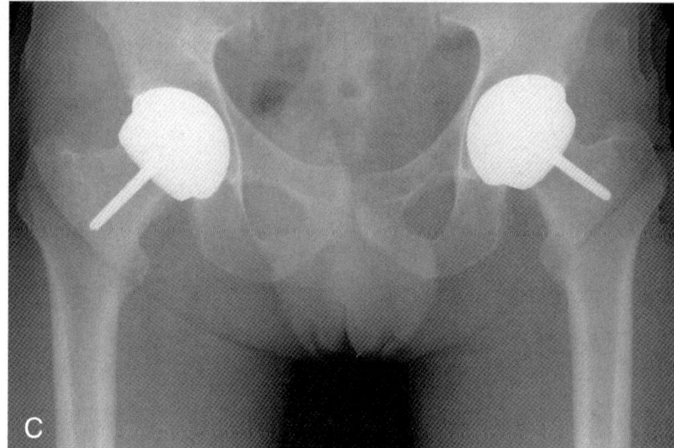

Figure 12-5 **A,** Anteroposterior radiograph of a 43-year-old ballet dancer with bilateral osteoarthritis. The insert shows the patient's extreme flexibility during a dancing exhibition. **B,** Anteroposterior radiograph of the patient 4 months after one-stage bilateral surgery. **C,** Anteroposterior radiograph taken 5 years after surgery. A remodeling of the lateral neck (more pronounced on the left side) is visible when compared to the 4-month film. The patient returned to principal ballet roles 10 months postoperatively, and after 9 years, continues with high activity. His University of California-Los Angeles hip scores are 10 for both hips in pain, walking, function, and activity.

Table 12-2 Preoperative and Postoperative Range-of-Motion Measurements

	Preoperative Flexion	Preoperative Flexion Contracture	Preoperative Abduction (in Extension)	Preoperative Adduction (in Extension)	Preoperative Rotation Arc (in Extension)	Postoperative Flexion	Postoperative Flexion Contracture	Postoperative Abduction (in Extension)	Postoperative Adduction (in Extension)	Postoperative Rotation Arc (in Extension)
Whole series (1000 hips)	105.6	16.1	23.2	14.5	23.5	125.9	1.9	45.2	27.9	76.6
Osteoarthritis (n = 696)	105.1	16.1	22.9	14.1	21.9	125.7	1.9	44.8	27.7	75.7
Other etiologies (n = 304)	106.8	16.2	23.7	15.6	27.1	126.3	1.8	46.0	28.5	78.4
P	0.159	0.839	0.434	0.026	0.000	0.553	0.870	0.060	0.080	0.044

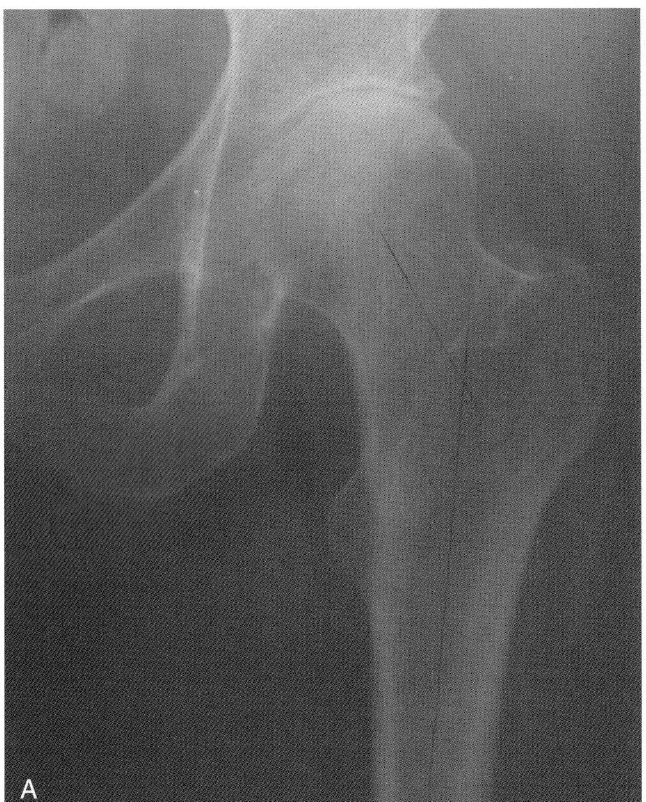

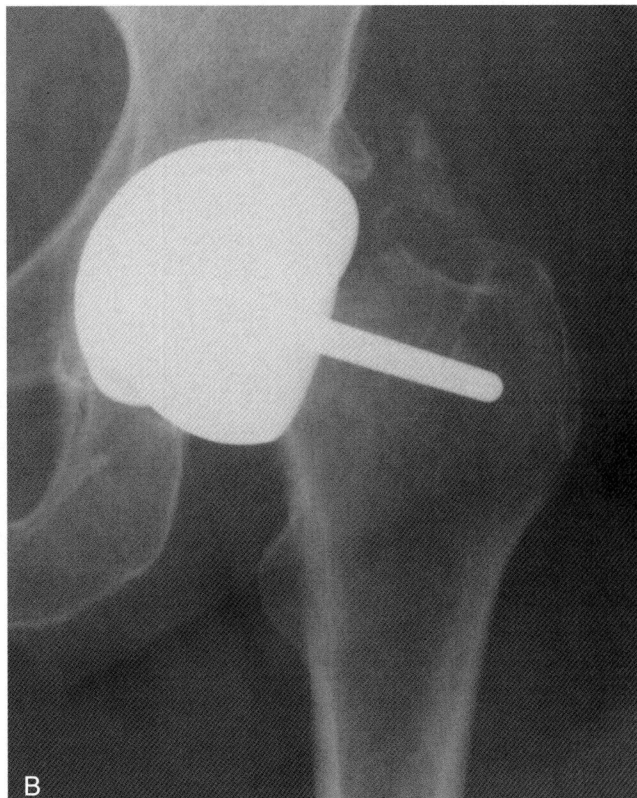

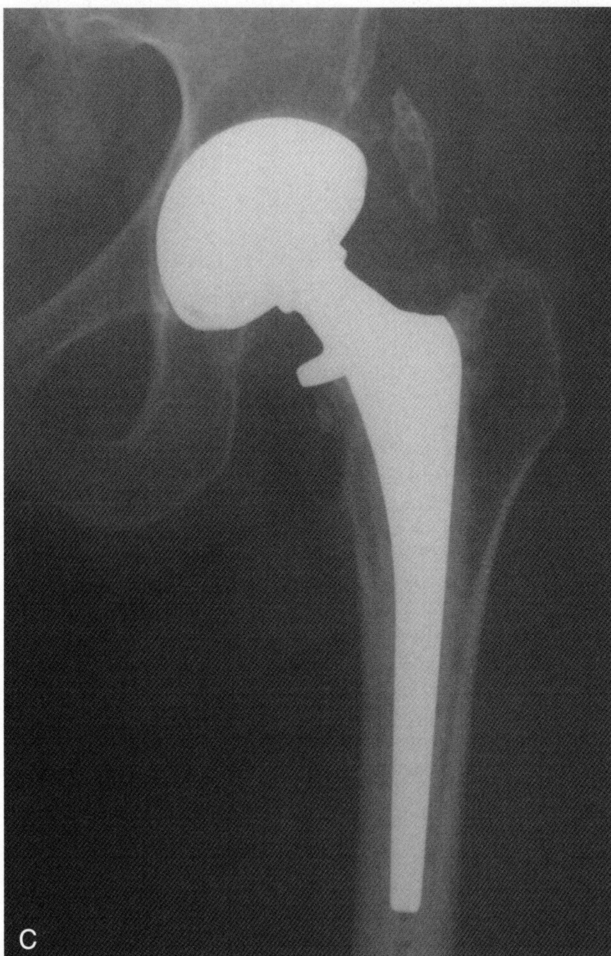

Figure 12-6 **A,** Preoperative anteroposterior radiograph of a 71-year-old woman with osteoarthritis who had prior contralateral total hip replacement, remained symptomatic, and requested a hip resurfacing on the other side. **B,** Six weeks after surgery, the patient sustained a fracture of the femoral neck. **C,** The well-fixed acetabular component was left in place, and the femoral component revised to a cemented Perfecta stem (Wright Medical Technology, Inc., Arlington, TN) with a unipolar head matching the acetabular component inside diameter. The patient has been symptom free for 10 years, with University of California-Los Angeles scores of 9, 8, 6, and 5 for pain, walking, function, and activity, respectively.

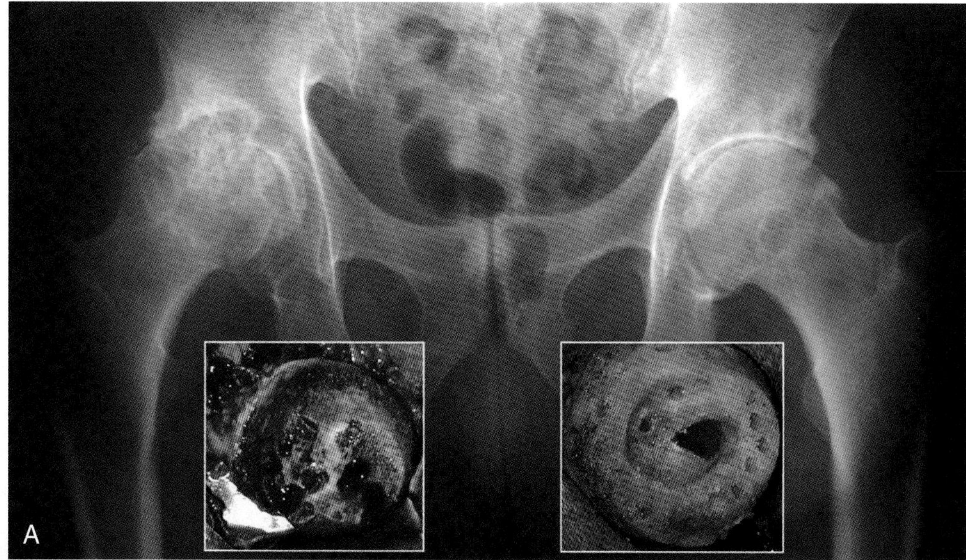

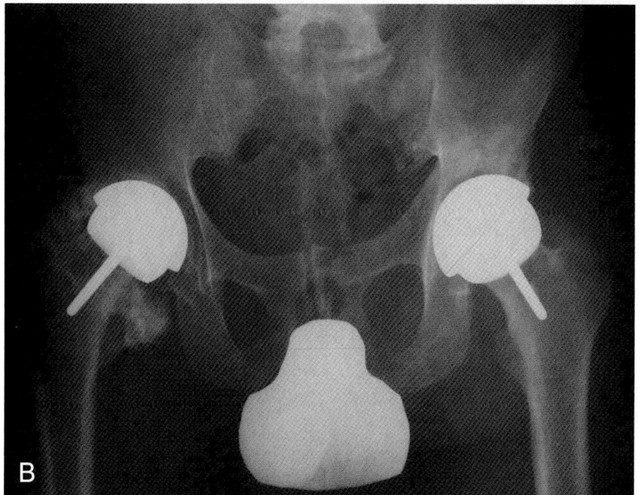

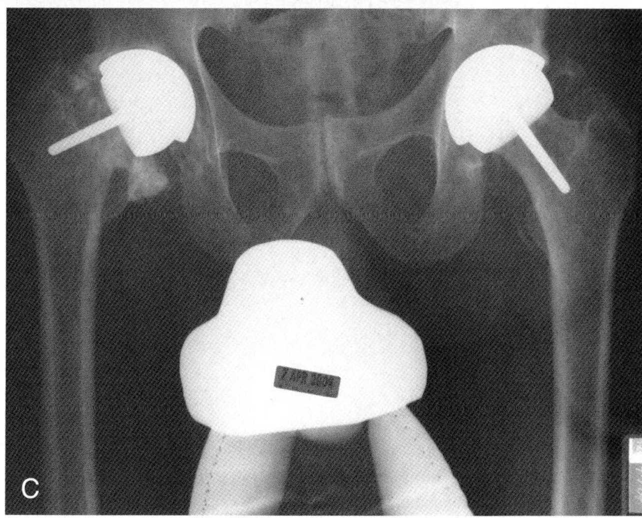

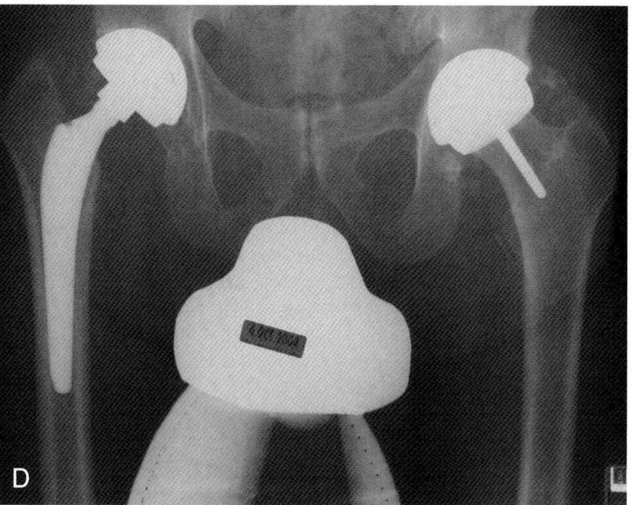

Figure 12-7 A, Anteroposterior radiograph of a 66-year-old half-marathon runner with severe osteoarthritis and cystic changes of the right hip, and although he was asymptomatic on the left side, showed nonetheless definite arthritic changes. Bone preparation was not optimal (first generation), as shown in the right hip insert. Despite our recommendation to the contrary because of cystic degeneration present at surgery, he returned to long distance running. **B,** The patient formed Brooker grade III heterotopic ossification and had slight reduction in range of motion. The left hip developed cystic changes and was resurfaced 4 years after the right with much better bone preparation (second generation). **C,** Five years after right hip resurfacing, the femoral component loosened as a result of a combination of poor bone quality, inadequate early fixation technique, small component size (46 mm) and high activity. The left hip formed grade II HO despite prophylactic radiation therapy but the hip range of motion is not restricted. **D,** The right hip was converted to a total hip replacement with a 46-mm Big Femoral Head and a standard anthropometric total hip (ATH) grit-blasted size 8. Radiation therapy plus indomethacin prophylaxis, and resection of heterotopic ossification (HO) were performed at the same setting. Minimal HO formed postoperatively. The patient now cycles for exercise.

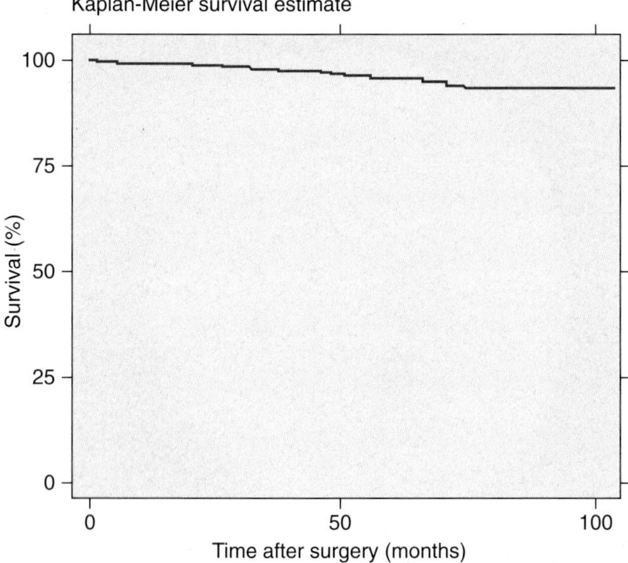

Figure 12-8 Kaplan-Meier survivorship curve of Conserve®Plus in patients with primary osteoarthritis, using any revision as an endpoint.

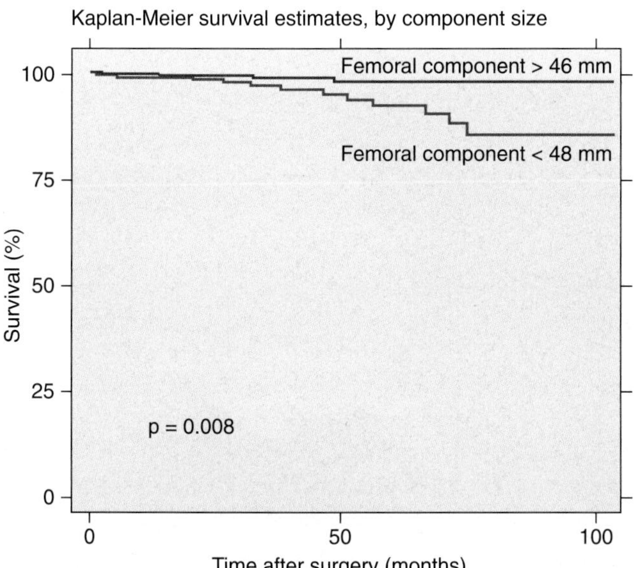

Figure 12-9 Kaplan-Meier survivorship curves of small (<48 mm) versus large (>46 mm) femoral components in the primary osteoarthritis cohort. The curves are significantly different, illustrating the importance of a large area for fixation in the durability of the prosthesis.

(<48 mm) femoral components. We found that the Kaplan-Meier survivorship curves were significantly different (log rank test: $P = 0.008$), as illustrated in Figure 12-9. The 5-year survivorship of the small components (<48 mm) was 92.2% (95% CI, 85.0 to 96.1) and the 5-year survivorship of the large components (>46 mm) was 98.1% (95% CI, 95.1 to 99.3).

In this group of patients, similarly to the results presented in Chapter 9, the most significant improvement in survivorship has been the result of improved bone preparation (Fig. 12-10) and cementing techniques (generation 2 and 3 over the first generation).

In the subgroup who were older than 65 years of age, there were two failures: one femoral neck fracture in a 71-year-old woman (hip #15) who failed to comply with postoperative weight-bearing instructions and one femoral component loosening in a 66-year-old half-marathon runner (hip #111). The 5-year survivorship of this group of patients was 98.4% (95% CI, 89.3% to 99.8%) and was higher than that of the younger patients with 95.7% (95% CI, 92.5% to 97.6%), but this difference was not significant (log rank test $p = 0.760$).

Complications

There were a total of 34 complications in this series for an overall incidence rate of 4.9%, which is similar to the overall group.

These adverse events were distributed as follows:

- Five dislocations (0.7%), three secondary to traumatic events and two associated with an excessive abduction angle of the acetabular component (>55 degrees). All were treated with closed reduction and are free of recurrence. We believe that dislocations due to component positioning can be prevented by accurately assessing the stability after implantation (range of motion and testing for stability are presented in detail in Chapter 7).
- Four hematogenous sepses (0.5%). One was converted to THR in a two-stage reoperation, and the other three were treated with urgent, thorough débridement of the infected tissues surrounding the prosthesis and antibiotics. They are now free of sepsis 5, 6, and 8 years postoperatively.
- Twelve nerve palsies (1.7%), 11 femoral and one peroneal (associated with compartment syndrome). All femoral nerve palsies recovered fully with no treatment in the months following surgery, whereas some sequelae remained with the peroneal nerve palsy. Nine of these nerve palsies are thought to be associated with the use of a particular pelvic stabilizer as described in Chapter 9.
- Eleven blood-related complications (1.6%), including two thromboembolic events, six hematomas, and three bleeds. All recovered with standard management techniques, except for the common femoral artery thrombus, which leads to the development of compartment syndrome. It was treated with thrombectomy of the vessel and surgical release (see Chapter 9). This is an extremely rare complication that may have been the result of a migrating anterior pubic support mentioned earlier increasing the pressure or even injuring the vessel. Pelvic positioning and stabilization are very important for resurfacing, and the device used to stabilize the pelvis must remain rigid.
- Two other unusual events were recorded (0.3%): the first one was the entrapment of bone debris in the joint space that required immediate reoperation after this problem was

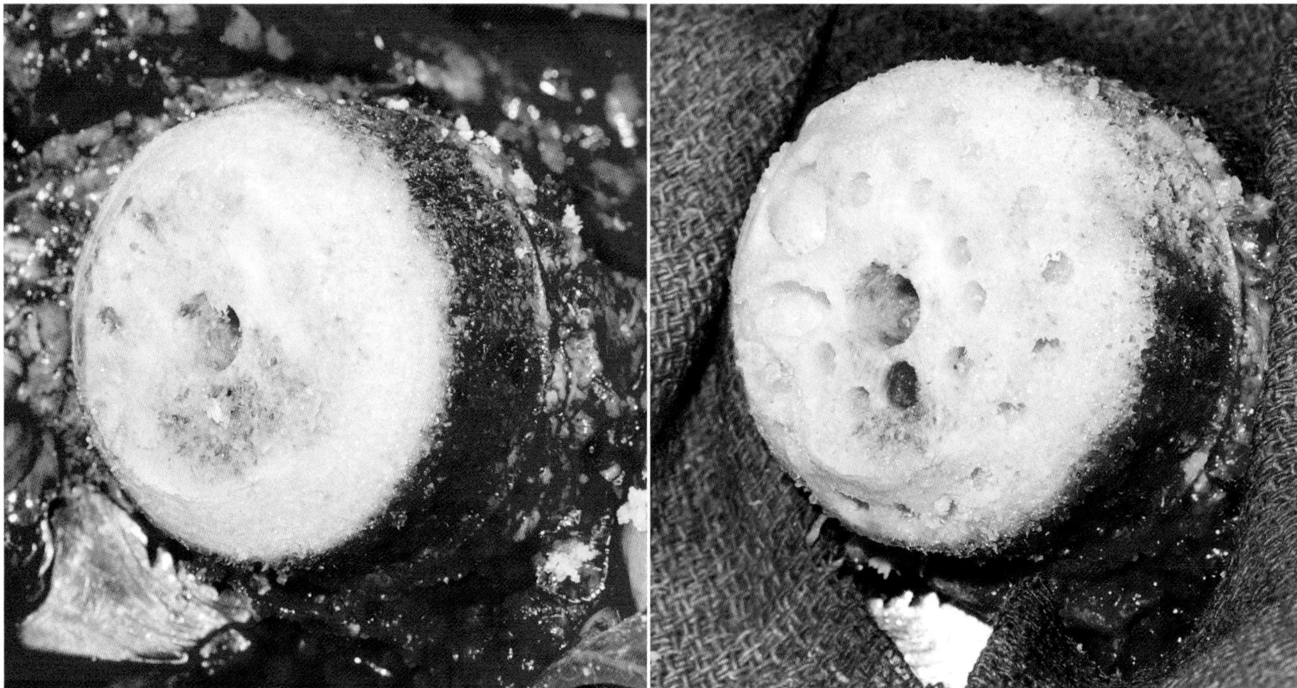

Figure 12-10 Intraoperative photographs of the femoral head of a 64-year-old man with primary osteoarthritis. On the left is the head immediately after chamfer reaming. On the right, all cystic material has been removed with a curette and a high-speed burr. Numerous drill holes were also added to increase the bone-cement contact area and facilitate interlocking of the two materials.

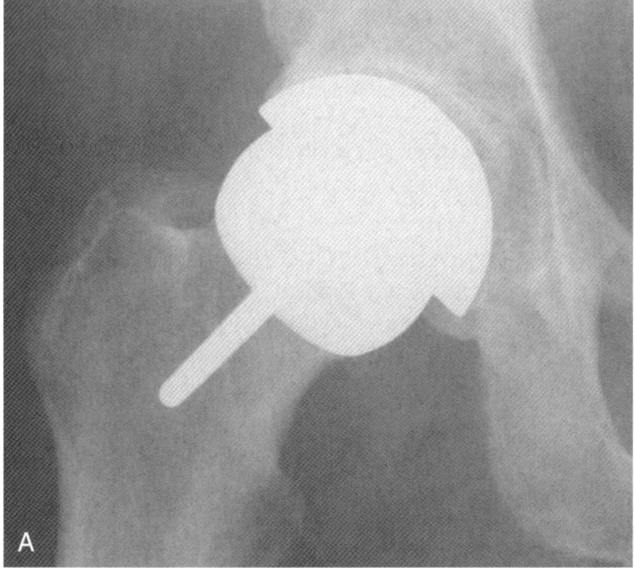

Figure 12-11 **A,** Immediate postoperative anteroposterior radiograph of a 57-year-old man with osteoarthritis. At first glance, the geometric centers of the acetabular and femoral components do not seem to coincide. **B,** The application of the template confirms the likelihood of the presence of a foreign body within the joint space. The patient was brought back to the operating room, and a piece of osteophyte from the anterior neck was removed.

identified from the postoperative AP radiograph. In this case, the range of motion checked after component insertion revealed limited internal rotation in flexion due to impingement, so the anterior neck osteophyte was removed. A portion of it fell unnoticed into the socket. It is important to make sure that there is nothing in the socket by searching with a good light just before hip reduction (Fig. 12-11).

- The second event was the reorientation of a malpositioned acetabular component immediately after surgery without any dislocation or subluxation when it was identified on the AP pelvis radiograph that the abduction angle of the cup was too large.

Two of these complications (3.1%) occurred in the age group who were older than 65 years of age: one femoral nerve palsy and one hematoma, both of which were resolved without treatment.

Summary

The results measured by our outcome clinical scores are better than the other etiologic groups combined, possibly in part because the patients with OA tend to resume a more active lifestyle. This was a predominately male population, slightly older than the rest of the cohort, with a larger femoral component size (48.2 mm versus 45.8 mm, $P < .0001$). In terms of risk factors for revision, the OA group presented a lower prevalence of femoral defects greater than 1 cm in size: 27.5% versus 53.1%, $P < .0001$. Also, the OA group had fewer hips with high SARI scores: 12.8% versus 39.1%, $P < .0001$. These characteristics make OA patients ideal for the procedure. However, these differences do not seem to have affected the survivorship of the prosthesis in favor of OA versus the other etiologic groups, at least not at this level of follow-up. Furthermore, all etiologic groups have benefited from the second- and third-generation bone preparation and cementing techniques to the extent that there have been fewer failures or radiolucencies in any group. The OA group did not differ in overall complication rate from the rest of the cohort (5.0% versus 4.9%). All complications encountered are largely preventable, and the overall rate of complication has dropped from 6.1% to 3.6% in the last 300 hips for the OA group (after we stopped using a pelvic positioner, which was at least partially responsible for several nerve palsies).

References

1. Eijer H, Leunig M, Mahomed N, Ganz R: Cross-table lateral radiographs for screening of anterior femoral head-neck offset in patients with femoro-acetabular impingement. Hip International 2001;11:37-41.
2. Murray R: The aetiology of primary osteoarthritis of the hip. Br J Radiol 1965;38:810-824.
3. Ganz R, Parvizi J, Beck M, Leunig M, Notzli H, Siebenrock K: Femoroacetabular impingement: a cause for osteoarthritis of the hip. Clin Orthop Relat Res 2003;417:112-120.
4. Ito K, Minka M, Leunig M, Werlen S, Ganz R: Femoroacetabular impingement and the cam-effect. A MRI-based quantitative anatomical study of the femoral head-neck offset. J Bone Joint Surg Br 2001;83:171-176.
5. Beaulé P, Zaragoza E, Motamedi K, Copelan N, Dorey F: Three-dimensional computed tomography of the hip in the assessment of femoroacetabular impingement. J Orthop Res 2005; 23:1286-1292.
6. Tanzer M, Noiseux N: Osseous abnormalities and early osteoarthritis: the role of hip impingement. Clin Orthop Relat Res 2004;429:170-177.
7. Beaulé P, Le Duff M, Zaragoza E: Quality of life following femoral head-neck osteochondroplasty for femoroacetabular impingement. J Bone Joint Surg Am 2007;89:773-779.
8. Ganz R, Gill T, Gautier E, Ganz K, Krügel N, Berlemann U: Surgical dislocation of the adult hip: A technique with full access to the femoral head and acetabulum without the risk of avascular necrosis. J Bone Joint Surg Br 2001;83:1119-1124.
9. Mardones R, Gonzalez C, Chen Q, Zobitz M, Kaufman K, Trousdale R: Surgical treatment of femoroacetabular impingement: evaluation of the effect of the size of the resection. J Bone Joint Surg Am 2006;88:84-91.

CHAPTER 13

Osteonecrosis of the Hip

Harlan C. Amstutz
Michel J. Le Duff
Paul D. Boitano

Introduction

Osteonecrosis (ON) of the hip is the correct term for death of the bone due to compromised circulation, and it replaces terms used in the past such as avascular necrosis, aseptic necrosis, and ischemic necrosis. ON refers to death of fat and hematopoietic cells of the marrow as well as osteocytes in a localized region of the bone. ON of the femoral head was initially described by Konig[1] in 1888. ON has received a considerable amount of attention in the recent literature, with an increasing number of cases due to the prolonged survival of patients with diseases associated with the development of ON, such as sickle cell anemia, systemic lupus erythematosis (SLE), and renal failure, and of patients who receive commonly associated drugs (e.g., steroids) for a variety of reasons including immunosuppression for organ transplantation.

Despite recent advances in joint replacement, ON of the femoral head remains a particularly challenging condition to treat because the patients are often very young,

In addition, the disease is frequently bilateral, and when there is collapse, it is progressive, leading to secondary degenerative arthritis. The vastly different causes lead to the condition that has a remarkably constant radiographic and clinical expression.

Except in the case of direct traumatic injury to the blood supply, the exact biologic process that initiates the pathogenesis leading to ON of the other etiologies is still unknown and is controversial. However, it is important to probe the clinical history for one of the etiologic factors if the patient is between the third and sixth decades of life with a painful hip, as truly idiopathic ON is not common.

Although many diseases and drugs have been associated with ON, the variability in incidence strongly suggests that those patients who develop nontraumatic ON of the hip have some innate susceptibility that, when coupled with one or more other etiologic factors, the disease becomes manifest. Although Jones[2] and Ficat[3] divide causes into accepted and associated causes, or definite and possible categories, the supporting evidence for the etiology in the literature is circumstantial and not conclusive.[4] Even though the pathology in the various stages is known and remarkably constant, a clear understanding of the basic mechanisms that initiate the pathogenesis has yet to emerge.

Although the mechanism by which corticosteroids lead to the development of ON remains controversial, Felson and Anderson[5] found a strong correlation between the total oral daily dose of corticosteroids and the development of ON; they also found that bolus steroids pose little risk of producing ON, but the minimum amount remains controversial. Evidence for fatty liver, destabilization and coalescence of endogenous plasma lipoproteins, or disruption of fatty bone marrow or other adipose tissue depots, all resulting in continuous or intermittent fat embolism, is related to many clinical conditions, including alcoholism and hypercortisonism. These two common problems accounted for two thirds of nontraumatic ON cases in one study.[6] A related theory, not mutually exclusive to the fat emboli or compartment syndrome theory, suggests that an increase in marrow fat concentration by lipocyte hypertrophy produces a rise in bone marrow pressure within the intraosseous extravascular compartment of the proximal femur. The result is an alteration in blood flow,[7] leading to progressive ischemia of the femoral head.[8] Steroid intake increases the marrow lipocyte volume 25% and the total volume of the marrow compartment 15% owing to osteoporosis. Thus there is a greater increase in cell volume than in the compartment space, which may increase the intraosseous pressure and so reduce blood flow.

Dysbaric ON, also known as caisson disease, is thought to result from nitrogen or fatty emboli due to rapid decompression.[9]

The etiology of pregnancy-induced ON is thought to be due to fat emboli, because acute fatty liver often occurs during the third trimester of pregnancy and is associated with elevated plasma lipid levels during the third month of gestation. Similarly, Jacobs linked the use of oral contraceptives to femoral head ON.[10]

ON complicating renal transplantation has been reported in 13% of patients from 18 renal transplant centers.[11] However, the reported incidence of ON of the hip in renal transplant recipients has varied from 4% to 40%, with 50% of the cases being bilateral. Pre-existing renal osteodystrophy, manifested by osteoporosis, osteomalacia, and secondary hyperparathyroidism, is thought to play a role in the development of ON. However, cardiac transplantation recipients with ON do not have these coexistent bony changes, which further implicates corticosteroids as the etiology of ON in the transplant population. Moreover, there is no histologic evidence that renal osteodystrophy is more severe or persistent in patients with ON. As with the treatment of SLE, a correlation exists between the total steroid dose and the development of ON.[12] Nonetheless, ON of bone can occur in patients with SLE, even in those who never received cortisone and have no other associated diseases or risk factors. Thromboses involving multiple organ systems, including bone, are common in patients with SLE.

The mechanism by which sickle cell (SC) disease and its variants cause ON is not clear. Although the abnormal red blood cells may sickle, causing reduced flow and sludging, thereby leading to focal intravascular coagulation and an arterial infarct, intraosseous venous occlusion may also occur. Hip ON has been associated with sickle cell anemia (HgbSS disease), SC disease, sickle-thalassemia (S-Thal), hereditary persistence of fetal hemoglobin, and sickle cell trait. The reported incidence varies from 0 to 68% but is probably about 3%.[13]

In their large series of sickle cell anemia patients, Lee and associates[14] noted that almost one half of patients with sickle cell anemia had bilateral involvement of the hip. The age of onset of hip symptoms referable to ON was 9 to 45 years, with 82% between 10 and 29 years; 72% had associated acetabular changes. Hanker and Amstutz[15] noted epiphyseal infarcts most frequently in the proximal femur and humerus, usually bilaterally and commonly in adolescents and young adults aged 15 to 30 years. Sebes and Kraus[16] found a higher incidence of hip ON in patients with SS disease than in those with SC disease: 19% versus 9%, respectively. The average age of onset of necrosis was at 25.8 years (range 12 to 56 years); and, unexpectedly, 20 of 47 patients with ON did not have any hip symptoms.

Iwegbu and Fleming[13] reported on a large series of sickle cell disease patients from Nigeria, and they found a 3% incidence of hip ON among their population, with a male/female ratio of 1.0 : 1.6; 96.6% of patients with ON had Hgb SS and 3.4% (one patient) had Hgb SC. Those most susceptible for hip disease were 6 to 15 years of age. The type and severity of the roentgenographic pattern of necrosis varied widely but appeared to relate to the patient's age at the onset of hip symptoms. Also, the severity of a patient's hip symptoms did not correlate with age or sex but did correlate with the type of roentgenographic lesion. Moreover, Iwegbu and Fleming concluded that hip ON was not more common within Hgb SC than with Hgb SS, as previously believed, but that it occurred with all types of sickle cell disease in the same frequency, yielding a distribution proportional to the type of hemoglobin electrophoretic pattern in any given population or geographic area under study.

Gaucher's disease is the most common inherited metabolic disorder of lipid metabolism with type 1 disease following a relatively benign course, often without affecting life span but in past years producing significant morbidity especially relating to the skeletal system. However, with enzyme therapy, the skeletal manifestations seem less frequent and severe.

The pathogenesis of ON in patients is not clear but is associated with the infiltration of Gaucher cells with the abnormal cerebroside into the femoral neck, causing avascular necrosis of the femoral head as well as protean manifestations throughout the skeleton with osteolytic lesions and ON of the humeral head and talus.

We performed three hip resurfacings with polyethylene (PE) for patients with Gaucher's disease in the late 1980s and failures due to polyethylene induced osteolysis were similar to those observed with other etiologies. If the articular cartilage is normal, we prefer hemiresurfacing for Ficat II, III, or early IV in a young patient. However, full metal-on-metal resurfacing should be considered based on our success with ON from other etiologies, although we have not as yet had an appropriate candidate. For the older patient, we have been performing a conventional total hip replacement (THR) with a double wedge taper, grit-blasted stem, and the midterm results are excellent; we have operated on 12 hips in 11 patients with an average follow-up of 5.0 years (range 1.0 to 10.5), and there have been no revisions.

As early as 1993, Chevalier et al[17] had suggested that human immunodeficiency virus (HIV) infection could be a possible risk factor for ON. This has since been confirmed by the abundant literature on the topic.[18]

Finally, an association between a state of hypercoagulation and the development of ON has been demonstrated and should also be taken into account in establishing the risk factors for the disease.[19]

Pathology of Advanced Osteonecrosis

The crescent sign, pathognomonic for ON, is a circumferential fracture in the femoral head that occurs within the subchondral bone and usually terminates at the superior pole of the fovea.[20,21] It appears on roentgenograms as a subchondral radiolucent line before collapse, whereas the articular cartilage overlying this fracture is metabolically and functionally normal.

The necrotic portion of the head stands out as a yellowish white area, usually in the anterosuperior portion of the femoral head (see Fig. 13-2A). Later, proliferation of capillaries is observed in the cancellous bone, and new living bone is laminated onto dead trabeculae in conjunction with resorption of the dead bone. The repair process appears to be self-limited and, unfortunately, incompletely replaces dead bone with living bone. In the subchondral bone, bone formation occurs at a slower rate than does resorption, resulting in a net removal of bone, loss of structural integrity, subchondral fracture, and eventually collapse. The cancellous bone's stiffness and strength have been reported to decrease substantially, on the order of 50% to 70%.[22,23] Thus, resorption of bone is postulated to cause fractures deep in the femoral head, leading to segmental collapse. The area of collapse presumably is initiated at a point of stress concentration in the interface between resorbed and stiff bone.[24] This stress comes from weight bearing, and the collapse of the necrotic fragment leads to painful degenerative arthritis.[25] Once collapse occurs, the articular cartilage no longer functions as it should, and the process quickly and inexorably leads to secondary degenerative arthritis. At the base of the fracture, callous formation is seen in the form of irregular regions of cartilaginous and bony proliferation. Reparative tissues invade the subchondral plate from the synovia and reach the joint tissue and spread across it like a pannus, destroying the underlying articular cartilage. Osteophyte formation and remodeling of the external contours of the femoral head are late events. In the most advanced lesions, the articular surfaces become deformed and the joint space is narrowed radiographically, resembling degenerative arthritis. Once radiographic changes of ON are noted, advanced changes may be seen within 2 years. The most useful distinguishing pathologic difference between primary osteoarthritis and osteoarthritis secondary to ON is that the eburnation found in primary osteoarthritis is characteristically absent in secondary osteoarthritis due to ON, except for the viable bone at the margin of the old infarct.[26]

Clinical Presentation

The prototypical ON patient ranges in age from 20 to 50 years.[27] Men are more commonly affected with idiopathic ON.[28] Merle D'Aubigné et al noted 50% bilateral involvement in patients with ON without a history of corticosteroid use.[29] Ficat noted that up to 80% of patients with ON due to steroid intake have the disorder in both hips.[30] Hanzeur et al[31] reported an 89% incidence of bilateral ON in patients with nontraumatic ON. In and of itself, ON usually does not always cause symptoms. However, acute discomfort is felt by the patient when necrotic bone no longer performs its support function and a subchondral fracture or collapse occurs.[32] Thus, most patients present with an unexplained onset of hip pain that is usually located in the groin, radiates over the thigh, or is referred to the knee. In the early stages, the pain is worse with weight bearing or strenuous activities and may produce an antalgic gait.[21] The pain is progressive and eventually constant, including at rest and at night.

The patient's history must be carefully obtained, looking for one or more associated etiologic factors or a history of major trauma to the hip.

Initially, the physical examination may be within normal limits, with no limitation of hip range of motion. However, depending on the degree of severity, stage of the disease, or presence of synovitis, varying degrees of decreased range of motion are noted, especially with internal rotation.[33] Loss of rotation, primarily internal rotation, with pain on range of motion is usually found in patients with stage II ON and all patients with stage III ON. This is the one condition in which hip rotation should be evaluated in both flexion and extension with a protractor, because the changes in motion may be subtle. Because the disease advances in stages, there is increasing loss on internal rotation to a greater degree than flexion and abduction.

Radiographic Classification and Evaluation

Staging of the disease is of paramount importance in order to select the appropriate treatment option. Many surgical procedures exist for ON of the femoral head, but the procedures may be appropriate for certain stages and not for others. Several staging systems exist for this purpose,[3,34-36] but for the purposes of evaluating indications for hemisurface and full resurfacing, the Ficat and Arlet scheme is sufficient.

Ficat and Arlet have divided the radiographic progression of ON of the femoral head into four stages that permit clinical, prognostic, and therapeutic interpretation.[35] Their system was based solely on plain anteroposterior and lateral roentgenograms. This classification system is preferred by many investigators and clinicians because of its simplicity. It was later modified by Ficat to include a fifth, additional stage 0, describing the silent (asymptomatic), usually contralateral, hip (roentgenogram normal) in a patient with an established diagnosis of ON of the femoral head on one side.[30]

With stage I disease, a patient may or may not be symptomatic. Standard anteroposterior and frog lateral roentgenograms of the hip may be within normal limits or reveal minimal osteopenic changes with or without mottled densities that may be evident in the femoral head, especially if compared with the contralateral, normal hip. However, the magnetic resonance imaging (MRI) shows changes of ON.

Stage II ON presents with constant or increasing pain and limitation of motion with roentgenographic subchondral sclerosis, osteoporosis, or both. A well-demarcated wedge of infarction in the anterosuperior or anterolateral segment of the femoral head is usually seen. The absence of collapse is verified with the frog lateral projection, which is the preferred lateral projection for this disease.

Stage III ON is characterized by the pathognomonic crescent sign, with flattening of the femoral head on the frog or modified table down, lateral radiograph. The joint width still appears normal without degenerative changes present on the acetabulum side of the joint.

Stage IV ON shows in addition to collapse of the avascular sequestrum, secondary acetabular degenerative changes.

Current Treatment Recommendations

(Table 13-1)

Stage I: Observation is advised if the hip is asymptomatic.

Stage II: If asymptomatic, continue with observation.

Stage III or IV: For those older than 30 up to approximately 55 years, full resurfacing is recommended.

If symptomatic, the practical options are core decompression or hemisurfacing. Because the results of core decompression are variable and there are potential adverse effects with loss of valuable bone stock, a resurfacing procedure may be compromised if needed later. Despite the lack of uniform success, there remain advocates (Hungerford, Mont, Steinberg).[37,38] Coring may relieve pain, but progression is likely if the lesion is large, especially and/or if a large core is made. Multiple small core tracks are potentially less likely to weaken the head and lead to collapse.

When we began our MM Hybrid resurfacing, our age indications for a hemisurface procedure included patients up to 50 years of age. However with increasing success and durability of full metal-on-metal hip resurfacing, we have been more selective and have lowered the age for hemisurfacing to less than 30 years. For those young patients, our preference is hemiresurfacing rather than coring because of the more predictable result in our experience and because it is now possible to convert at least some patients to a full resurfacing when the cartilage wears out by inserting the thin acetabular shell.

Total hip arthroplasty is the treatment of choice for older patients (65+ years) or in case of an extensive total head necrosis in a slightly younger patient. However, if our good results continue to hold up with longer follow-up in hips with extensive necrosis, resurfacing may be acceptable in somewhat older patients as well.

Grafting procedures and osteotomies are not recommended. Although in theory a collapsed anterosuperior portion of the femoral head can be rotated out of the weight-bearing contact region by an osteotomy, the results have been unpredictable, even with small lesions. A poor result may diminish the success of a resurfacing procedure. Another approach involves the use of a vascularized or nonvascularized graft to support the defect area. Unfortunately, the results of these surgical treatments are also unpredictable and the pain relief and functional results as measured by a variety of outcome measures (Harris hip score [HHS] score and so on) are less than those achieved by resurfacing or THR, even in the more successful cases.[38] Furthermore, there is also donor site morbidity with the free vascularized fibular graft (FVFG). Further collapse and degeneration are inevitable in hips that have already collapsed. I do not believe either osteotomy or grafting procedures are ever indicated today because of the predictability of success with full hip resurfacing, total hip replacement and in some cases hemiresurfacing, which has the lowest associated morbidity of all these procedures.

One 32-year-old medical student with SLE requiring steroids had bilateral FVFG performed after collapse of the femoral heads (Fig. 13-1). The patient had significant pain and morbidity and was on crutches for 1 year after surgery before a bilateral hemiresurfacing procedure was performed.[39] The patient has done surprisingly well for 8 years despite prior extensive cartilage damage due to the delay in performing the hemiresurfacing procedures. The right hip now has a pain score of 6 (the left a score of 8) and may require conversion to a THR soon (both components are 45-mm Conserve and were not superfinished and, therefore, cannot be maintained for a conversion to a full resurfacing). Although complete pain relief after hemiresurfacing is not as predictable as with the full-surface procedure or THR, there are a group of similarly young patients whose results have been sufficiently comparable to continue this option as a method to postpone a more drastic procedure.

Technique for Femoral Bone Preparation and Cementation

The technique of bone preparation and cementation is critical with osteonecrotic hips to promote long-term durability of hip hemisurfacing or full resurfacing. All of the dead yellowish friable necrotic bone must be removed with a curette and high-speed burr down to the normal or dense white reactive

Table 13-1 Treatment Algorithm for Osteonecrosis

Acetabular Cartilage Grading[41]	I or II		III to IV	
Patient age	<30	>30	<30	>30
Ficat stage I[3]	Observation	Observation	N/A	N/A
Ficat stage II	Hemiresurfacing core–small lesions only (<one third)	Hemiresurfacing core–small lesions only (<one third)	N/A	N/A
Ficat stage III	Hemiresurfacing	Full resurfacing	Full resurfacing	Full resurfacing
Ficat stage IV	Full resurfacing or THR if femoral head not resurfaceable	Full resurfacing or THR if patient older than 65 or head not resurfaceable	Full resurfacing or THR if femoral head not resurfaceable	Full resurfacing or THR if patient older than 65 or head not resurfaceable

N/A, not applicable; THR, total hip replacement.

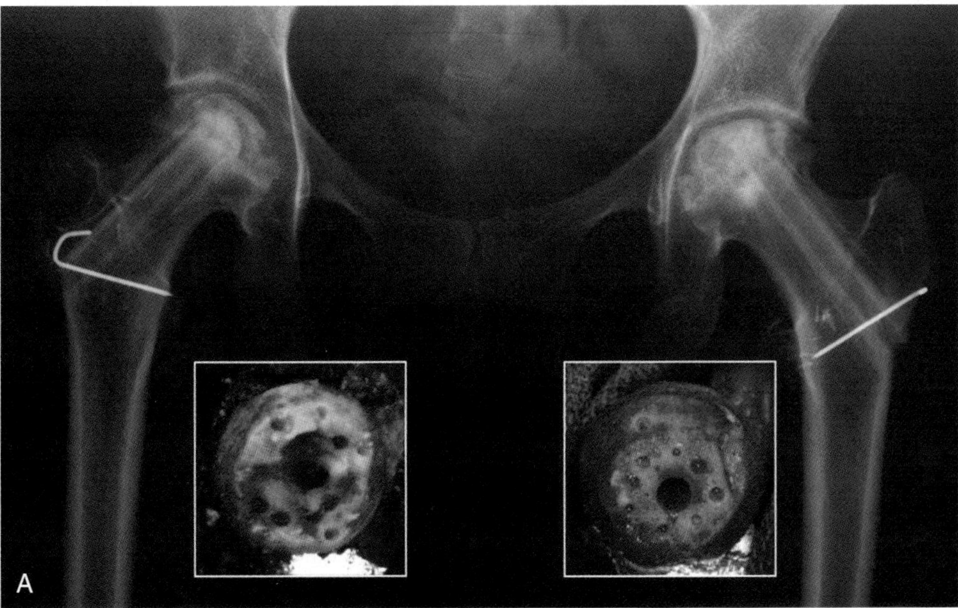

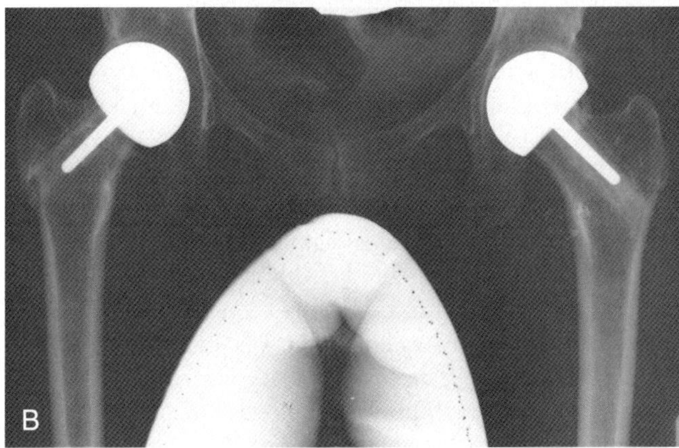

Figure 13-1 A, Preoperative anteroposterior radiograph of a 32-year-old medical student with systemic lupus erythematosus 1 year after bilateral free vascularized fibula grafts. The patient had undergone this procedure for steroid induced osteonecrosis Ficat stage III on both hips. Both heads have collapsed, and the patient was unable to walk without assisting devices at her clinical evaluation. The inserts show the femoral heads after reaming for hemi-resurfacing. Note the failed incorporation of the graft on the right side. The stem of the left hemiresurfacing was placed down the intramedullary canal of the fibular graft. **B,** Eight years after bilateral hemiresurfacing, the femoral components are well fixed but the patient's postoperative University of California-Los Angeles pain scores have decreased from 9 to 8 on the left and 9 to 6 on the right because the remaining articular cartilage has narrowed, but she has become a practicing physician in the meantime. A right hip conversion to total hip replacement may be needed in the near future.

bone. This is achieved by alternating burring, irrigation, and drying. This may lead to substantial loss of the head, but even in severe cases, some portion of the circumferential cylindrically reamed bone generally remains, which is essential. Once this débridement has been completed, the bone should be penetrated with multiple 3-mm drill holes to increase the surface area for acrylic fixation (Fig. 13-2). When the bone has been optimally prepared, then cementation is equally important. Pressurized acrylic is inserted into the available cylindrical reamed cancellous bone, into the stem hole, and you must make certain to seat the component fully. We do not recommend bone grafting these large defects because of the loss of fixation area due to the interpositional graft and in the unlikely event that the cement will be able to contact host bone. In addition, there is no retrieval evidence that the grafts will be incorporated. However, we grafted four hips in our full-resurfacing series for ON for the following reasons: Two hips presented failed coring with large cylindrical defects in the neck and trochanteric areas, and two hips had post-traumatic ON and had large residual pin defects. The grafts were inserted and impacted distally into the neck and intertrochanteric areas with a small round impactor so as not to lose acrylic fixation area in the head (except in one case in which 50% of the defect in the head was grafted). These four patients have relatively low University of California-Los Angeles (UCLA) activity score levels ranging from 4 to 7 with a current follow-up time of 7 to 8 years.

Hemiresurfacing

Rationale for Hemiresurfacing

As outlined in Chapter 1, we began to use hemiresurfacing (femoral head only) in 1981 because of the high failure rate of metal-on-polyethylene resurfacings, especially in patients with Ficat stage III or early stage IV ON, in which the acetabular cartilage damage was not severe. Loosening of the device has been extremely rare, and no adverse outcomes (besides the lower pain relief in poorly selected patients and the inevitable acetabular cartilage wear over time) have been observed in our 25-year experience.[40,41] Revision of the femoral component became necessary mainly when the acetabular cartilage wore out (see Fig. 1-15). In 1987, Sedel et al[42] reported good results

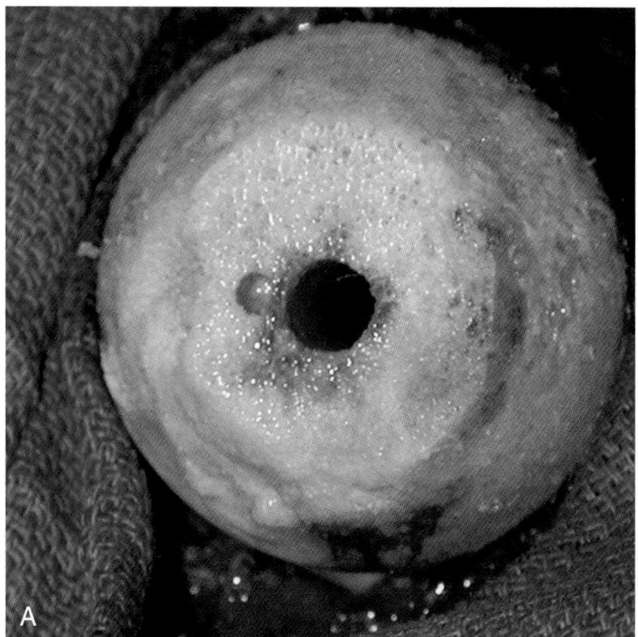

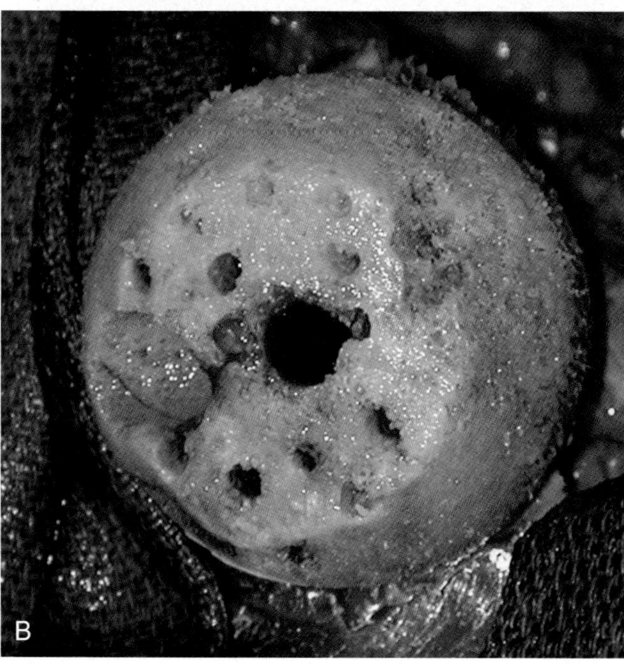

Figure 13-2 A, Intraoperative photograph of the right femoral head in a 40-year-old man with bilateral steroid-induced osteonecrosis. The photograph was taken immediately after chamfer reaming. Note the residual yellowish necrotic bone extensively covering the reamed bone. **B,** Intraoperative photograph of the same femoral head after completion of the preparation. All of the necrotic bone was curetted out and numerous 3-mm drill holes were added to enhance cement fixation.

in 82% of hips at an average 7-year follow-up after Luck cup arthroplasty for ON.

De Meulemeester and Rosing[43] reported only 8% failure at an average of 8 years using the Thomine cup. In 1987 Scott et al[44] also reported a 13% revision rate at an average of 3 years in a series of total articular replacement arthroplasty (TARA) surface hemiarthroplasties performed for stage III and IV ON. Krackow et al[45] reported 84% good or excellent results in nine hips with the TARA, with an average patient age of 41 years at an average of 3 years postoperatively. In 1978, Wagner reported no revisions at 4 years maximum follow-up in a series of ceramic surface hemiarthroplasties.[46] Using a hemispherical titanium alloy component for femoral head resurfacing, Nelson presented a survivorship of 82% at 5 years in patients whose ON was either idiopathic or caused by etiologies other than sickle cell disease.[47] Wear of the acetabular cartilage was the cause for revision in all cases. In our experience at the time of conversion of the hemiresurfacing, the histologic response has been very benign, with a few macrophages and some metallic debris scattered throughout a predominantly loose connective tissue despite significant burnishing of the soft titanium alloy components. It is surprising how well the articular cartilage space has been preserved in some patients for more than 20 years, even though soft titanium alloy femoral components were used with the presence of rather advanced articular cartilage fibrillations in some areas of the acetabulum at surgery. It is our belief that a harder bearing surface such as cobalt-chromium or alumina might produce even longer durability by minimizing the friction and metallic debris due to the relatively soft titanium alloy component. One of our patients now counts 25.5 years of follow-up after a THARIES cobalt-chromium femoral component was implanted, which seemed to have the best fit within the acetabulum rather than any of three custom titanium components that had been made because of a more optimal diameter and fit. Although her joint space has somewhat narrowed, her UCLA hip scores remain high with 9, 7, 8, and 6 for pain, walking, function, and activity, respectively (Fig. 13-3). We believe that the favorable survival of these prostheses was due to the "precision" fitting of these custom implants to the remaining normal acetabular cartilage in suitable patients with relatively low activity levels.

For those requiring reoperation, revision to either full surface or total hip replacement was easy and much like a primary replacement because of bone stock preservation and intact intramedullary canals and because there was no debris incited granuloma. Because the quality of the articular cartilage, once collapse has occurred, is related to long-term durability, we recommend non-weight bearing when a stage III ON has been identified in order to minimize secondary acetabular articular cartilage changes. Surgical delay caused by the need for custom components was overcome with the introduction of the Conserve in millimeter increments beginning in 1995. However, because of the improved success of full resurfacing for ON with the Conserve®Plus, the indications for hemisurfacing have narrowed. With the age group lowered and usage declining, the decision was made to discontinue the 1-mm increments when the thin socket shells were introduced in 2003. The rationale included the possibility that the hemiresurfacing procedure could be converted to full resurfacing by the addition of a thin acetabular shell, and the manufacturing of matching 1-mm increment sockets was not practical or cost-efficient. We now use the hemiresurfacing devices in 2-mm increments. Although the 2-mm increments midterm

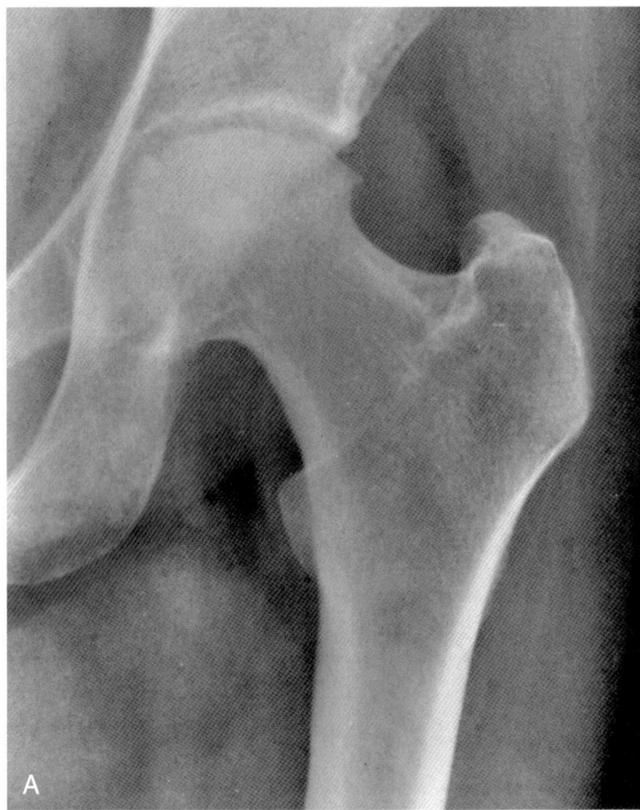

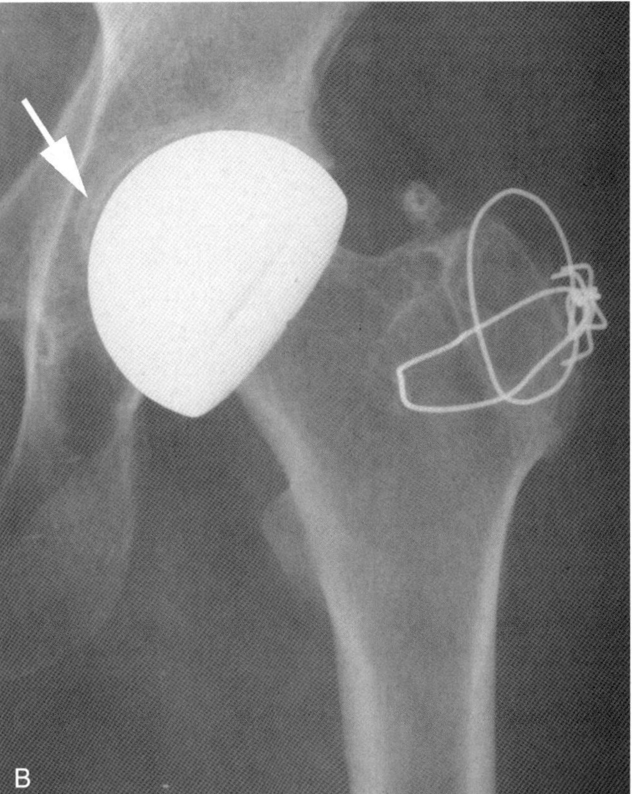

Figure 13-3 **A,** Preoperative anteroposterior radiograph of a 35-year-old woman with systemic lupus erythematosus/steroid-induced osteonecrosis Ficat stage III of the left hip. **B,** Twenty-five and a half years after hemiresurfacing. There is new bone formation in the acetabular fossa (*arrow*), and although the acetabular cartilage has narrowed, the patient continues to do well clinically with high University of California-Los Angeles hip scores.

results are not yet available to determine if the results will be as good as with the 1-mm increments, there is precedent and past experience of others using 2- and 3-mm increments for hemisurfacing with the TARA (2- and 3-mm)[44,45] and our porous surface replacement (PSR) femoral components manufactured by DePuy (2-mm) in the 1980s. The survivorship reported by others was similar to ours with approximately 80% at 5 years, 60% at 10 years, and 45% at 15 years.[48] Grecula et al[49] evaluated the benefits of the presence of a metaphyseal stem in the more recent designs and concluded in favor of a better alignment and a reduction in femoral neck fracture rate with components which had a stem. More recently, lower survivorship rates was reported by Cuckler et al,[50] who also reported an association of early failure with a lower preoperative HHS. Similarly, Adili et al[51] reported only a 76% survivorship at 3 years, although the indications in that series as well as in Cuckler's were broadened to include a higher percentage of post-transplant and patients on steroids than in our experience.

Indications for Hemiresurfacing

Surface hemiarthroplasty offers an attractive, bone preserving, and "time buying" alternative to very young selected patients with stage II and III and, occasionally, in a very young patient with early stage IV (minimal acetabular cartilage changes) ON of the femoral head. This method should be considered as part of a lifetime treatment plan in the young patient despite the potentially better initial performance of full resurfacing or conventional total hip arthroplasties that will probably require revision.

The indications include young patients who have normal, grade I or no more than grade II cartilage changes (absence of any full thickness cartilage loss). We include hips with whole head lesions, which, after subsequent débridement, retains at least some circumferential cylindrically reamed portion of the head. Bone preparation and cement technique including cementing the stem are critical. From our experience, hemiresurfacing is not indicated in heavy patients (bone mass index [BMI] > 30), workman's compensation cases, or those who must work standing and walking on hard cement floors. Our early unsatisfactory results with these patients are the justification for such exclusion criteria.

Hemiresurfacing Patient Demographics

A series of 30 hips in 25 patients received a Conserve hemiresurfacing procedure for ON of the femoral head and have a 2.5- to 11-year follow-up. Factors for the development of ON were diverse in this group and distributed as follows:

- Steroids 15 (50%)
- Alcohol 6 (20%)

Table 13-2 Demographics of the Patients Operated with Hemiresurfacing for Arthritis Secondary to Osteonecrosis

	Men and Women Combined
Age (years)	36.1 (21-52)
Weight (kg)	71.9 (40-117)
Femoral component size (mm)	48.7 (40-54)
Charnley class	
A	8 (32%)
B	13 (52%)
C	4 (16%)

- Trauma 3 (10%)
- No dominant risk factor (Idiopathic ON) 3 (10%)
- Gaucher's disease 2 (6.7%)
- Degenerative OA 1 (3.3%)

There were 4 hips rated Ficat stage II, 24 hips rated Ficat stage III, and 2 hips rated Ficat stage IV. The average age of the patients was 36.1 years (range, 21-52 years). Most of the patients were men (16/25, 64%). Seventeen patients had bilateral disease (68%), six of whom had lateral hemiresurfacings including one with a contralateral alumina component. Four patients had a contralateral full resurfacing. Four hips (13.3%) had undergone at least one previous surgery: two had failed core decompressions, and two hips in one patient had FVFG.

The demographics of this group of patients are shown in Table 13-2.

Results of Hemiresurfacing

Clinical Scores

The average UCLA hip scores all improved significantly ($P < .001$) between preoperative and last follow-up visits. The pain score increased from 4.9 ± 2.1 to 7.9 ± 1.5, the walking score from 5.7 ± 1.8 to 9.0 ± 1.3, the function score from 5.1 ± 1.8 to 7.8 ± 2.2, and the activity score from 4.1 ± 1.4 to 5.5 ± 1.3. The Short Form-12 (SF-12) scores also improved significantly ($P < .001$). The average physical component was 29.6 ± 8.4 preoperatively and 36.0 ± 8.6 at the last follow-up examination, and the mental component increased from 45.8 ± 13.6 to 51.5 ± 11.3. The mean postoperative HHS was 75.9 (62-93). The wide standard deviations reflect considerable variability, which has been observed by others.[50] For example, in our series, there were four patients who reported a pain score of 6 and three with a pain score of 7, but three reported no pain (10). These clinical scores are lower on average than those obtained with full resurfacing ($P < .004$), except for the UCLA walking and the SF-12 mental scores, which were not significantly different ($P = .141$ and $P = .380$, respectively).

One patient, a 35-year-old physician with SLE who developed severe malignant hypertension necessitating steroids, had one hip resurfaced with a Conserve and the contralateral with a similar size alumina component (Fig. 13-4). Our prior experience with alumina components has been successful but not necessarily better than with metal as a mating material for the acetabular cartilage, although further follow-up may show some differences. Until this case we had not implanted the two materials in the same patient for comparison. One advantage of the alumina relates to its brittleness and the subsequent ability to remove the component easily when the acetabular cartilage wears out. The alumina shell can be cracked and removed without further damage to the femoral head so that the conversion to full resurfacing becomes possible without having to maintain the femoral component. This type of conversion to full-surface arthroplasty has been performed in two young patients, and both are functioning well 10 years after the conversion surgery. The bone loss would be more substantial with the removal of the metallic femoral component of the current design, precluding a conversion to full resurfacing, so our hope is that at least some hemiresurfacing devices can be converted without removing the femoral component by simple insertion of a matching acetabular component (Fig. 13-5).

Range of Motion

The preoperative and postoperative range-of-motion measurements are summarized in Table 13-3.

ON patients (in particular patients who have had a short duration of symptoms, as is generally the case with patients undergoing hemiresurfacing) typically present a relatively large range of motion preoperatively, except for a consistent loss of internal rotation and some abduction-adduction, which does normalize after surgery.

Conversions

There were five revisions in this series. The reasons for revision were the following: one sepsis, one enigmatic pain, and three acetabular cartilage wear. Three hips were revised to total hip replacements; one was converted to a metal-on-metal surface replacement, keeping the femoral component; and one was revised to a metal on cross-linked polyethylene surface replacement, again retaining the original femoral component. Both are doing well 1.5 and 6 years after revision with UCLA scores of 10, 10, 8, 7 and 10, 9, 10, 7, respectively, for pain, walking, function, and activity. The patients' HHS are 93 and 94.

The patient revised for sepsis underwent a two-stage conversion at another facility to a cementless THR and is doing well 6 years later.

Complications

One patient suffered deep vein thrombosis of the contralateral leg 11 weeks after surgery, which resolved with heparin and coumadin. (The patient was initially treated post-operatively with dalteparin [Fragmin] rather than our usual postoperative coumadin.) There were no other complications.

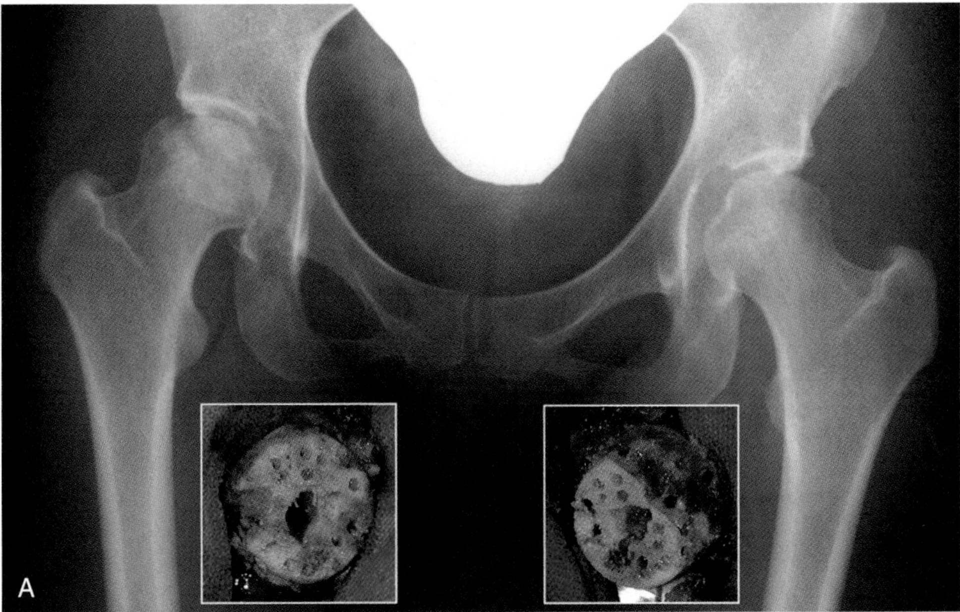

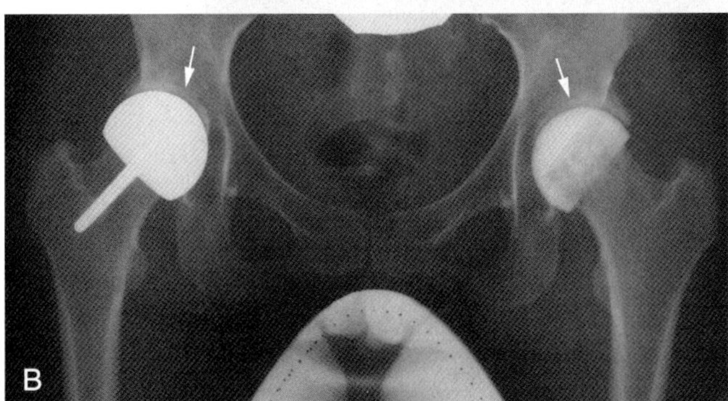

Figure 13-4 **A,** Preoperative anteroposterior radiograph of a 35-year-old woman with steroid-induced bilateral osteonecrosis Ficat stage early IV on the right and Ficat stage II on the left. The inserts show the femoral heads after preparation with the extensive defects typically associated with femoral head necrosis. **B,** Postoperative radiograph taken 77 months after Conserve (*right*) and 73 months after custom alumina (*left*). The patient has comparable University of California-Los Angeles pain scores of 8 on both hips despite the use of two different designs and materials. Note the meniscus of bone within the superior acetabular fossa (*arrows*).

Table 13-3 Preoperative and Postoperative Range of Motion Measurements in Hemiresurfacing

	Flexion	Flexion Contracture	Abduction (in extension)	Adduction (in extension)	Rotation Arc (in extension)
Preoperative score	125.2	4.7	39.3	23.7	59.3
Postoperative score	126.0	1.0	47.0	30.7	79.7
P	0.825	0.237	0.106	0.026	0.080

Summary for Hemiresurfacing

The clinical results and survivorship of this group of hemiresurfacing with the Conserve component are similar to our previously published results obtained with earlier generations of hemisurface with implantation dating back to 1981.[41,52] Although the clinical results are not as good as those of full resurfacing, they are comparable to our experience with osteotomy and reported results of grafting procedures. Furthermore, most patients are satisfied with the results. Two of our patients who are less satisfied had bilateral disease in which one side received a hemiresurfacing device and the contralateral a full resurfacing (HHSs of 69 and 65 on the hemiresurfacing sides). However, when reminded of the objectives of the decision to do one hemiresurfacing, the patients seem to understand the reason for not implanting two full-bearing couples in both hips at a very young age. With our experience and that of others, it is unrealistic to expect a pain relief comparable to full resurfacing in every case. These patients should be fully informed and accept the "time-buying" objectives before undergoing surgery. However, a surprisingly long durability has been demonstrated in some patients who have kept their activity level in the nonsporting, normal range.

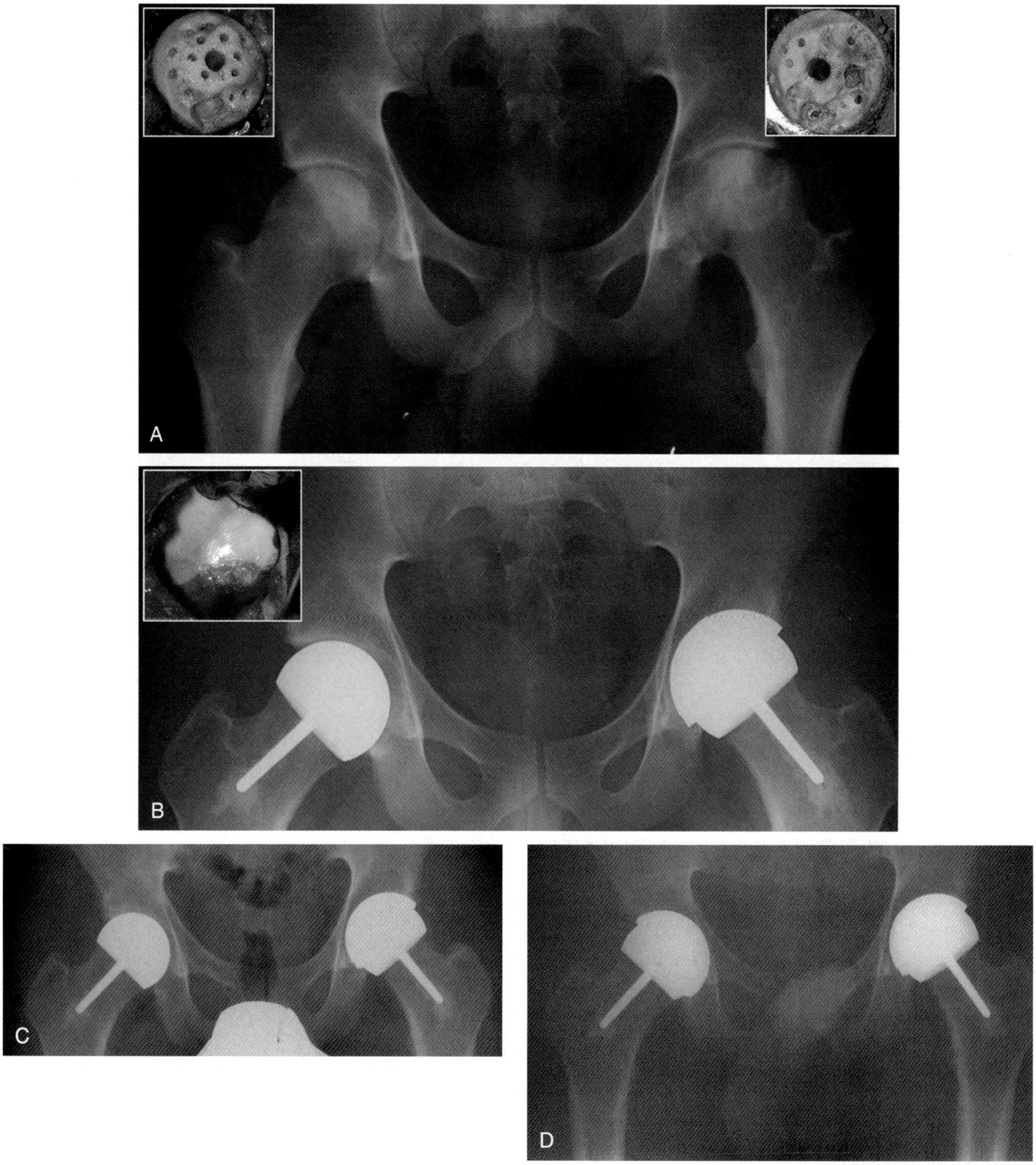

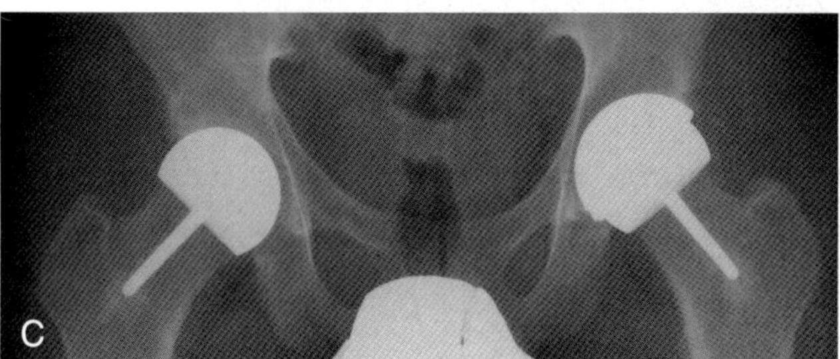

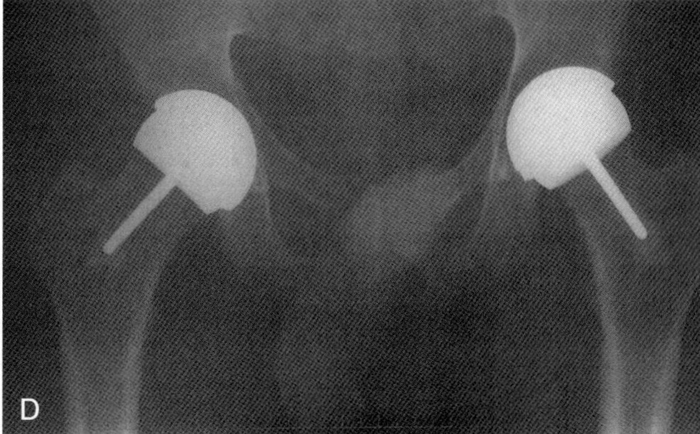

Figure 13-5 A, Twenty-four-year-old man with bilateral osteonecrosis (Ficat III, *right*; Ficat IV, *left*) of the hips. Inserts show intraoperative photographs taken at the end of the preparation phase of the femoral head. **B,** One month postoperative one-stage bilateral hip arthroplasty; the left hip, a total hip resurfacing 50 to 56 mm; the right hip, a hemiresurfacing 50 mm (slightly undersized). The insert shows grade III acetabular cartilage of the right hip intraoperatively. Note preosteophytes inferiorly. Both stems were cemented. **C,** Eleven months postoperatively, the right hip indicates oblitered acetabular cartilage, University of California-Los Angeles scores of 5, 7, 7, 6, for pain, walking, function, and activity, respectively. In retrospect, the acetabular cartilage of the right hip was probably too damaged to anticipate buying a significant amount of time before conversion and reoperation was needed after only a year. **D,** The patient is shown 9 months following conversion of right hip to full resurfacing, and 20 months postoperatively on the left. He has returned to a normal quality of life with University of California-Los Angeles hip scores for both hips of 10, 10, 8, and 7 for pain, walking, function, and activity, respectively.

Full Hip Resurfacing

Indications for Full Hip Resurfacing

Full hip resurfacing should be considered in somewhat older patients, generally those older than 35 with Ficat III or younger for advanced Ficat III with grade III cartilage damage. As with hemiresurfacing, our indications include very large lesions as long as the cylindrically reamed bone was intact circumferentially. Our choice was primarily age-based for the very young or older, but otherwise healthy (<61), irrespective of the size of the lesion. Figure 13-6 shows examples of large defects associated with longstanding ON of the femoral head in patients younger than the age of 52 who have undergone a resurfacing procedure with Conserve®Plus and had successful midterm results.

Demographics of Full Hip Resurfacing for Osteonecrosis

From our series of 1000 hips (838 patients), 84 hips (70 patients) received a Conserve®Plus resurfacing for arthritis secondary to ON of the femoral head. The risk factors for the development of ON were diverse in this group and distributed as follows:

- Steroids 31 (36.9%)
- Trauma 19 (22.6%)
- Alcohol 6 (7.1%)
- Sickle cell disease 1 (1.2%)
- No dominant risk factor (idiopathic ON) 27 (32.1%)

There were 19 hips rated ON Ficat stage III and 65 rated Ficat stage IV.

The average age of the patients was 40.1 years (range, 14 to 61 years). Most of the patients were men (51/70, 81.4%), a proportion even greater than the overall resurfacing population.

From this cohort, 33 patients (47.1%) had bilateral disease. However, excluding the 19 patients with post traumatic defects (all unilateral), the incidence of bilaterality was 64.7%. There were four patients with a contralateral hemiresurfacing, 15 with bilateral full metal-on-metal resurfacing (one of them with one device from another manufacturer), three with a contralateral conventional THR, and seven with a contralateral core decompression. Twenty-eight hips (33.3%) had undergone at least one previous surgery: 17 had a core decompression, three had a hemiresurfacing, five had been pinned, two had previous FVFG, and one had a Judet graft.

The demographics of this group of patients are shown in Tables 13-4 and 13-5.

The percentage of large defects was the highest of any etiologic group undergoing metal-on-metal hip resurfacing, with only 21% having none or a defect size of 1 cm or less. In this series, 43 hips (52.2%) were implanted with the femoral metaphyseal stem cemented, the highest percent of all the etiologic groups. This included four in the first 37 (11%) and 39 of the remaining 47 (83%).

Results of Full Hip Resurfacing

Clinical Scores

The average UCLA hip scores all improved significantly ($P < .0001$) between preoperative and last follow-up visits. The pain score increased from 3.5 ± 1.5 to 9.4 ± 0.9, the walking score from 5.7 ± 1.5 to 9.4 ± 1.1, the function score from 5.2 ± 1.5 to 9.3 ± 1.4, and the activity score from 4.3 ± 1.3 to 7.0 ± 1.7.

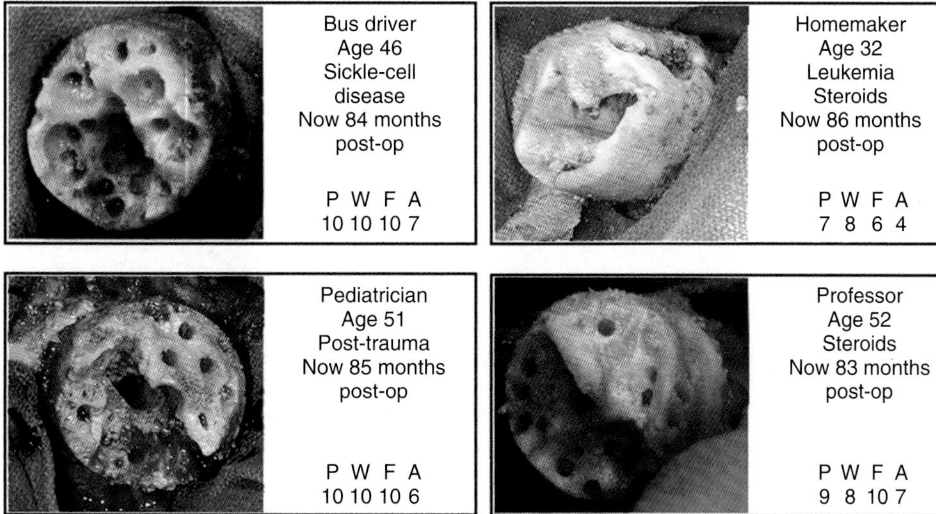

Figure 13-6 Four intra-operative photographic examples of challenging resurfacings performed by the senior author on patients with osteonecrosis of the femoral head. The photographs were taken before cementing of the femoral component. These patients have now had a follow-up greater than 7 years since their reconstruction with a Conserve®Plus metal-on-metal hybrid resurfacing. The intraoperative photo of the lower left hip reveals some residual cystic material, which we believe had required further cleaning of debris with a high-speed burr.

Table 13-4 Demographics of the Patients Operated with Full Resurfacing for Arthritis Secondary to Osteonecrosis

	Males	Females	Combined
Age (years)	42.4 (16-61)	30.3 (14-49)	40.1 (14-61)
Weight (kg)	85.1 (57-114)	61.4 (46-92)	80.6 (46-114)
Height (cm)	179.5 (165-198)	161.9 (148-175)	176.2 (148-198)
BMI	26.4 (19.2-38.6)	23.3 (17.6-30.0)	25.8 (17.8-38.6)
Femoral component size (mm)	47.7 (42-56)	40.4 (36-44)	46.3 (36-56)
Cysts >1 cm	57 (83.8%)	14 (87.5%)	71 (84.5%)
Charnley class			
A	26 (45.6%)	8 (61.5%)	34 (48.6%)
B	27 (47.4%)	2 (15.4%)	29 (41.4%)
C	4 (7.0%)	3 (23.1%)	7 (10.0%)

BMI, body mass index.

Table 13-5 Distribution of Hip Bone Quality by Femoral Single or Multiple Defect Size

	n	Percentage of Hips
Good Bone—no defect	9	10.7
Defects 0 to 1 cm	9	10.7
Defects 1 to 2 cm	30	35.7
Defects 2 to 3 cm	36	42.9

The SF-12 scores also improved significantly ($P < .0001$). The average physical component was 31.1 ± 7.9 preoperatively and 48.5 ± 9.8 at the last follow-up, and the mental component increased from 43.8 ± 13.0 to 49.1 ± 12.3. The post-operative HHS was 91.8 ± 11.3. The clinical scores were comparable to that of the rest of the cohort except for the activity score, which was lower in average (7.0 versus 7.5, $P = .0015$) and, as previously noted, higher on average than for hemiresurfacing except for the walking and SF-12 mental scores.

Range of Motion

The preoperative and postoperative range-of-motion measurements are summarized in Table 13-6.

As previously stated in the section reporting the range of motion of patients treated with hemiresurfacing, ON patients presented less limitation in range of motion preoperatively (larger than the rest of the cohort in flexion, adduction and rotation). Postoperatively, the hip range of motion normalized.

Case Histories

Case #1: Metal-on-metal resurfacing was performed on a 14-year-old student who sustained a femoral neck fracture in 2003. After internal fixation, the patient had developed ON and she received an FVFG in October of 2004. She failed to get pain relief and presented in our office with Ficat stage IV ON in July 2005 (Fig. 13-7). Two years after surgery, the patient has resumed a normal student lifestyle with UCLA scores of 10, 10, 10, and 7 for pain, walking, function, and activity, respectively.

Case #2: The patient is a 48-year-old resort developer who had a fracture of the femoral neck consecutive to a bicycling accident. The fracture was reduced and pinned, but the femoral head developed ON Ficat stage IV (Fig. 13-8). One year after Conserve®Plus metal-on-metal resurfacing, the patient had resumed his usual physical activities including competitive skiing. Ten years after surgery, his UCLA scores are 10, 10, 10, and 9 for pain, walking, function, and activity, respectively.

Case #3: The patient is a 48-year-old police officer who sustained a hip injury after a fall during work-related exercise in February of 1996. The femoral head developed ON, and the patient underwent coring and bone grafting procedures. The coring attempt failed, and the patient presented in our office 1 year later with Ficat stage IV ON (Fig. 13-9). The patient is

Table 13-6 The Pre-operative and Postoperative Range of Motion Measurements in Full Hip Resurfacing

	Pre-op Flexion	Pre-op Flexion Contracture	Pre-op Abduction (in extension)	Pre-op Adduction (in extension)	Pre-op Rotation arc (in extension)	Post-op Flexion	Post-op Flexion Contracture	Post-op Abduction (in extension)	Post-op Adduction (in extension)	Post-op Rotation Arc (in extension)
Whole series (1000 hips)	105.6	16.1	23.2	14.5	23.5	125.9	1.9	45.2	27.9	76.6
Osteonecrosis (n = 84)	111.0	13.7	24.1	16.7	30.0	126.7	1.3	46.5	28.9	78.1
Other etiologies (n = 16)	105.1	16.3	23.1	14.3	22.9	125.8	1.9	45.0	27.8	76.4
P	0.003	0.091	0.539	0.042	0.001	0.567	0.347	0.168	0.191	0.428

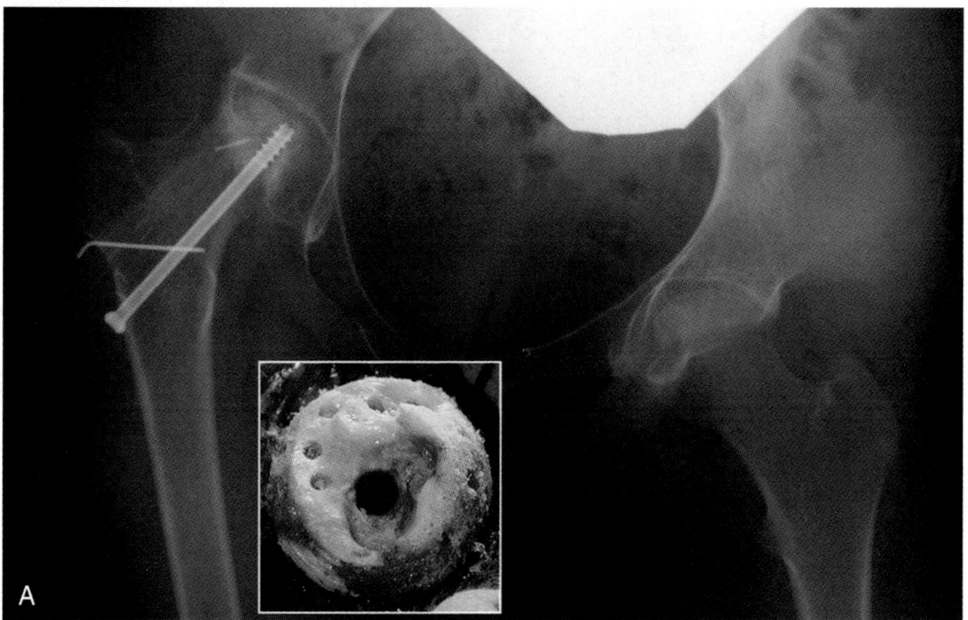

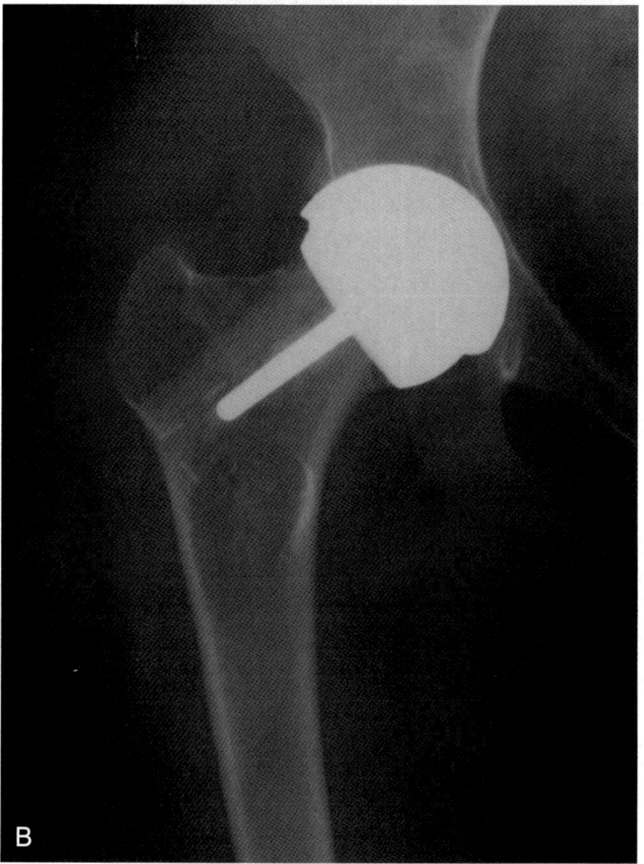

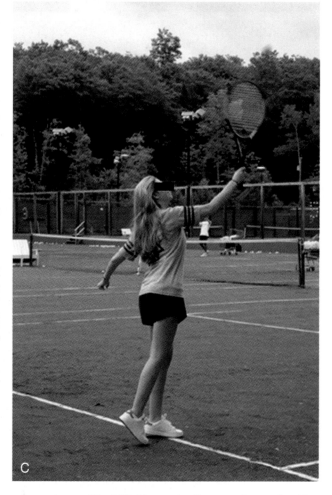

Figure 13-7 A, Preoperative radiograph of a 14-year-old student with post-traumatic osteonecrosis Ficat stage IV of the right hip, 1 year after unsuccessful free vascularized fibular graft. The insert shows the femoral head after preparation for cementation of the Conserve®Plus component. The graft had healed but did not prevent further collapse. **B,** Two years after surgery, the components are well fixed. All of the vascular clips were not removed, and the graft remains superior to the stem. **C,** The patient has resumed a normal lifestyle, participating occasionally in sporting activities, although caution has been advised.

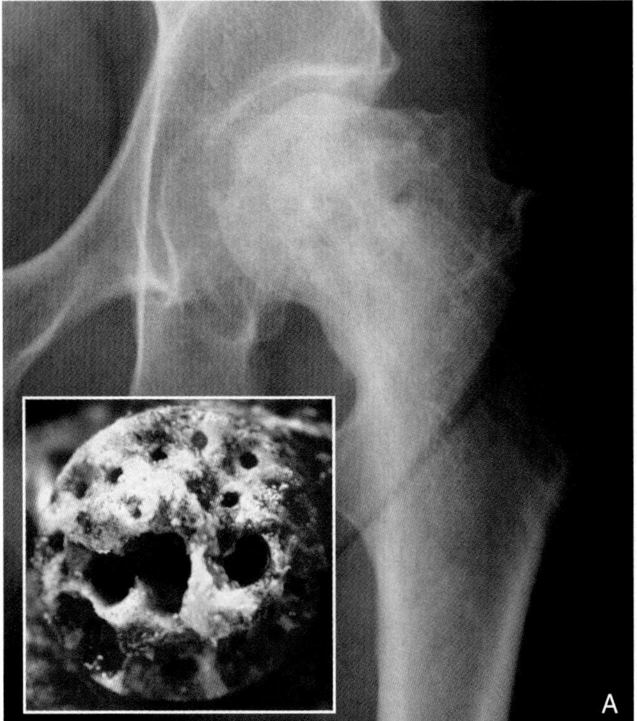

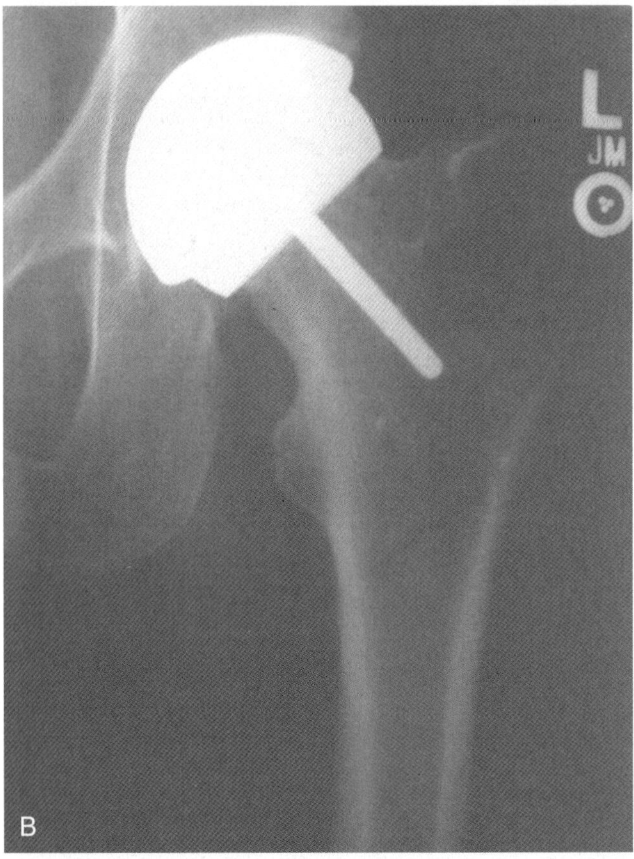

Figure 13-8 A, Forty-eight-year-old man with osteonecrosis of the left hip due to trauma. Insert shows an intraoperative photograph of the femoral head after preparation for a total hip resurfacing. Note the extensive defects due to the pin tracts and necrosis. The preparation of the bone was satisfactory (hip #18 in the overall series—50-mm head size), although more bone cleaning and drying would be in order today. **B,** Radiograph of the patient 74 months following resurfacing. University of California-Los Angeles hip scores were 10, 10, 10, and 9 for pain, walking, function, and activity, respectively, and are unchanged 10 years postoperatively. *(Reprinted with permission from Amstutz H, Le Duff M, Dorey F: Hip resurfacing: indications, results, and prevention of complications. In Sofue M, Endo N (eds): Treatment of Osteoarthritic Change in the Hip. Shinano, Japan, Springer; 2007, pp 195-204.)*

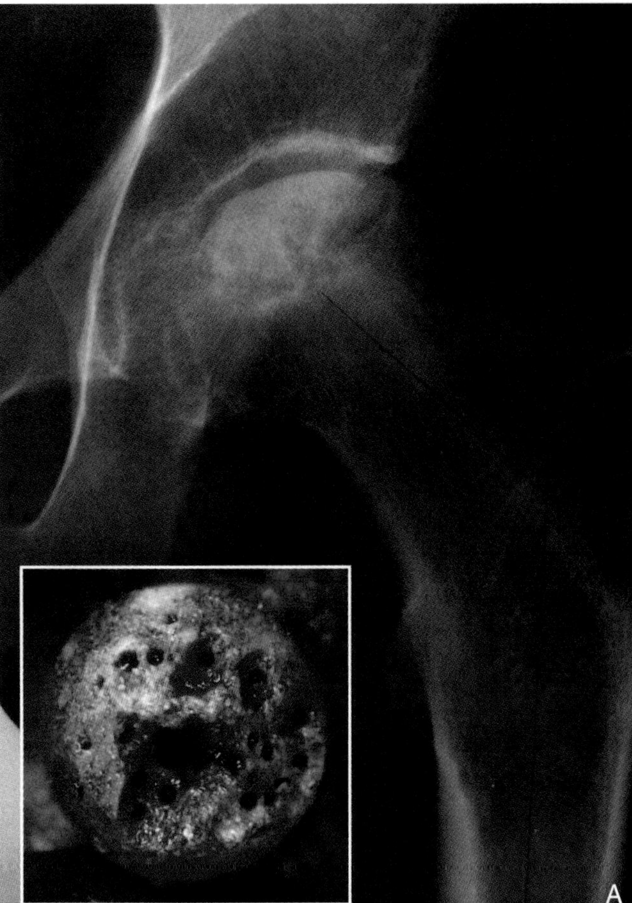

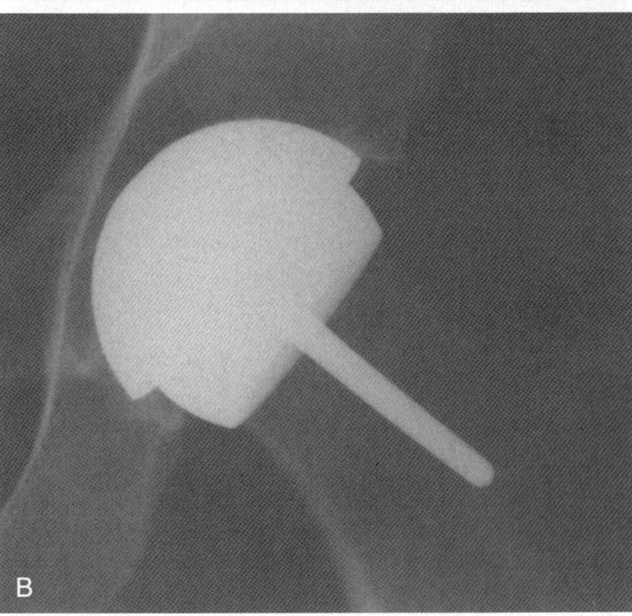

Figure 13-9 A, Forty-eight-year-old man with osteonecrosis Ficat stage IV of the hip that had undergone a previous core decompression; insert is an interoperative photograph of the femoral head with a large defect after preparation for a total resurfacing (hip #32 in the overall series). Despite relatively large defects (one > 2 cm) with a 50-mm femoral component, the stem was not cemented in at that time. **B,** Radiograph of the patient at 9.5 years following metal-on-metal resurfacing. University of California-Los Angeles hip scores for pain, walking, function, and activity are 10, 9, 10, and 8, respectively.

still fairly active, playing golf occasionally and was recently seen 9.5 years after surgery. His UCLA scores are 10, 9, 10, and 8 for pain, walking, function, and activity, respectively.

Conversions to Total Hip Replacement

There were two conversions to THR in this series. Both were consecutive to loosening of the femoral component at 23 and 61 months. Both of these patients were operated on early in our series (hips #6 and 25) with crude bone preparation and implant techniques relative to our current technique and one had a gross seating error and was in severe varus (Fig. 13-10).

In addition, one simultaneous bilateral patient with poor bone quality required a reoperation to reconstruct the acetabular wall, and the revision of the acetabular component after this one protruded 3 days after surgery. This was associated with over-reaming and due to new very sharp "bear claw" reamers.

Using any cause for revision as endpoint, the Kaplan-Meier survivorship results for this group of patients was the following (Fig. 13-11):

3 years: 97.1% (95% confidence interval (CI), 88.7 to 99.2)

4 years: 97.1% (95% CI, 88.7 to 99.2)

5 years: 97.1% (95% CI, 88.7 to 99.2)

8 years: 93.1% (95% CI, 76.9 to 98.0)

We also computed the Kaplan-Meier survivorship results for this group of patients using femoral failure only as end point. This analysis yielded a 98.4% survivorship at 5 years (95% CI, 88.9 to 99.8).

Complications

There were no complications in this series.

Discussion

The results and especially the durability of our series of patients already far surpass those of our previous generations of metal-polyethylene resurfacings[53] and rival survivorship of THR.[54] Even with our early technique, there have been no revisions in hips performed in the last 10 years. However, three hips from our first-generation technique have radiolucencies, but

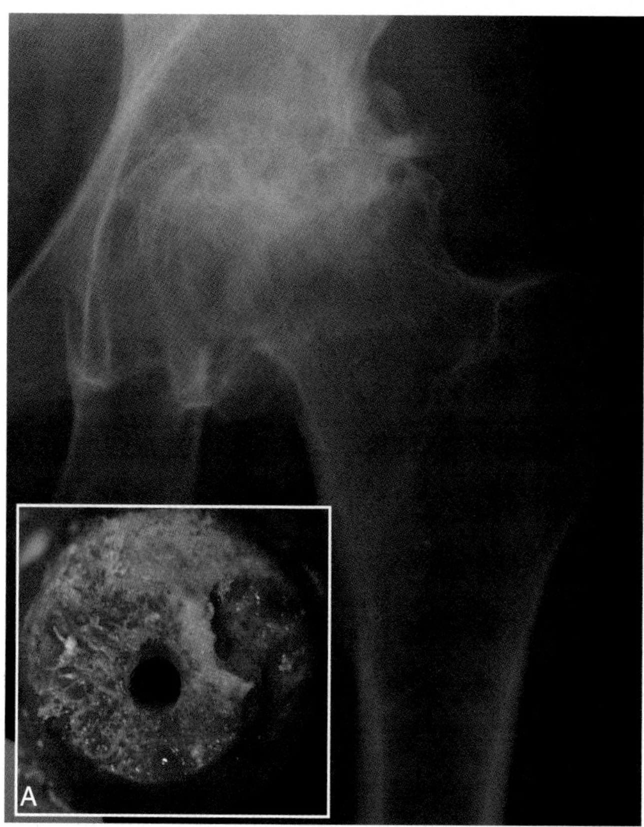

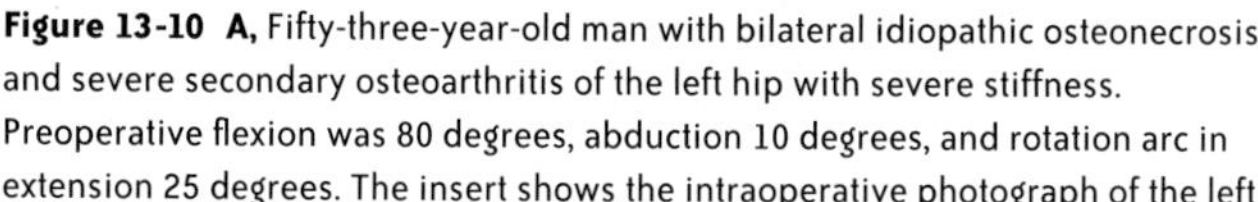

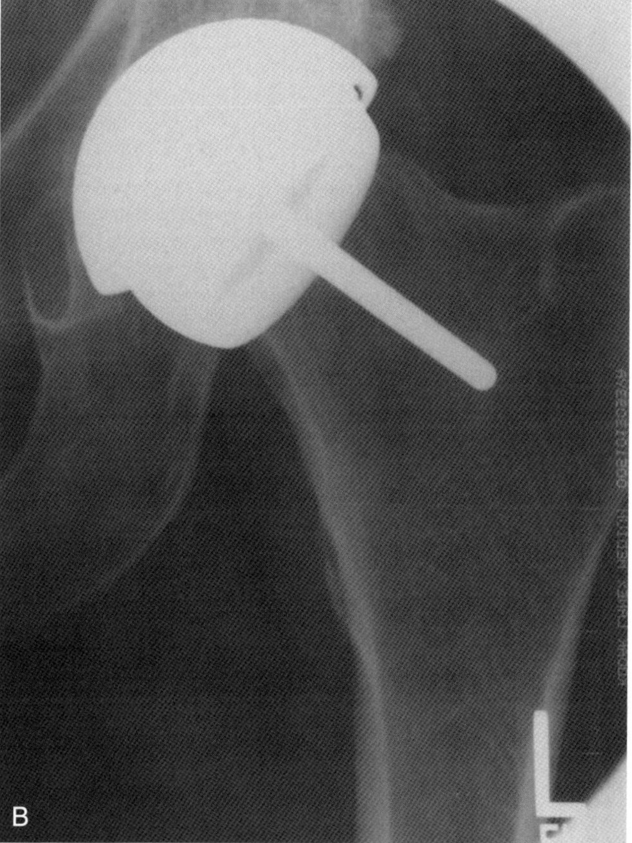

Figure 13-10 A, Fifty-three-year-old man with bilateral idiopathic osteonecrosis and severe secondary osteoarthritis of the left hip with severe stiffness. Preoperative flexion was 80 degrees, abduction 10 degrees, and rotation arc in extension 25 degrees. The insert shows the intraoperative photograph of the left femoral head at the end of preparation phase for total resurfacing, with a defect of 1 cm and some osteopenia. **B,** Immediate postoperative radiograph resurfaced with poor technique (hip #6 in our series). The femoral component was inserted in varus (124 degrees).

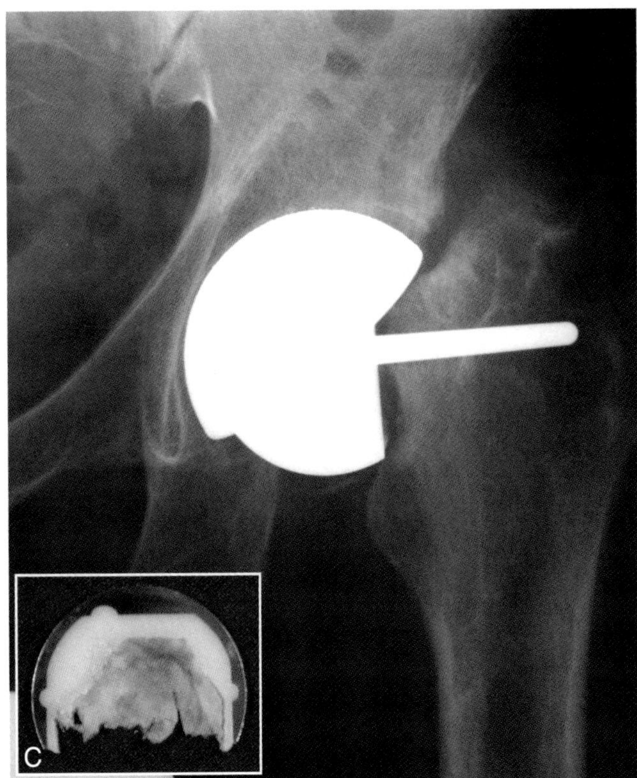

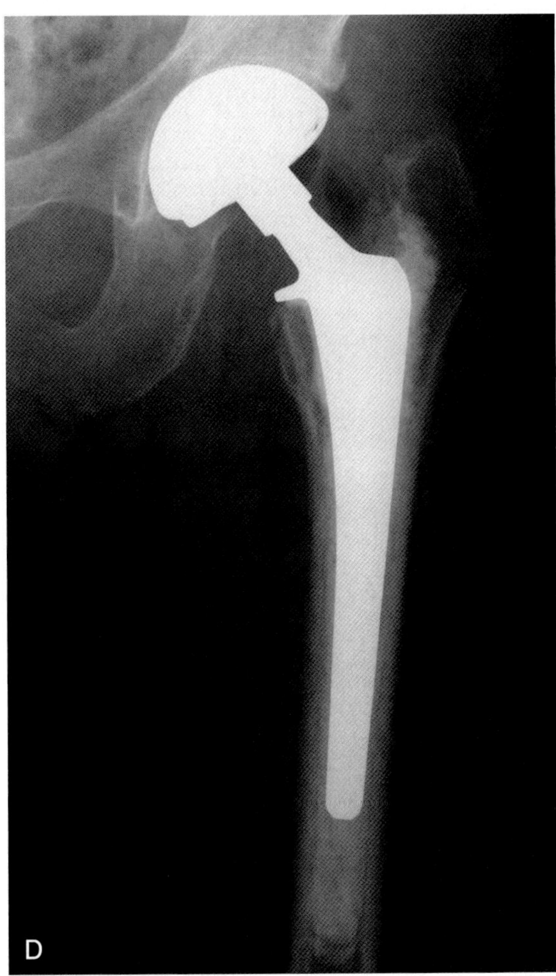

Figure 13-10 *Continued* **C,** Radiograph of the patient at 23 months shows a failed total resurfacing. The mode of failure determined to be aseptic loosening of the femoral component. The sections (*insert*) showed incomplete seating of the component. Histologic analysis revealed features consistent with loss of cement fixation and loosening, resulting in fibrous replacement of the head. **D,** Anteroposterior radiograph shows the left hip converted to a total hip replacement with a cemented Perfecta stem (Wright Medical Technology, Arlington, TN) and a unipolar head matching the inner diameter of the well-fixed acetabular shell, which was left in situ. The University of California-Los Angeles hip scores at the last follow-up were 9, 9, 8, 5 for pain, walking, function, and activity, respectively. The hip has now been converted to total hip replacement for 8.5 years.

Table 13-7 Recent Reports on the Treatment of Osteonecrosis with Hip Resurfacing

					INDICATIONS										
Surgeon	# Cases	# Patients	Age in Years (Range)	M/F	Alcohol	Chemotherapy	Idiopathic	Sickle Cell	Corticosteroid Use	Trauma	Not Documented	Tumor	SLE	LCP
Treacy (Revell)[56]	73	60	43 (17–69)	42/18 70%/30%	3 (4%)	2 (3%)	34 (47%)	1 (1%)	20 (27%)	8 (11%)	5 (7%)	N/A	N/A	N/A
Mont[57]	42	36	40 (18–64)	25/11 69%/31%	N/A	N/A	3 (7%)	1 (2%)	11 (26%)	11 (26%)	6 (14%)	4 (10%)	3 (7%)	3 (7%)
McMinn[55]	104	94	44 (16–68)	N/D	8%	included with steroids	43%		25%	20%				4%
Amstutz Current Results	84	70	42 (14–61)	68/16 81%/19%	6 (7%)	included with steroids	27 (32%)	1 (1.2%)	31 (37%)	19 (22.6%)	N/A	N/A	N/A	N/A

N/A, not applicable; N/D, not determined.

they have been stable and asymptomatic for over 7 years (Fig. 13-12). There have been no loosenings in the 46 hips where the stem was cemented. There are three other recent reports on resurfacing for ON, two with the Birmingham Hip Resurfacing (BHR)[55,56] and one with the Conserve®Plus.[57] The indications for surgery differed in these publications in that only defects of less than 33% were accepted. McMinn, with a 6.7% failure rate at 4.5 years of average follow-up, was concerned that failures were due to advancing necrosis but did not provide supporting data. He now prefers a midhead resection and using a prosthesis with a larger and longer stem, filling the metaphysis. Our results strongly suggest that a midhead prosthesis is not necessary with optimal resurfacing bone preparation and cementing technique. Treacy and Mont also expressed optimism regarding their resurfacing results although they are more conservative in their patient selection and select heads with less than one third involvement (Table 13-7).

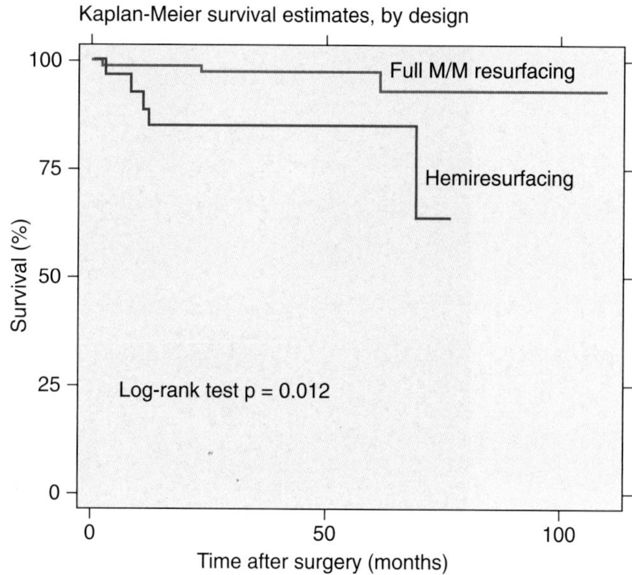

Figure 13-11 Kaplan-Meier survivorship curve of Conserve®Plus full resurfacing plotted against Conserve hemiresurfacing in osteonecrosis patients, using any revision as an endpoint.

Summary

Patients with ON of the hip present specific challenges because of the large defects often present and filled initially with extensive yellowish, friable necrotic bone. This necrotic bone must be completely removed down to the underlying white hard reparative bone to ensure proper component fixation and durability. The residual defects, which are often large, should not be grafted and the stem should be cemented to maximize the fixation area. Patients with large defects that have been filled with cement should not, in our view, engage in impact activities if optimal durability of the prosthesis is to be achieved. Our results with the Conserve®Plus highlight that the etiology of ON itself does not constitute a contraindication for resurfacing, and the risk factors for the procedure are similar to that of primary osteoarthritis. The femoral survivorship has been comparable to other etiologies from the initiation of the series and 100% for patients implanted after August of 1997. The complication rate has been lower than that of other etiologies. We have not recorded any heterotopic ossification, dislocation, nerve palsy, or blood-related adverse events. There were no early or late hematogenous sepses in full resurfacing and only one late post-operative sepsis in a patient with Gaucher's disease in our hemiresurfacing series.

	FICAT STAGE								
Surgeon	II	III	IV	% of Head Necrotic	Implant Type	# Bilaterals (Percent of Cohort)	AVG Follow Up in Months (Range)	# Revisions (%), AVG Time to Revision in Months (Range)	Complications (Type)
Treacy (Revell)[56]	2 (3%)	12 (34%)	46 (63%)	<35%	18 Corin (25%), 55 BHR (75%)	13 (10 male, 3 female, 22%)	73.2 (24–144)	5 (6.8% include 1 pending)	2
		2 revised	3 revised					57.5 (3–86)	(dvt, broken guidewires)
Mont[57]	N/D	N/D	N/D	N/D	42 Conserve®Plus	6 (unknown breakdown, 17%)	41 (24–61)	2 (5%) 17 (3–30)	N/D
McMinn[55]	N/A	"all were either III or IV"	Mid Head resection used in "large" lesions	McMinn Resurfacing Hip, BHR (unknown breakdown)	10 (unknown breakdown, 11%)	52 (14–126)	48 (5–81)	7 (6.7%)	N/D
Amstutz Current Results		19 (23%)	65 (77%)	Up to 100% on the dome	84 Conserve®Plus	14 (11 male, 3 female, 20%)	72 (7.2–123.6)	3 (3.5%) 29 (3–62)	None
		1 revised	2 revised						

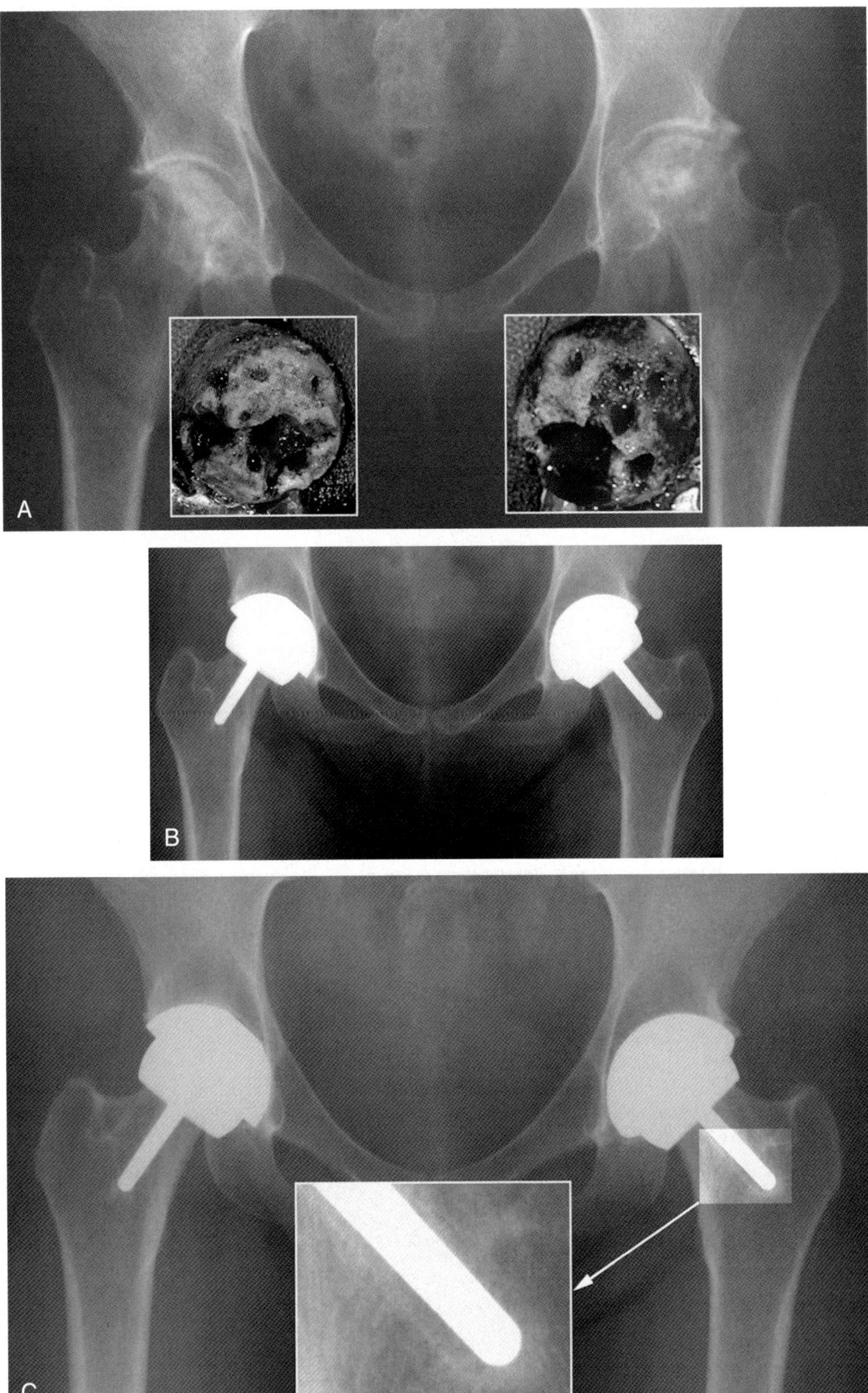

Figure 13-12 A, Thirty-one-year-old woman with systemic erythematosus and bilateral osteonecrosis of the hip secondary to steroid use. Inserts show the femoral heads after preparation for a total hip resurfacing, with larger defects on the right hip than the left. **B,** The patient is shown 4 months after undergoing single stage, bilateral metal-on-metal total hip resurfacing (hips #306 and 307 in our series). The metaphyseal stem on the right side was cemented into place, whereas the left was press-fit without cement. **C,** At 27 months after surgery, a complete radiolucency around the metaphyseal stem on the left hip is noted. Note the reactive bone around the tip of the stem. The patient was still asymptomatic at the last follow-up (84 months postoperatively), and her University of California-Los Angeles hip scores were 9 on the right side and 10 on the left side for pain, 10 for walking, 10 for function, and 6 for activity. *(Reprinted with permission from Amstutz H, Le Duff M, Campbell P, Dorey F: The effects of technique changes on aseptic loosening of the femoral component in hip resurfacing. Results of 600 Conserve Plus with a 3-9 year follow-up. J Arthroplasty 2007;22:481-489.)*

References

1. Konig F: Ueber freie korper in der gezenken z. Beitrage Zoe Aetiologic Der Cordora Mobilia. Entstehung Derselben Durch Osteochondritis dissecans. Dtsch Z Chir 1888;27:90-109.
2. Jones JP Jr: Fat embolism, intravascular coagulation, and osteonecrosis. Clin Orthop 1993;292:294-308.
3. Ficat RP: Idiopathic bone necrosis of the femoral head. Early diagnosis and treatment. J Bone Joint Surg Br 1985;67:3-9.
4. Meyers M: Osteonecrosis of the femoral head: pathogenesis and long-term results of treatment. Clin Orthop Relat Res 1988;231:51-61.
5. Felson D, Anderson J: A cross study evaluation of association between steroid dose and bolus steroids and avascular necrosis of the bone. Lancet 1987;1:902-906.
6. Jones JJ: Fat embolism and osteonecrosis. Orthop Clin North Am 1985;16:595-633.
7. Wang G, Sweet D, Reger S, Thompson R: Fat cell changes as a mechanism of avascular necrosis of the femoral head in cortisone-treated rabbits. J Bone Joint Surg Am 1977;59:729-735.
8. Johnson L: Histogenesis of avascular necrosis. In Proceedings of the Conference on Aseptic Necrosis of the Femoral Head. St Louis, 1964.
9. Miyanishi K, Kamo Y, Ihara H, Naka T, Hirakawa M, Sugioka Y: Risk factors for dysbaric osteonecrosis. Rheumatology 2006;45:855-858.
10. Jacobs B: Epidemiology of traumatic and nontraumatic osteonecrosis. Clin Orthop Relat Res 1978;130:51-67.
11. Harrington K, Murray W, Kountz S, Belzer F: Avascular necrosis of bone after renal transplantation. J Bone Joint Surg Am 1971;53:203-215.
12. Klipper A, Stevens M, Zizic T, Hungerford D: Ischemic necrosis of bone in systemic lupus erythematosus. Medicine 1976;55:251-257.
13. Iwegbu C, Fleming A: Avascular necrosis of the femoral head in sickle-cell disease. A series from the Guinea Savannah of Nigeria. J Bone Joint Surg Br 1985;67:29-32.
14. Lee R, Golding J, Serjeant G: The radiological features of avascular necrosis of the femoral head in homozygous sickle cell disease. Clin Radiol 1981;32:205-214.
15. Hanker GJ, Amstutz HC: Osteonecrosis of the hip in the sickle-cell diseases. Treatment and complications. J Bone Joint Surg Am 1988;70:499-506.
16. Sebes J, Kraus A: Avascular necrosis of the hip in the sickle cell hemoglobinopathies. J Can Assoc Radiol 1983;34:136-139.
17. Chevalier X, Larget-Piet B, Hernigou P, Gherardi R: Avascular necrosis of the femoral head in HIV-infected patients. J Bone Joint Surg Br 1993;75:160.
18. Mahoney C, Glesby M, DiCarlo E, Peterson M, Bostrom M: Total hip arthroplasty in patients with human immunodeficiency virus infection: pathologic findings and surgical outcomes. Acta Orthop 2005;76:198-203.
19. Korompilias A, Ortel T, Urbaniak J: Coagulation abnormalities in patients with hip osteonecrosis. Orthop Clin North Am 2004;35:265-271.
20. Kenzora J, Glimcher M: Accumulative cell stress: the multifactorial etiology of idiopathic osteonecrosis. Orthop Clin North Am 1985;16:669-679.
21. Mango E: Ischemic necrosis of the femoral head. In Dee R, Mango E, Hurst L (eds): Principles of Orthopaedic Practice. San Francisco, McGraw Hill, 1989, p 1357.
22. Brown T, Way M, Ferguson A: Mechanical characteristics of bone in femoral capital aseptic necrosis. Clin Orthop 1981;156: 240-247.
23. Favenesi J, Gardeniers J, Huiskes R, Sloof T: Mechanical properties of normal and avascular cancellous bone. In Ducheyne P, Vander Perre G, Aubert A: Biomaterials and Biomechanics 1983. Amsterdam, Elsevier Biomedical, 1984, p 121.
24. Glimcher M, Kenzora J: The biology of osteonecrosis of the human femoral head and its clinical implications: II. The pathological changes in the femoral head as an organ and in the hip joint. Clin Orthop Relat Res 1979;139:283-312.
25. Bonfiglio M, Bardenstein M: Treatment by bone-grafting of aseptic necrosis of the femoral head and non-union of the femoral neck (Phemister technique). 1: J Bone Joint Surg Am 1958;40-A:1329-1346.
26. Ilardi C, Sokoloff L: Secondary osteonecrosis in osteoarthritis of the femoral head. Hum Pathol 1984;15:79-83.
27. Hungerford DS: Treatment of osteonecrosis of the femoral head: everything's new. J Arthroplasty 2007;22(4 Suppl 1):91-94.
28. Taylor L: Multifocal avascular necrosis after short-term high-dose steroid therapy. A report of three cases. J Bone Joint Surg Br 1984;66:431-433.
29. Merle D'Aubigné R, Postel M, Mazabraud A, Massias P, Gueguen J, France P: Idiopathic necrosis of the femoral head in adults. J Bone Joint Surg Br 1965;47:612-633.
30. Ficat R: Treatment of avascular necrosis of the femoral head. Hip 1983;279-295.
31. Hauzeur J, Pasteels J, Orloff S: Bilateral non-traumatic aseptic osteonecrosis in the femoral head. An experimental study of incidence. J Bone Joint Surg Am 1987;69:1221-1225.
32. Hedley A, Kim W: Prosthetic replacement in osteonecrosis of the hip. Instr Course Lect 1983;32:265-271.
33. Meyers M: Surgical treatment of osteonecrosis of the femoral head. Instr Course Lect 1983;32:260-265.
34. Marcus N, Enneking W, Massam R: The silent hip in idiopathic aseptic necrosis. Treatment by bone-grafting. J Bone Joint Surg Am 1973;55:1351-1366.
35. Ficat R, Arlet J: Ischaemia and Necrosis of Bone. Baltimore, Williams & Wilkins, 1980.
36. Steinberg ME, Hayken GD, Steinberg DR: A quantitative system for staging avascular necrosis. J Bone Joint Surg Br 1995;77: 34-41.
37. Steinberg M, Larcom P, Strafford B, Hosick W, Corces A, Bands R, Hartman K: Core decompression with bone grafting for osteonecrosis of the femoral head. Clin Orthop Relat Res 2001;386:71-78.
38. Mont M, Jones L, Hungerford D: Nontraumatic osteonecrosis of the femoral head: ten years later. J Bone Joint Surg Am 2006;88:1117-1132.
39. Beaulé P, Le Duff M, Amstutz H: Hemiresurfacing arthroplasty of the hip for failed free-vascularized fibular graft. J Arthroplasty 2003;18:519-523.
40. Beaulé P, Amstutz H, Le Duff M, Dorey F: Surface arthroplasty for osteonecrosis of the hip: Hemiresurfacing versus metal-on-metal hybrid resurfacing. J Arthroplasty 2004;19:54-58.
41. Beaulé P, Schmalzried T, Campbell P, Dorey F, Amstutz H: Duration of symptoms and outcome of hemiresurfacing for hip osteonecrosis. Clin Orthop 2001;385:104-117.
42. Sedel L, Travers V, Witvoet J: Spherocylindric (Luck) cup arthroplasty for osteonecrosis of the hip. Clin Orthop 1987;219:127-135.

43. Meulemeester FRAJ, Rosing PM: Uncemented surface replacement for osteonecrosis of the femoral head. Acta Orthop Scand 1989;60:425-429.
44. Scott R, Urse J, Schmidt R, Bierbaum B: Use of TARA hemiarthroplasty in advanced osteonecrosis. J Arthroplasty 1987; 2:225-232.
45. Krackow KA, Mont MA, Maar DC: Limited femoral endoprosthesis for avascular necrosis of the femoral head. Orthop Rev 1993;22:457-463.
46. Wagner H: Surface replacement arthroplasty of the hip. Clin Orthop 1978;134:102-130.
47. Nelson CL, Walz BH, Gruenwald JM: Resurfacing of only the femoral head for osteonecrosis. Long-term follow-up study. J Arthroplasty 1997;12:736-740.
48. Amstutz H, Grigoris P, Dorey F: Evolution and future of surface replacement of the hip. J Orthop Sci 1998;3:169-186.
49. Grecula M, Thomas J, Kreuzer S: Impact of implant design on femoral head hemiresurfacing arthroplasty. Clin Orthop Relat Res 2004;418:41-47.
50. Cuckler J, Moore K, Estrada L: Outcome of hemiresurfacing in osteonecrosis of the femoral head. Clin Orthop Relat Res 2004;429:146-150.
51. Adili A, Trousdale R: Femoral head resurfacing for the treatment of osteonecrosis in the young patient. Clin Orthop Relat Res 2003;417:93-101.
52. Amstutz HC, Noordin S, Campbell PA, Schmalzried TP: Precision fit surface hemiarthroplasty for femoral head osteonecrosis. In Urbaniak JR, Jones JP Jr (ed): Osteonecrosis: Etiology, Diagnosis, and Treatment. Rosemont IL: American Academy of Orthopaedic Surgeons; 1997, pp 373-383.
53. Amstutz HC, Dorey F, O'Carroll PF: THARIES resurfacing arthroplasty. Evolution and long-term results. Clin Orthop Rel Res 1986;92-114.
54. Ortiguera C, Pulliam I, Cabanela M: Total hip arthroplasty for osteonecrosis. Matched-pair analysis of 188 hips with long-term follow-up. J Arthroplasty 1999;14:21-28.
55. McMinn D, Daniel J, Pradhan C, Ziaee H: Avascular necrosis in the young patient: a trilogy of arthroplasty options. Orthopedics 2005;28:945-947.
56. Revell M, McBryde C, Bhatnagar S, Pynsent P, Treacy R: Metal-on-metal hip resurfacing in osteonecrosis of the femoral head. J Bone Joint Surg Am 2006;88:98-103.
57. Mont M, Seyler T, Marker D, Marulanda G, Delanois R: Use of metal-on-metal total hip resurfacing for the treatment of osteonecrosis of the femoral head. J Bone Joint Surg Am 2006; 88:90-97.

CHAPTER 14

Childhood Disorders

Harlan C. Amstutz

Michel J. Le Duff

Edwin P. Su

Introduction

In the present chapter, four separate etiologies were regrouped under the category of childhood disorders. These disorders include developmental dysplasia of the hip (DDH), slipped capital femoral epiphysis (SCFE), Legg-Calvé-Perthes disease (LCP), and multiple epiphyseal dysplasia (ED) involving the hips. Although there are some similar anatomic abnormalities, performing hip resurfacing for arthritis secondary to these disorders presents distinct challenges in creating a more normal anatomy and efficient biomechanics for hips with particular individual characteristics. These unique reconstructive challenges include deficient acetabular bone stock, aberrant proximal femoral (head and neck) geometry, leg-length discrepancy, abductor insufficiency, muscle contractures, all occurring in a younger patient population.[1-4]

Legg-Calve-Perthes Disease and Slipped Capital Femoral Epiphysis

LCP disease and SCFE are disorders of the hip that occur in children and adolescents, which may result in degenerative joint disease in adulthood. Both LCP and SCFE often cause alterations in proximal femoral anatomy that affect joint mechanics, create impingement, and lead to the development of degenerative joint disease. LCP often results in a broad, flattened, retroversion head (coxa plana) and short, wide, anteverted femoral neck in association with relative acetabular dysplasia. The resultant mismatch in congruity between the head and the socket typically leads to degenerative arthritis in a patient's 3rd to 5th decades, depending upon the degree of severity. In a recent publication, we described quantitatively the head-neck relationship of the hips from our series of patients who received a Conserve®Plus prosthesis for osteoarthritis secondary to LCP or SCFE.[5]

The wide femoral neck poses a challenge to hip resurfacing because of the possibility of damaging the femoral neck while preparing the femoral head. Furthermore, LCP anatomy leads to biomechanical considerations as well, with the need to orient the femoral component in such a way to preserve leg length and avoid impingement. Coxa magna, another residual deformity seen after LCP in which the femoral head is enlarged, may result in a larger acetabulum. Thus, careful planning of the acetabular and femoral component sizes is required when contemplating hip resurfacing.

SCFE is characterized by displacement of the femoral head through the upper femoral epiphyseal growth plate. The displacement usually results in a varus and external rotation orientation between the epiphysis and the metaphysis. When the deformity is severe or there are secondary complications such as chondrolysis or osteonecrosis (ON), osteoarthritis becomes an early secondary outcome.

This deformity can occur even after minor, asymptomatic slips. Of patients who develop degenerative osteoarthritis, about 5% have known SCFE[6]; however, a larger number of patients may have had an "asymptomatic" slip, predisposing them to secondary osteoarthritis. Several investigators have reported on long-term follow-up results of SCFE as it relates to the onset of degenerative osteoarthritis.[7-9] In general, the more severe the deformity of the hip, the worse the prognosis with earlier onset of debilitating osteoarthritis. Jerre[10] found that the results worsened with longer follow-up and with severe slips. Oram[11] also described earlier and more severe degeneration with severe slips. Ross et al[12] found increasing deterioration of the hip joint with time and noted that it occurred even with mild slips. The onset of osteoarthritis may be preceded by avascular necrosis and chondrolysis leading to arthrofibrosis. Chondrolysis, the rapid, progressive loss of articular cartilage, has been noted even in the hips of patients with SCFE without prior treatment. Avascular necrosis (AVN) of the femoral head is rare in patients with untreated SCFE. Unfortunately, this complication appears to be related to treatment, especially manipulative reduction and pinning as well as from corrective osteotomies of the femoral neck. Some special cases of SCFE exist, such as in patients with metabolic disorders, endocrinopathies, and renal osteodystrophy,[13,14] and in those who have received radiation therapy.[15]

The residual deformities of SCFE include a pistol-grip deformity with a retroverted head on a wide femoral neck.[16]

Both Stulberg et al[17] and Murray[18] reported that 40% of patients without known prior hip disease undergoing total hip arthroplasty were noted to have a pistol-grip or tilting deformity characteristic of SCFE. As such, radiographic evaluation in two planes is necessary to evaluate a condition in which the posterior epiphyseal tilt is generally greater than that observed medially. The medial and posterior tilting of the femoral head results in a poorer head-neck offset anteriorly and superiorly[5]; this makes hip resurfacing more difficult, because there will be less clearance on the lateral or tension sides of the femoral neck.

Developmental Dysplasia of the Hip

DDH is generally defined as a condition of the hip characterized by abnormal sloping of the acetabulum roof and shallowness of the acetabulum. The deformity creates a secondary change, or molding, of the head to conform to the acetabulum, and is associated with increased anteversion of the femoral neck and abnormal muscle forces with a shortened lever arm. As the child grows to an adult, these abnormalities cause fatigue and pain before there is radiographic evidence of degenerative arthritis. The contact area between the femoral head and the acetabulum is diminished, with the head being uncovered, leading to high stress concentration and inevitably osteoarthritis. These high-contact stresses are undoubtedly related to the often rapid development of cystic changes latterly in the acetabulum and femoral head.

Hip dysplasia may also occur as a result of ED of the femoral head and, by definition, it also occurs with other acquired conditions, for example, congenital coxa vara, as well as aforementioned LCP disease, and SCFE, with resultant abnormal molding of the head and acetabulum.

There is a spectrum of disease severity from mild dysplasia with slight acetabulum sloping, to more severe dysplasia with a nearly uncovered femoral head, to complete dislocation. In the most severe situation, the femoral head, having been dislocated from birth, makes no contact with the true acetabulum and is completely displaced, lying proximally and posteriorly.

The femoral intramedullary canal is also dysplastic, smaller, and straighter. There is increased femoral neck anteversion, and because the femoral head does not contact a joint surface, the femoral head becomes atrophic and may be entirely cystic and devoid of structural bone.

Crowe and colleagues[19] classified dysplastic hips roentgenographically into four classes using the acetabular angle and the amount of proximal migration as the significant features. Although the center edge measurement of Wiberg[20] is useful for quantifying the degree of subluxation in children, it is not useful in adults because of the secondary arthritic changes and the fact that the lateral margin of the acetabulum is often eroded. However, the acetabulum angle, as described by Sharp,[21] is useful varying from 30 to 42 degrees in normal patients. Stulberg and Harris'[22] measurements were similar (33 degrees average; range 25 to 41 degrees). According to Crowe et al[19] the acetabulum angle in patients with dysplasia ranges from 41 to 63 degrees (average 52 degrees). They also found that the bony landmarks—height of pelvis, head and neck junction in the dysplastic hip, and inferior margin of the teardrop—were always identifiable, and that the head height is approximately 20% of the height of the pelvis from the ischium to the ilium. We recommend their method of quantifying proximal migration, which measures the distance from the bottom of the teardrop to the femoral head-neck-junction. In the normal hip, the head-neck junction is at or about the level of the bottom of the teardrop. If the percentage of the displaced head height due to proximal migration is less than 50%, it is class I, if it is 50% to 75%, it is class II. A displacement of 75% to 100% of the normal head height is Crowe class III, Crowe class IV would be more than 100%. Femoral dysplasia, especially in the mediolateral (coronal) plane with a small, straight diaphysis, is present to a varying degree, often even with the more minor degrees of dysplasia.

The dysplastic hip is challenging for hip resurfacing mainly because of the abnormal acetabular anatomy. The native acetabulum is more shallow, often with a deficient anterior wall. In hip resurfacing with the Conserve®Plus socket, adjuvant fixation is generally not used on the acetabulum, thus assessment of the acetabular reamed cavity and careful placement of the socket are paramount. Medialization of the socket is often necessary to improve lateral coverage. Furthermore, because both the femoral neck and acetabulum may be excessively anteverted, hip stability may be compromised unless adjustments are made. A socket with the ability to add up to three screws is available, but we have not had a problem obtaining initial stability and lasting fixation.

Epiphyseal Dysplasia

The nature and characteristics of ED have been described in detail by Hesse and Kohler,[23] who present EDs as a category of osteochondral dysplasias in a heterogenous group of skeletal dysplasias. These conditions are hereditary and are generally revealed by a short stature due to a dysplasia at more than one region of the body. There are several forms of EDs: the Fairbank, Ribbing, and Meyer forms, ranked in decreasing order of severity. The disease is related to an abnormality of cartilage growth secondary to a disruption of the bony structure of the epiphysis. The femoral head deformity is similar to that of LCP disease but often with bilateral hip involvement (Fig. 14-1). There are fewer cystic and sclerotic changes, and absence of subluxation. The bilateral symmetry of the hips and involvement of other joints to a varying degree helps to establish the diagnosis. Also the use of magnetic resonance imaging

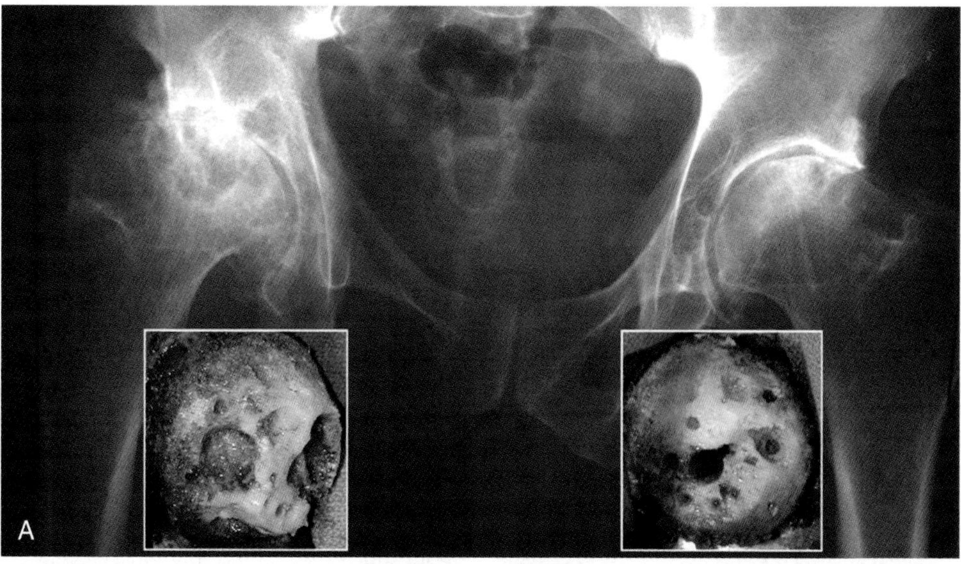

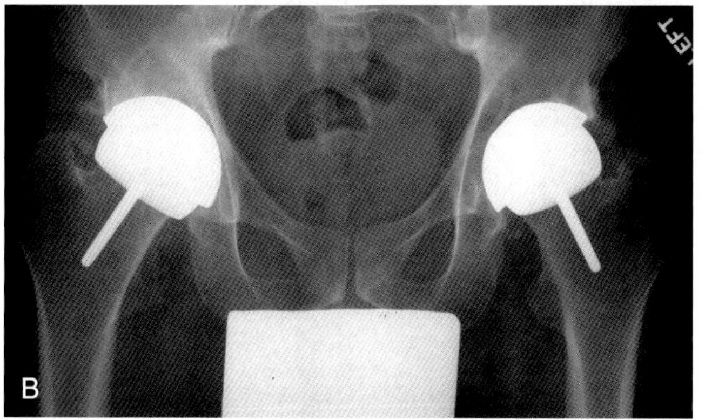

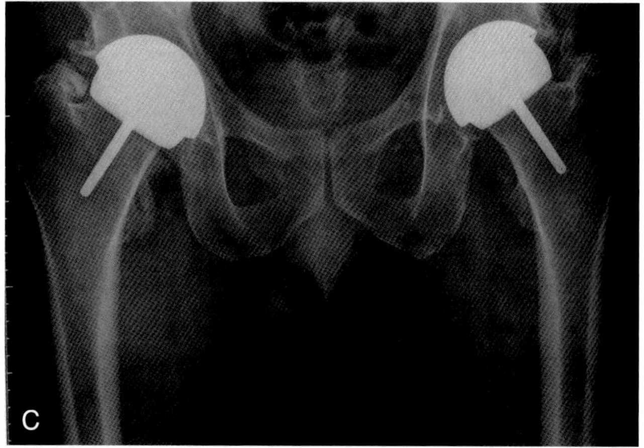

Figure 14-1 **A,** Anteroposterior radiograph of a 39-year-old male business owner with bilateral osteoarthritis of the hips secondary to epiphyseal dysplasia. Inserts show the femoral heads after preparation for total hip resurfacing and confirm the extensive cystic degeneration noticeable on the radiograph. **B,** Radiograph at 5 months after surgery after undergoing single stage bilateral metal-on-metal total hip resurfacing; the right was done before the left. **C,** Patient at 74 months after surgery. Brooker grade III heterotopic ossification has developed, but the patient is not restricted with University of California-Los Angeles hip scores of 10, 10, 9, and 7 for both hips for pain, walking, function, and activity, respectively.

(MRI) can be useful to clearly distinguish the two diagnoses.[24]

Khermosh and Wientroub[25] published in 1991 a prospective longitudinal clinical and radiologic study of 18 children diagnosed with dysplasia epiphysealis capitis femoris. They found that half the cases were bilateral and that boys were affected five times more often than girls. Their imaging studies suggest that the cartilaginous proximal femoral epiphysis is hypoplastic, with delayed appearance of single or multiple ossification centers. Progressive improvement occurred and at an average age of 5 years and 6 months, with complete fusion of all the ossific nuclei and normal density and texture of the epiphyseal bone. The end result was a round epiphysis with a slightly diminished height. The dysplasia is attributed to focal hypoplasia of the proximal femoral epiphysis.

ED will pose similar difficulties in hip resurfacing as with LCP, because the femoral neck is wide and short.

Joint-Preserving Surgeries of the Hip

In youthful patients with symptoms but with no or minimal degenerative changes, it is important to consider surgical alternatives such as pelvic osteotomy. Although it is technically more difficult to perform, the Ganz periacetabular osteotomy (PAO)[26] or other triple inominate osteotomy has the best opportunity to correct the deformity in three directions to provide greater anatomic coverage of the femoral head. A decision to undergo osteotomy is based on the age of the patient and absence of arthritic changes in order to have a more predictable outcome of significantly delaying osteoarthritis. Those age-related results must be equated with the marked improvement in results and durability after hip resurfacing and total hip replacement. In the past, varus or valgus femoral osteotomies played a role in management of some hips but are rarely indicated today. Femoral derotation osteotomy may be indicated with severe degrees of anteversion. For SCFE patients, the Dunn open replacement with cervical osteotomy,[27] the Kramer basilar neck osteotomy,[28] the Sugioka transtrochanteric rotational osteotomy,[29] and the Southwick[30] biplane osteotomy have been performed in the hope of slowing the development of early degenerative osteoarthritic changes. However, because of varying degrees of morbidity and unpredictable results, they are less frequently performed today.

Indications for MM hip resurfacing with DDH include patients with Crowe class I and II and, occasionally, Class III depending on the severity of leg-length discrepancy and other anatomic deformities. Because of the success of Conserve®Plus cementless sockets to date, we have not added bone graft to cover the lateral aspect of the socket, even though all of the acetabular socket is not always covered by bone. Bone grafting is not recommended although grafting the lateral acetabulum was traditionally included in cemented reconstructions and was beneficial. However, grafting was proven not to be beneficial in our previous experience with our earlier porous surface replacement (PSR) cementless resurfacings because of graft absorption. This, we believe, was due to good initial stability of the socket and rapid ingrowth of the host bone preceding the bony union and revascularization of the graft. The load needed for the graft incorporation and load transfer did not occur, and the graft absorbed.

Operative Technique

Preoperative Evaluation and Planning

Preoperative planning is essential to avoid intraoperative and postoperative complications and to promote long-term durability after replacement. Routine roentgenograms can be augmented by False Profile or Judet oblique views, but a more accurate way to evaluate the congenital dysplastic hip could be the use of a computed tomography (CT) scan. However, with the Conserve®Plus prosthesis 2-mm increments, this is rarely necessary. When considering the trade-offs of conventional total hip replacement (THR) versus hip resurfacing, it is important to evaluate the degree of anteversion by the cross-table lateral or, if necessary, with CT or special anteversion studies. More than 55 degrees may require a derotation osteotomy if resurfacing is to be performed, thereby increasing the magnitude of the procedure.

Operative planning also includes assessing the length of the femur by pelvic leveling, with various size blocks being placed under the short leg. It is not possible to lengthen more than 2 cm and this length must be obtained by bringing the socket as close as possible to the anatomic acetabulum. The femoral head can occasionally be prepared by not removing any dome bone to compensate for a shortened head or neck and cancellizing the dense bone for fixation with multiple small drill holes as described in Chapter 7.

For most Crowe III or IV, THR is preferable with an osteotomy to shorten or derotate the femur. We believe one should not plan to lengthen more than 10% of the femoral length. In general, the older the patient, the less ambitious the limb-length restoration is desirable because recovery from nerve palsy, should it occur, is less predictable. We do not recommend preliminary traction, as the contractures are generally severe and unrelenting, and attempted distraction has not been successful. Furthermore, it is not advisable to perform releasing procedures until the socket has been implanted and a trial reduction attempted, because it cannot be predicted how much or which muscles to release. With the dislocated hip, there is severe weakness of the hip after surgery, so it is important not to release any muscles that can be spared for a more rapid recovery.

Although the exact relationship of leg lengthening with the development of nerve palsies is not clear, our goal is to equalize the length of the lower extremities without placing undue tension on the nerve.

Disease-Specific Surgical Tips

Slipped Capital Femoral Epiphysis

It is important to have adequate exposure to be able to assess the head and neck and acetabular anatomy. Because of the wide neck and poor offset between the lateral head and neck, ream as close as possible to the inferior neck and identify the inferior subcapital recess under neck osteophytes. If the head is extremely large or eccentric, reduce the size of the femoral head medially gradually with an oscillating saw or osteotome. These measures will help avoid damage to the lateral femoral neck. However, if a neck notch is necessary to fit the acetabular component without sacrificing a large amount of anterior or posterior acetabular wall thickness and strength, consider notching medially where the cortex is generally thicker. A notch has not been necessary in our series because the thin acetabular sockets became available. In severe cases with posterior tilt and anterior erosion of the head, creating anterior offset is more difficult because it is important to preserve a circumferential cylindrical reamed area to optimize initial stability of the femoral component. In some cases, the resultant offset may be only as thick as the anterior wall of the component. Should impingement and lack of internal rotation be demonstrated on range-of-motion testing at surgery, then resect impinging bone from the acetabulum. This is one situation in which doing a trial reduction with the trial component on the head is helpful, for assessment and treatment.

Removal of retained internal fixation pins is sometimes problematic and was not possible in three hips, but by preoperative templating, it was believed that resurfacing could be performed. With a careful pin centering for reaming, the implantation was possible and hardware removal was not

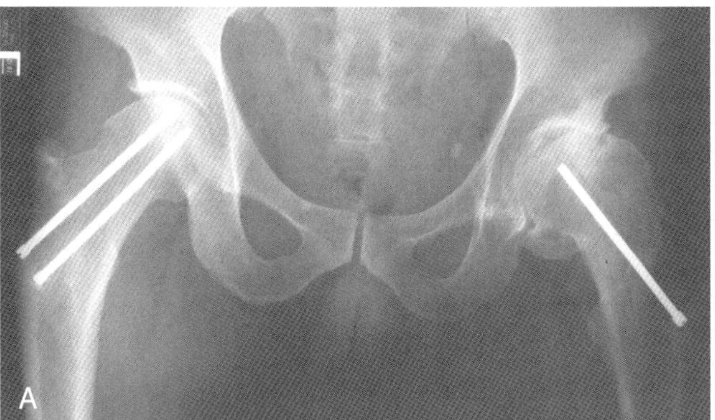

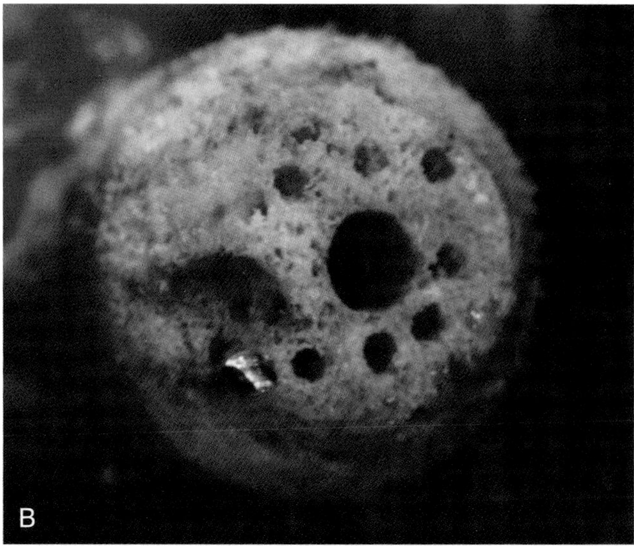

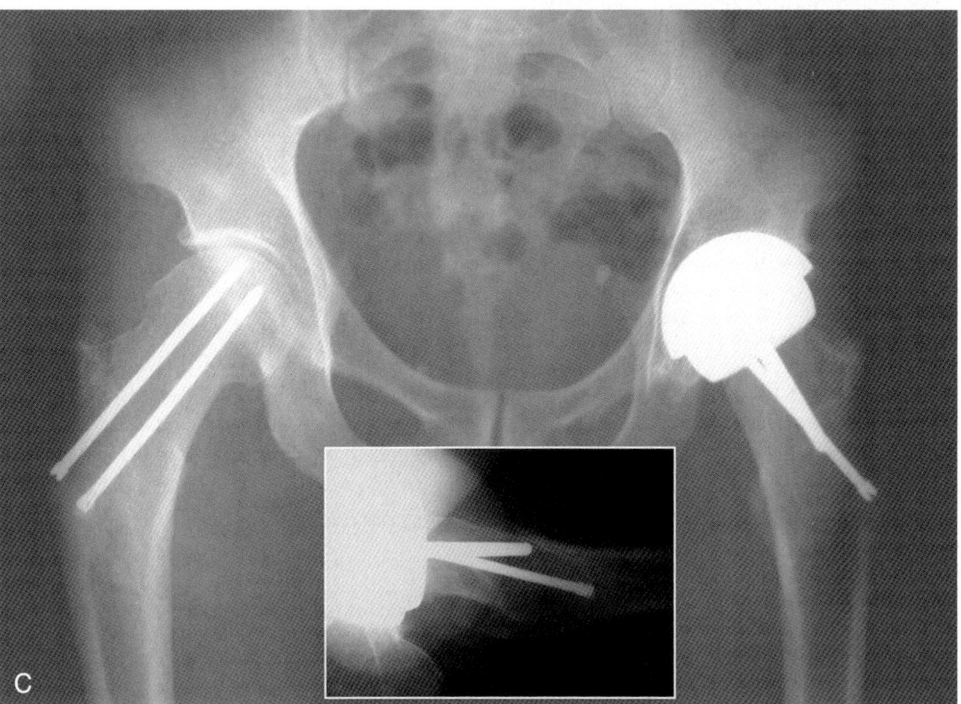

Figure 14-2 **A,** Anteroposterior view of the pelvis of a 37-year-old teacher with bilateral slipped capital femoral epiphysis (SCFE) and secondary osteoarthritis. Note the large inferior osteophyte, and the large, extruded, incongruent osteopenic head. There is minimal joint space narrowing of the right hip. **B,** Intraoperative photograph of the femoral head (6th hip operated for SCFE in the series, #325 overall). The pin, which could not be removed, was burred below the surface of the dome. There is a 2-cm adjacent cyst and some areas of osteopenia, especially inferiorly (*top left*). **C,** Seven years post-resurfacing with a 48-mm head and 58-mm socket. The insert shows the Johnson lateral view. Note the posterior-to-anterior orientation of the metaphyseal stem with respect to the residual pin and the anterior offset restoration

necessary. A 37-year-old teacher with bilateral SCFE and a 10-year history of left hip osteoarthritis and severe restriction of motion (flexion, 90 degrees; abduction, 10 degrees, and no rotation) presented in our office. Preoperative pain was 1 (left hip) and 10 (right hip), relieved by narcotics, walking (6), function (5), and activity (4). An attempt to remove the remaining pin during surgery was unsuccessful. Now 7 years after resurfacing with the hardware left in situ, his University of California-Los Angeles (UCLA) scores are 10, 10, 10, and 8 for pain, walking, function, and activity, respectively. His flexion is 105 degrees with no contracture, abduction-adduction arc 65 degrees, and rotation arc 75 degrees, and comparable to the more normal right hip (Fig. 14-2).

Legg-Calve-Perthes or Epiphyseal Dysplasia

In LCP, or ED, in which the head-neck segment is short or is associated with limb-length inequality or poor abductor lever arm, minimally resect the dome bone of the femoral head in order to preserve and restore as much length to the head and neck. Even if there are large osteophytes around the base of the neck, it may be impossible to attach the pin-centering guide. Alternatively the lollipop or a large cylindrical reamer can be used to estimate the location of the neck central axis. Then, place the pin close to the central axis and use the cylindrical reamer feeler gauges on the pin to accurately assess its location and provide guidance to make a change. If it is not optimally positioned, then relocate the pin with the relocator guide, as described in Chapter 7. It is always wise to ream by incrementally downsizing slowly so that you do not downsize too much and damage the neck.

Unless there is significant impingement after trial reduction, do not remove osteophytes anteriorly or laterally, especially when the osteophyte contains structural bone and in absence of the normal cortex. Furthermore, if there is osteopenia of the lateral neck, it is important to ream the head into a valgus position to minimize the tensile stresses across the neck. If it is possible, use a cylindrical reamer size large enough to clear the osteophyte, because this may be preferable to removing it, assuming there is enough acetabular bone stock and you do not thin the acetabular walls unnecessarily while reaming for the socket.

If the socket does not have enough stability after impaction, remove it and ream deeper with a 1-mm smaller reamer. In general, a 1-mm interference fit is optimal, especially in young patients.

In the LCP and SCFE groups with a short neck, evaluate the external rotation of the hip in extension. Limitation of motion may be due to impingement of the greater trochanter against the ischium. In our series, the posterior ridges of three greater trochanters were removed flush with the neck with an osteotome to increase the external rotation. An 18-year-old male student with osteoarthritis of the left hip secondary to LCP disease was treated with metal-on-metal resurfacing (Fig. 14-3). The head was flat, and the femoral neck very wide with a low head-neck ratio. The patient had a severely restricted motion. Now 7 years after surgery, the patient's UCLA scores are 10, 10, 10, and 8 for pain, walking, function, and activity, respectively. His flexion arc improved from 100 degrees preoperatively to 125 degrees, abduction-adduction arc from 30 to 75 degrees, and rotation arc from 25 to 70 degrees. Leg length was preserved. The patient is now a graduate student doing well despite a Surface Arthroplasty Risk Index (SARI) score of 5.

Developmental Dysplasia of the Hip Crowe Class II

In Crowe class II DDH, the femoral head is subluxed superiorly. The acetabular component should be generally reconstructed at or near the anatomic acetabulum. Direct the reamer inferiorly in order to save all of the remaining superior (lateral) acetabular wall, which is often eroded. It is possible to leave approximately 5 to 10 mm (depending on size) of the socket uncovered laterally and still obtain rigid initial fixation. However, it is vitally important to protect the anterior wall of the acetabulum in order to obtain fixation. There should be at least 60% coverage in the frontal plane. In order to deepen the acetabulum, it may be necessary on occasion to ream to the medial wall. One 40-year-old woman with Crowe class III DDH and secondary osteoarthritis had a leg-length discrepancy of 1 cm before resurfacing (Fig. 14-4). The socket could not be reconstructed at the anatomic acetabular location due to superior erosion. However, good initial stability was achieved in the more proximal location despite the fact that the socket was uncovered by bone laterally. She is active with nonimpact activities, mostly skiing. UCLA hip scores are 10,

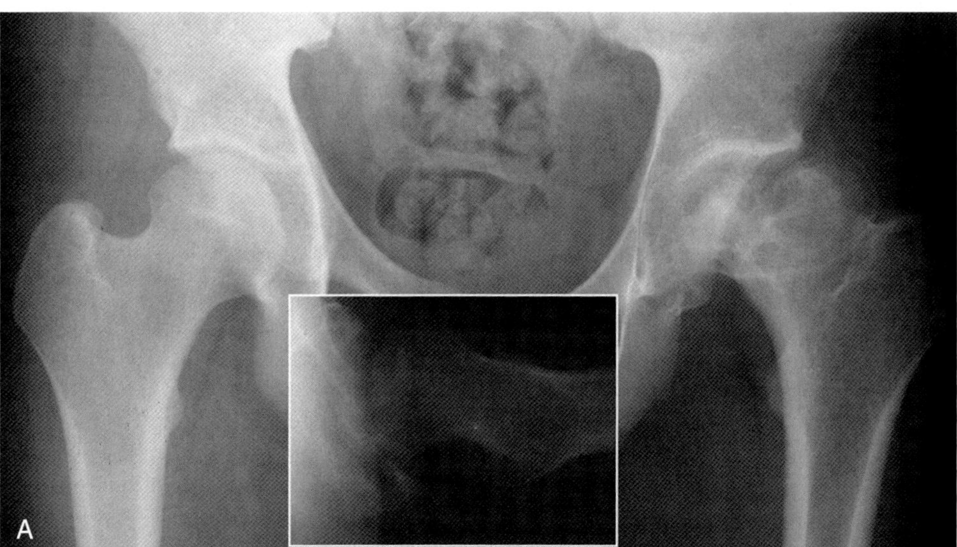

Figure 14-3 **A,** Anteroposterior view of the pelvis of an 18-year-old male student with osteoarthritis of the left hip secondary to Legg-Calvé-Perthes disease. The head is flattened, and the femoral neck is very wide. The insert shows the Johnson lateral view and confirms the deformity of the head and the presence of large femoral cysts.

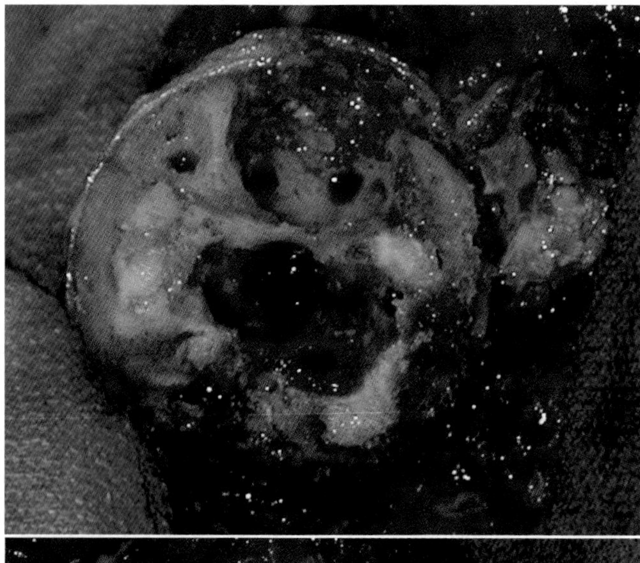

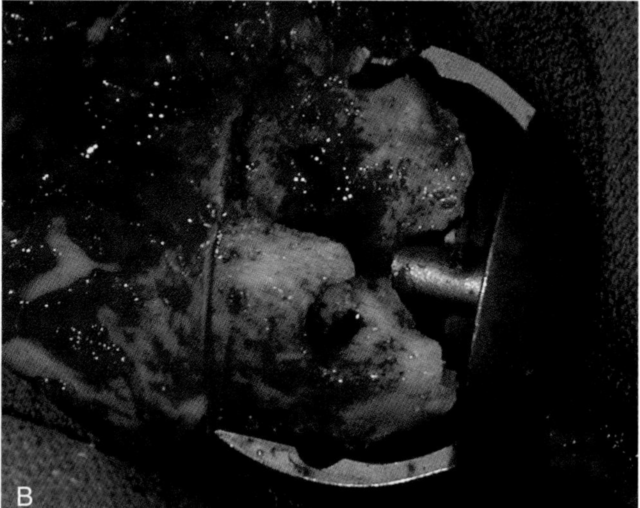

Figure 14-3, cont'd B, Intraoperative photographs showing the femoral head after preparation. As evidenced by the template before cementation, there was considerable bone loss. The large femoral cysts (>3 cm with erosion into the cylindrical area, which is ordinarily a contraindication, except that the patient was so young) were curetted out, and the femoral neck notched inferiorly to accommodate a 46-mm component compatible with the size of the acetabular component of 56 mm (5-mm thick socket shell). **C,** Postoperative anteroposterior radiograph showing the slight inferior notch of the femoral neck and the posterior-to-anterior positioning of the femoral component observed on the lateral view.

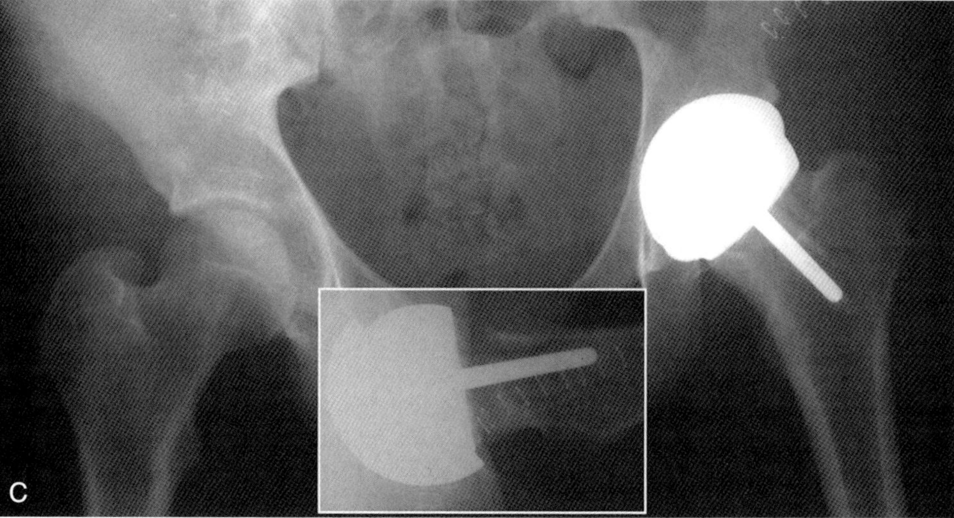

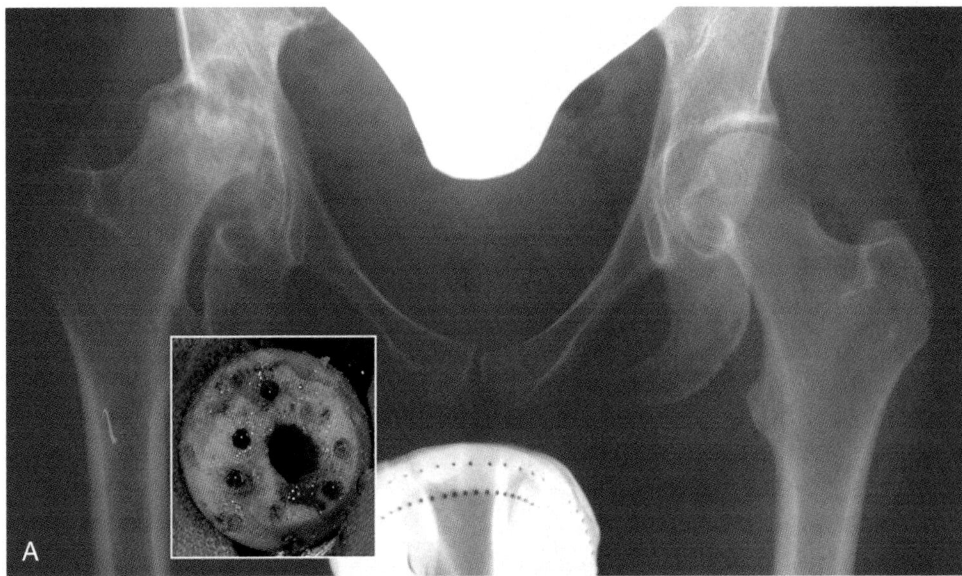

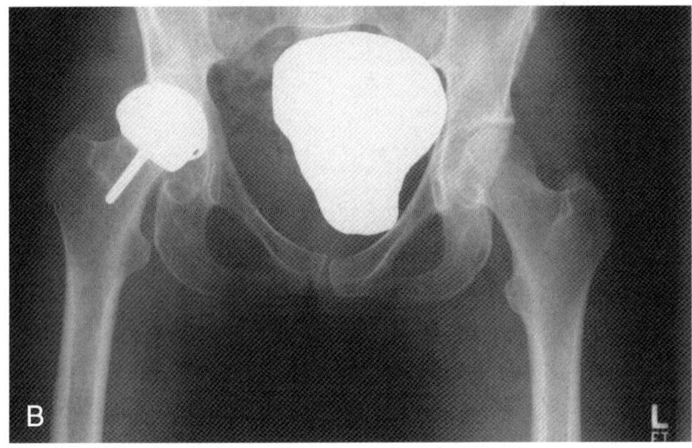

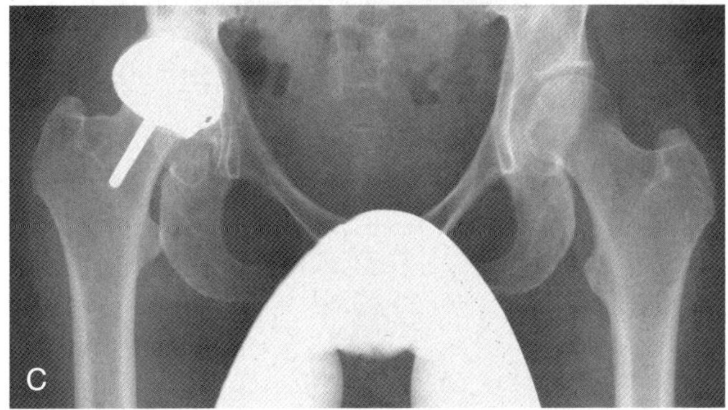

Figure 14-4 **A,** Anteroposterior view of the pelvis of a 40-year-old woman with osteoarthritis of the right hip secondary to developmental dysplasia of the hip, Crowe class III. Insert shows the femoral head after preparation for a metal-on-metal total hip resurfacing. **B,** Immediate postoperative radiograph following total hip resurfacing. The lateral aspect of the socket was left partially uncovered. The initial leg-length discrepancy could not be compensated during surgery and remained 1 cm. **C,** Radiograph at 64.6 months after surgery. A slight remodeling of the lateral aspect of the femoral neck is visible, possibly related to some neck impingement with the patient's above-normal flexibility (Flexion arc, 170 degrees; abduction-adduction arc, 95 degrees; Rot arc, 105 degrees).

10, 10, and 9 for pain, walking, function, and activity, respectively.

Patient Demographics

From our initial series of 1000 hips (838 patients), 145 hips (127 patients) received a Conserve®Plus resurfacing for arthritis secondary to the four above-mentioned childhood disorders. The average age of the patients was 44.9 (range, 15 to 68 years). Most of the patients were women (74/127, 58.3%). One hundred and three hips had an etiology of DDH, four ED, 21 LCP disease, and 17 SCFE. Twenty-two hips (15.2%) had undergone previous surgery before resurfacing, including 12 osteotomies, nine pinnings, and one free vascularized fibular graft. There were 18 with bilateral resurfacings (10 one-stage, and 8 two-stage), with an average of 23 months between surgeries (range 3.9-95.3 months).

There have been nine healthy babies born to five mothers resurfaced after osteoarthritis secondary to DDH, and the average age at time of surgery for these women was 34.0 years (range 23.0-39.1 years). In this group of patients, there are 18 other women of childbearing age (40 years old and younger at the time of surgery). One woman who was resurfaced at age 23 years has given birth to three healthy children who are now 1, 3.5, and 5.5 years old. She underwent a successful Ganz osteotomy when her right hip became painful before the last pregnancy. Her UCLA scores for pain, walking, function, and activity are now 10 (right hip and left hip), 8, 6, and 5, respectively (Fig. 14-5).

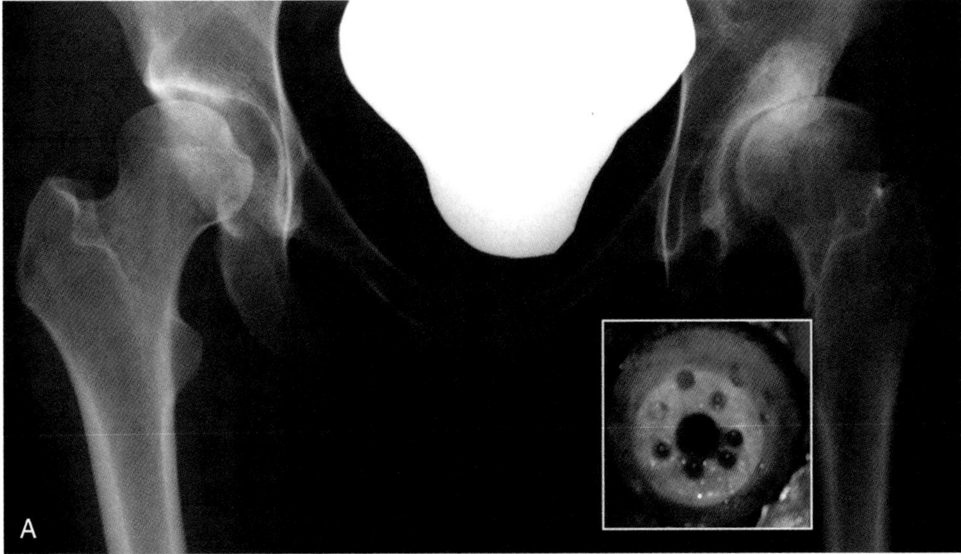

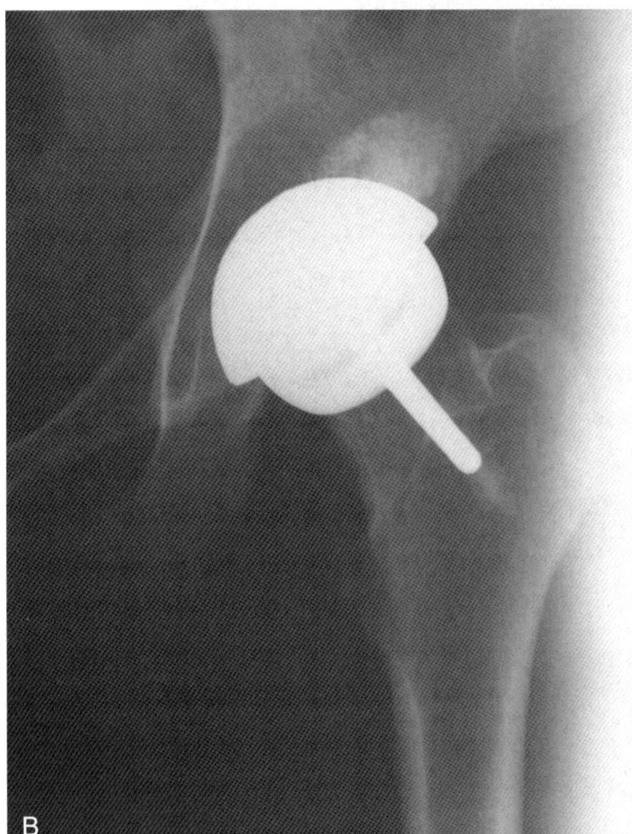

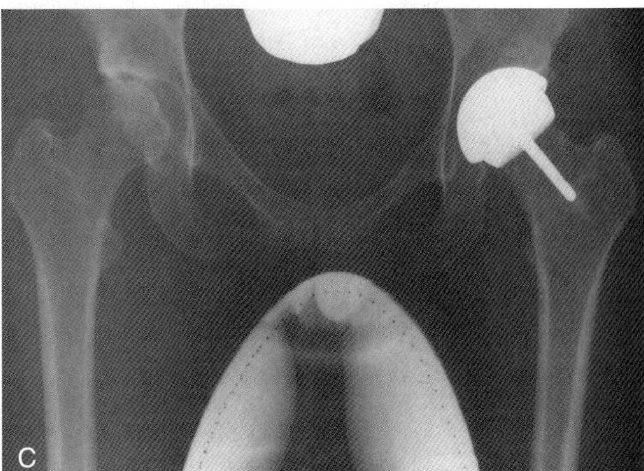

Figure 14-5 **A,** Anteroposterior radiograph of a 23-year-old homemaker with osteoarthritis secondary to developmental dysplasia of the left hip. The femoral head is subluxed laterally, which further reduces the area of contact with the acetabulum. Insert shows very good bone quality of the femoral head after preparation for total metal-on-metal resurfacing. **B,** Immediate postoperative radiograph following surgery. **C,** Anteroposterior radiograph taken 52 months after resurfacing.

The demographics of this group of patients are shown in Tables 14-1 to 14-4.

Among the four hips that were resurfaced with a 5-mm shell, one was in a male patient with DDH, one a female patient with DDH who had undergone a prior pelvic osteotomy, and two were patients with SCFE.

The incidence and size of cystic defects was higher than the overall cohort and, except for ON, higher than other etiologies (highest being ED > LCP > SCFE >DDH).

Results

Clinical Scores

The average UCLA hip scores all improved significantly ($P < .0001$) between preoperative and last follow-up visits. The pain score increased from 3.3 ± 1.1 to 9.2 ± 1.3, the walking score from 6.3 ± 1.4 to 9.5 ± 1.0, the function score from 5.8 ± 1.6

Table 14-1 Demographics of the Patients Operated for Osteoarthritis Secondary to Childhood Disorders

	Men (n = 53)	Women (n = 74)	Combined (n = 127)
Age (years)	44.3 (15-68)	45.3 (15-63)	44.9 (15-68)
Weight (kg)	88.1 (61-136)	65.3 (42-103)	75.2 (42-136)
Height (cm)	177.1 (157-193)	165.0 (140-178)	170.2 (140-193)
BMI	28.1 (18.4-43.4)	24.0 (17.6-34.3)	25.8 (17.6-43.4)
Femoral component size (mm)	49.1 (36-58)	42.7 (36-48)	45.5 (36-58)
Cysts >1 cm	34 (54.0%)	33 (40.2%)	67 (46.2%)
Charnley class			
A	32 (50.8%)	52 (70.3%)	84 (66.1%)
B	29 (46.0%)	21 (28.4%)	40 (31.5%)
C	2 (3.2%)	1 (1.3%)	3 (2.4%)

BMI, body mass index.

Table 14-2 Proportion of Male and Female Patients in Each Etiologic Category

	DDH	LCP	SCFE	Epiphyseal Dysplasia
Men	23.3% (21/90)	94.4% (17/18)	75% (12/16)	100% (3/3)
Women	76.7% (69/90)	5.6% (1/18)	25% (4/16)	0% (0/3)

DDH, developmental dyplasia of the hip; LCP, Legg-Calve-Perthes disease; SCFE, slipped capital femoral epiphysis.

Table 14-3 Proportion of Original (5-mm) and Thin (3.5-mm) Shells Used with Patients Operated for Osteoarthritis Secondary to Childhood Disorders Since 11-03, Introduction of the Conserve®Plus Thin Shell for Resurfacing*

Original (5-mm) Shells	8.3% (4/48)
Thin (3.5-mm) Shells	91.7% (44/48)

**Prior to 11-03, all had 5-mm shells.*

to 9.4 ± 1.2, and the activity score from 4.7 ± 1.4 to 7.2 ± 1.7. The tight standard deviations reflect the overall uniform good quality of results. The average physical component was 32.5 ± 7.7 preoperatively and 51.9 ± 8.5 at the last follow-up (P = .0001), and the mental component increased from 46.6 ± 13.0 to 52.1 ± 10.7 (P = .0002). The postoperative Harris hip score (HHS) was 92.6 ± 10.0.

Range of Motion

The range of motion of each etiologic group is summarized in Tables 14-5 to 14-7.

In comparing the hip range of motion of SCFE patients to other etiologic groups, preoperative flexion was found to be significantly less (93.5 versus 105.8 degrees, $p < 0.003$), with a similar preoperative flexion contracture (17.4 versus 16.1 degrees, P = .707). The postoperative flexion was also less in our study population (116.7 versus 126.1 degrees, P = 0.004), but the net gain in flexion arc was comparable (38.7 versus 34.7 degrees, P = 0.525).

Table 14-4 Proportion of Hips by Etiology with Femoral Head Defects Greater Than 1 cm

	Number of Hips with >1-cm Defects	Percentage
DDH	43	41.7
ED	3	75.0
LCP	12	57.1
SCFE	9	52.9

DDH, developmental dysplasia of the hip; ED, epiphyseal dysplasia; LCP, Legg-Calvé-Perthes disease; SCFE, slipped capital femoral epiphysis.

	DDH		ED		LCP		SCFE	
	n	%	n	%	n	%	n	%
Good bone (no defect)	31	30.1%	0	0.0%	3	14.3%	3	17.6%
Defect 0 to 1 cm	29	28.2%	1	25.0%	6	28.6%	5	29.4%
Defect 1 to 2 cm	32	31.1%	3	75.0%	10	47.6%	6	35.3%
Defect >2 cm	11	10.7%	0	0.0%	2	9.5%	3	17.6%

Leg Length Restoration

Please see Tables 14-8 and 14-9 for a preoperative and postoperative summary of leg-length discrepancies.

Limb-length discrepancies were present before surgery for 59 hips. The discrepancy was less than 1 cm in 34 cases, 1 to 2 cm in 20 cases, and 2 to 3 cm in five cases. Of these 59 hips, the limb lengths were postoperatively equalized in 43 cases, nine were maintained with the same amount of discrepancy, and seven decreased their discrepancy by at least 1 cm.

Table 14-5 DDH Patients

	PRE FLX	Flexion Contracture	Abd	Add	Rot Arc	LFU FLX	Flexion Contracture	Abd	Add	Rot Arc
Whole 1000	105.6	16.1	23.2	14.5	23.5	125.9	1.9	45.2	27.9	76.6
DDH	109.4	15.6	27.3	17.5	32.5	130.3	2.0	47.9	29.9	83.9
Others	105.2	16.2	22.7	14.2	22.3	125.4	1.8	44.8	27.7	75.7
P	0.015	0.687	0.001	0.001	0.000	0.000	0.850	0.002	0.003	0.000

Abd, abduction; Add, adduction; DDH, developmental dyplasia of the hip; PRE FLX, preoperative flexion; LFU FLX, last follow-up flexion.

Table 14-6 SCFE Patients

	PRE FLX	Flexion Contracture	Abd	Add	Rot Arc	LFU FLX	Flexion Contracture	Abd	Add	Rot Arc
Whole 1000	105.6	16.1	23.2	14.5	23.5	125.9	1.9	45.2	27.9	76.6
SCFE	93.5	17.4	23.8	9.7	17.1	116.7	4.3	43.3	25.7	72.7
Others	105.8	16.1	23.2	14.6	23.6	126.1	1.8	45.2	28.0	76.6
P	0.003	0.707	0.851	0.046	0.173	0.004	0.066	0.401	0.187	0.388

Abd, abduction; Add, adduction; PRE FLX, preoperative flexion; LFU FLX, last follow-up flexion; SCFE, slipped capital femoral epiphysis.

Table 14-7 LCP Patients

	PRE FLX	Flexion Contracture	Abd	Add	Rot Arc	LFU FLX	Flexion Contracture	Abd	Add	Rot Arc
Whole 1000	105.6	16.1	23.2	14.5	23.5	125.9	1.9	45.2	27.9	76.6
LCP	106.2	18.6	23.1	16.2	23.1	117.3	1.3	41.0	25.7	67.3
Others	105.6	16.1	23.2	14.5	23.5	126.1	1.9	45.2	28.0	76.7
P	0.880	0.406	0.978	0.447	0.929	0.008	0.700	0.056	0.187	0.040

Abd, abduction; Add, adduction; LCP, Legg-Calve-Perthes disease; PRE FLX, preoperative flexion; LFU FLX, last follow-up flexion.

Table 14-8 Preoperative Summary of Leg-length Discrepancies

Preoperative	Equal	0-1 cm	1.1-2 cm	2.1-3 cm
DDH (n = 103)	65	23	12	3
ED (n = 4)	1	3	0	0
LCP (n = 21)	10	5	5	1
SCFE (n = 17)	10	3	3	1

DDH, developmental dysplasia of the hip; ED, epiphyseal dysplasia; LCP, Legg-Calvé-Perthes disease; SCFE, slipped capital femoral epiphysis.

Table 14-9 Postoperative Summary of Leg Length Discrepancies

Postopertive	Equal	0-1 cm	1.1-2 cm	2.1-3 cm
DDH (n = 103)	93	9	0	1*
ED (n = 4)	4	0	0	0
LCP (n = 21)	19	2	0	0
SCFE (n = 17)	13	3	0	1

DDH, developmental dysplasia of the hip; ED, epiphyseal dysplasia; LCP, Legg-Calvé-Perthes disease; SCFE, slipped capital femoral epiphysis.

**Crowe class 4 developmental dysplasia of the hip on the contralateral side.*

None of the patients showed any obvious gait disturbances at last follow-up.

Case Histories

- Case #1 presents a 52-year-old teacher with osteoarthritis secondary to LCP who underwent hip resurfacing of the left hip despite extreme proximal femoral deformity (Fig. 14-6). Six years postoperatively, the UCLA scores are 10, 10, 10, and 8 for pain, walking, function, and activity, respectively. Despite the short femoral neck, the patient's range of motion is relatively normal and entirely functional with a flexion arc of 130 degrees and no flexion contracture (compared with 105 degrees minus 5 degrees preoperatively), abduction-adduction arc of 85 degrees and rotation arc of 70 degrees.
- Case #2 presents a 38-year-old computer programmer with SCFE who underwent hip resurfacing of the left hip despite severe proximal femoral deformity who had been informed that his hip could not be corrected with a resurfacing (Fig. 14-7). Based on our prior experience with 12 patients (12 hips) who were universally satisfied with their outcome, we proceeded with resurfacing. The deformity was among the worst and the result surprising with nearly equal leg lengths. The hip had to be reconstructed in varus in order to have a

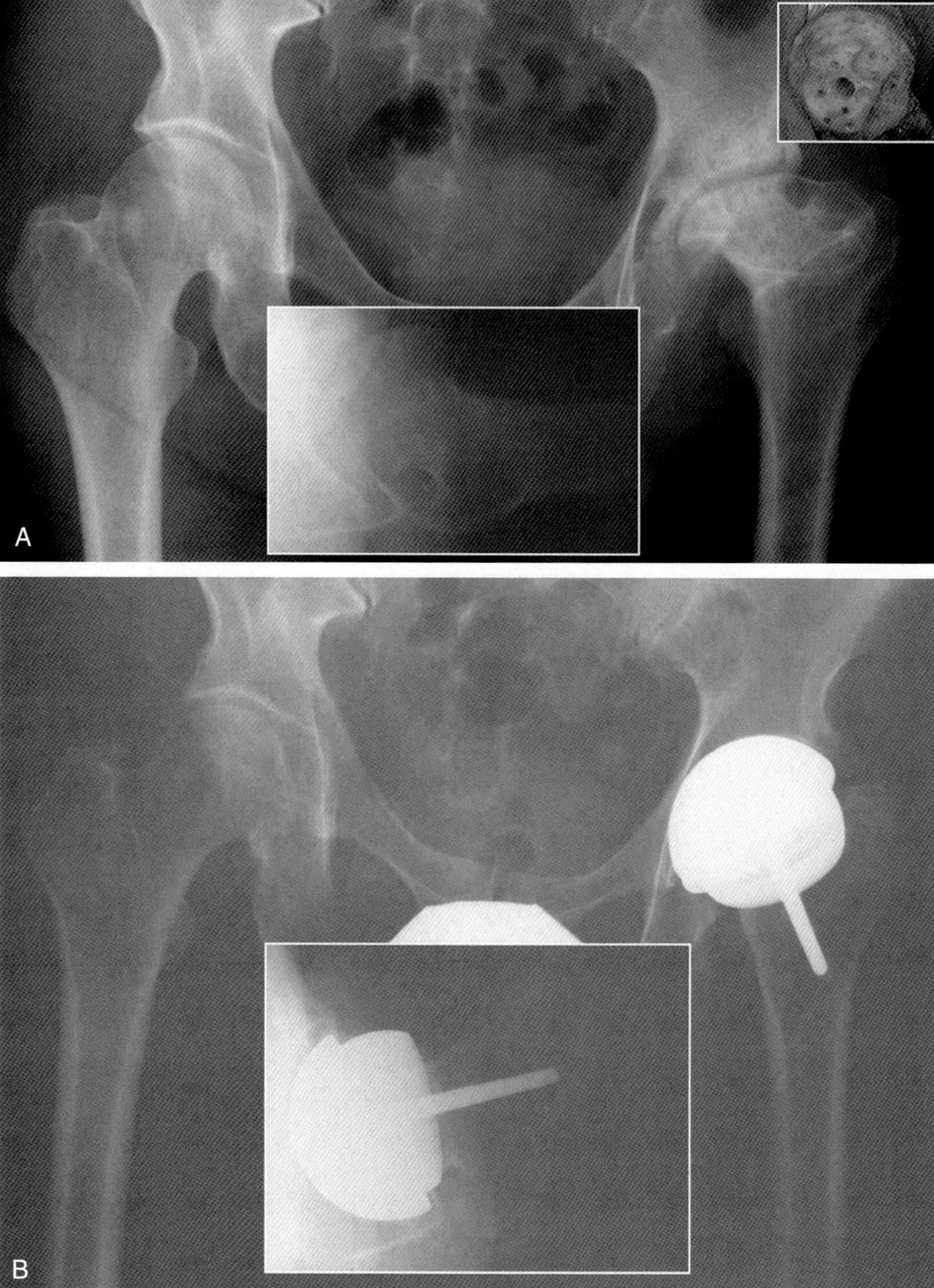

Figure 14-6 **A,** Anteroposterior radiograph of a 52-year-old man with osteoarthritis secondary to Legg-Calvé-Perthes disease. The femoral head is extremely flattened and anteverted (insert of Johnson lateral view). There is a large femoral head cyst in the superior portion of the head that is shown on the intraoperative photograph taken at the end of the femoral head preparation (*insert*). **B,** Six years after surgery, the component was positioned low on the femoral neck and in an anterior-to-posterior orientation (Johnson lateral insert) as dictated by the unusual configuration of the proximal femur. There is a good balance of anterior and posterior offset.

wider cylindrical area for fixation. The patient's UCLA scores are 10 for pain, walking, function, and 8 for activity, although the patient admits participating occasionally in basketball games. His range of motion is remarkable despite the short femoral neck and similar to the opposite hip with a flexion arc of 150 degrees (no flexion contracture), a rotation arc of 80 degrees, and an abduction-adduction arc of 70 degrees (which is within 10 degrees of the right hip). Video footage of this case is included in the DVD provided with this volume.

- Case #3 presents a 37-year-old carpenter with multiple ED who underwent hip resurfacing with two successive generations of implants (Fig. 14-8). The left hip was resurfaced in 1992 with a hybrid Porous Surface Replacement (PSR) (DePuy, Warsaw, IN) using an alumina femoral component through our transtrochanteric approach. Six years postoperatively, he became symptomatic on the contralateral (right) hip with secondary osteoarthritis and was resurfaced using the posterior

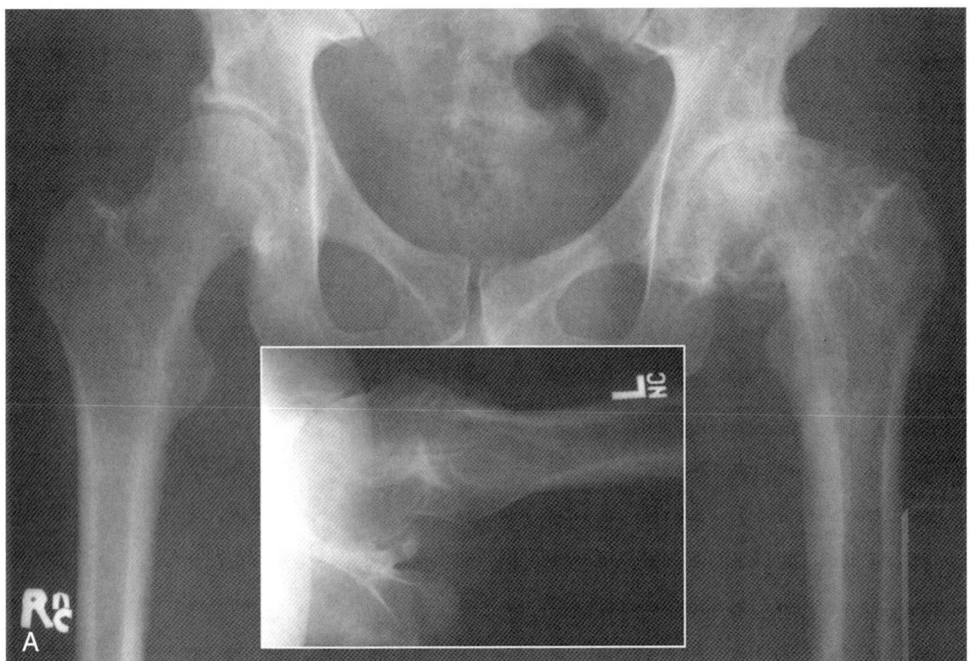

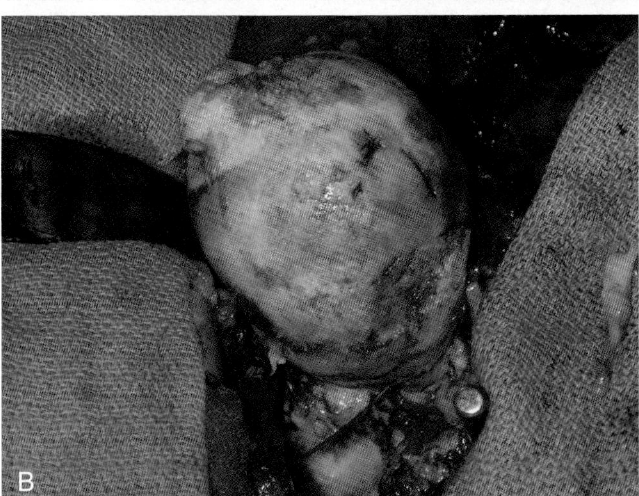

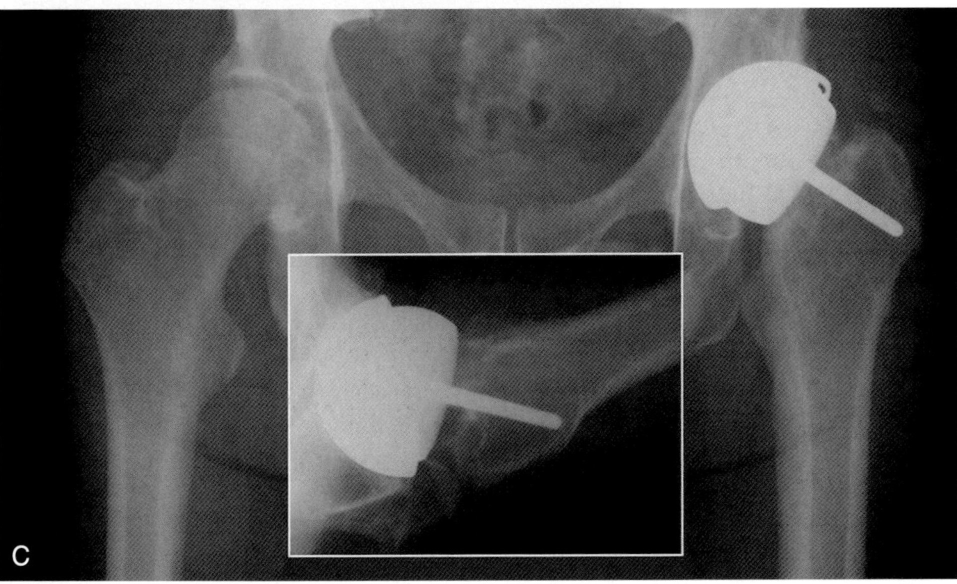

Figure 14-7 **A,** Anteroposterior radiograph of a 38-year-old man with osteoarthritis secondary to slipped capital femoral epiphysis and previous pinning of the femoral head. **B,** Intraoperative photograph of the femoral head before reaming, showing the severe flattening and erosion superiorly. The combined head-neck was short. **C,** Three and a half years after surgery, the positioning of the femoral component in varus and in an anterior to posterior orientation was dictated by the head-neck anatomy. Video footage of the patient's 2-year follow-up visit is available on the DVD provided with this volume.

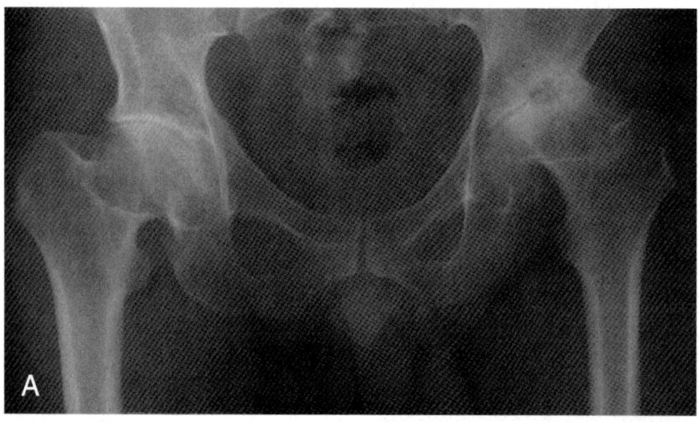

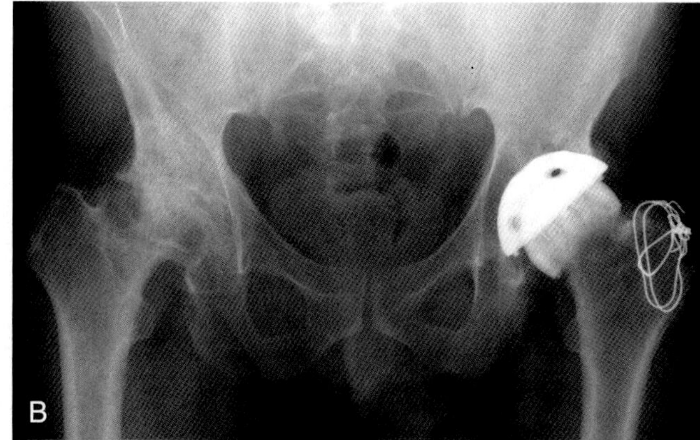

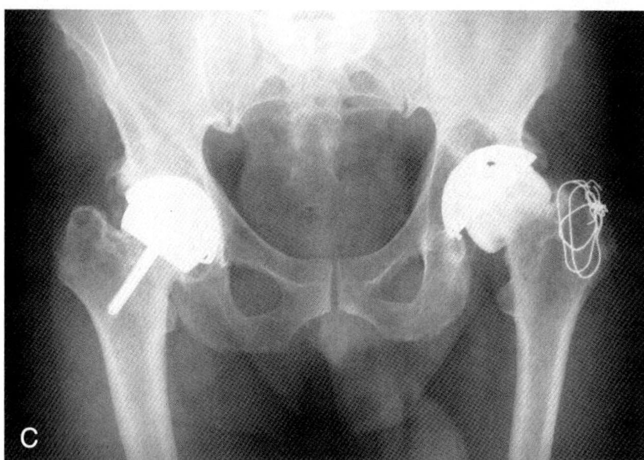

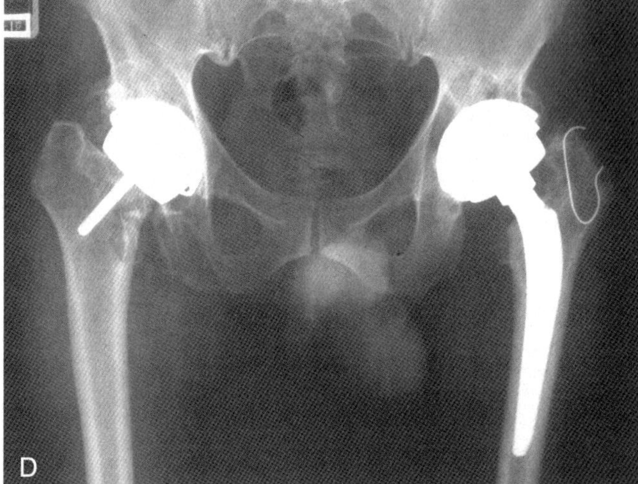

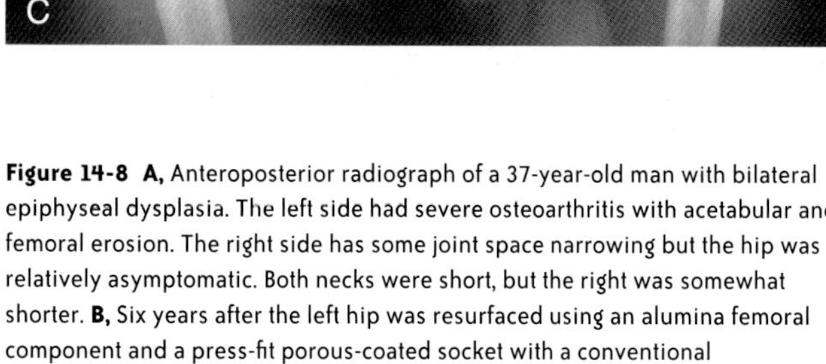

Figure 14-8 **A,** Anteroposterior radiograph of a 37-year-old man with bilateral epiphyseal dysplasia. The left side had severe osteoarthritis with acetabular and femoral erosion. The right side has some joint space narrowing but the hip was relatively asymptomatic. Both necks were short, but the right was somewhat shorter. **B,** Six years after the left hip was resurfaced using an alumina femoral component and a press-fit porous-coated socket with a conventional polyethylene liner. There is now secondary osteoarthritis of the right hip and complete obliteration of the joint space. **C,** The right hip was resurfaced with a modern metal-on-metal hybrid resurfacing device (Conserve®Plus). **D,** Anteroposterior view of the pelvis 9 years after right hip resurfacing and 2.5 years after left hip conversion to total hip replacement with a 44-mm Big Femoral Head and a grit-blasted standard anthropometric total hip (ATH) size 5. The porous surface replacement (PSR) resurfacing was revised at 12 years owing to femoral loosening of the femoral component and osteolysis. A double-socket technique was used, cementing a Conserve®Plus thin shell into the retained well-fixed PSR socket.

approach with a Conserve®Plus prosthesis. At 12 years, the left hip was revised with a 44-mm Big Femoral Head (BFH), a grit-blasted standard ATH size 5, and a Conserve®Plus 50-mm thin shell cemented into the well-fixed PSR porous-coated socket. He continues to work on his feet as a carpenter and has the following UCLA scores: pain 10 (right hip), 8 (left hip), walking 10, function 10, activity 6. His range of motion is comparable between the two hips with 95 degrees of flexion, 50 degrees (right) and 45 degrees (left) of abduction-adduction arc, and 45 degrees (right) and 35 degrees (left) of rotation arc. He has mild symptoms from bilateral knee and ankle dysplasia. He is of short stature (158 cm), similar to other patients with multiple ED.

Conversions to Total Hip Replacement

In this series, there were 8 conversions to THR, for the following reasons:

- Two due to a femoral neck fracture at 2 and 5 months after surgery
- Five secondary to aseptic loosening of the femoral component at an average of 64.6 months (range, 39 to 100). A 32-year-old woman with osteoarthritis secondary to DDH, Crowe II with 2 cm of leg length discrepancy of the left hip was treated with resurfacing (Fig. 14-9). To maintain leg length, no bone was removed from the dome area. She delivered a healthy infant, but 74 months after surgery, the femoral component loosened. The component was not completely seated, and fibrous tissue developed at the bone-cement interface requiring conversion to THR with a grit-blasted ATH long-stem size 5 and a 44-mm BFH.
- One due to recurrent subluxations 50 months after resurfacing in a 39-year-old woman who had right hip osteoarthritis secondary to developmental dysplasia (Fig. 14-10). She had undergone prior pelvic and femoral osteotomies

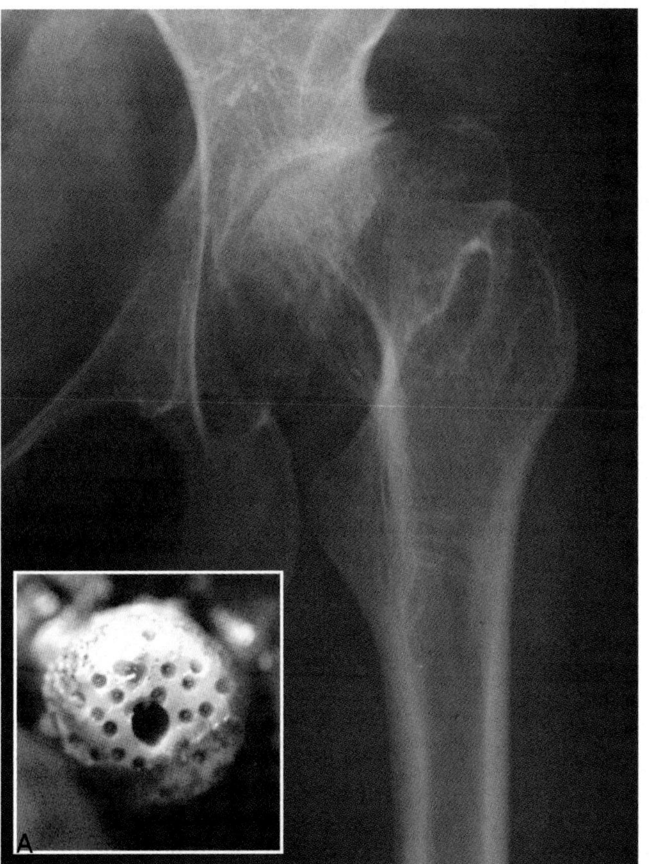

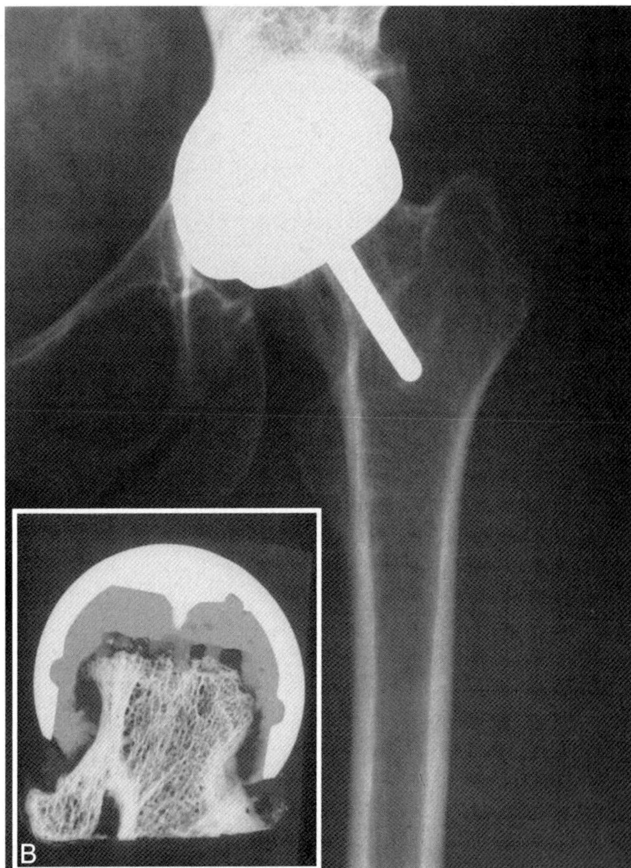

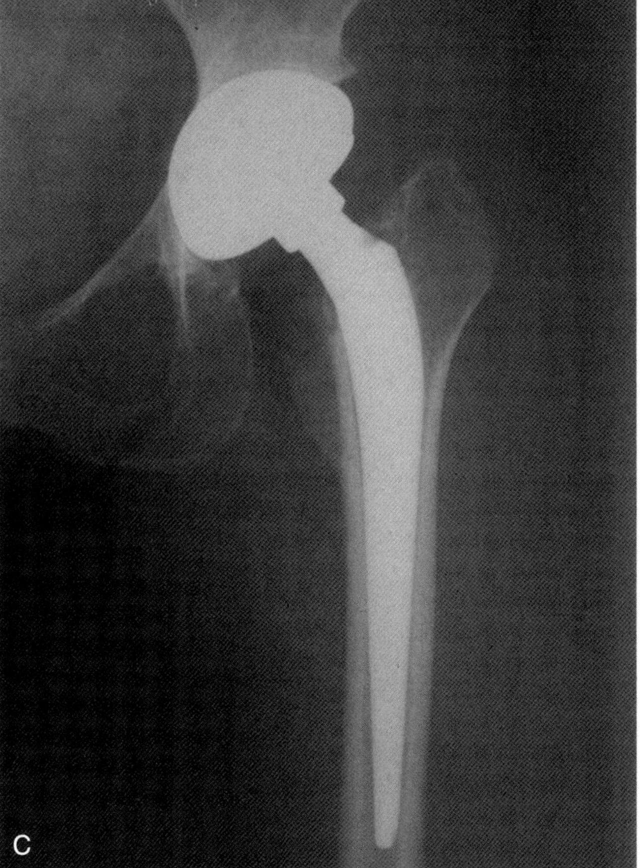

Figure 14-9 **A,** Preoperative anteroposterior radiograph of a 32-year-old woman with developmental dysplasia of the left hip. The insert shows the femoral head after preparation. No bone was removed from the dome area in an attempt to compensate for the 2 cm of leg-length discrepancy. **B,** Seventy-four months after surgery, the femoral component loosened. The insert shows a microradiograph of a cut section of the retrieved component. The component was incompletely seated, and fibrous tissue had developed at the bone-cement interface. **C,** The femoral component was revised to a grit-blasted anthropometric total hip (ATH) long stem size 5 and a 44-mm Big Femoral Head articulating with the well-fixed acetabular component left in situ.

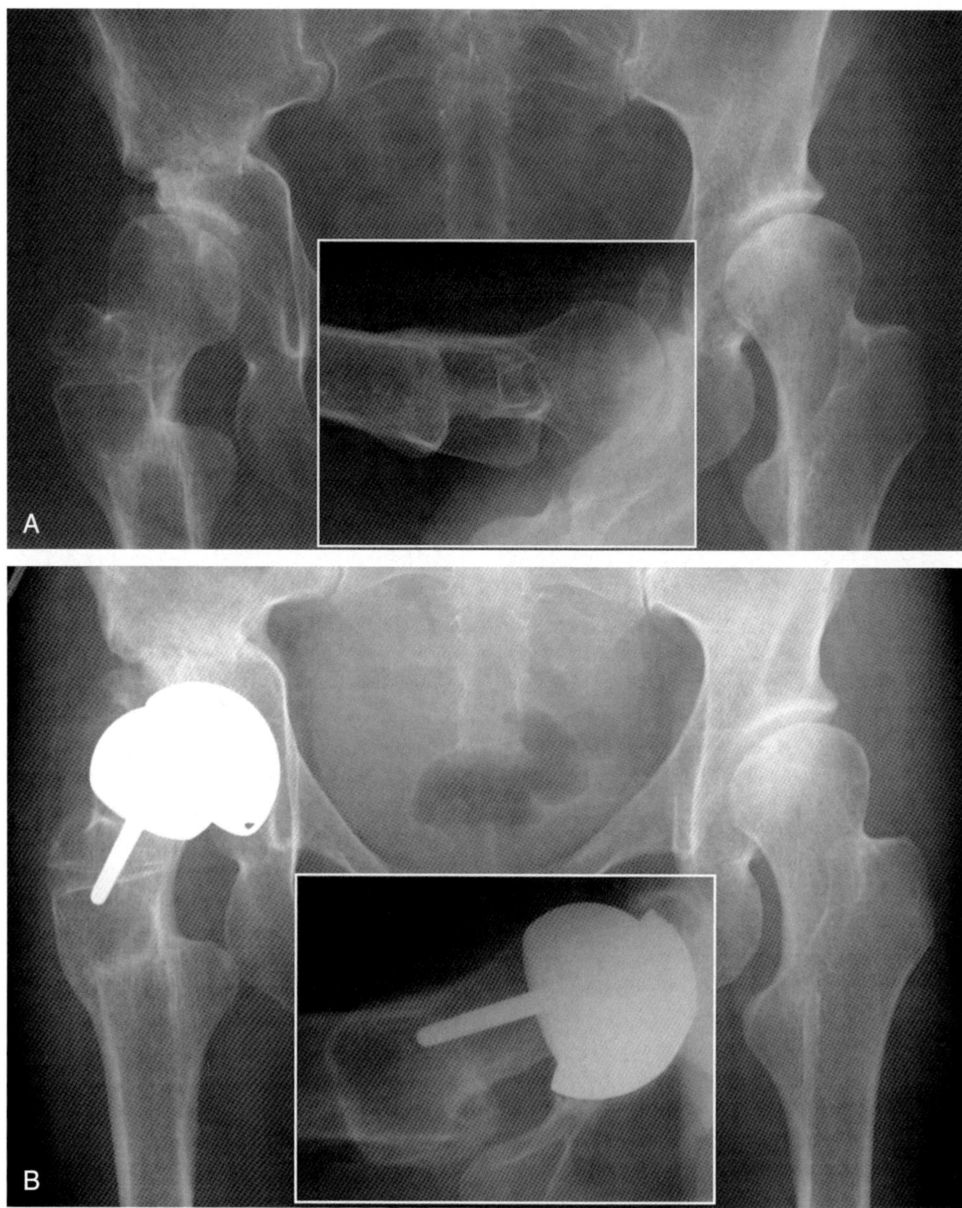

Figure 14-10 **A,** Anteroposterior view of the pelvis of a 39-year-old woman with right hip osteoarthritis secondary to developmental dysplasia of the hip. The patient had undergone both pelvic and femoral osteotomies before resurfacing, resulting in severe valgus and poor offset. Insert shows the Johnson lateral preoperative view. **B,** One-year postoperative anteroposterior radiograph. The altered proximal femoral geometry created a bone on bone impingement between the lesser trochanter and the ischial tuberosity, responsible for recurrent subluxations. The patient was converted to total hip replacement 4 years after surgery at another institution despite an attempt to surgically correct the impingement problem.

resulting in severe valgus and poor offset. The altered proximal femoral geometry created a bone on bone impingement between the lesser trochanter and the ischial tuberosity responsible for recurrent subluxations. This was our first Conserve®Plus resurfacing. Intraoperative range of motion check as described in Chapter 7 could have identified and allowed correction of the problem, possibly by ischial resection or intraoperative conversion to THR, although this was before BFH was available. The patient was converted to THR 4 years after surgery at another institution despite an attempt to surgically correct the impingement problem.

Two of the remaining hips show a radiolucency about the metaphyseal femoral stem. These radiolucencies have been visible on the patients' anteroposterior (AP) radiographs for 34 and 94 months, respectively, and do not have any clinical symptoms of component loosening.

Using any cause for revision as endpoint, the Kaplan-Meier overall survivorship results for this group of patients with childhood disorders were the following:

3 years: 98.4% (95% confidence interval [CI], 93.7 to 99.6)

4 years: 97.0% (95% CI, 90.7 to 99.1)

5 years: 91.3% (95% CI, 80.7 to 96.2)

8 years: 85.9% (95% CI, 67.9 to 94.2)

In comparison, for the patients operated on with second- and third-generation technique, the Kaplan-Meier survivorship results at 5 years were 98.7% (95% CI, 90.9 to 99.8).

Complications

There were a total of 12 complications in this group of patients, for an overall incidence rate of 8.3%.

These adverse events were distributed as follows:

- Four dislocations (2.8%): one secondary to a traumatic event (patient fell lighting up a barbecue); one associated with an excessive abduction angle of the acetabular component, which was reoriented surgically; one due to extensive soft tissue dissection to retrieve a broken scalpel blade in a 55-year-old female with osteoarthritis of the right hip secondary to developmental dysplasia (Fig. 14-11). After resurfacing of the right hip, she had a subluxation in the recovery room, consecutive to extensive dissection of the surrounding tissues to retrieve a broken scalpel blade.[31] The hip was reduced by internally rotating and abducting the leg. Fourteen days after surgery, the patient bent forward and the hip dislocated anteriorly, which was reduced and the patient placed in a one-leg spica cast for 4 weeks. The patient has recovered without sequelae or recurrence (9 years). Subsequently, the left hip developed secondary osteoarthritis and was resurfaced with a femoral component of the same size as the right side (42 mm), but the use of the thin shell allowed for a gain of 3 mm on the acetabular component size. The patient UCLA hip scores are now 10, 10, 10, and 6 for pain, walking, function, and activity, respectively, for both hips. The last case of dislocation was described in the previous section devoted to conversions to THR.
- One trochanteric bursitis (0.7%) in a hip that had been implanted with a transtrochanteric approach early in the series.
- Four femoral nerve palsies (2.8%), which recovered fully with no treatment in the months following surgery.
- One deep vein thrombosis (0.7%) complicated with a bleed due to the use of heparin to treat it.
- Two other unusual events were recorded (1.4%): The first one was a mismatch of the acetabular and femoral component sizes, which happened before sterilized packaging became routine. At this time, based on templating estimates, several sizes were sterilized in preparation for surgery. The acetabular component was revised 1 year after surgery because of the 2-mm mismatch and high metal ion levels (36.46 ppb and 14.98 ppb for serum cobalt and chromium, respectively). A custom socket with the correct inside diameter was manufactured with a 2-mm increase in outer diameter. The second event was the entrapment of cement in the joint space that required immediate reoperation after this problem was identified from the postoperative AP radiograph.

Summary

Initial experiences of surface arthroplasty with polyethylene featuring cemented one-piece acetabular components required more extensive reaming of the acetabulum than for conventional total hip arthroplasty (THA). Consequently, the results in patients with DDH and other childhood disorders featuring some type of acetabular dysplasia were inferior to the results in other conditions,[32] especially in combination with a low head-neck ratio. Acetabular failures due to loss of fixation and wear debris-induced periprosthetic osteolysis were more prevalent than failures on the femoral side (71%), often with considerable bone loss. New hip resurfacing implants, with metal-on-metal bearing surfaces and thinner non-cemented acetabular cups, alleviate the problems of osteolysis secondary to polyethylene debris. Improved surgical technique also has been associated with markedly improved survivorship.[33] There have been no socket failures, and there are no radiographic signs of acetabular component loosening so far in this series despite the absence of adjunct fixation and incomplete bone coverage laterally.

In this series of DDH patients, the hip center was routinely medialized, possibly enhancing cup fixation. The rough porous beaded surface locks the socket into the bone with impaction and provides rigid initial stability when the cavity is reamed correctly 1 mm under the outside dimension of the component. The initial stability of the acetabular component is obtained primarily from an interference fit between the anterior and posterior columns.[34,35] The acetabular component is inserted below the anterior pubic wall to enhance fixation and avoid iliopsoas irritation. Because of this very secure stability, it is possible to leave the component uncovered laterally by as much as 20%. Deformities of the proximal femur are more difficult to alter and therefore long-term results need to be evaluated.

The clinical results (pain, walking, function, and HHS) of the patients from this series improved significantly in all patients and are similar to those reported for other patients treated with this resurfacing arthroplasty,[36,37] regardless of etiology. The two femoral neck fractures in this series were previously reported and analyzed in retrieval studies from a group of more than 600 implants.[38] The risk factors included poor bone quality with large cysts and inadequate component seating. Because of poor bone quality, both patients would have been better served with a primary conventional THA, but both have done well after uncomplicated conversions to stemmed-type devices.

Three of the femoral components that loosened or had a radiolucency had severe cystic disease.[37] In another, the bone quality was sclerotic due to reconstruction without removing any dome bone and the femoral component was left proud with a thick cement mantle. These cases all were performed with first-generation bone preparation technique.

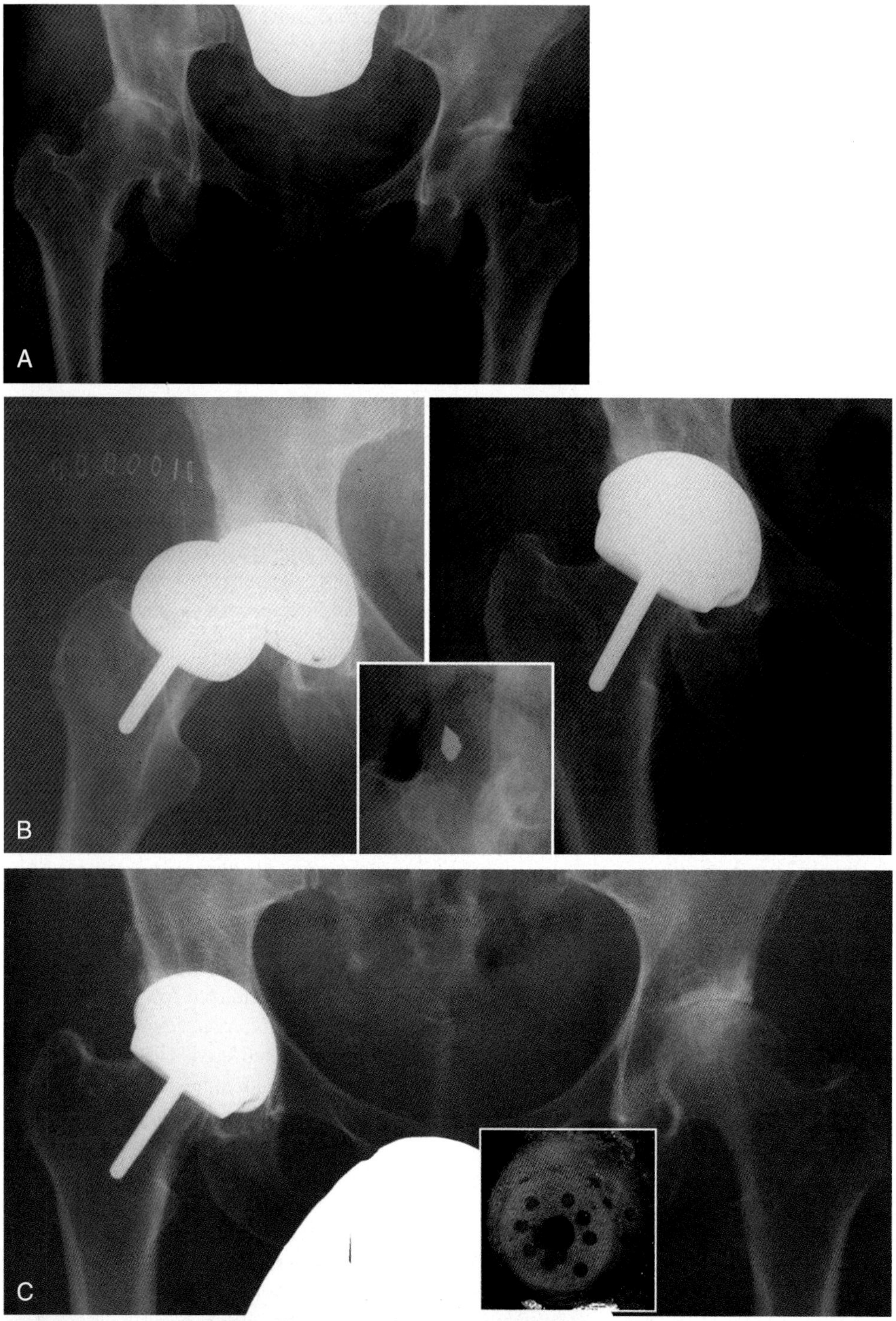

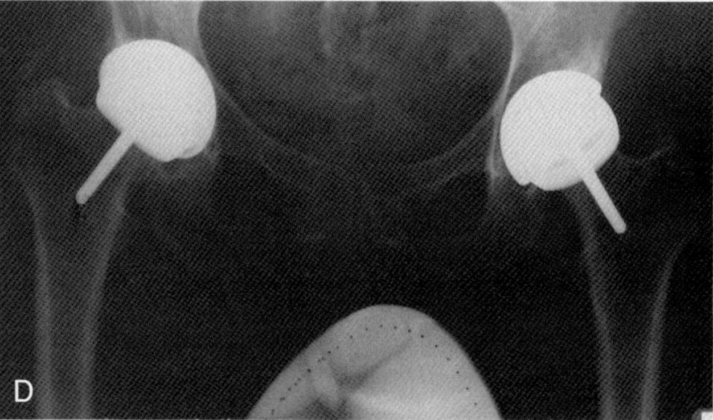

Figure 14-11 **A,** Anteroposterior view of the pelvis of a 55-year-old woman with osteoarthritis of the right hip secondary to developmental dysplasia of the hip. The left hip is also dysplastic but was not osteoarthritic. **B,** The resurfaced hip was subluxed in the recovery room and was reduced by internally rotating and abducting the leg. **C,** Eight years after surgery, the right resurfaced hip has been stable, but the left hip is painful, with complete obliteration of the joint space. Insert shows the left femoral head after the preparation phase for metal-on-metal resurfacing. **D,** Radiograph at 9 years follow-up on the right, and 1 year following metal-on-metal resurfacing on the left. The left side was resurfaced with a femoral component of the same size as the right side (42 mm), but the use of the thin shell allows for a gain of 3 mm on the acetabular component size.

Since that time, there have been no loosening and components have remained stable using second- and third-generation techniques despite high activity levels (UCLA activity > 7) in 22 patients (43%), including a 38-year-old woman who returned to playing competitive beach volleyball 1 year after resurfacing. She also gave birth to a healthy child 4 years after having metal-on-metal resurfacing surgery (Fig. 14-12). Seven years after surgery, her UCLA hip scores are 10, 10, 10, and 9 for pain, walking, function, and activity respectively. Her current range of motion is also exceptional, with 150 degrees for flexion with no flexion contracture, 95 degrees for the abduction-adduction arc, and 80 degrees for the rotation arc.

In our first 59 hips treated for DDH,[37] the dislocation incidence was a disappointing 5% despite the inherent stability of the larger head size (average 42 mm). However, the patient selection and technique issues have now been eliminated with no dislocations in the last 44 DDH cases. The intraoperative stability assessment after component insertion were modified to include a better assessment of anterior stability[35] so that the socket position could be corrected at surgery (see Chapter 7). Initially, we increased the anteversion of the socket to 20 to 30 degrees to favor the internal rotation for this largely female group of patients that, in some cases with increased femoral neck anteversion, was too much and resulted in anterior instability. In case of severe anteversion of the femoral head (>20 degrees), the anteversion of the socket should be lessened. Forty degrees of external rotation in extension are desirable and any sources of impingement should be corrected.

Leg-length equalization was achieved in the majority of our patients. Of 145 hips, only two could not be brought within 1 cm of the contralateral limb, including one patient who had a contralateral Crowe class IV DDH treated by THR (see Tables 14-8 and 14-9). In general, full normalization of leg lengths and hip biomechanics are more challenging with resurfacing than with a THR. When the anatomy is severely abnormal, it is unusual to be able to safely gain more than 1 cm of length, and it can only be accomplished by reaming and implanting the socket distally from the location of the dysplastic acetabulum, at the location of the true acetabulum, and most certainly not by leaving the femoral component proud on the reamed femoral head.[38]

There has been some concern regarding the advisability of implanting metal-on-metal implants in women of childbearing age because of a concern that the ion levels may cause birth defects. Brodner et al[39] reported on three women who had elevated serum ion levels with metal-on-metal total hip arthroplasties and reported no detectable cobalt or chromium ion levels in the cord blood at the level of detection of the testing facility used. Since that time, ions have been detected with Inductively coupled plasma mass spectroscopy equipment in the cord blood in children (see Chapter 11). At present, there are insufficient data to determine the level of risk, and studies are currently ongoing to establish baseline levels in women of childbearing age, and to monitor ion levels in their children.

The medium-term clinical results with the Conserve®Plus metal-on-metal surface arthroplasty in Crowe I and II DDH did not meet our initial expectations, although the porous-coated socket fixation has been excellent. Although the incidence of femoral neck fracture and femoral component loosening was higher than desired in our initial report, we have been able to lessen the risk of femoral loosening and neck fractures by improved patient selection, and with femoral bone preparation and fixation including cementing the stem in patients at risk for loosening.

In the LCP group, the head was often enlarged and flattened, resulting in a shorter femoral neck and head length. The shorter length of the femoral neck and head, along with the loss of height, made it difficult to restore limb length during surgery and prepare the bone to allow proper seating of the femoral component, without damaging the neck. The head-to-neck ratio and offset of the head did not seem to be affected.[5]

With the SCFE patients, the head was offset medially and posteriorly. The anterior offset ratio, as described by Eijer et al[40] averaged 0.20 preoperatively in our previously published study[5] and does not seem to confirm anterior femoroacetabular impingement as a contributing factor to the development of arthritis. We also looked at the lateral offset ratio, which averaged only 0.12, a confirmation of a tilting of the head medially. At this point, there is no published data for comparison of this number, but we found it useful to characterize the relationship of the head to the neck in the SCFE group. Despite these anatomic abnormalities, hip resurfacing was successfully performed in all of the patients.

Johnson lateral radiographs revealed three hips in which the femoral component stem abutted, and two hips in which the stem penetrated the anterior femoral cortex. These deviations from the central axis of the neck were related to the difficulty in visualizing the head to neck relationship in our early experience especially in heavy patients, inadvertently directing the stem along the contours of the head. In spite of these findings, the patients were asymptomatic with up to 10 years of follow-up and maintained high UCLA hip scores.

Although hip resurfacing is a technically difficult operation in these patients, the results to date have been encouraging. By taking extra care to avoid notching the neck on the anterior and lateral tension sides, satisfactory results can be achieved with a low incidence of complications.

Hip resurfacing is emerging as a treatment option for younger patients with end-stage arthritis secondary to childhood disorders because of its bone-conserving nature, stability, and the ability to easily convert to a THR should there be a femoral failure especially when the anatomy is relatively normal.[41] The low head-to-neck ratio, short neck length, and abnormal position of the head relative to the neck make it a challenge to perform resurfacing without violating the integrity of the neck. Other difficulties include increasing leg length and orienting the components to minimize impingement. The biomechanics and leg length discrepancy can be more simply corrected with a conventional THR, but the problems of

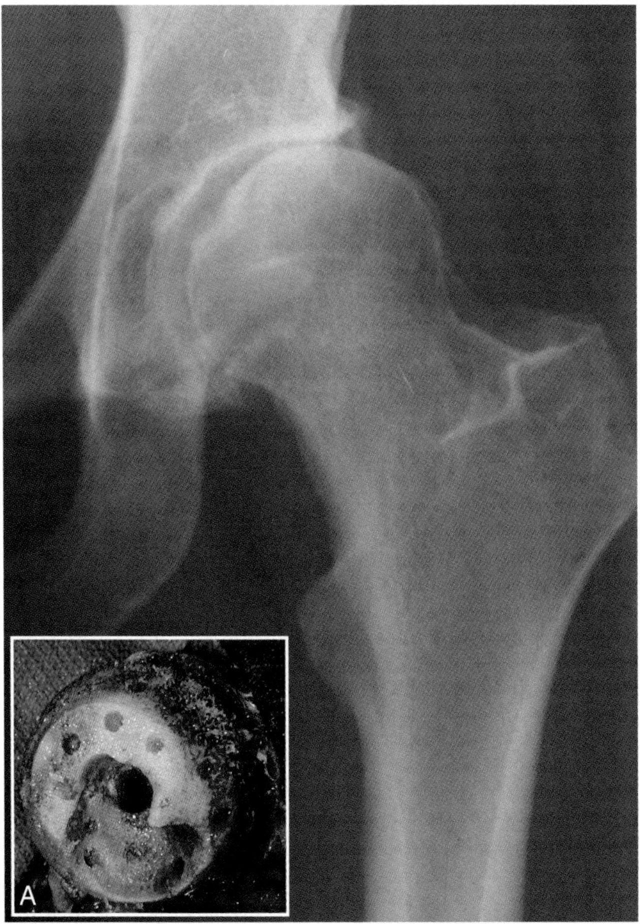

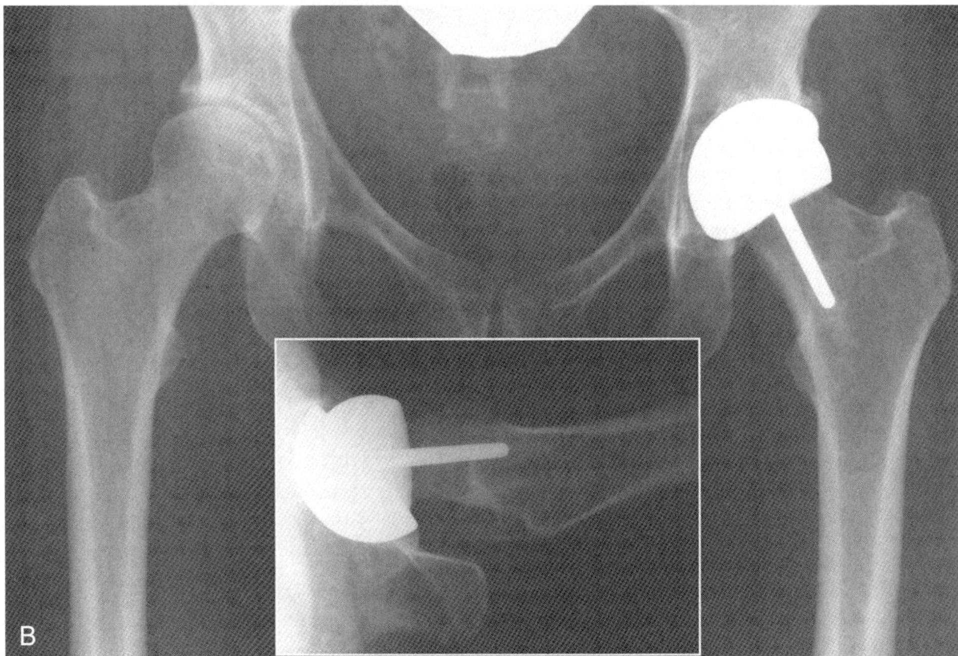

Figure 14-12 A, Anteroposterior radiograph of a 38-year-old beach volleyball player with osteoarthritis secondary to developmental dysplasia of the left hip. Note the large cystic defect in the femoral head, also visible on the intraoperative photograph of the femoral head after preparation for metal-on-metal resurfacing. **B,** Seven years after surgery, the patient has been very active playing competitive beach volleyball, as well as skiing or running for recreation. Component fixation and positioning are excellent; the metaphyseal stem was cemented.

proximal stress shielding and revision of stem type devices remain. For LCP and SCFE, full leg equalization was not always possible, but only one patient required a lift. Although one surgeon has recommended concurrent osteotomy or trochanteric osteotomy with advancement in an attempt to normalize the anatomy before undertaking resurfacing either as a two stage or one stage procedure,[42] we have concentrated on optimizing as much as possible the biomechanics and restoring normal leg length with resurfacing alone and have been surprised at the quality of clinical results even though it is not always possible to normalize the proximal femoral anatomy. Despite the inability to normalize the anatomy with short femoral necks and less than normal motion, the patients were uniformly satisfied and the most grateful of all of the etiologic groups. This is reflected by the high postoperative Short Form-12 (SF-12) mental scores. This elation is due, we suspect, to the length of time since childhood that the patients have endured considerable disability and restricted motion combined with pain relief and marked functional improvement. Hip resurfacing often requires downsizing the femoral head diameter to the margins of the femoral neck, especially when the neck is wide to save acetabular bone stock. Occasionally, it may be necessary to notch the femoral neck in order to perform resurfacing without removing excessive acetabular bone, although this has not been necessary since the thin (3.5-mm) shells have been available.

References

1. Paavilainen T, Hoikka V, Solonen K: Cementless total replacement for severly dysplastic or dislocated hips. J Bone Joint Surg Br 1990;72-B:205-211.
2. Charnley J, Feagin J: Low friction arthroplasty in congenital subluxation of the hip. Clin Orthop 1973;91:98-113.
3. Haddad F, Masri B, Garbuz D, Duncan C: Primary total replacement of the dysplastic hip. J Bone Joint Surg Am 1999;81-A:1462-1482.
4. Jasty M, Anderson M, Harris W: Total hip replacement for developmental dysplasia of the hip. Clin Orthop 1995;331:40-45.
5. Amstutz H, Su E, Le Duff M: Surface arthroplasty in young patients with hip arthritis secondary to childhood disorders. Orthop Clin North Am 2005;36:223-230.
6. Solomon L: Patterns of osteoarthritis of the hip. J Bone Joint Surg Br 1976;58:176-183.
7. Catterall A: Legg-Calve-Perthes syndrome. Clin Orthop Rel Res 1981;158:41-52.
8. Leunig M, Casillas MM, Hamlet M, Hersche O, Notzli H, Slongo T, Ganz R: Slipped capital femoral epiphysis: early mechanical damage to the acetabular cartilage by a prominent femoral metaphysis. Acta Orthop Scand 2000;71:370-375.
9. Stulberg SD, Cooperman DR, Wallensten R: The natural history of Legg-Calve-Perthes disease. J Bone Joint Surg Am 1981;63:1095-1108.
10. Jerre T: A study in slipped upper femora epiphysis with special reference to late function and roentgenological results and the value of closed reduction. Acta Orthop Scand 1950;(Suppl 6).
11. Oram V: Epiphysiolysis of the head of the femur; a follow-up examination with special reference to end results and the social prognosis. Acta Orthop Scand 1953;23:100-120.
12. Ross P, Lyne E, Morawa L: Slipped capital femoral epiphysis long-term results after 10-38 years. Clin Orthop Relat Res 1979;141: 176-180.
13. Goldman A, Lane J, Salvati E: Slipped capital femoral epiphyses complicating renal osteodystrophy: a report of three cases. Radiology 1978;126:333-339.
14. Shea D, Mankin H: Slipped capital femoral epiphysis in renal rickets. Report of three cases. J Bone Joint Surg Am 1966;48: 349-355.
15. Chapman J, Deakin D, Green J: Slipped upper femoral epiphysis after radiotherapy. J Bone Joint Surg Br 1980;62:337-339.
16. Goodman D, Feighan J, Smith A, Latimer B, Buly R, Cooperman D: Subclinical slipped capital femoral epiphysis. Relationship to osteoarthrosis of the hip. J Bone Joint Surg Am 1997;79: 1489-1497.
17. Stulberg S, Cordell L, Harris W, Ramsey P, MacEwen G: Unrecognized childhood hip disease: a major cause of idiopathic osteoarthritis of the hip. The Otto E. Aufranc Award Paper. The Hip: Open Scientific Meeting of the Hip Society, 1975, pp 212-228.
18. Murray R: The aetiology of primary osteoarthritis of the hip. Br J Radiol 1965;38:810-824.
19. Crowe J, Mani V, Ranawat C: Total hip replacement in congenital dislocation and dysplasia of the hip. J Bone Joint Surgery Am 1979;61-A:15-23.
20. Wiberg G: Studies on dysplastic acetabula and congenital subluxation of the hip joint. Acta Chir Scand 1939;(Suppl 58).
21. Sharp I: Acetabular dysplasia: acetabular angle. J Bone Joint Surg Br 1961;43:268-272.
22. Stulberg S, Harris W: Acetabular dysplasia and the development of osteoarthritis of the hip. The Hip: Open Scientific Meeting of the Hip Society, 1974.
23. Hesse B, Kohler G: Does it always have to be Perthes' disease? What is epiphyseal dysplasia? Clin Orthop Relat Res 2003;414:219-227.
24. Grimm J, Just M: Epiphyseal dysplasia of the hip joint, its diagnosis and differential diagnosis with MRI. Rofo 1992; 157:47-52.
25. Khermosh O, Wientroub S: Dysplasia epiphysealis capitis femoris. Meyer's dysplasia. J Bone Joint Surg Br 1991;73:621-625.
26. Ganz R, Klaue K, Vinh T, Mast J: A new periacetabular osteotomy for the treatment of hip dysplasias: technique and preliminary results. 1988. Clin Orthop Relat Res 2004;418:3-8.
27. Dunn D: Severe slipped capital femoral epiphysis and open replacement by cervical osteotomy. The Hip: Open Scientific Meeting of the Hip Society, 1975, pp 115-126.
28. Kramer W, Craig W, Noel S: Compensating osteotomy at the base of the femoral neck for slipped capital femoral epiphysis. J Bone Joint Surg Am 1976;58:796-800.
29. Sugioka Y: Transtrochanteric rotational osteotomy in the treatment of idiopathic and steroid-induced femoral head necrosis, Perthes' disease, slipped capital femoral epiphysis, and osteoarthritis of the hip. Indications and results. Clin Orthop Relat Res 1984;184:12-23.
30. Southwick W: Biplane osteotomy for very severe slipped capital femoral epiphysis. The Hip: Open Scientific Meeting of the Hip Society, 1975, pp 105-114.
31. Prasad R, Amstutz HC, Sparling EA: Use of a magnet to retrieve a broken scalpel blade. J Arthroplasty 2000;15:806-808.

32. Amstutz HC, Dorey F, O'Carroll PF: THARIES resurfacing arthroplasty. Evolution and long-term results. Clin Orthop Rel Res 1986;213:92-114.
33. Amstutz H, Le Duff M, Campbell P, Dorey F: The effects of technique changes on aseptic loosening of the femoral component in hip resurfacing. Results of 600 Conserve Plus with a 3-9 year follow-up. J Arthroplasty 2007;22:481-489.
34. Amstutz H, Beaulé P, Le Duff M: Hybrid metal-on-metal surface arthroplasty of the hip. Operative Techniques in Orthopedics 2001;11:1-10.
35. Amstutz H, Beaulé P, Dorey F, Le Duff M, Campbell P, Gruen T: Metal-on-metal hybrid surface arthroplasty—Surgical technique. J Bone Joint Surg 2006;88 A:234-249.
36. Amstutz H, Beaulé P, Dorey F, Le Duff M, Campbell P, Gruen T: Metal-on-metal hybrid surface arthroplasty: two to six year follow-up. J Bone Joint Surg 2004;86-A:28-39.
37. Amstutz H, Antoniades J, Le Duff M: Results of metal-on-metal hybrid hip resurfacing for Crowe type I and II developmental dysplasia. J Bone Joint Surg Am 2007;89:339-346.
38. Amstutz H, Campbell P, Le Duff M: Fracture of the neck of the femur after surface arthroplasty of the hip. J Bone Joint Surg 2004;86 A:1874-1877.
39. Brodner W, Grohs J, Bancher-Todesca D, Dorotka R, Meisinger V, Gottsauner-Wolf F, Kotz R: Does the placenta inhibit the passage of chromium and cobalt after metal-on-metal total hip arthroplasty? J Arthroplasty 2004;19:102-106.
40. Eijer H, Leunig M, Mahomed N, Ganz R: Cross-table lateral radiographs for screening of anterior femoral head-neck offset in patients with femoro-acetabular impingement. Hip International 2001;11:37-41.
41. Ball S, Le Duff M, Amstutz H: Early results of conversion of a failed femoral component in hip resurfacing arthroplasty. J Bone Joint Surg Am 2007;89:735-741.
42. O'Hara J: Hip resurfacing and femoral osteotomy in the treatment of complex hip deformity. In Combined Orthopaedic Associations, 2004 October 24-29; Sydney, Australia.

CHAPTER 15

Post-Traumatic Arthritis

Harlan C. Amstutz
Michel J. Le Duff

Introduction

Post-traumatic arthritis (PTA) is osteoarthritis that develops as a result of prior hip trauma. In general, the development is related to the severity of the initial trauma to the skeletal structure and articular cartilage, and the efficacy of treatment.[1] Although the ability to acutely treat major hip injuries is improving, if anatomic distortion or bone loss is severe, reconstruction can be challenging and many patients require reconstructive surgical procedures. Bhandari et al[2] reviewed a series of 1076 fractures of the acetabulum and found that, among several variables, the quality of the reduction of the fracture was the most powerful predictor of the outcome of the procedure. Arthritis may develop due to joint surface incongruities that result from unreduced or incompletely reduced fractures of the acetabulum, femoral head, or cartilage defects or chondrocyte death leading to degeneration of cartilage and arthritis.[3] Finally osteonecrosis (ON) of the femoral head after hip dislocation or femoral neck fractures can lead to femoral head subchondral bone collapse and osteoarthritis.[4]

Although primary arthroplasty has been advocated by some when the damage is severe, it is preferable to do the best possible reconstruction, keeping the fixation screws as far away as possible from the articular surface so as not to interfere with subsequent arthroplasty sockets, if needed. The use of prophylaxis to prevent heterotopic ossification is recommended, especially if the surgery occurs between 3 and 14 days after the injury. Allow sufficient time for fracture healing and adaptation to residual incongruities. Prediction as to the outcome is imprecise and recommendation for arthroplasty should be based on overall disability, age, and other patient demographics.

In addition, PTA is typically considered by surgeons a difficult etiology on which to perform hip arthroplasty. With a 78% survivorship at 10 years Weber and colleagues[5] showed that the results of total hip replacement (THR) for PTA, due to the treatment of an acetabular fracture, are lower than for other indications. However, uncemented acetabular components seem to be performing well and showing a low rate of loosening in this challenging patient population.[6]

Current Indications and Techniques of Hip Resurfacing for Post-Traumatic Arthritis

Treatment recommendations for isolated acetabulum PTA are not different from those for "primary" osteoarthritis (see Chapter 12). However, Cuckler[7] cautions the surgeons about the similarities of treating PTA hips with a THR and performing a revision surgery. Hip resurfacing is our preference, especially for the young patient, and with increased durability of hip resurfacing, there may be a potential to get patients through their lifetime with one operation. The stability of hip resurfacing is an advantage, and if no osteotomy is performed, routine postoperative mobilization is possible. The procedure does not preclude future osteotomy or conversion to a conventional total hip replacement if needed. If there is a limb shortening of more than 2 cm, consideration might include a resurfacing and an osteotomy with a plate or other more traditional form of internal fixation. Then the bone stock available for a conventional THR at a later date in the presence of PTA with femoral deformity is not compromised by an interim surface replacement.

Technique Considerations

Conventional templating and routine techniques are sufficient for those with minimal acetabulum deformity. Those acetabular fractures that healed with significant deformity often have a cavernous acetabulum that can accommodate a standard acetabular component. However, if the diameter is even larger and there is an associated leg-length discrepancy (LLD), consider using the Conserve®Plus Superfix (+10-mm–eccentric) socket (Fig. 15-1).

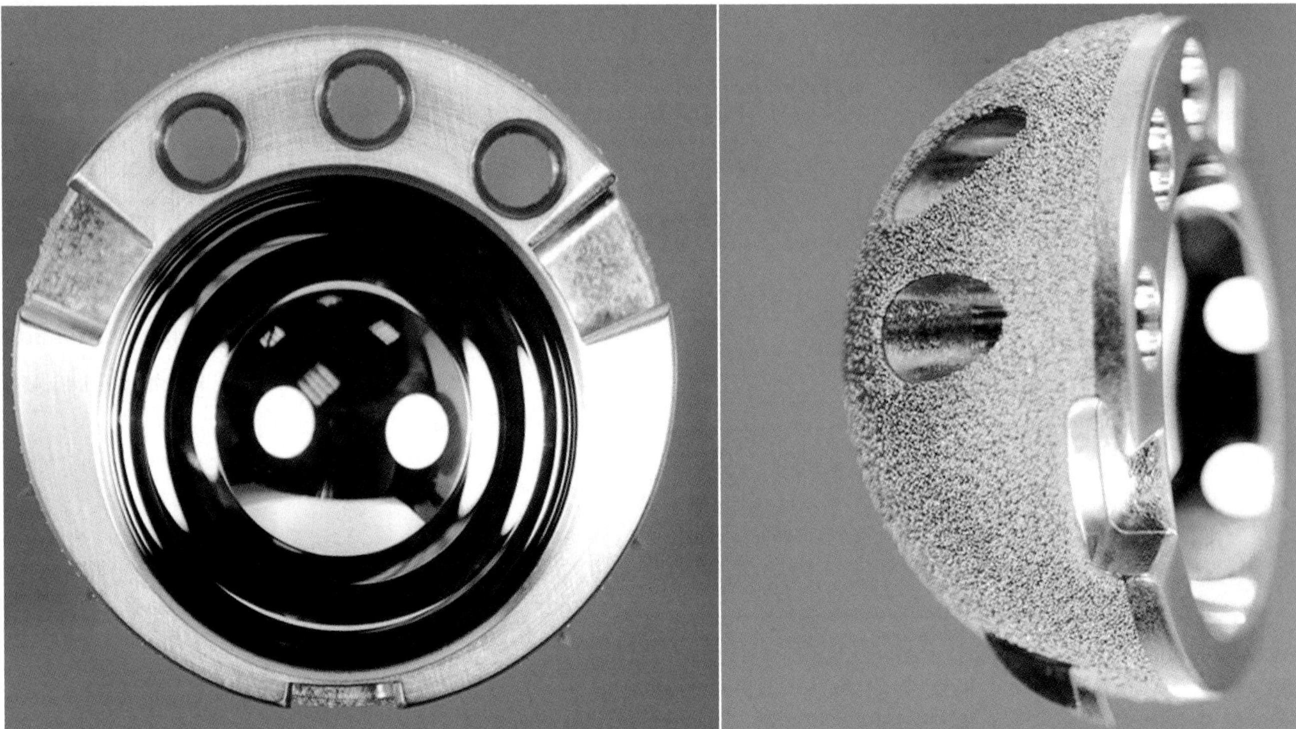

Figure 15-1 The Conserve®Plus Superfix cup (Wright Medical Technology Inc., Arlington, TN).

In our series, we did not have to remove any fixation plate devices, but we did have to burr several screw tips below the acetabular bony surface and remove several other screws so that they would not prevent the seating of the socket component and achieve the necessary initial stability for osseointegration. For this reason, it is important to recess all metal projections below the acetabular surface.

A 13-year-old student who sustained bilateral acetabular fractures in a bicycle collision with a car presented in our office 5 years after the accident with secondary osteoarthritis (OA) of the left hip and a LLD of 2.5 cm (Fig. 15-2A). Although the right hip fracture was not displaced, the left sustained a fracture dislocation, and had been treated with open reduction/internal fixation using a posterior ilioischial plate. His preoperative University of California-Los Angeles (UCLA) hip scores for pain, walking, function, and activity were 5, 6, 5, 3; and the range of motion included 70 degrees of flexion with a 45-degree contracture, 35 degrees in abduction, 15 degrees in adduction, and rotational arc of 15 degrees. Judet obliques were obtained, which suggested that the hardware did not have to be removed in order to perform the resurfacing, which was carried out at 18 years of age. Although the offset was reduced, he has a negative Trendelenburg sign with a 1.5 cm LLD (Fig. 15-2B). The patient uses a lift but not on a regular basis. His current UCLA hip scores are 9, 9, 10, and 8 for pain, walking, function, and activity, respectively.

A computed tomography (CT) scan was not necessary preoperatively in this case but has been helpful in others to assess bony defects or limb length discrepancy due to proximal acetabulum migration, and assist in determining socket size and the possible need for hardware removal.

The indications for hip resurfacing for patients who develop post-traumatic ON with or without acetabulum deformity are similar to those described in Chapter 13.

PTA in the presence of a severely deformed proximal femur may create additional technical complexity. The magnitude of complexity depends on the degree and location of the deformity and limb-length shortening. One option could be a corrective osteotomy of the deformed femur with simultaneous or staged conventional total hip replacement. However, we have not found it necessary to perform a two-stage procedure in our series. Grafting and acetabular reconstruction of untreated fracture-dislocations with implantation of both femoral and acetabulum components can generally be carried out in one operation.

Soft tissue defects should be evaluated preoperatively with a plastic surgeon so that the operative area has both good coverage and no tension on the wound margins with skin and subcutaneous closure. It is important to assess whether the defect requires a staged procedure or if it is possible to transfer a flap at the time of resurfacing. We had one wound area breakdown in a 44-year-old machinist who had a large soft tissue deficit in the hip area (Fig. 15-3). The patient initially had multiple fractures of the proximal femur consecutive to an automobile accident and had been treated with a nail plate combination. He developed postoperative sepsis requiring six débridements. The hip became arthritic with preoperative UCLA hip scores of 3, 5, 5, and 3 for pain, walking, function,

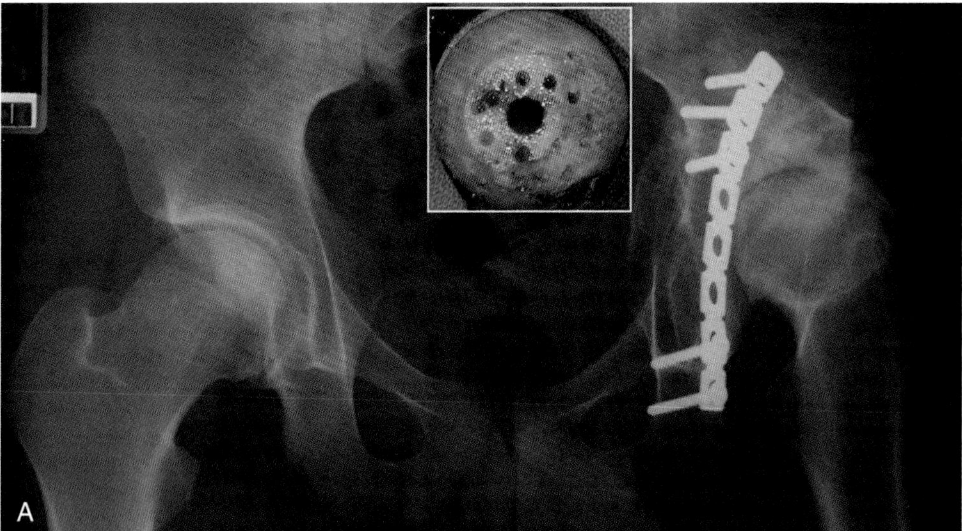

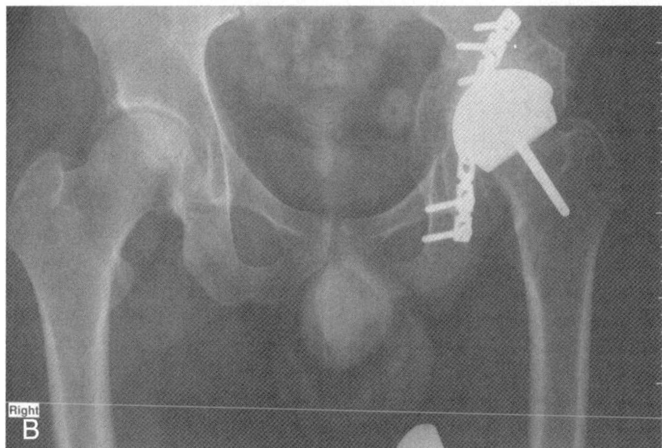

Figure 15-2 **A,** Radiograph of an 18-year-old man with osteoarthritis of the left hip, secondary to a pelvic fracture dislocation and reduction with a posterior plate. There is a thick medial wall and lateral subluxation. The lateral radiograph showed grade II heterotopic bone. Insert shows the femoral head with overall good bone quality, although there are several small cystic areas smaller than 1 cm in size and a sclerotic area superiorly. **B,** The patient is shown at 79.7 months following metal-on-metal resurfacing, with an acetabular cup of 58 mm, and femoral component of 48 mm. At the time of surgery, the patient had heterotopic ossification that was excised and the hip was medialized but the hardware did not have to be removed. The socket was fully covered by the acetabular bone.

and activity, respectively. The patient's range of motion was 40 degrees in flexion, with a 45 degree flexion contracture, a 10-degree adduction contracture, and no rotation. In addition, the patient had an apparent LLD of 2 cm (due to an adduction contracture), with the affected leg being shorter. After resurfacing of the hip, the wound closure was tight, and there was a breakdown at the distal portion of the incision with persistent drainage and ultimately secondary enterococcus sepsis. His erythrocyte sedimentation rate (ESR) was 70, and C-reative protein (CRP) was 46. Fortunately, the resurfacing was salvaged with a thorough débridement and vastus lateralis flap transfer performed after all of the necrotic and septic tissue was removed, 1 month after resurfacing. There was no detectable interface defect under the femoral component or involvement of the intramedullary canal. He required 6 weeks of intravenous of vancomycin and rocephin, followed by oral amoxicillin and bactrim for 1 year. The patient has now been free of recurrent sepsis for 6 years with UCLA scores of 9 for pain and walking, 10 for function, and 6 for activity. The ESR and CRP are normal. Although limited, he has a serviceable range of motion with 90 degrees of flexion, 80 degrees of abduction-adduction arc, and a rotation arc of 40 degrees. The patient shows a marked improvement in Short Form-12 (SF-12) scores, with the physical component improving from 27 to 47 and the mental component from 45 to 54. He has a slight limp, but the Trendelenburg sign is negative. In retrospect, the flap transfer should have been done either before or at the time of the resurfacing.

Patient Demographics

From our series of 1000 hips (838 patients), 41 hips (41 patients) received a Conserve®Plus resurfacing for PTA that was not associated with ON. Those with post-traumatic ON were included in the series studied in Chapter 13.

The average age of the patients was 41.3 years of age (range, 16 to 65 years). Most of the patients were men (35/41, 85.4%). Sixteen hips (39.0%) had undergone at least one previous surgery before resurfacing, as testified by hardware present on the preoperative radiographs. Ten patients had undergone pelvic reconstruction only, four had a femoral reconstruction

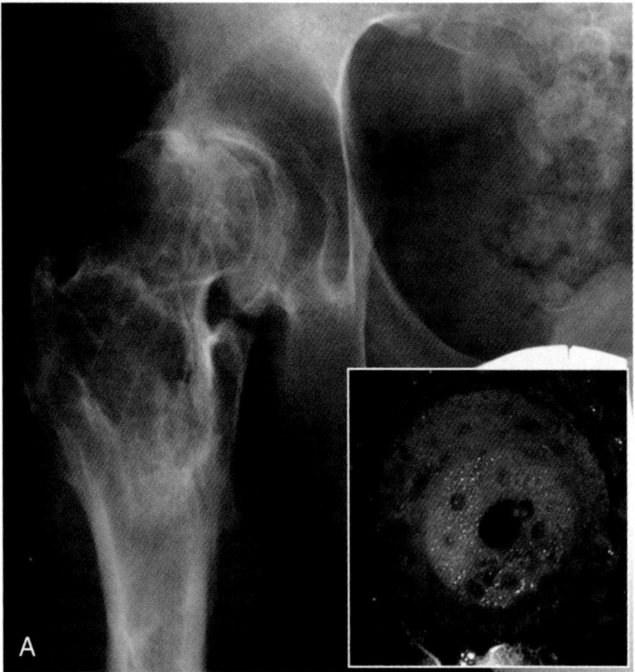

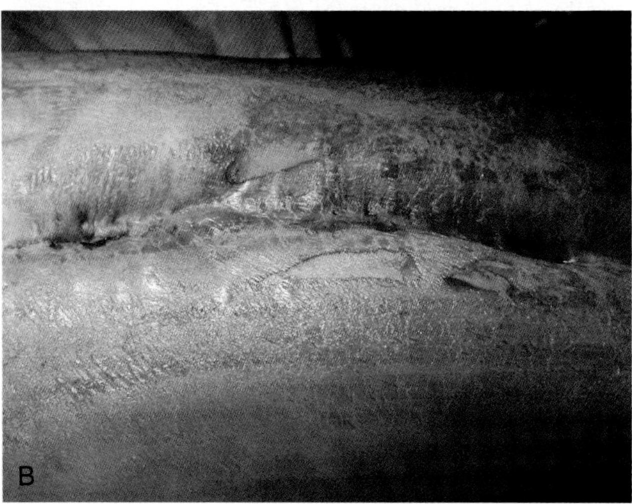

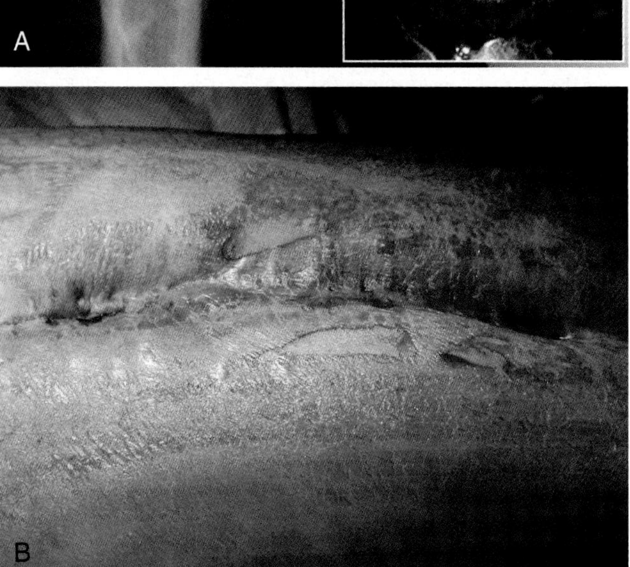

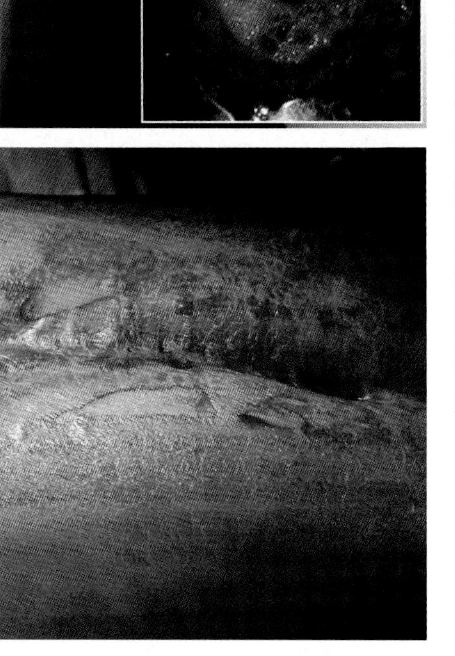

Figure 15-3 **A,** Radiograph of a 44-year-old man with osteoarthritis of the right hip, secondary to trauma in an accident that shattered his hip; Note the valgus of the neck residuals outline of previous nail in the femoral head and the cystic degeneration superiorly. Preoperative insert shows femoral head following preparation for resurfacing. The cystic superior area is at the bottom. **B,** The patient had a depressed scar from six operations to débride infected tissues post fracture reduction. The patient also had minimal soft tissue over the greater trochanter. One month after surface replacement, he required débridement owing to sepsis of the wound and antibiotics, and plastic surgery (vastus lateralis flap) to normalize the anterolateral aspect of his thigh. **C,** The resurfaced hip is well fixed, but there is neck shortening and reduced offset. However the patient is pleased to have had 70 septic-free months of follow-up. Note the residual screw holes in the proximal femur from the previous plate.

only and two had both a femoral and pelvic reconstruction. The vast majority of patients had unilateral disease.

The demographics of this group of patients are shown in Table 15-1.

At surgery, 13 (32%) patients showed femoral heads with good bone quality (no defects), 10 (24%) had defects less than 1 cm in size, 14 (34%) had defects 1 to 2 cm in size, and 4 (9.8%) had defects greater than 2 cm in size. The defects size and incidence was similar to the overall cohort and less than either ON or childhood disorders.

Results

Clinical Scores

The average UCLA hip scores improved significantly ($P <$ .0001) between preoperative and last follow-up visits. The pain score increased from 3.6 ± 1.2 to 9.1 ± 1.4, the walking score from 6.3 ± 1.5 to 9.4 ± 1.3, the function score from 5.6 ± 1.6 to 9.3 ± 1.5, and the activity score from 4.4 ± 1.3 to 7.3 ± 1.6. The average physical component was 32.6 ± 7.2 preoperatively

Table 15-1 Demographics of the Patients Operated for Osteoarthritis Secondary to Trauma

	Men n = 35	Women n = 6	Combined n = 41
Age (years)	41.8 (16-65)	38.4 (18-54)	41.3 (16-65)
Weight (kg)	87.4 (63-164)	67.2 (56-84)	84.4 (56-164)
Height (cm)	180.1 (162-195)	165.8 (157-170)	178.0 (157-195)
BMI	26.8 (19.9-46.4)	24.4 (20.5-30.9)	26.4 (19.9-46.4)
Femoral component size (mm)	48.3 (40-54)	43.3 (38-46)	47.6 (38-54)
Cysts > 1 cm	14 (40.0%)	4 (66.7%)	18 (43.9%)
Charnley class			
A	30 (85.7%)	4 (66.7%)	34 (82.9%)
B	1 (2.9%)	2 (33.3%)	3 (7.3%)
C	4 (11.4%)	0 (0.0%)	4 (9.8%)

BMI, body mass index.

and 52.1 ± 6.9 at the last follow-up ($P < .0001$), and the mental component increased from 51.5 ± 11.8 to 54.3 ± 9.1 ($P = .166$). The postoperative Harris hip score was 93.7 ± 4.7. These scores are not different than our entire cohort. One patient exceeded the average scores for seven years before succumbing to rapidly advancing amyotrophic lateral sclerosis at the age of 48 years.

Retention of Hardware

The pre-existing hardware was retained during the resurfacing procedure in 10 hips out of 12 (83.3%) for the acetabular side and one hip out of 6 (16.7%) for the femoral side.

Leg-Length Equalization

In this group of 41 patients, one patient was an amputee of the contralateral leg, six had a preoperative leg-length discrepancy (LLD) of 0 to 1 cm, two had LLD of 1 to 2 cm, five had LLD of 2 to 3 cm, one had LLD of greater than 3 cm, and 26 presented equal leg lengths. Post-operatively, three patients had remaining LLD, but these had been reduced by either 1 or 2 cm.

Case Histories

- Case #1. A 44-year-old speech therapist who developed PTA after a gunshot wound to the abdomen and thigh also had a severe muscle weakness with an absence of any flexor power and weak abductors (Fig. 15-4A). UCLA preoperative hip scores were 4, 6, 5, and 4 for pain, walking, function, and activity, respectively. At resurfacing, 12 buck shots were removed during the exposure and two were located adjacent to the acetabulum, which were encased in greenish discolored tissue. The large iliac defect was approximately 10 cm proximal to the acetabulum. Postoperatively, the hip has remained stable. The patient's lack of flexor power is unchanged, but there is a slight improvement in the abduction strength; UCLA hip scores are 8, 9, 10, 4 for pain, walking, function, and activity. Although the patient's overall activity is modest, she is able, on occasion, to take a horseback ride and dance (Fig. 15-4B).
- Case #2. At the time of his first visit to our office, a 25-year-old man had a chief complaint of right hip pain from osteoarthritis secondary to multiple pelvic and acetabular fractures sustained in a bicycling accident (the patient was hit by a truck). A complex pelvic reconstruction was performed, which left a considerable amount of hardware in the area of the affected hip (Fig. 15-5). The patient's hip muscle strength was low; grade 2 to 3 for flexors, abductors and extensors. UCLA preoperative hip scores were 4, 6, 6, 4 for pain, walking, function, and activity, respectively. It was impossible to remove the three screws proximally, which were found to be protruding into the acetabulum because they were buried under the recon plate. They were removed from within the cavity with a high-speed burr, and the defects were filled with bone graft. It was then possible to optimize the orientation and initial stability of the acetabular component. The patient has now enjoyed his hip resurfacing for 9.5 years with his 6.5-year UCLA scores marked at 10 for pain, walking, and function, and 8 for activity. The muscle strength improved, but his Trendelenburg sign was negative. The range of motion (flexion 140 degrees without contracture, abduction-adduction arc 85 degrees, and rotation arc 65 degrees) has been minimally affected by the Brooker grade III heterotopic ossification.
- Case #3. A 52-year-old data processor came to our office with progressive hip pain and PTA (Fig. 15-6). At age 17 the patient had sustained a fracture-dislocation of the right hip, and was then treated with a Thompson Z-nail. The cross-section was a Z, and the bone grew through the holes, making it nearly impossible to remove without destroying the head and neck. The patient's preoperative UCLA scores

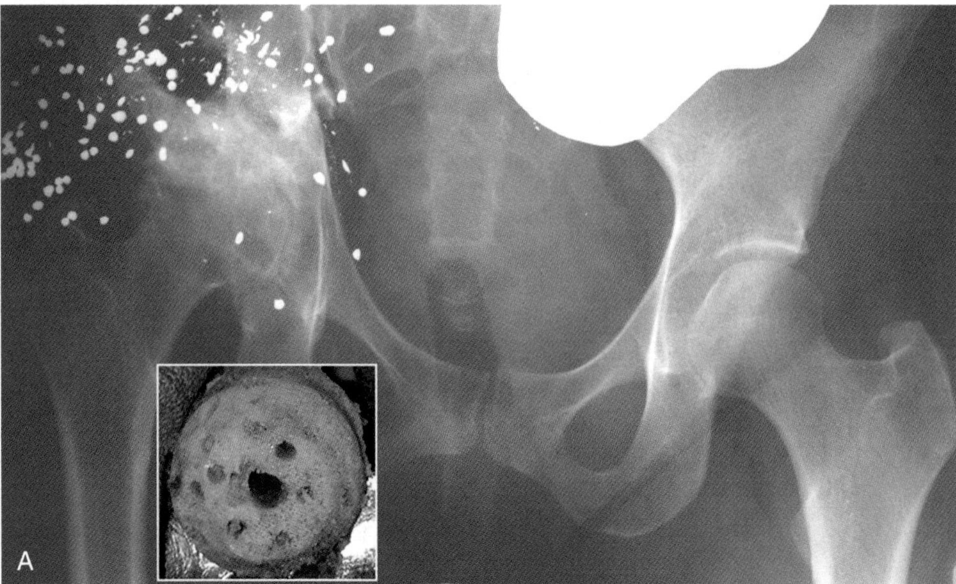

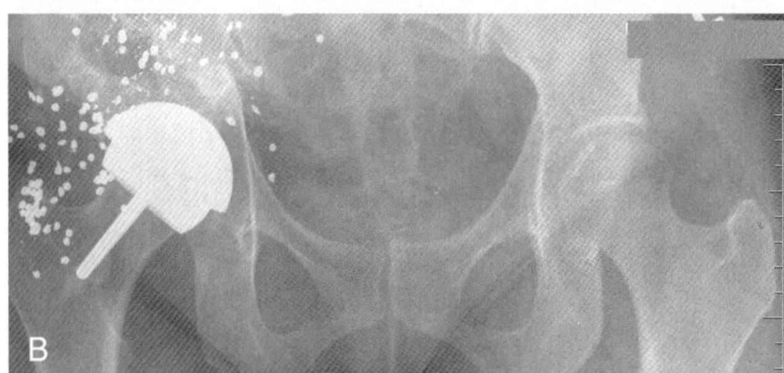

Figure 15-4 A, Radiograph of a 44-year-old woman with osteoarthritis of the right hip secondary to trauma, a gunshot wound. Note the large spherical defect in the ilium above the acetabulum and the retained buckshot. Insert shows femoral head following preparation for a total hip resurfacing. **B,** Patient at 38 months following metal-on-metal resurfacing.

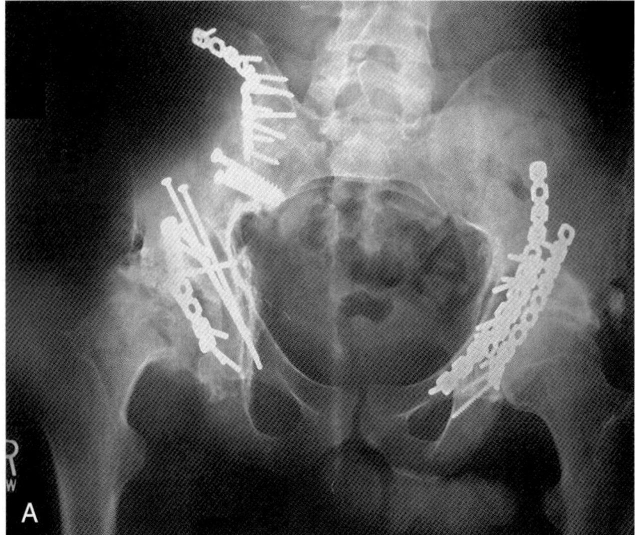

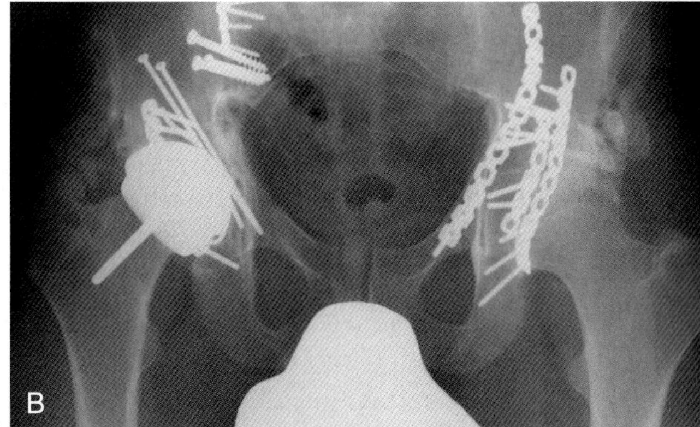

Figure 15-5 A, Anteroposterior pelvis radiograph of a 25-year-old man with osteoarthritis of the right hip, secondary to a previous fracture and dislocation. The acetabular and pelvic fractures were fixed with recon plates and screws. **B,** Anteroposterior pelvis radiograph 78 months postoperatively following metal-on-metal resurfacing. Three screws were removed during surgery to accommodate the seating of the acetabular component, and acetabular defects were bone grafted.

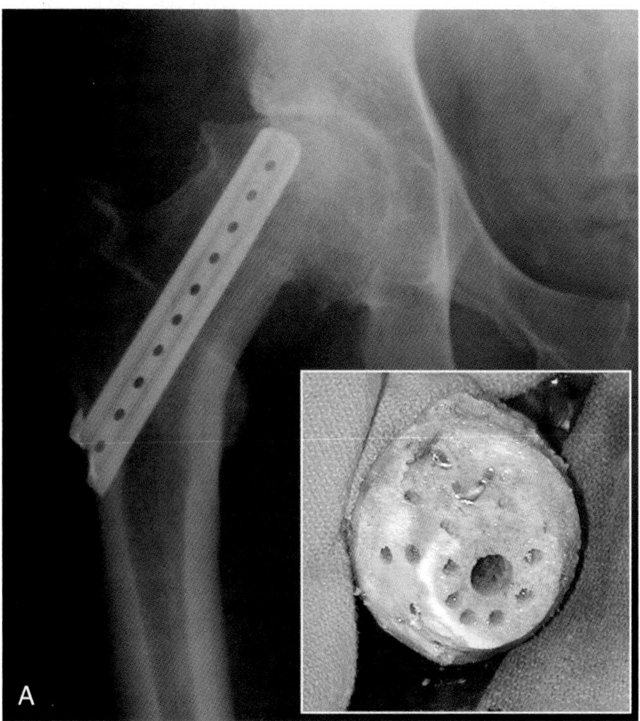

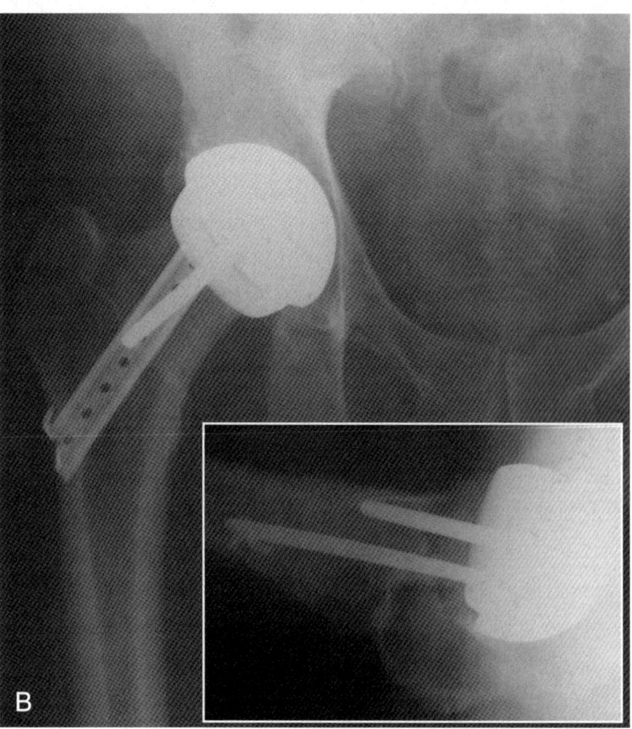

Figure 15-6 **A,** Anteroposterior radiograph of a 52-year-old man with post-traumatic osteoarthritis and in situ Thompson Z-nail. The insert shows an intraoperative photograph of the femoral head after preparation and the burred protruding nail to allow seating of the femoral component. **B,** The patient is shown 7 years after surgery. The metaphyseal stem of the femoral component was inserted anteriorly compared with the retained hardware and oriented on a posterior to anterior axis to parallel the path of the Z-nail.

were 4 for pain, 6 for walking and function, and 5 for activity. His range of motion was restricted with 115 degrees of flexion and a 5-degree contracture, 20 degrees of abduction-adduction arc and 20 degrees of rotation. It was elected to leave the nail in situ and insert the pin to guide the reamers a sufficient distance from it in order to preserve space for the metaphyseal stem. It was necessary to burr the prominence, which would have interfered with the femoral component seating. With a follow-up of 7 years, the UCLA scores are 10 for pain, walking, and function, and 8 for activity.

Conversions to Total Hip Replacement

In this series, there was one conversion to THR in a 29-year-old electrician who was resurfaced with first-generation technique (hip #156 in our overall series). The large cyst (>3 cm) extended into the cylindrical area of the component. This risk factor would dictate stem cementation today. The patient did well initially, but the femoral component loosened 29 months after surgery (Fig. 15-7).

In addition, one patient (hip #105) had a radiographically loose femoral component at his last visit (19 months), but was lost to follow-up because he was deported.

Using revision for any cause as an endpoint, the Kaplan-Meier survivorship results at 7 years for this group of patients was 95.8% (95% confidence interval, 73.9 to 99.4).

Complications

There were two complications in this series (4.9%). One dislocation occurred in a 59-year-old patient who had a contralateral hip disarticulation. A double socket reconstruction was necessary because of the cavernous acetabulum (the superfix socket was not available at that time). The socket was excessively open laterally (72 degrees for the Conserve+ inside shell, 67 degrees for the Interference PSR shell). He dislocated his hip in the postoperative period at home, but has remained stable after closed reduction.

There was one case of postoperative sepsis described earlier in a 44-year-old machinist who had a tight skin closure due to a large, soft tissue defect anterior in the hip area. He required débridement, antibiotics, and a plastic surgery flap to cover the defect area (see Fig. 15-3). It would have been preferable in this case to have had plastic surgery consultation in advance so that the flap transfer could be performed before hip resurfacing or at the same time to minimize the risk of wound problems.

Summary

The results in this group of patients are comparable to those of primary osteoarthritis despite a higher incidence of previous surgeries and prior muscle damage. Both failures occurred

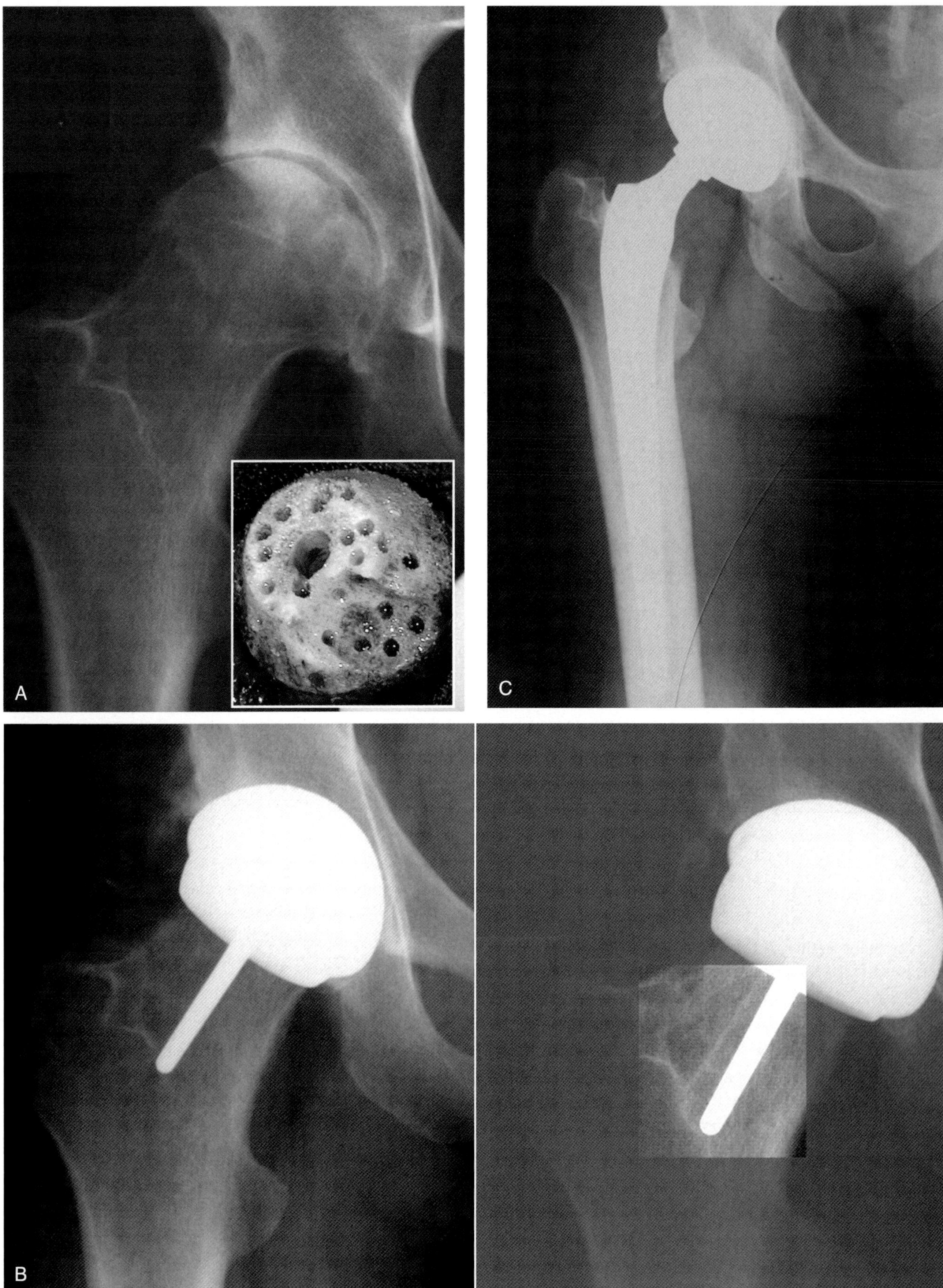

Figure 15-7 A, Anteroposterior radiograph of a 28-year-old man with osteoarthritis of the right hip, secondary to trauma. Insert shows the femoral head after preparation for resurfacing. Notice the large cyst that extends into the cylindrical area. **B,** On the left, the patient is 3 months postoperative metal-on-metal resurfacing. The right radiograph shows the components 29 months after surgery. The large radiolucency around the metaphyseal stem is indicative of loosening and migration of the femoral component. **C,** (Top right) Radiograph at 38 months following conversion to a total hip replacement. Only the femoral component was revised to an anthropometric total hip (ATH) long-stem grit-blasted size 11 and a 50-mm Big Femoral Head matching the well-fixed Conserve® Plus socket.

early in our series with first generation femoral bone preparation and fixation techniques. Fifteen other hips (13 men and two women) were operated on with first-generation femoral head preparation techniques that have a follow-up of 7 to 10 years. A lower prevalence of cyst formation and large component size were the balancing favorable factors that enabled good initial fixation of the femoral component. There have been no such complications in the past 8 years, with no revision pending.

References

1. Matta J: Fractures of the acetabulum: accuracy of reduction and clinical results in patients managed operatively within three weeks after the injury. J Bone Joint Surg Am 1996;78:1632-1645.
2. Bhandari M, Matta J, Ferguson T, Matthys G: Predictors of clinical and radiological outcome in patients with fractures of the acetabulum and concomitant posterior dislocation of the hip. J Bone Joint Surg Br 2006;88:1618-1624.
3. John T, Stahel P, Morgan S, Schulze-Tanzil G: Impact of the complement cascade on posttraumatic cartilage inflammation and degradation. Histol Histopathol 2007;22:781-790.
4. Bonfiglio M, Bardenstein M: Treatment by bone-grafting of aseptic necrosis of the femoral head and non-union of the femoral neck (Phemister technique). J Bone Joint Surg Am 1958; 40-A:1329-1346.
5. Weber M, Berry D, Harmsen W: Total hip arthroplasty after operative treatment of an acetabular fracture. J Bone Joint Surg Am 1998;80:1295-1305.
6. Berry D, Halasy M: Uncemented acetabular components for arthritis after acetabular fracture. Clin Orthop Relat Res 2002; 405:164-167.
7. Cuckler J: Dealing with post-traumatic arthrosis of the hip. Orthopedics 2001;24:867-868.

CHAPTER 16

Rheumatoid Arthritis and Related Disorders

Harlan C. Amstutz

Michel J. Le Duff

Introduction

Because the indications for hip resurfacing for rheumatoid disorders may be more controversial than for other etiologies, considerable background material is herewith provided. Rheumatoid arthritis (RA) is a chronic, inflammatory systemic disease, at times remitting, but if it continues, it usually results in progressive joint destruction and deformity. The many extra-articular features of neuropathy, rheumatoid nodules, pleurisy, pericarditis, lymphadenopathy, and splenomegaly occur with varying frequency and emphasize the systemic nature. Although the etiology of this disease is still unknown, the susceptibility to most rheumatic diseases is strongly influenced by human leukocyte antigens (HLAs).

The radiographic signs of RA of the hip depend on the clinical activity and the stage of the disease. Classically, the involvement is bilateral and symmetric, although recently we have observed more cases with predominately unilateral involvement. Loss of joint space due to loss of articular cartilage from both the femoral head and the acetabulum and some degree of osteoporosis may be the earliest and most reliable signs. Next the femoral head may be noted to migrate either axially or superiorly due to progressive loss of articular cartilage. Later a protrusio acetabuli may develop. Erosions and cysts develop usually in the subchondral bone and are present more often in the femoral head, but they are also observed in the acetabulum representing the invasion of pannus tissue. In general the rheumatoid hip shows evidence of an inflammatory disease, with the joint not having a capacity to repair itself. Osteophytes, the hallmark of osteoarthritis, are not classically observed.

In time, acetabular sclerosis and small osteophytes may appear, but bony ankylosis of the hip joint is rare. Occasionally, osteonecrosis of the femoral head may be seen in rheumatoid patients who have received high doses of corticosteroids.

Total hip arthroplasty has been successful in relieving pain and improving function in most patients with RA, with some having achieved lifetime durability. Others have required revision with varying results.[1] Hip arthroplasty for patients with RA presents a particular challenge because the bone quality is diminished secondary to osteopenia and bone resorption. On the other hand, these patients are generally much less active than other patients because of multiple joint involvement and the associated systemic disabilities caused by this disease. Patients with RA may also have an increased incidence of delayed wound healing, sepsis, and general overall complications due to their disease and their drug treatment. Juvenile RA (JRA) occurs in children and adolescence and, like the adult form, has a varying degree of severity and pleomorphism.

Fortunately, medical treatment today is much more successful in minimizing severe manifestations of RA and its inherent disabilities than in the past so that the numbers of patients requiring a hip arthroplasty have diminished. However, when the degree of hip pain significantly interferes with sleeping or the activities of daily living, then arthroplasty should be considered. The decision for resurfacing or total hip replacement (THR) is based on the experience of the surgeon, who realizes that there may be an increased risk of neck fracture after resurfacing due to relative osteopenia or osteporosis. This chapter also includes a discussion of ankylosing spondylitis (AS).

Evaluation of the Rheumatoid Patient for Hip Replacement Surgery

Hematologic Factors

Most rheumatoid patients show a normocytic or normochromic anemia of moderate degree that is usually associated with low serum iron and a normal or low iron-binding capacity.

Patients with significant anemia may not be able to donate blood for autologous transfusions. Some patients have Felty syndrome (a chronic RA associated with splenomegaly and leukopenia) and a splenectomy may rarely be advised for some to obtain a reversal of the neutropenia.

Infections

RA patients who take glucocorticoids are more susceptible to infections than RA patients who were not taking such medications. Furthermore, they are more susceptible to multiple infections. Poss et al[2] concluded that the incidence of sepsis in RA patients is 1.8 times that of osteoarthritic patients.

Drugs

Although high-dose oral corticosteroid treatment for RA is rarely used today, some patients still receive prednisone at a dose of more than 10 mg per day.

Other patients receive immunosuppressive therapy. Such drugs may depress the patients' bone marrow, causing abnormal blood counts. Patients who have received corticosteroids within a few years of their surgery may not be able to increase their normal corticosteroid response to the stress of surgery, and they should receive booster doses of corticosteroids perioperatively, which are then tapered to their baseline dose.

Other Extra-articular Factors

Rheumatoid patients have a fragile atrophic skin that is easily traumatized; thus, ecchymoses are frequently seen as are skin ulcerations. Vasculitis also occurs in some RA patients, and large ischemic ulcers may develop in the lower legs. In such patients, it may be wise to obtain Doppler flow studies preoperatively.

Involvement of the Cervical Spine

Cervical spine involvement in a patient with RA is common, and it must be evaluated in all patients requiring a general anesthetic given by endotracheal intubation. Standard roentgenograms of the cervical spine should be obtained, as should an open-mouth frontal projection and a lateral view in flexion and extension, assessing the stability of the cervical spine.

Subluxation of 6 to 7 mm mandates a careful neurologic examination. This subluxation is variable and must be dealt with on an individual basis. Additional studies, such as computed tomography (CT) and magnetic resonance imaging (MRI) scans, are also helpful for evaluating these patients. Some RA patients and most JRA patients have a stiff cervical spine, and some will have limited jaw motion as well. Such patients may require nasotracheal intubation.

Ankylosing Spondylitis

AS is a seronegative spondyloarthropathy that has a variety of clinical and pathologic features. Although it is now universally recognized as a distinct and separate entity from RA, these patients are included here because of their traditional relationship.

There is an increased rate of occurrence of the histocompatibility antigen HLA-B27 in patients with AS (as in 90% of white patients with AS). There is more equal balance between men and women, but a higher rate of clinical expression in men.

The most important clinical criteria to establish the diagnosis of AS are

1. The clinical history of low back pain
2. The limitation of chest expansion and back motion on physical examination
3. The radiographic severity of sacroiliitis

Typically, the age of onset of clinical symptoms is during the late 20s. Because of the inflammatory nature of the condition, it is frequently associated with morning stiffness that improves over the course of the day and with exercise. Low-grade fever, weight loss, and fatigue may be accompanying signs. Patients sometimes complain of tenderness at the points of insertion of major muscles to bone and at major ligamentous attachments.

Loss of spinal mobility and progressive lumbar lordosis are also typical of AS. Medical management is crucial in preventing severe kyphosis, which often required spinal osteotomy in the past. Late involvement of the cervical spine can be associated with a fixed flexion deformity, C1-C2 subluxation or dislocation, and in severe cases neurologic symptoms similar to those seen with RA (e.g., the cauda equine syndrome).

Ankylosis or subluxation of the temporomandibular joint can be common, but peripheral involvement tends to involve the larger joints of the lower extremities and is frequently asymmetric. Progressive limitation of motion at the costovertebral joints leads to progressive loss of chest expansion. Restriction of motion to less than 2.5 cm can decrease vital capacity and compromise pulmonary function significantly.

Technical Considerations

Previously, a transtrochanteric approach was preferred in surgery to avoid undue manipulative force, which may fracture the weakened bone. However, most can be mobilized and dislocated carefully by the posterior approach. Often, the femoral intramedullary canal has a "stove pipe" appearance with straight lateral walls.

The occurrence of heterotopic bone formation following THR in these patients has been a major concern. Yet a review of the literature on this subject and a careful analysis of our own patients suggests that the occurrence rate of heterotopic bone formation is not significantly greater than that observed following THR in male patients who have osteoarthritis. Those who have developed clinically significant heterotopic bone following one hip operation are at high risk to do so again after hip surgery on the contralateral hip or repeat surgery on the same hip. We recommend some form of prophylactic treatment, such as indomethacin or low-dose radiation therapy, to prevent the formation of heterotopic bone.

Total Hip Replacement in Rheumatoid Arthritis

Because some surgeons regard resurfacing as contraindicated in patients with RA, it is important to review our experience and relevant literature with THR. Comparable results have been reported with THR either with cemented[3-5] or cementless devices,[6] and Kirk and associates[7] did not find any midterm difference in clinical scores or implant fixation between these two options. Interestingly, a recent article by Eskelinen and coworkers[8] highlights better results of cemented cups versus cementless acetabular components in young patients with RA, and concludes that proximally porous-coated stems and all polyethylene cemented cups should be the implants of choice for these patients.

Cemented Total Hip Replacement

In a University of California-Los Angeles (UCLA) series reported by Severt et al,[9] satisfactory results were obtained in 88% of the hips replaced, with significant improvement in pain, walking, and function. The average age was 49.9 years (range, 17 to 73 years) at the time of the index operation with a follow-up averaging 7.4 years (range, 4 to 14 years).

The revision rate for aseptic loosening was 7% (four acetabular implants and one femoral implant). Our radiographic analysis indicated that another 13% were at risk to loosen (six acetabular implants, three femoral implants, and one hip with both sides showing loosening). Because of the restriction of activities imposed by this systemic disease, these patients had not become symptomatic enough to request a revision arthroplasty. We noted that some of the RA patients who were young and heavy showed increased evidence of loosening. Other published results suggest a higher incidence of cup versus stem loosening.[10]

Deep sepsis occurred in 5.3% of patients who had THR, with one occurring early and three late. Hematogenous infection occurred in hips on an average of 4.9 years postoperatively. Additionally, wound healing problems occurred in 19%, with one developing deep sepsis. Two RA patients in our THR series initially had successful bilateral conventional THR and total knee replacement but eventually required removal of all of the implants because of hematogenous sepsis. Fortunately, similar observations have not been made in recent years, perhaps due to better medical follow-up including infectious disease consultants and surgical management. However, other authors have suggested an increased susceptibility to operative and postoperative hematogenous sepsis and an increased difficulty in eradication of infection.

Cementless Total Hip Replacement

Because of the known failure rate of implants fixed with acrylic cement, cementless implants have advanced and have been increasingly successful. Cracchiolo and associates[11] analyzed 40 primary THRs in 34 patients with RA disease using first-generation cementless implants (Harris-Galante [HG], porous coated anatomic [PCA], and anatomic modular locking [AML]) at a 2- to 6-year follow-up.

The overall clinical results were good in this group, although the thigh pain incidence was 7.5%. Only one patient with a femoral fracture had radiolucencies in three of seven femoral zones. Moreover, radiolucent and sclerotic lines developed around areas of porous coating in only one hip and in another patient with an intraoperative femoral fracture with subsequent subsidence of 10 mm. The acetabular implants also appeared to be stable, and only rarely were radiolucencies and sclerotic lines seen (13%).

Recently Effenberger et al[6] reported on 70 longer term, very successful results using second-generation, cementless, double-wedge taper titanium stem designs with either a threaded socket or HG socket with a 1- to 10-year follow-up (mean of 49 months). They did not report on their thigh pain incidence. One socket was revised, and there was one serious femoral fracture. There were three dislocations. Both socket and the stem appeared to be osseointegrated, with some showing severe remodeling changes around the stem but without midterm consequences.

Total Hip Replacement in Patients with Protrusio Acetabulae

Before the availability of porous ingrowth acetabular components, we designed a special protrusio polyethylene socket in order to restore hip biomechanics by lateralizing the acetabulum component without the use of excessive acrylic cement. Cracchiolo and colleagues[1] reviewed our experience with patients who had protrusio acetabuli and found fewer radiolucencies with the protrusio socket at an average of 3 years (range, 2 to 8 years).

Nonetheless, bone grafting and the use of porous ingrowth components is the current treatment of choice for patients with these difficult acetabulum reconstructions. Although patients with protrusio sockets appeared to do better overall than those operated on using regular acetabular implants and thick acrylic cement, a comparable study has not been done with cementless sockets.

Hip Resurfacing

Because many patients with RA of the hip requiring arthroplasty are young, we implanted The Total Hip Articular Replacement with Internal Eccentric Shells (THARIES, Zimmer, Warsaw, IN) prostheses in our early experience. Survivorship at 6 years was approximately 75%, and the failures were mostly due to aseptic acetabular loosening. A few of these hips survived beyond 15 years in patients who were less active. We performed seven porous in-growth surface replacements with titanium alloy femoral components. Like the results with other etiologies, cementless sockets outperformed those that were cemented, but wear debris–induced osteolysis became a more significant problem on the femoral side. However, there was sufficient promise with our resurfacing experience that if fixation could be improved and osteolysis from debris reduced or eliminated with the metal-on-metal (MM) bearing, successful long-term durability would become more realistic.

Indications for Metal-on-Metal Hybrid Metal-on-Metal Hip Resurfacing

Although many patients do well with THR because of anticipated low overall activity so that wear consequences may not be a problem with current bearing materials, the risk of sepsis in the immune-compromised patient makes resurfacing an attractive alternative because a septic joint that does not involve the intramedullary canal is more easily and possibly more successively treated. There are also the other advantages to resurfacing, such as a more precise anatomical replacement without leg-length inequality, a physiologic loading of the metaphysis and diaphysis with absence of stress shielding, and the greater stability with the large ball size.

Technical Features

It is of utmost importance to be careful in bone preparation because generally there is some degree of osteopenia in the femoral neck and acetabulum. There are often small miliary cysts in the dome area of the femoral head and acetabulum. Fortunately, these are generally removed with the normal head and socket preparation. The incidence of large cyst degeneration is less than with other etiologies. When the head-neck ratio is large, the risk of violation of the lateral cortex is less, and the stem-shaft valgus may be increased more than 140 degrees to lessen forces on the neck, especially in cases with osteopenia. Figure 16-1 shows the case of a 37-year-old woman, a teacher, who developed JRA at the age of 2. She became disabled initially because of her right hip and subsequently 6 years later because of the left hip. She is now 10 and 7 years post MM resurfacing with Conserve®Plus. She has multiple joint arthropathy and is a Charnley class C patient. Her current UCLA hip scores are pain right 9, pain left 8, walking 7, function 6, activity 5. She has 110 degrees of flexion, 70 degrees of abduction-adduction arc, and 60 degrees of rotation arc. Her last Harris hip scores were 72 for the right hip and 62 for the left. The patient is taking Enbrel, Plaquenil, and Ecotrin and had right-hand metacarpal-phalangeal (MP) replacements and has bilateral knee involvement. On the preoperative radiograph, the apparent neck shaft angle (NSA) on the right was 160 degrees, on the left, 155 degrees, but the externally rotated position of the femur certainly inflates those figures. Postoperatively, the stem-shaft angle (SSA) was 145 degrees for the right hip and 155 degrees for the left.

With hips in patients with AS, it is important to make sure that the capsule is released posteriorly, and as far as possible superiorly and inferiorly to lessen the trauma associated with the dislocation of the hip. A 35-year-old male ferry operator with bilateral inflammatory AS was treated with MM resurfacing (Fig. 16-2). Preoperatively, the patient had 105 degrees of flexion with a 20-degree flexion contracture, 45 degrees of abduction-adduction arc, and 45 degrees of rotation arc. His UCLA hip scores were 4, 7, 7, and 5 for pain, walking, function, and activity, respectively. He had single-stage bilateral hip resurfacing and has been pain free for 9 years. His UCLA scores for both hips are 10, 10, 10, and 6.

Patient Demographics (4/05/07)

From our series of 1000 hips (838 patients), 17 hips (13 patients) received a Conserve®Plus resurfacing for arthritis secondary to rheumatoid disease.

The average age of the patients was 35.3 years (range, 16 to 47 years). Surprisingly, most of the patients were male (9/13, 69.2%). Five hips had an etiology of inflammatory AS, four JRA, and 8 RA. No hips had undergone any surgery before resurfacing.

The patients were very young and lightweight, and all but two had multiple arthropathy (Charnley Class C) at the time of surgery and all but one at the last follow-up. The demographics of this group of patients are shown in Table 16-1.

The incidence of cystic degeneration was considerably lower than that observed with any other etiology, with none after bone preparation in the nine male patients. The femoral head size was also smaller, with an average of 43.5 mm (range, 36 to 52 mm). The stem was not cemented in for the first nine hips but was cemented in the last eight hips.

Results

Clinical Scores

Their average UCLA hip scores all improved significantly ($P < .001$) between preoperative and their last follow-up visit. The average follow-up was 6.4 years, with a range of 1.5 to 10 years. The outcomes were comparable to our overall series as far as pain relief, walking, and function, whereas the activity level and physical component of the Short Form-12 (SF-12) was less. The pain score increased from 2.9 ± 1.0 to 9.6 ± 0.6, the walking score from 5.9 ± 1.4 to 9.5 ± 1.2, the function score from 5.1 ± 1.5 to 9.3 ± 1.6, and the activity score from 4.1 ± 1.2 to 6.7 ± 1.5. The average physical component was 28.3 ± 5.1 preoperatively and 43.8 ± 11.2 at the last follow-up ($P = .002$), and the mental component increased from 43.0 ± 12.7 to 50.6 ± 9.1 ($P = .021$). The postoperative Harris hip score was 92.3 ± 12.0. The average pain, walking, and function scores were comparable to those of our overall cohort, whereas the activity score was lower ($P = .0455$). The average SF-12 physi-

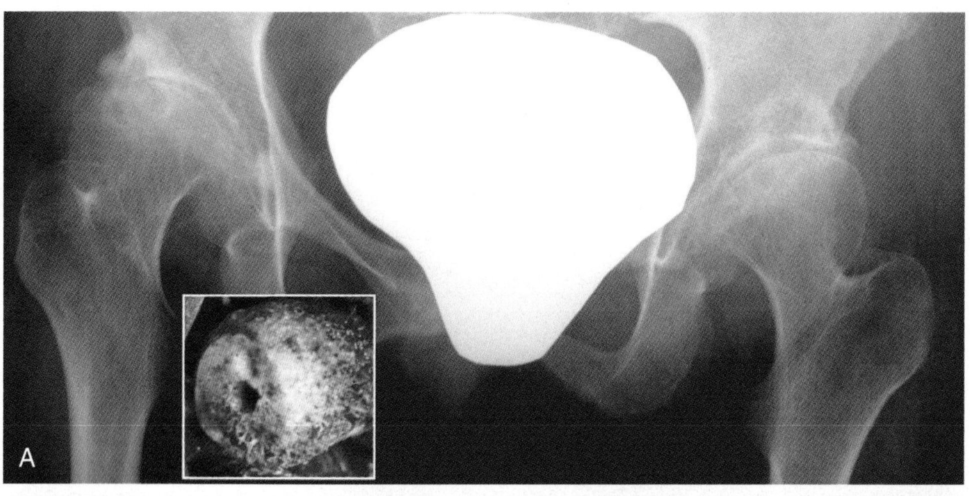

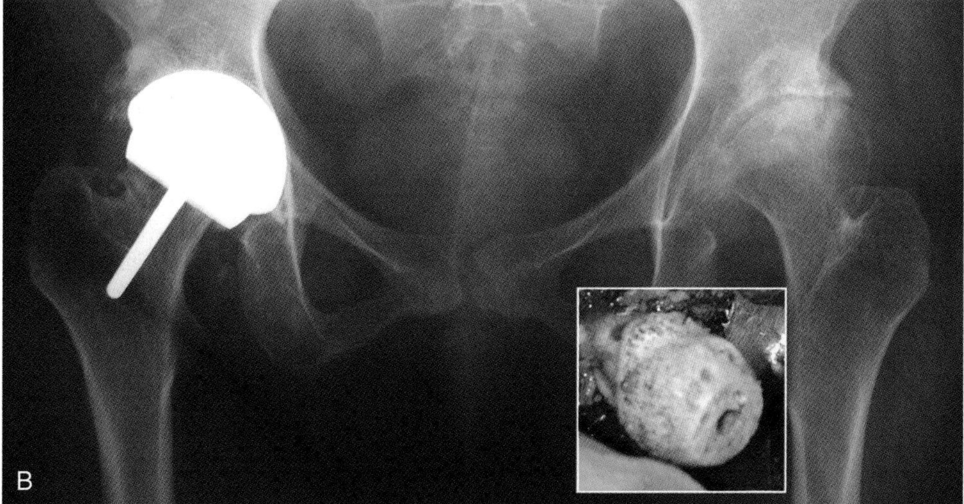

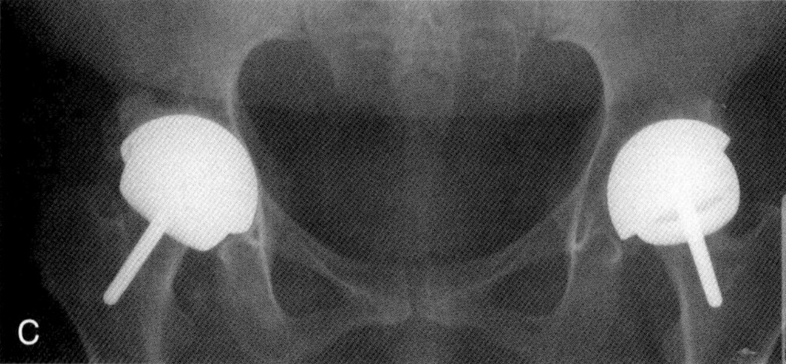

Figure 16-1 **A,** A 37-year-old female patient with bilateral osteoarthritis of the hip, secondary to juvenile rheumatoid arthritis; the right hip with more severe disease than the left. The insert shows the right femoral head after preparation for resurfacing. Note the osteopenia inferiorly. **B,** Thirty-four months following metal-on-metal hip resurfacing on the right, the left hip disease has progressed and is to undergo the same procedure. Insert shows the prepared femoral head with one small cyst and some reamed bone posteriorly, which was not entirely covered by the component. **C,** The patient is shown 7 years postoperatively on the right and 4 years on the left. Her University of California-Los Angeles hip scores are pain right 9, left 8, walking 7, function 6, and activity 5.

Table 16-1 Demographics of the Patients Operated for Osteoarthritis Secondary to Rheumatoid Disease

	Men	Women	Combined
Age (years)	37.8 (27–47)	29.2 (16–39)	35.3 (16–47)
Weight (kg)	78.5 (55–105)	66.4 (47–80)	74.9 (47–105)
Height (cm)	174.8 (160–187)	165.8 (164–168)	172.1 (160–187)
BMI	25.5 (20.2–30.0)	24.1 (17.5–28.3)	25.1 (17.5–30.0)
Femoral component size (mm)	45.5 (42–52)	38.8 (36–42)	43.5 (36–52)
Cysts >1 cm	0 (0.0%)	2 (40.0%)	2 (11.8%)
Charnley class (at surgery)			
A	1 (11.1%)	1 (25.0%)	2 (15.4%)
B	0 (0.0%)	0 (0.0%)	0 (0.0%)
C	8 (88.9%)	3 (75.0%)	11 (84.6%)

BMI, body mass index.

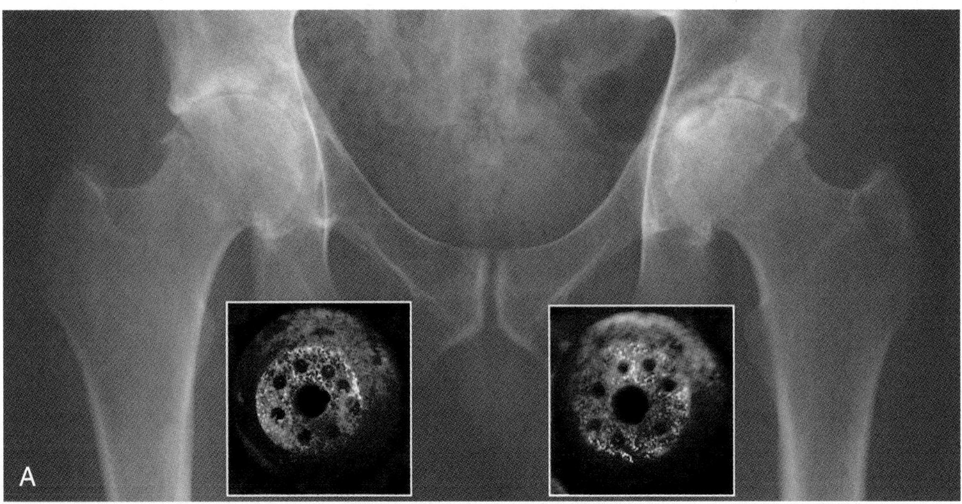

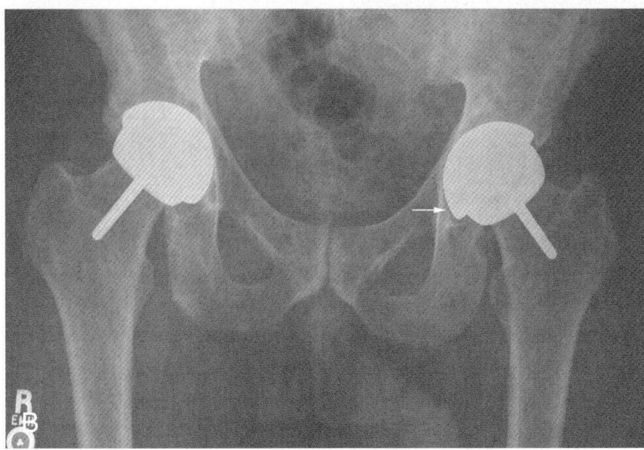

Figure 16-2 A, Anteroposterior radiograph of a 35-year-old man with bilateral inflammatory ankylosing spondylitis. The inserts show the femoral heads after preparation (first-generation technique, hips #65 and #66 in the overall series). The bone quality was good, and only a few drilled holes in the dome have been sufficient for long-term durability of the fixation. **B,** The patient is shown 9 years postoperatively, following bilateral single-stage metal-on-metal hip resurfacing. Fixation of all components is secure. There is a small radiolucency at the bone-acetabular component interface, in the inferior aspect of Charnley and De Lee Zone 3.

Table 16-2 Summary of Range-of-motion Measurements

	PRE FLX	Flexion Contracture	Abd	Add	Rot Arc	LFU FLX	Flexion Contracture	Abd	Add	Rot Arc
Whole 1000	105.6	16.2	23.2	14.5	23.5	125.9	1.9	45.2	27.9	76.6
Rheumatoids	99.5	20.5	16.2	10.2	17.1	124.8	0.0	42.2	27.7	70.0
Others	105.8	16.0	23.4	14.7	23.7	125.9	1.9	45.2	27.9	76.7
P	0.050	0.081	0.007	0.018	0.074	0.669	0.087	0.087	0.886	0.076

Abd, abduction; Add, adduction; LFU FLX, last follow-up flexion; PRE FLX, preoperative flexion; Rot, rotation.

cal scores were lower ($P = .0044$), reflecting the high percentage of Charnley B and C patients, but the scores improved by a comparable margin from pre- to postoperative scores.

Range of Motion

Table 16-2 presents a summary of the range-of-motion measurements for this group of patients. The flexion, abduction, and adduction were significantly reduced preoperatively. However the postoperative range-of-motion measurements were not different for this group compared with the rest of the cohort. A 23-year-old patient with AS recently underwent hip resurfacing. He had only a jog of motion (<5 degrees) and a 65-degree flexion contracture, and now has near-complete range of motion at short follow-up.

Conversions to Total Hip Replacement

In this series, there were two conversions to THR. The first was a 32-year-old woman with RA who had articular erosions and a moderate protrusio (Fig. 16-3). Her pain, walking, function, and activity scores were 2, 4, 4, and 2, respectively. She was doing well (UCLA scores of 10 for pain, walking, and function, and 8 for activity) when she developed a late hematogenous sepsis at 36 months after resurfacing. The treatment was delayed for 1 month after the symptoms occurred. At surgery, although the femoral component seemed well fixed, some granulation tissue was found under the rim and it would have been impossible to perform a thorough débridement without removing the component.

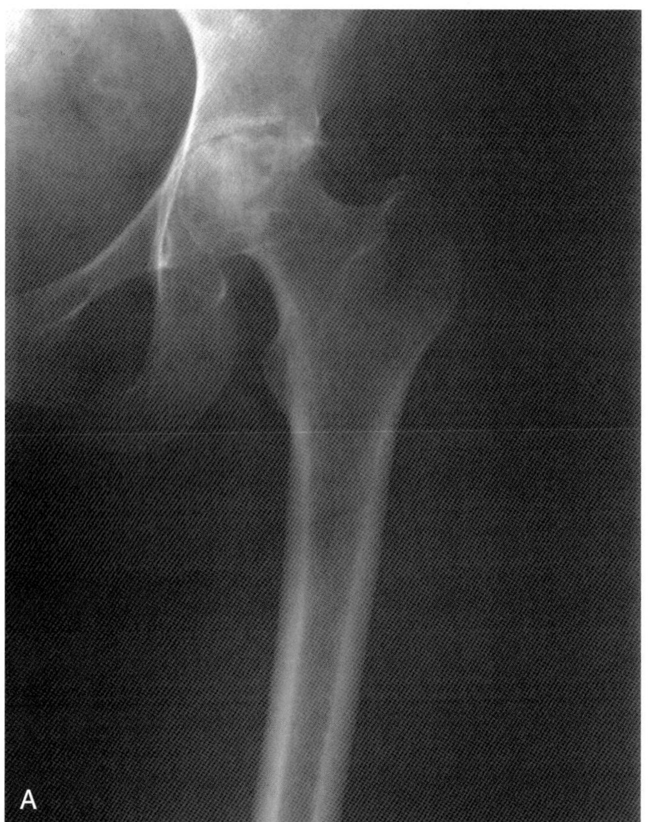

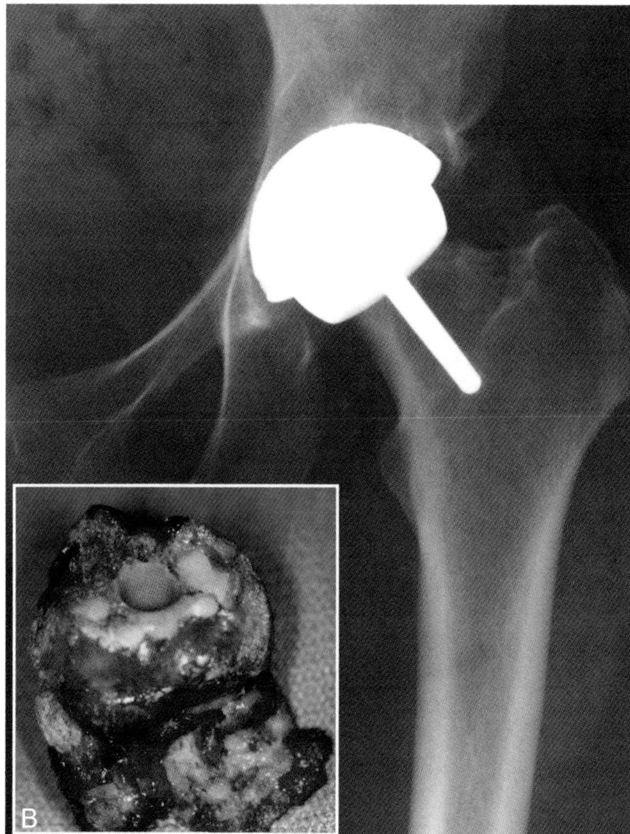

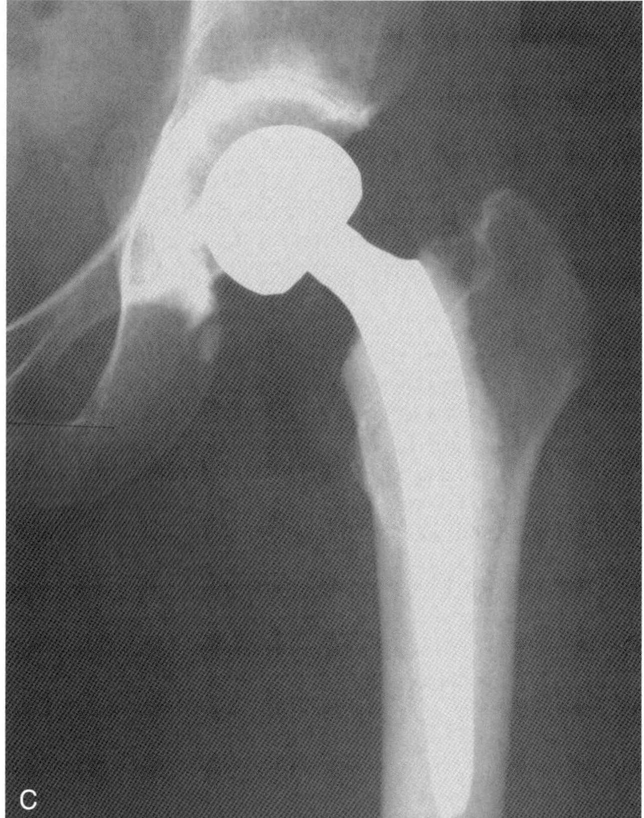

Figure 16-3 **A,** A 31-year-old woman with protrusio of the left hip secondary to rheumatoid disease and subsequent osteoarthritis. Note the cystic erosions and the "geode" in the neck. **B,** Thirty-six months after resurfacing the patient developed a late hematogenous sepsis. At surgery, some granulation tissue was found under the rim of the well-fixed femoral component and could be pried off without too much bone destruction (*insert*). **C,** The total hip replacement was a direct exchange using a cemented cross-linked polyethylene acetabular component (Longevity, Zimmer, Warsaw, IN), a cemented stem (CTN, Kinamed, Newbury Park, CA) with a 36-mm cobalt-chromium ball with antibiotics (Vancomycin) mixed in the acrylic.

After thorough débridement it was elected to convert the hip to a THR in a direct exchange, using a cemented stem (CTN, Kinamed, Newbury Park, CA) with a 36-mm cobalt-chromium ball. In addition to antibiotics (vancomycin) mixed in the acrylic, she had a 6-week course of intravenous antibiotics (ceftriaxone [Rocephin]). She is currently 5 years post-conversion to THR. Her hip scores are 10, 10, 10, and 6 for pain, walking, function, and activity, respectively.

The other revision was performed outside our control in a patient with AS at 43 months, and it was presumed to be secondary to loosening of the femoral component. Unfortunately, the patient did not have serial follow-ups, and we did not receive the specimen, so the exact cause is unknown. None of the remaining hips in any of the patients show any radiolucency about the metaphyseal femoral stem, indicating enduring good fixation.

There are no apparent differences in survivorship with the other etiologies, but the size of the sample (n = 17) is too small to provide a meaningful Kaplan-Meier survivorship analysis.

Complications

There have been no neck fractures or no other intra- or post-operative complications in this series.

Discussion

There is one published short-term report of 20 resurfacings in 17 patients with an average follow-up of 3 years (range, 1 to 5 years) with the hybrid Cormet 2000 device (Corin Medical, Cirencester, UK). One 27-year-old female patient sustained a neck fracture 1 year postoperatively, but the others were reported to be doing well as reflected by an average postoperative Harris hip score of 89.[12]

There have been no neck fractures in this series despite varying degrees of osteopenia. All of the components were pressed into the seated final position by hand pressure on the component (see Technique in Chapter 7). Similarly, but at longer follow-up, our series does not show any predisposition of rheumatoid patients for a higher revision rate due to loosening than other etiologies with MM hybrid resurfacing. In fact, even with the first-generation technique, the fixation achieved has been durable despite a smaller femoral component size. Possible explanations for the initial and enduring fixation include the very low incidence of cystic disease and lower postoperative activity scores. Although THR performs well in the majority of RA patients, a definite advantage goes to resurfacing versus any kind of THR because of the young age of this patient population (average 35.3 years in our series), its conservative nature, and the normal loading of the proximal femur avoiding stress shielding. As expected, the postoperative activity level of these patients on average does not match that of other etiologies. This can be explained by a lifestyle that is often altered by the disease long before a surgical solution is needed.

Summary

Our results justify continuing to perform hip resurfacing in RA. With the increased susceptibility of sepsis in these patients, it is beneficial not to invade the femoral canal. With one failure in a patient with AS and although our experience now consists of five patients and six hips, this sample is too small to warrant any conclusions regarding safety and efficacy of the procedure at this time. We continue to conduct implant surgery in all groups but are extremely careful with our intraoperative technique.

References

1. Cracchiolo A: Rheumatoid arthritis. In Amstutz HC (ed): Hip Arthroplasty. New York, Churchill Livingstone, 1991, pp 745-765.
2. Poss R, Maloney J, Ewald F, Thomas W, Batte N, Hartness C, Sledge C: Six- to 11-year results of total hip arthroplasty in rheumatoid arthritis. Clin Orthop Relat Res 1984;182:109-116.
3. Chmell M, Scott R, Thomas W, Sledge C: Total hip arthroplasty with cement for juvenile rheumatoid arthritis. Results at a minimum of ten years in patients less than thirty years old. J Bone Joint Surg Am 1997;79:44-52.
4. Lehtimaki M, Lehto M, Kautiainen H, Lehtinen K, Hamalainen M: Charnley total hip arthroplasty in ankylosing spondylitis: survivorship analysis of 76 patients followed for 8-28 years. Acta Orthop Scand 2001;72:233-236.
5. Lehtimaki M, Kautiainen H, Lehto U, Hamalainen M: Charnley low-friction arthroplasty in rheumatoid patients: a survival study up to 20 years. J Arthroplasty 1999;14:657-661.
6. Effenberger H, Ramsauer T, Bohm G, Hilzensauer G, Dorn U, Lintner F: Successful hip arthroplasty using cementless titanium implants in rheumatoid arthritis. Arch Orthop Trauma Surg 2002;122:80-87.
7. Kirk P, Rorabeck C, Bourne R, Burkart B: Total hip arthroplasty in rheumatoid arthritis: comparison of cemented and uncemented implants. Can J Surg 1993;36:229-232.
8. Eskelinen A, Paavolainen P, Helenius I, Pulkkinen P, Remes V: Total hip arthroplasty for rheumatoid arthritis in younger patients: 2,557 replacements in the Finnish Arthroplasty Register followed for 0-24 years. Acta Orthop 2006;77:853-865.
9. Severt R, Wood R, Cracchiolo A, Amstutz H: Long-term follow-up of cemented total hip arthroplasty in rheumatoid arthritis. Clin Orthop Relat Res 1991;265:137-145.
10. Onsten I, Bengner U, Besjakov J: Socket migration after Charnley arthroplasty in rheumatoid arthritis and osteoarthritis. A roentgen stereophotogrammetric study. J Bone Joint Surg Br 1993;75:677-680.
11. Cracchiolo A, Severt R, Moreland J: Uncemented total hip arthroplasty in rheumatoid arthritis diseases. A two- to six-year follow-up study. Clin Orthop Relat Res 1992;277:166-174.
12. Abdel Shafi T, El Koussy N, El Said A, Zafaan S: Resurfacing hip arthroplasty in rheumatoid arthritis. Med J Cairo Univ 2006;74:77-84.

CHAPTER 17

Hip Resurfacing for Other Conditions and Etiologies

Harlan C. Amstutz

Michel J. Le Duff

Introduction

This chapter's purpose is to highlight less common etiologies or diagnoses that we have encountered during the course of the various series studied and reviewed in this book, some of which constitute special indications for hip resurfacing and were previously mentioned as such in Chapter 8. The present chapter also discusses diagnostic techniques, suitability, surgical technique, and results for each of these conditions.

Melorheostosis

Melorheostosis is a rare form of hyperostosis characterized by a linear pattern distributed along major axes of bones. It was initially described by Leri and Joanny[1a] because of the pattern's appearance that resembled melting wax dripping down one side of a candle. The disease is usually in the long bones, but it is not always monomelic. It can involve any bone in the body. It tends to progress more quickly during childhood and less quickly in adult life. The extent of the involvement may be monostotic, polyostotic, or monomelic, or more rarely, it may include limbs and trunk. The affected extremity may be shorter or, less frequently, longer than normal, but usually larger in circumference, angulated or curved.

The patient seeks medical attention for relief of pain, stiffness, limitation of joint motion, or deformity. The pain is present in almost every patient ranging from a dull ache to a sharp and penetrating pain, which is constant, rarely severe, and often aggravated by activity. The location of pain is usually over the affected bone or joint and occasionally radiates along the extremity. The joints are often restricted in motion as a result of contracture and fibrosis in the soft tissues on the extremity. Extension of the bone abnormality can be found into the joint, including periarticular masses of ectopic bone and deformity of the articular surface or nonspecific synovitis. Osteoarthritis was not mentioned in the excellent review of this malady by Campbell et al.[1] There are no reports of a hip joint replacement having been performed for this condition in the literature.

Case History

A 45-year-old woman came to our office with a chief complaint of 10 years of hip pain and a history of melorheostosis diagnosed at the age of 19 (Fig. 17-1). Her disease involved only her right lower limb. She was using anti-inflammatory agents for pain relief, with her preoperative University of California-Los Angeles (UCLA) hip scores calculated at 5 for pain and walking, 4 for function, and 3 for activity. The computed tomography (CT) study revealed a severe hyperostosis with some irregularity under the cartilage of the acetabulum (Fig. 17-1B). Her range of motion (ROM) was severely affected, with only 65 degrees of flexion from a 65-degree contracture, no abduction-adduction arc, and 15 degrees of rotation arc (all external). In addition, the patient had a history of low back pain secondary to a severe lumbar lordosis aggravated by her hip flexion contracture. Based on the CT, we envisioned bone preparation difficulties, which was confirmed by the very dense and hard bone.

The patient's young age and the absence of a femoral canal made hip resurfacing a practical prosthetic solution. Several sets of new sharp instruments, especially reamers, were helpful in acetabular reaming. There was no problem with insertion nor obtaining stability with the Conserve®Plus porous-beaded socket. One year after hip resurfacing, she had no hip pain, and her back pain was markedly improved. The patient returned to working full time as a legal secretary. Her flexion contracture was reduced initially to approximately 20 degrees. The patient was recently seen in follow-up at 8.5 years postoperatively with a UCLA score of 8 for pain, 7 for walking, 6 for function, and 6 for activity, which scores are diminished by a recurrent pain in her low back and the ankle that are very stiff with arthrofibrosis. Although in our experience, ROM rarely changes after 1 or 2 years postoperatively with hip

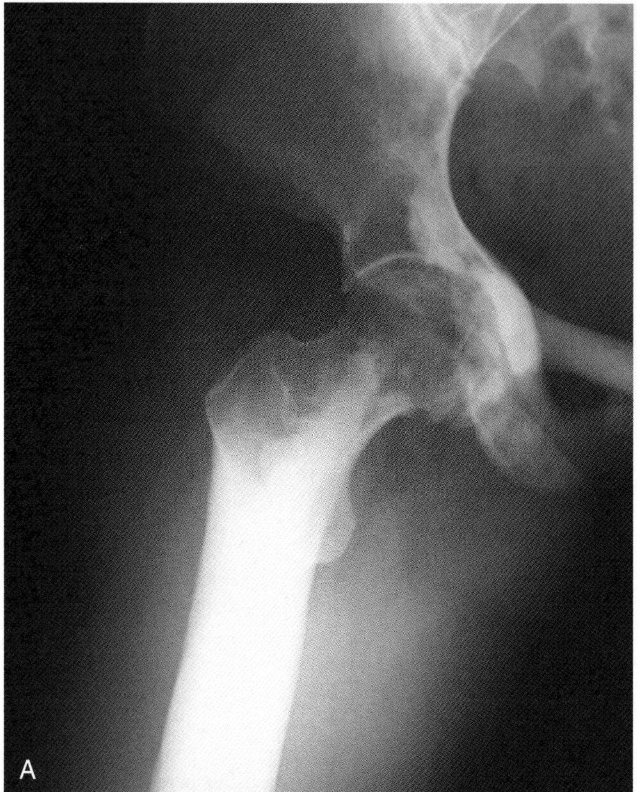

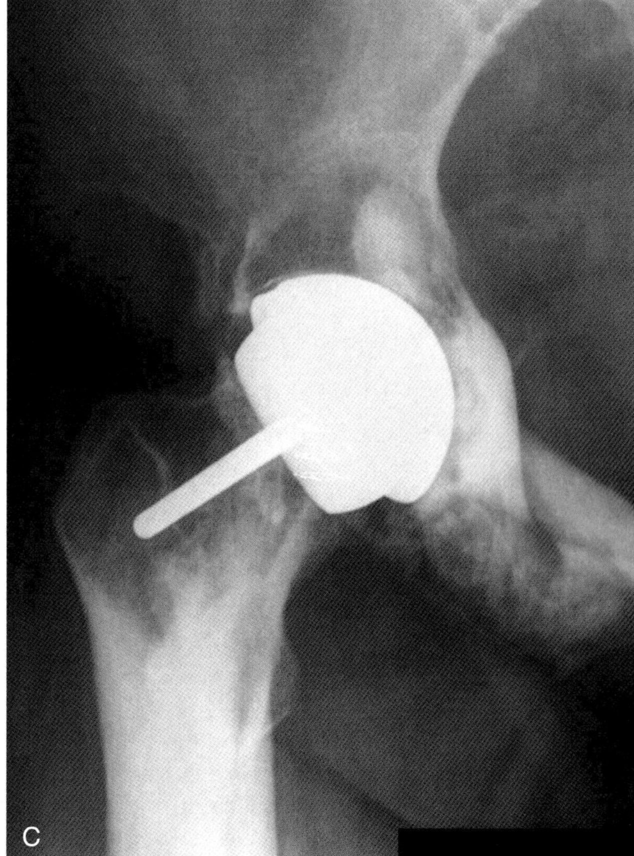

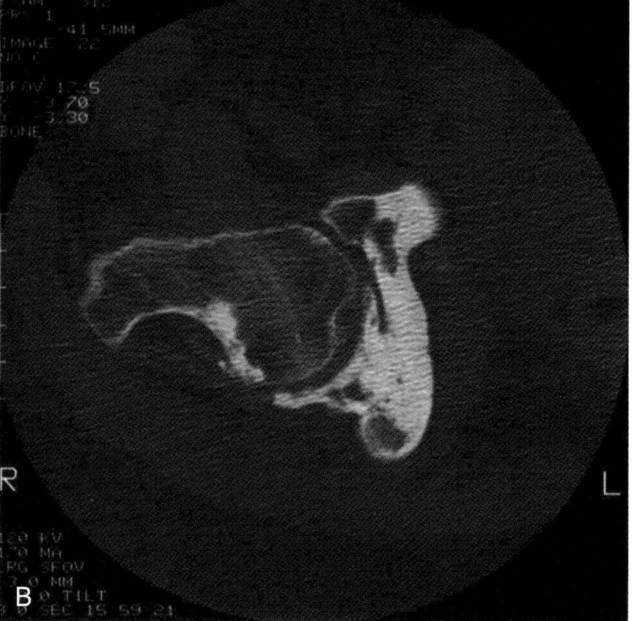

Figure 17-1 **A,** A 45-year-old woman with monomelic melorheostosis and severe joint contractures. The joint space is relatively well preserved, although not well delineated in Zone 3. **B,** Preoperative computed tomography scan showing the extent of the hyperostosis disease in the acetabulum, relatively well-preserved joint space with some lack of sphericity of the head, and an osteophyte in the acetabular fossa arising inferiorly. **C,** Eight and a half years after surgery. An increase in heterotopic ossification has been observed adjacent to the neck. A zone one femoral stem radiolucency has been visible for 6 years without change.

resurfacing in patients followed up now to 10.5 years. However, in this patient the hip contracture increased from 20 to 35 degrees and the rotation arc had decreased from 40 to 20 degrees, whereas the abduction-adduction arc remained unchanged with 50 degrees of motion. There had been an increase in heterotopic ossification (HO), which was first noticed 3 years after surgery, at a Brooker grade III in the area of femoral component neck junction, and again, the back symptoms have progressed. The cause of the increase in HO observed in this condition is unknown. With other etiologies, an increase in HO 3 to 6 years after hip resurfacing has not been observed in my experience.

Osteopetrosis

Osteopetrosis is an inherited skeletal condition characterized by an increased bone density. There are three clinical types of osteopetrosis:

1. Infantile malignant autosomal recessive, which is generally fatal within the first few years of life in the absence of effective therapy.
2. An intermediate autosomal recessive type that appears during the first decade but that does not follow a malignant course.
3. An autosomal dominant form that has a full life expectancy but with many associated orthopaedic problems.

In all three types, there is a lack of osteoclast function, resulting in decreased bone resorption and with increased cortical bone and calcified cartilage.

The major problem is the occurrence of pathologic fractures in 40% of the involved patients. Some patients have extreme fragility of bone and multiple fractures. The fractures are often transverse, demonstrating the typical characteristics of fractures through pathologic bone. Bone pain, especially in the lumbar area, is reported in 25% of the patients. Two other specific problems are cranial nerve palsy and osteomyelitis, especially of the mandible. Coxa vara is typical. Radiographic features show increased radiodensity throughout the skeleton. The metaphyses are wider than normal because of a failure of metaphyseal remodeling. The metaphyseal regions often show alternating transfer bands of both radiodense and radiolucent bands indicative of periods of exacerbation and remission. Periosteal elevation caused by trauma and bleeding can be inferred from the longitudinal peridiaphyseal alternating bands of radiodensity and radiolucency, often referred to as "the onion skin" phenomenon. A bone biopsy to quantitate osteoclast activity is useful. Check the preoperative platelet count before biopsy. Attempts have been made to try to increase osteoclasts. The coxa vara appears to be caused by a stress fracture of the proximal femoral neck. Osteotomy has been fraught with difficulty because the hardness of the bone makes stabilization technique difficult.[2] Other orthopaedic problems include osteoarthritis, nonunion of fractures, and osteomyelitis. Both osteoarthritis and periarticular nonunions have been treated successfully with stem-type total hip replacement (THR). High-speed burrs are used to create a cavity for the stem with fluoroscopic control being helpful. Cemented small or mini components, or components of developmental dysplasia of the hip (DDH) have been used most frequently.[3,4] The acetabular components have been generally cemented, but cementless sockets with screw fixation have been also used successfully. These procedures were reported as challenging with long operative times. More recently, thin-stem, cementless femoral components were successfully implanted with a threaded expansion socket.[5] A single, hybrid metal-on-metal hip resurfacing procedure was also successful using a cementless acetabular component with a side bar and screw fixation.[6]

Case History

A 36-year-old technician with bilateral hip pain contacted our office. The patient had a known history of osteopetrosis, and had had approximately 40 fractures spread throughout his body, mostly affecting his fingers and toes. The patient was normally active without playing sports. His pre-operative UCLA hip scores were 4 on the right and 2 on the left for pain, walking 5, function 6, and activity 3. The density of the bony structure was evident on the x-ray studies (Fig. 17-2). It was elected to proceed with resurfacing on the left side initially as the first step of a staged bilateral resurfacing. After precise templating, special very sharp new instrumentation was ordered to aid in bone preparation of the dense, sclerotic, and brittle material. The head of the femur was small and the neck wide with a low head-neck ratio. A CT scan was performed to precisely measure the head, neck and acetabulum in order to determine the optimal size and to minimize the amount of reaming that would be necessary. Femoral preparation began with "pin centering" using a carbide steel 1/8th inch drill (K-wire would not penetrate this dense bone), and reaming was done slowly and carefully in incremental steps. The standard bear claw–type of reamers were used to create the acetabular cavity for the Conserve®Plus socket. Unfortunately during impaction to seat the component, two stress fractures occurred in the acetabulum despite a reduction of the press fit to less than 0.1 mm. These were noted on the postoperative radiograph. For this brittle bone, the hoop stresses were too severe and had resulted in the fractures. As a result, the patient had an unusual amount of pain postoperatively, and he was placed on a non–weight-bearing regimen. The pain subsided gradually over the next several weeks, the acetabular fractures healed without further intervention, and the socket is now stable. Five months after the left hip resurfacing, the patient underwent right hip resurfacing. For this surgery, three custom sockets were obtained from Wright Medical Technology and precisely measured to provide a range of 0.04 mm with a Shadow Graph Comparator with a 5 power lens (Model #20-1600, made by Scherrtumico). The cavity was carefully prepared and checked with ring gauges so that it was precisely 0.5 mm undersized. The second surgery was uneventful, and the patient now has a follow-up of 7 months on the right side and 1 year on the left. His current UCLA scores are 9 (left) and 10 (right) for pain, 9 for walking, function 10, and activity 6. The patient admits participating occasionally in softball batting practice.

Pigmented Villonodular Synovitis

Pigmented villonodular synovitis (PVNS) was the proposed term by Jaffé[7] for a locally aggressive disease, with the joint destruction believed to be inflammatory in origin. However, a tendency for recurrence as well as recent studies describing chromosomal abnormalities and monoclonality have led some investigators to believe it to be of a neoplastic origin.[8-11] The disease and its symptoms are slowly progressive and generally confined to the joint; however, there can be masses extending beyond the articular capsule compressing the femoral or sciatic nerve. The arthropathy is characterized by circumferential joint space narrowing, which lacks specificity. The syno-

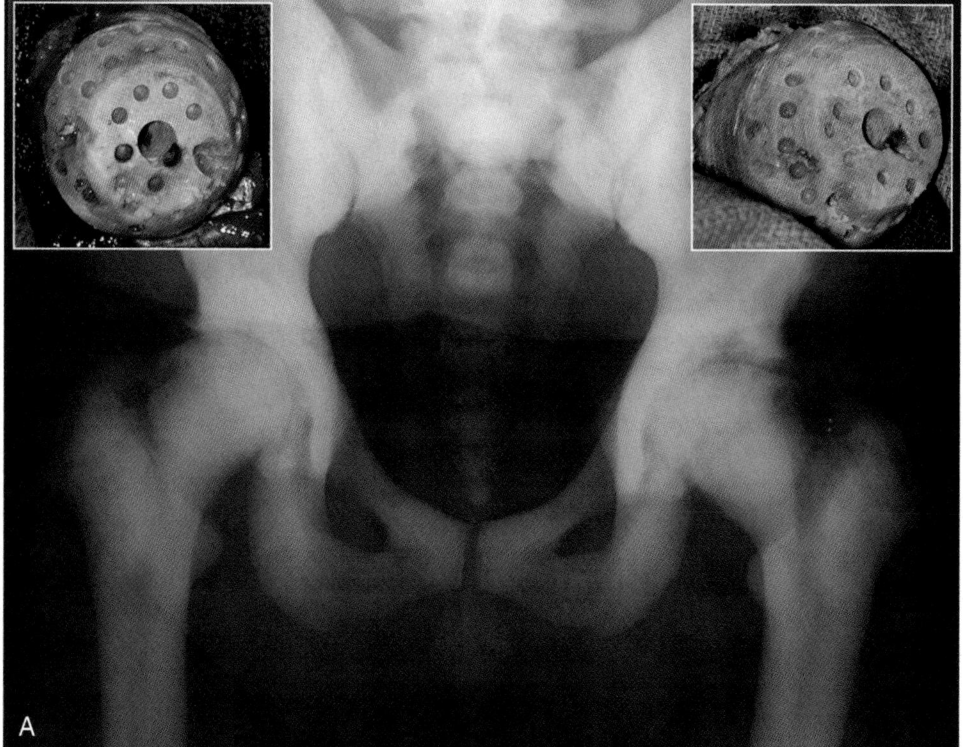

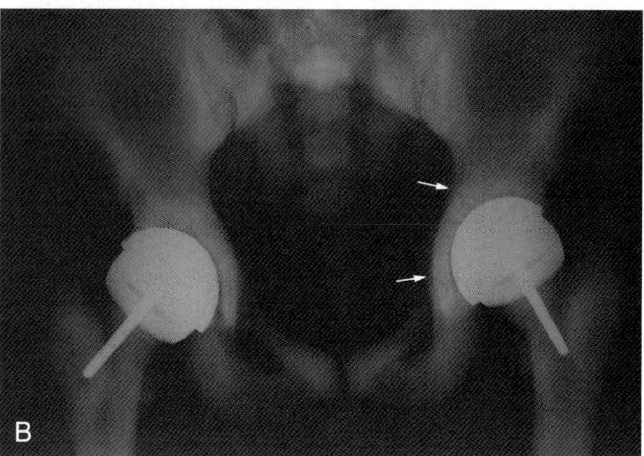

Figure 17-2 **A,** Anteroposterior pelvis radiograph of a 36-year-old man with osteopetrosis. Inserts show intraoperative photographs taken at the end of the preparation phase of the femoral head. The bone is densely sclerotic with no cancellous bone. **B,** The patient underwent staged bilateral procedures 5 months apart. The bone of this type of patient is extremely dense and brittle. A nondisplaced fracture of the left acetabular wall occurred intraoperatively, which was more obvious on the radiographs taken a few days postoperatively. The patient was placed on a non–weight-bearing regimen, and the fracture has now healed without any reoperation.

vial lesions cause erosion of the acetabulum and femoral head, and in the late stages, degenerative changes and marked joint space narrowing occur. Osteophytes are seldom observed. The lytic lesions in the femoral head, acetabulum, and trochanter may mimic a tumor or even tuberculosis.

A CT scan is useful in determining the extension of the bone lesions. A magnetic resonance imaging (MRI) scan on T2-weighted or gradient-echo images may define the lesion as a PVNS. The nodules are attributable to the paramagnetic effect, which is reduced by hemosiderin, which, in turn, causes rapid T2 decay, yielding diminished signal intensity. Gradient-echo sequences have little correction for field inhomogeneities, including paramagnetic effects and, therefore, are very sensitive to PVNS deposits. The MRI scan provides a noninvasive method for early detection of recurrences. Blood tests are within normal limits. A biopsy is effective in diagnosis 90% of the time.

Young patients without compromise of the articular cartilage should be treated with extensive synovectomy by an anterior approach or trochanteric flip. When the joint cartilage is compromised, treatment in the past has been provided with a THR or arthrodesis. Radiation has often been administered before or after surgery or as a sole treatment, but this is highly controversial, and there are many questions concerning the efficacy of radiation.

Synovectomy alone is associated with a higher recurrence rate than synovectomy plus THR, as was concluded in a recent study in which all the patients who were treated with synovectomy alone developed secondary arthritis requiring arthroplasty.[12] Although there have been no prior reports of hip

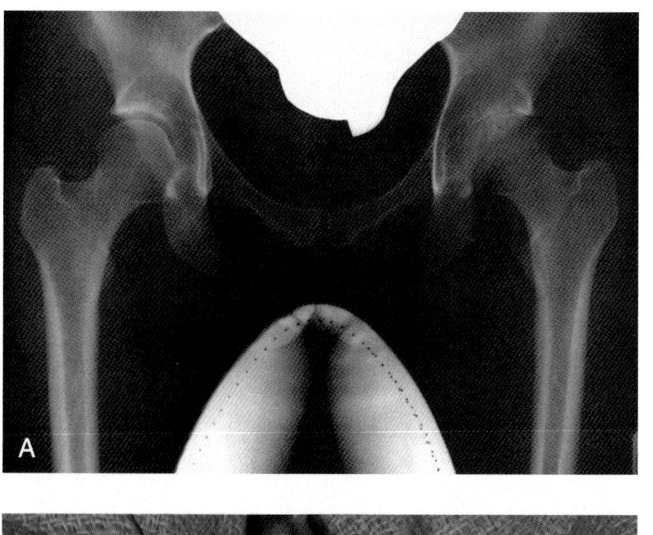

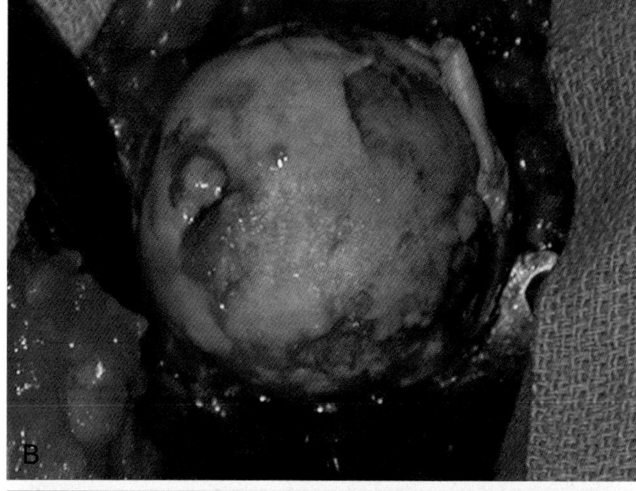

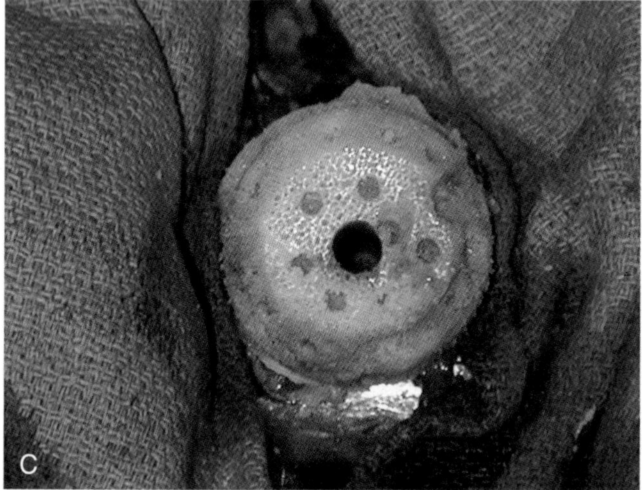

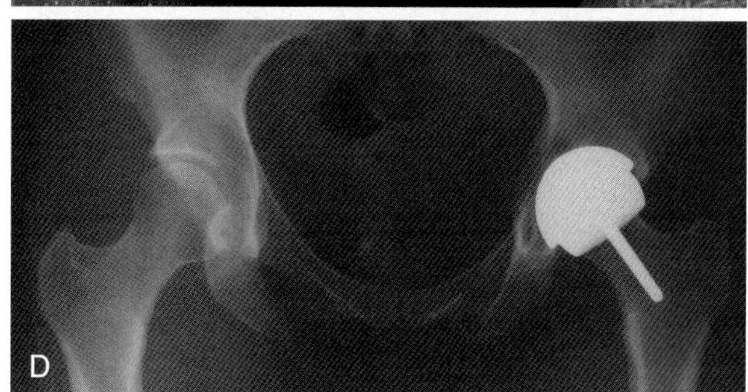

Figure 17-3 **A,** Preoperative anteroposterior radiograph of a 26-year-old woman with pigmented villonodular synovitis. The joint space is obliterated with small periarticular erosions and suggestive osteopenia. Note the absence of osteophytes. **B,** Femoral head cartilage destruction due to pigmented villonodular synovitis. **C,** Femoral head after preparation. **D,** Postoperative anteroposterior radiograph taken 2 years after the resurfacing procedure. There has not been a recurrence.

resurfacing for PVNS, our series now includes two successfully treated patients without recurrence, including one with a follow-up of 5.5 years.

Case History

A 26-year-old attorney presented with a 4-year history of hip pain. She was always very active, particularly in running and dancing ballet. Six months after her symptoms began, as she noted a worsening of symptoms, the hip was examined through an arthroscope and degenerative changes were observed. Her preoperative UCLA scores were 4, 7, 6, and 4 for pain, walking, function, and activity, respectively. The patient is naturally very flexible, but her ROM was restricted (compared with her healthy, contralateral side) to 135 degrees (150 degrees) in flexion, 80 degrees (135 degrees) in abduction-adduction arc, and 50 degrees (100 degrees) in rotation arc. Hip resurfacing was performed combined with excision of an extensive PVNS located around the joint (Fig. 17-3). Two years after surgery, the patient has recovered a near-normal ROM with 140 degrees of flexion, 120 degrees abduction-adduction arc, and 105 degrees of rotation arc, which is comparable to her contralateral normal hip. Her current UCLA hip scores are 9, 10, 10, and 8 for pain, walking, function, and activity, respectively.

Failed Osteochondroplasty

Femoral osteochondroplasty has emerged as a possible "time buying" procedure for femoroacetabular impingement in order to alleviate symptoms and perhaps forestall progression of advancing osteoarthritis.[13] Ganz has popularized the trochanteric flip[14] as the preferred approach for chondro-osteoplasty, whereas some surgeons have performed the procedure arthroscopically. We have observed patients who have not been relieved or regressed after an initial period of

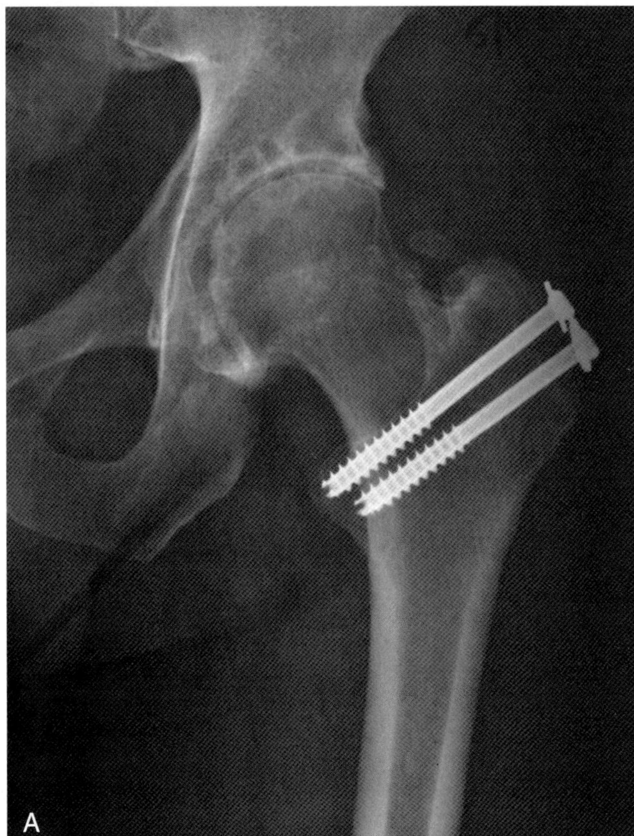

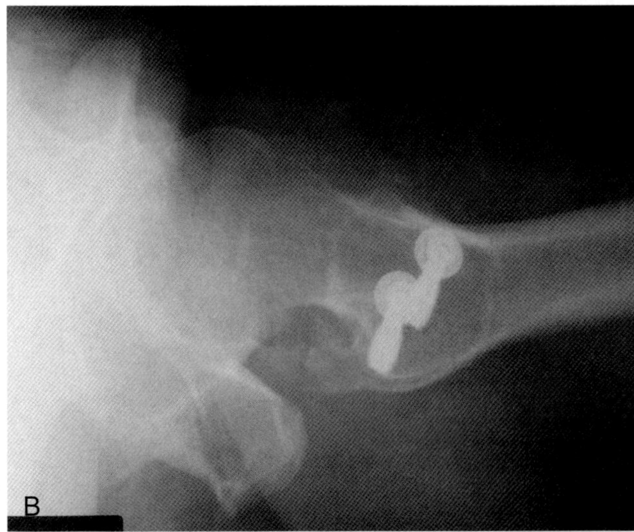

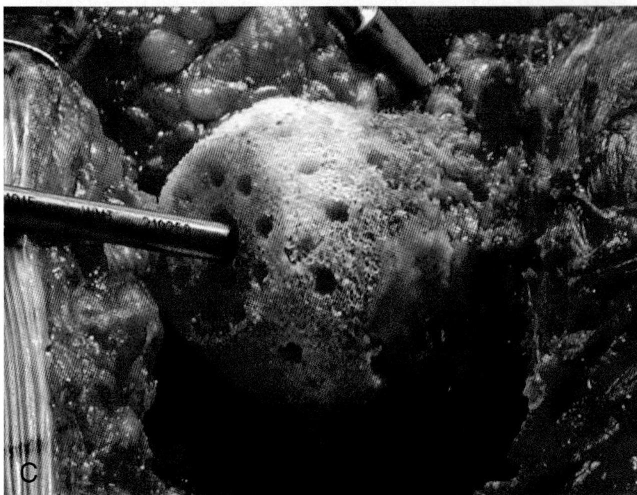

Figure 17-4 **A,** Preoperative anteroposterior radiograph of a 44-year-old systems analyst with osteoarthritis. The patient had a prior chondro-osteoplasty through a trochanteric flip to remove a cam-type impingement of the femoral neck. The patient had substantial pain relief at first, but after 5 years, the procedure was unsuccessful in stopping the osteoarthritic process, and the patient acknowledged the return of the original symptoms. **B,** Preoperative Johnson lateral view. The anterior portion of the head-neck junction does not seem to have been reshaped during the chondro-osteoplasty. **C,** The femoral head is shown after reaming and final preparation for cementation. The chondro-osteoplasty performed 6.5 years before resurfacing had healed. The bone quality was good, devoid of any cystic defect.

improvement sufficient enough to consult us for further treatment.

Case History

A 44-year-old system analyst had a 12-year history of hip pain. The patient was initially treated arthroscopically and showed clinical improvement. He then underwent osteochondroplasty, but 5 years later was seriously disabled. His UCLA scores were 4, 7, 7, 4 for pain, walking, function and activity. His ROM was 75 degrees in flexion with a contracture of 25 degrees, abduction-adduction arc of 40 degrees, and rotation arc of 30 degrees. Four years before the onset of the hip symptoms, the patient had had back surgery, which provided considerable relief. Inspection at surgery showed that the contoured defect had healed, but there were arthritic changes and a hip resurfacing was performed (Fig. 17-4). There are no previous reports of hip resurfacing after this type of surgery. His pain, walking, function and activity scores 1.5 years after surgery are 9, 10, 10, and 8 with normalization of ROM.

Femoral Canal Deformity, Post Sepsis or Both

Hip resurfacing should be considered when there is a deformity of the proximal femur in the subtrochanteric region so that insertion of a conventional stem would be impossible or require an osteotomy to realign the femur before an arthroplasty. In addition, patients who have had previous septic arthritis or sepsis in the subtrochanteric region, such as from

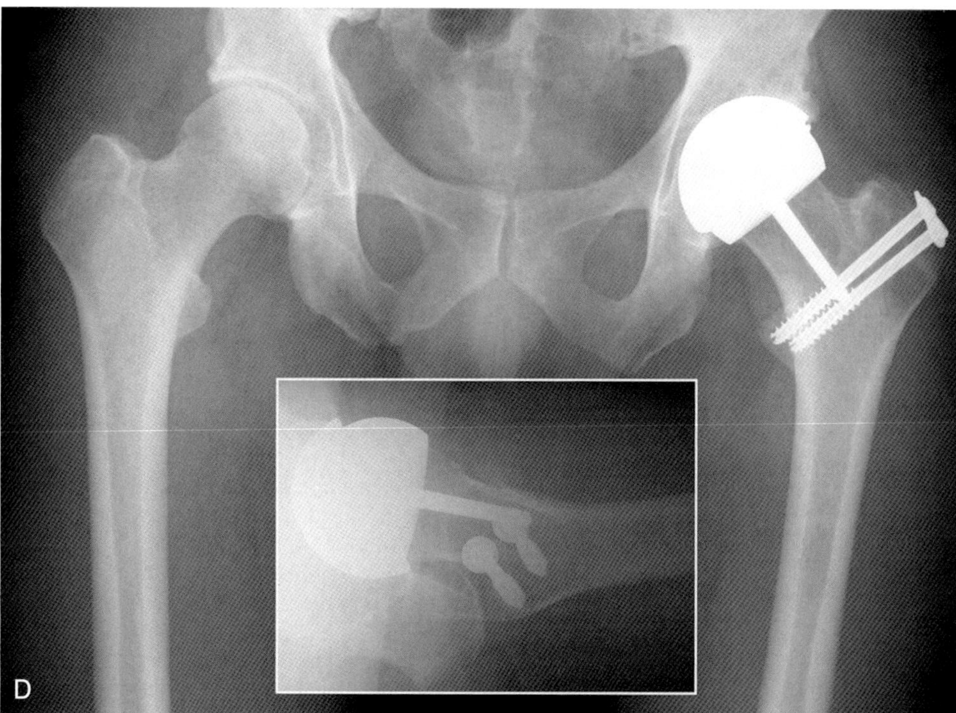

Figure 17-4, cont'd D, Anteroposterior radiograph of the patient 14 months after resurfacing. The screws from the prior trochanteric slide were retained because they were not in the way of the metaphyseal stem. The insert shows the Johnson lateral postoperative film. The patient's current University of California-Los Angeles hip scores are 9 for pain, 10 for walking and function, and 8 for activity.

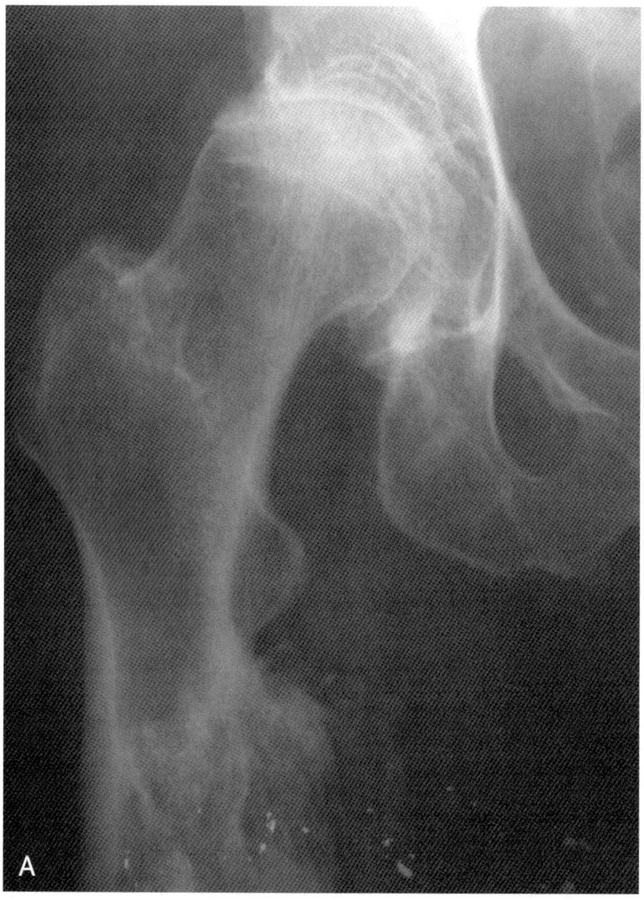

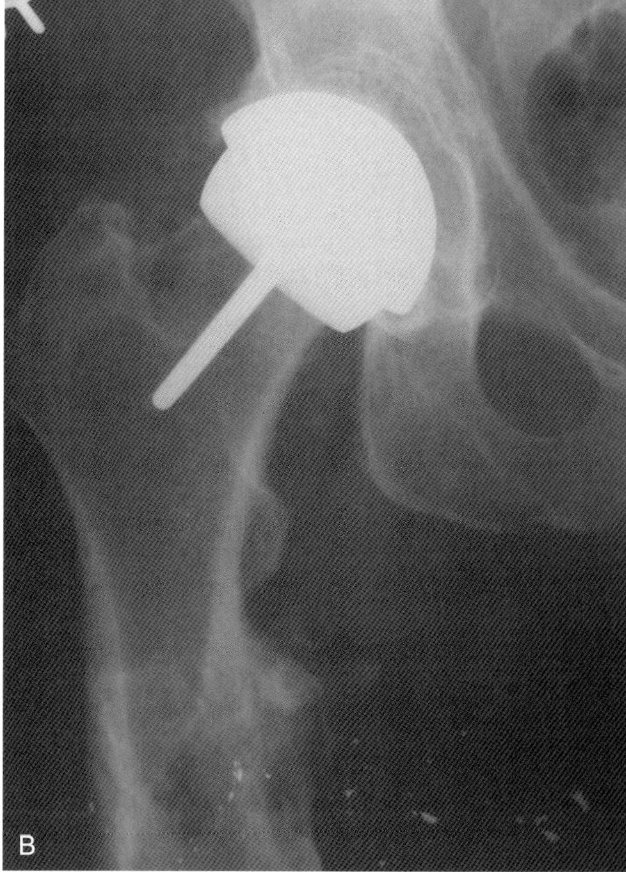

Figure 17-5 A, A 77-year-old male with osteoarthritis of the right hip. The femoral shaft was previously damaged by a gunshot so that the femoral canal is unsuitable for a conventional stemmed total hip replacement. **B,** Five years after resurfacing, the patient's quality of life has returned to normal. His University of California-Los Angeles hip scores are 9, 10, 10, and 6 for pain, walking, function, and activity respectively.

a prior trauma, or patients who have a high risk for sepsis are also logical candidates. Resurfacing in these situations poses less risk because the intramediary canal is not violated. If a recurrence of infection occurs, it can be more easily dealt with.

Case History

A 77-year-old retired engineer presented with a two-year history of progressive hip pain and osteoarthritis of the right hip. The femoral shaft had been previously shattered by a machine gun during World War II. He developed osteomyelitis and underwent multiple operations, but had not experienced drainage from the wound for 40 years. His UCLA scores were 3, 6, 4, and 3 for pain, walking, function, and activity. His ROM records showed 110 degrees of flexion with a 25-degree contracture, 25 degrees of abduction-adduction arc, and 5 degrees of rotation arc. He had a 20-degree flexion contracture of the knee with further flexion to 90 degrees, and low back symptoms. His thigh was seriously scarred, but with only a slight depression laterally and no erythemia. The radiograph revealed a severe femoral deformity with no intramedullary canal suitable for a conventional, stemmed THR (Fig. 17-5).

Five years after resurfacing, the patient's quality of life has returned to normal, with a postoperative Short Form-12 (SF-12) physical component score of 50.1 compared with a preoperative score of 32.1. The patient has subsequently had both knees replaced. His UCLA hip scores assessments were 9, 10, 10 and 6 for pain, walking, function, and activity, respectively.

References

1. Campbell C, Papademetriou T, Bonfiglio M: Melorheostosis. A report of the clinical, roentgenographic, and pathological findings in fourteen cases. J Bone Joint Surg Am 1968;50:1281-1304.

1a. Léri A, Joanny J: Une affection non décrite des os: hyperostose "en coulée" sur toute la longueur d'un membre ou "mélorhéostose". Bull Mem Soc Med Hosp Paris 1922;46:1141-1145.

2. Shapiro F: Osteopetrosis. Current clinical considerations. Clin Orthop Relat Res 1993;294:34-44.
3. Matsuno T, Katayama N: Osteopetrosis and total hip arthroplasty. Report of two cases. Int Orthop 1997;21:409-411.
4. Strickland J, Berry D: Total joint arthroplasty in patients with osteopetrosis: a report of 5 cases and review of the literature. J Arthroplasty 2005;20:815-820.
5. Gwynne Jones DP, Hodgson HB, Hung NA: Bilateral, uncemented total hip arthroplasty in osteopetrosis. J Bone Joint Surg Br 2004;86:276-278.
6. Girard J, Lavigne M, Vendittoli P, Roy A: Resurfacing arthroplasty of the hip in osteopetrosis. J Bone Joint Surg Br 2006;88:818-821.
7. Jaffé H, Lichtenstein L, Sutro C: Pigmented villonodular synovitis, bursitis and tenosynovitits: a discussion of the synovial and bursal equivalents of the tenosynovial lesion commonly denoted as xantoma, xantogranuloma, giant cell tumor or myeloplaxoma of the tendon sheath itself. Arch Pathol Lab Med 1941;31:731-765.
8. Rao A, Vigorita V: Pigmented villonodular synovitis (giant-cell tumor of the tendon sheath and synovial membrane). A review of eighty-one cases. J Bone Joint Surg Am 1984;66:76-94.
9. Choong P, Willen H, Nilbert M, Mertens F, Mandahl N, Carlen B, Rydholm A: Pigmented villonodular synovitis. Monoclonality and metastasis—a case for neoplastic origin? Acta Orthop Scand 1995;66:64-68.
10. Enzinger F, Weiss S: Benign tumors and tumorlike lesions of synovial tissue. In: Enzinger F, Weiss S (eds). Soft tissue tumors, ed 3. St Louis, Mosby, 1995, pp 742-749.
11. Jones F, Soule E, Coventry M: Fibrous xanthoma of synovium (giant-cell tumor of tendon sheath, pigmented nodular synovitis). A study of one hundred and eighteen cases. J Bone Joint Surg Am 969;51:76-86.
12. Gonzalez Della Valle A, Piccaluga F, Potter H, Salvati E, Pusso R: Pigmented villonodular synovitis of the hip: 2- to 23-year followup study. Clin Orthop Relat Res 2001;388:187-199.
13. Beaulé P, Le Duff M, Zaragoza E: Quality of life following femoral head-neck osteochondroplasty for femoroacetabular impingement. J Bone Joint Surg Am 2007;89:773-779.
14. Ganz R, Gill T, Gautier E, Ganz K, Krügel N, Berlemann U: Surgical dislocation of the adult hip: A technique with full access to the femoral head and acetabulum without the risk of avascular necrosis. J Bone Joint Surg Br 2001;83:1119-1124.

CHAPTER 18

Assessment of the Failed or Poorly Performing Hip Resurfacing: Lessons from a Lifetime of Experience

Harlan C. Amstutz

Introduction

The following is my personal accumulated experience of managing thousands of patients with total hip replacements (THRs) and nearly 2000 with resurfacing arthroplasties for more than 40 years.

Treatment and evaluation starts with a careful history based on a chronologic analysis of previous surgeries, including the immediate result, any intrahospital complications, intermediate and later results, and any subsequent surgeries. It is important to obtain records from previous hospitalizations including the operative notes, discharge summary, and any specific events that might have directly or indirectly affected the outcome.

The most difficult patient to evaluate is one in whom there is no obvious reason for failure but in whom the result is unsatisfactory. The result may be unsatisfactory for a variety of reasons, but the problem may be influenced by the patient's psychological make-up. The use and abuse of pain medications must be carefully recorded and evaluated. Patients who have emotional disturbances require careful psychological assessment, questioning of family members, and examination of the temporal relations and their progression in relation to their physical disabilities. Pain that persists unrelieved with no obvious complications after replacement arthroplasty also raises the possibility that the preoperative pain was not actually arising in the hip and emphasizes the importance in all cases of addressing the fundamental question of the origin of the pain. Pain that is not directly related to the arthroplasty may arise from the spine. The various sources of pain following hip resurfacing are summarized in Table 18-1. Fracture of the femoral neck and component loosening are two common causes of failure, and these are discussed in more detail in Chapter 10 in this book.

Pain: The First Clinical Indicator

Pain of sudden or relatively sudden onset in the immediate postoperative period, especially while the patient is on anticoagulants, may be due to bleeding. Rapid swelling and falling hematocrit levels are suggestive of this problem. Treatment includes a compressive bandage and ice application, and reversing the anticoagulation level. If increasing pain, swelling, or drainage ensues, this situation may warrant evacuation.

Pain persisting unchanged after the operation suggests that either the original pain was not in the hip, there is inadequate initial stability and fixation of the implant, or the presence of a postoperative infection. With infection, there are usually manifestations at the operative site including erythema, warmth, or drainage and possibly fever. Last, C-reactive protein and sedimentation rates are typically elevated and trending upward as opposed to normalizing.

Pain arising from the arthroplasty that is of gradual onset following a postoperative pain-free period of variable duration suggests mechanical loosening, hematogenous sepsis, or both. If the pain is present at rest, infection may be the cause. Acute pain with motion arising from a previously well-functioning arthroplasty suggests either neck fracture or mechanical loosening. Pain that is felt in the groin and in the lateral part of the buttock is often associated with socket loosening, with or without deep infection. Loosening and infection of the femoral component are more often associated with a deep pain in the entire thigh or in the groin that is aggravated by weight bearing on the affected limb. Pain and tenderness particularly over the greater trochanter suggest trochanteric bursitis and is frequently aggravated when the patient lies on the hip. Pain on internal rotation with flexion may be the result of impingement or iliopsoas bursitis especially if the pain is aggravated by resisted flexion. Although not frequent, pain arising from

Table 18-1 Summary of Modes of Failures and Associated Findings

Mode of Failure	Clinical Symptoms	Radiologic Features	Other
Femoral neck fracture	Pain—possible loss of leg length	Femoral component tipped in varus—fracture line visible	
Loosening of the femoral component	Pain—clicking of the device	Femoral component tipped in varus—radiolucency around the stem	
Loosening of the acetabular component	Pain—clicking of the device	Cup migration—complete radiolucency >1 mm in all three zones	
Infection	Pain—fever	—	Positive cultures
Dislocation/subluxation	Pain—deformation of the joint	Femoral and acetabular components have different geometric centers	
Heterotopic ossification	Possible limitation of range of motion	Radiodense formations around the joint (see Brooker grading system)	
Trochanteric Bursitis	Pain—lateral	—	
Iliopsoas Bursitis	Pain—location?	—	
Impingement		Remodeling of the femoral neck consistent with contact from the cup	
Metal sensitivity	Pain—Usually starting shortly after surgery	—	
Osteonecrosis	Pain—commensurate with the extent of the lesion	—	

the lumbar spine may mimic pain arising in the hip but is generally accompanied by paresthesias or neurologic findings. Rarely, groin pain may be caused by metal sensitivity.

Key points to evaluate in the history of patients who have had previous surgery are postoperative pyrexia, temporary or persisting wound drainage, and persistent leg swelling. Symptoms or signs of a clicking sensation of the hip or a sense of instability suggest subluxation, especially if there is an accompanying re-entry click or clunk as the hip is rotated or extended in the opposite direction. However, postoperative clicking after a hip resurfacing is common in patients with well-functioning hips and appears to have no pathologic significance. In the authors' experience, clicking may occur in approximately 20% of patients in the first few months after surgery, and then gradually resolves. The exact cause is unknown. We have speculated that it persists until the capsule heals and tightens and the muscles of the hip girdle, particularly the abductors, recover to a normal tone and strength. This sensation has also been observed in a small subset of our patients after a THR with a metal-on-metal bearing. A hip that has been silent begins to click months to years after the surgery, may represent loosening, particularly if it is accompanied by pain.

Physical Examination

Clinical evidence of past or present inflammatory changes, including healed sinus, is important. It is well to note the location of all previous incisions when there have been several operations and to identify which incision was related to which procedure. Local tenderness over the trochanter often is related to trochanteric bursitis and is occasionally present with painful nonunion of the greater trochanter. Pain due to heterotopic ossification is uncommon. Forced internal rotation in flexion indicates capsular swelling indicative of infection, loosening, or impingement.

The presence of Trendelenburg sign is indicative of a painful hip, which could be caused by one of a variety of causes, including mechanical muscle insufficiency. Patients who have back pain should be appropriately evaluated, including palpation of the interspinous, paravertebral, and sacroiliac areas with the patient relaxed and flexed over an examining table. Straight-leg raising and femoral nerve stretch maneuvers may give important information for the differential diagnosis. It is important to evaluate the circulation of the extremity and to determine if claudication exists. The venous stasis changes should be noted with the patient upright. The arterial system should be evaluated with palpation of the pulses while the patient is in the supine position and with the limb elevated. If elevation of the extremity obliterates or diminishes pulses, it is a warning sign of impaired arterial flow. The patient should be referred to a vascular surgeon for further evaluation and potential surgical treatment.

Investigations

Hematologic Studies

1. Erythrocyte sedimentation rate (ESR). Normal values are 0 to 19 mm/hour for men and 0 to 28 mm/hour for women. An elevated ESR is an indication of sepsis, but the patient's general medical condition must be evaluated to make an appropriate diagnosis. The ESR may be only slightly ele-

vated or normal with low-grade infections but is rarely elevated with mixed or more virulent organism infections. The ESR will become elevated from the stress of surgery but typically normalizes over the first 1 to 2 months after surgery. If the ESR is climbing after surgery, this is worrisome for infection.

2. White blood cell count and differential. These tests are generally normal unless there is acute, more obvious sepsis.
3. C-Reactive Protein (CRP). The CRP is an acute-phase protein produced by the liver and is a nonspecific test for sepsis that may indicate sepsis in combination with an elevated ESR. The normal values for the CRP vary from laboratory to laboratory. There is a high sensitivity test and a routine test that will provide very different normal ranges. The normal range must be known, and trends of this laboratory value should be followed with only one testing laboratory. The CRP level normalizes much more quickly after surgery than the ESR and, therefore, is a better predictor of early postoperative infections. When used in combination, the CRP and ESR are very sensitive for detecting and following infections. It should be noted that the CRP and ESR levels are reported to be slightly elevated in cases of metal sensitivity.
4. Ion studies. These studies are useful in evaluating a high wear situation, and as surgeons gain more experience with them, they may become more useful in evaluation of other conditions. At the present time we have been unable to explain the cause of the unusually high ions (outlier) in a well performing hip resurfacing (see Fig. 11-1).
5. Patch testing for reaction to metals has limited clinical diagnostic application to a problem hip. In our experience, patients can have a dermal sensitivity with no problem of metal sensitivity in the hip (see Fig. 11-3).
6. Leukocyte inhibition studies. These are mostly performed in a research situation, and there is currently insufficient data to determine their validity or diagnostic potential. The results do not necessarily diagnose a metal sensitivity or other problem in the hip. A case example is presented later in this chapter.

Routine Roentgenography

Good quality new anteroposterior and cross-table lateral x-ray films aid in assessing the implant status. Analog radiographs are preferred. Detailed evaluation of these films is outlined in Chapter 5. Has there been a change in component orientation to indicate loosening? This question can be answered correctly only after careful serial evaluation of all of the previous radiographs dating from the time of the resurfacing. The importance of this assessment cannot be overemphasized.

If the components are well fixed, is the component orientation acceptable? European surgeons who have considerable experience with failed resurfacings in Europe, especially with the Birmingham Hip Resurfacing, have established that there is a relationship between high wear and excessive abduction angle (higher than 55 degrees) which has been associated with increased ion levels and in some cases, bone destruction requiring revision (see the discussion on Implant Position in Chapter 11). The bone destruction may be secondary to loosening, but more likely is due to high wear causing osteolysis rather than loosening, although both may be present eventually.

It is essential to evaluate the progression of the signs of scalloping that may indicate osteolysis. Is there sufficient loss of bone to place the patient in danger of a fracture? In our experience malorientation in the lateral plane has not been specifically associated with loosening. In fact, severe posterior to anterior orientation of the component, with the tip of the stem juxtaposed to the anterior cortex or even penetrating the cortex, has not been associated with loosening, even with our first generation of cementing technique. Actual penetration occurred in three cases (all in heavy patients) in which there was difficulty in exposure of the femoral side.

The areas adjacent to the stem must be carefully evaluated for radiolucencies and for reaction of bone around the stem especially at the tip (see Chapter 5). Pedestal formation around the tip is a result of load transfer and represents a reaction to the loosening process. We have observed this phenomenon to be initially progressive and then on occasion become nonprogressive. Probably this then represents a stable fibrous fixation. However it is unlikely that the condition will withstand impact sports or other high activity for a prolonged period.

Heterotopic ossification (HO) is commonly observed after hip surgery, in particular in male patients with osteoarthritis. Most are Brooker grades I and II, which do not impair the patient's ability to function. Even the Brooker grades III and IV rarely cause sufficient impairment of motion or function to necessitate re-operation and removal.

Aspiration and Injection

Aspiration of the hip joint is mainly used for the diagnosis of sepsis. An initial attempt at aspiration may be done in the office setting without image assistance. If an adequate quantity of fluid is attained, no further aspiration is needed. However, a dry tap is not uncommon, and the patient should then be sent for fluoroscopy-assisted aspiration with or without arthrography to prove that the needle entered the joint. An 18-gauge needle is recommended. The most useful information is derived from the characteristics of the aspirate, including its color, cell count, and differential, and the 7-day culture results for aerobic and anaerobic growth.

If the signs and symptoms indicate aseptic loosening, the decision about aspiration must be made based on the experience of the surgeon and his or her accuracy in determining if the prosthesis is septic. When the signs and symptoms of sepsis are obvious, aspiration is mandatory. If radiolucencies are differentially present on one side of the replacement (i.e., socket or around the stem of the femoral component) sepsis is less likely unless the patient has an acute sepsis from hematogenous spread to the hip joint.

In the absence of sepsis, a very useful test is the injection of 1% bupivicaine (Marcaine) into the joint to confirm that the source of pain is indeed coming from the joint and may indicate a very subtle loosening process. In the absence of sepsis, injecting a steroid may be helpful. Injection of iliopsoas bursa and tendon sheath may also be helpful in the diagnosis and therapy. This should be done with a radiologist under image control.

Imaging Techniques

With the imaging techniques available today, magnetic resonance imaging (MRI) and computed tomography (CT) may be of assistance. However, the scatter associated with metallic devices sometimes confounds the ability to assess pathology in close proximity to the component. MRIs are sometimes helpful for evaluating a fluid collection, soft tissue mass, or the iliopsoas or other bursae. It has not been useful for identifying the continuity of the sciatic nerve or perineural edema in the evaluation of a postoperative nerve palsy.

Isotope Studies

The most successful study for evaluating a patient who may have sepsis is the indium white blood cell (WBC) study performed at 24 hours after injecting the patient's own WBCs labeled with indium 111 (^{111}In). Sensitivity and specificity, based on our studies of patients with septic THR, were 83 and 94 percent, respectively.

Technetium Tc 99m diphosphonate scans and technetium Tc 99m sulfur colloid scans can be useful. In the past, Tc 99m sulfur colloid scans were useful for evaluating failure of earlier generation resurfacing procedures without a metaphyseal stem, but we have not used them with these generation devices because the careful evaluation of radioluciences around the stem have replaced the need for isotopic scans.

Gallium citrate Ga 67 scanning has not been helpful in our evaluations of patients with sepsis. There are many false-positive and false-negative results, whereas the ^{111}In-WBC technique has been much more satisfactory. We previously also evaluated ^{99m}Tc-WBC scans with a three-dimensional analysis, but they have proved to be of no particular benefit.

Composite Evaluation to Establish a Diagnosis and Treatment Plan

The pain associated with loosening is often relieved by returning the patient to crutches and unloading the prosthesis. Pain due to sepsis may not be relieved. The decision for exploratory surgery in a case of suspected loosening must be based on whether the symptoms can be sufficiently relieved by protected non–weight-bearing status or protected limited weight-bearing and the use of an intrarticular injection of marcaine. It must also take into consideration the quality of the bone. Most patients who have suspected loosening do not require immediate revision surgery. If the bone loss is minimal, it is unlikely that a delay will be responsible for any deleterious effect. It may be sufficient to examine the patient at periodic intervals as long as the patient is functional and be certain of the diagnosis and to optimize treatment. A delay also enables the surgeon to have more time to evaluate new technologies. Treatment of loosening and neck fractures is detailed in Chapter 19.

Treatment of Subluxation—Dislocation

Dislocation can occur after resurfacing arthroplasty. However, unlike dislocations with older generation THRs with smaller ball sizes, a dislocation after a resurfacing tends to be an isolated, traumatic event as opposed to recurrent instability. Therefore, we have not had to reoperate on any Conserve®Plus hip for dislocation. (see Chapter 9 for details) If recurrent instability occurs, this is most likely an anatomic problem (such as a very low offset femur or pre-existing pelvic or femoral deformity), or it is due to significant component malposition. In these cases, the causative factor needs to be carefully assessed before any surgical intervention.

If the cup is adequately positioned and the source is a low-offset femur, for instance, the cup can be retained and conversion to a total hip stem with adequate offset and a large femoral head matching the inner diameter of the shell may be used. More commonly, with recurrent instability it is related to cup malposition into retroversion or a vertical opening angle. In this situation, the cup must be revised, and frequently, the femoral component needs to be revised as well because it will otherwise dictate the sizing of the new acetabular component (see Fig. 14-10 and Chapter 19).

Infection

In the case of chronic low-grade sepsis that is essentially asymptomatic, one could consider using antibiotics to suppress the infection. However, because patients who undergo resurfacing tend to be younger, it is preferable to attempt a cure of the infection so that they are not subjected to a lifetime of antibiotic suppression. With chronic infections, this typically requires resection of implants, placement of an interval antibiotic-loaded methyl methacrylate spacer followed by delayed re-implantation of a THR (two-stage revision). Direct exchange (one-stage revision) may also be attempted. There is insufficient literature related specifically to infections in hip resurfacing to determine which is the preferable course of action. However, extrapolating the total hip literature, a two-stage revision should be considered the standard of care. Our experience is detailed in Chapter 19 and our one direct exchange in Chapter 16.

Metal Sensitivity

If the patient has pain and there is no obvious reason for the pain and no demonstrable evidence of failure, it is unlikely that revision surgery is going to successfully relieve that patient's pain unless it is a case of metal sensitivity. However, in this case, there will likely be diagnostic fluid or a groin mass. At present, we have not identified any case of metal sensitivity requiring revision in my series of Conserve®Plus, although we have observed two of 44 McMinn resurfacings that developed fluid accumulations or fibrin masses which were, surprisingly not diagnostic of metal sensitivity. One patient remains with a functional prosthesis 12 years postoperatively and 8 years following aspiration of 400 mL of bloody or dark brown joint fluid. There is marked remodeling and neck narrowing and some residual swelling, but the patient is reluctant to proceed with revision. The other case was revised and is presented below.

Case History

At her first visit to our office, the patient was a 19-year-old woman who developed hip and thigh pain. She had x-ray evidence of joint space narrowing (Fig. 18-1). There were cystic lesions in the dome and surrounding sclerosis, representing atypical osteonecrosis versus atypical osteoarthritis with a possible origin of osteochondritis diseccans. The cystic areas on CT were in the anterior portion of the femoral head. She had a Sugioka rotational osteotomy, rotating the posterior portion of the femoral head anteriorly (Fig. 18-1A). A McMinn resurfacing with a double-socket technique was performed 15 years later due to secondary degenerative changes (Fig. 18-1B).

Nine years after resurfacing, she was doing well with minimal pain ($P = 9$) in the hip joint area, swimming regularly, and being active as a teacher with two children. She developed cruciform swelling of the left thigh. The neck had been observed to progressively narrow following the McMinn resurfacing (Fig. 18-1C). An MRI showed three distinct masses with a high fluid content (Fig. 18-1D). The patient had ion studies and sensitivity studies performed before resection at 116 months postoperatively. Ion levels in serum were 1.13 for cobalt, 0.52 for chromium, and urine chromium was 1.08 (relatively normal). The fluid collection was also verified by ultrasound, and 450 mL of brownish fluid was removed.

A week later, she underwent revision surgery elsewhere because of insurance difficulties. The soft tissue mass in the

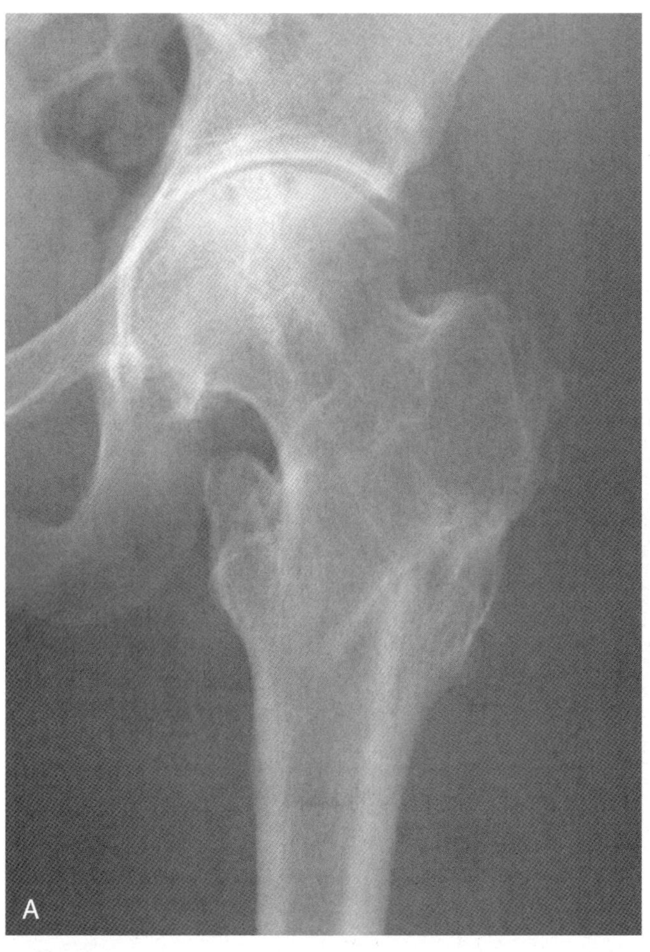

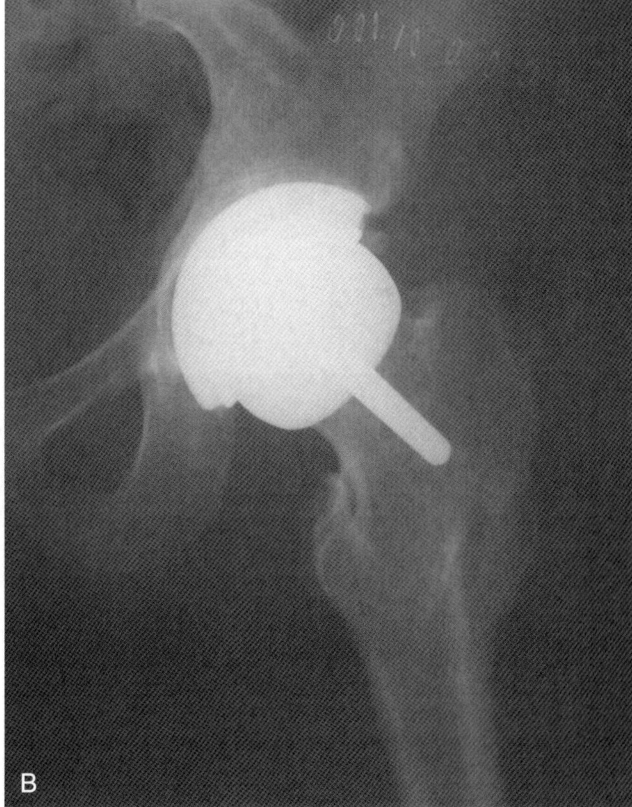

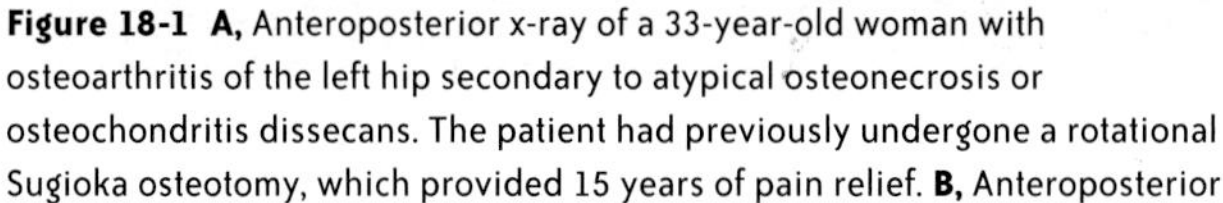
Figure 18-1 **A,** Anteroposterior x-ray of a 33-year-old woman with osteoarthritis of the left hip secondary to atypical osteonecrosis or osteochondritis dissecans. The patient had previously undergone a rotational Sugioka osteotomy, which provided 15 years of pain relief. **B,** Anteroposterior x-ray showing the patient immediately after metal-on-metal resurfacing with a McMinn cemented device (Corin Medical, Cirencester, UK) which acetabular component was cemented into a DePuy PSR hemispherical cementless shell (double socket technique).

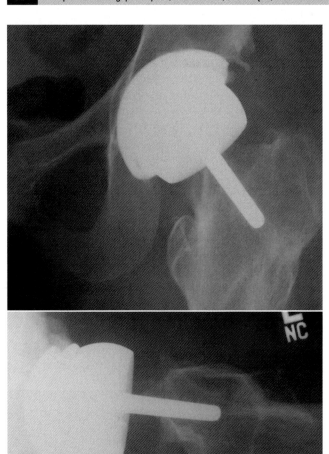

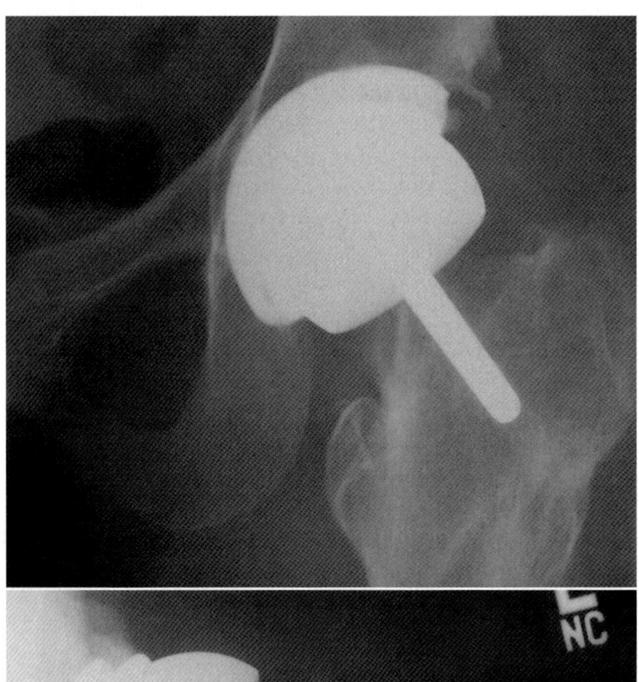

Figure 18-1, cont'd C, Nine years after resurfacing, there is considerable bone resorption at the junction of the neck and the femoral component, both on the anteroposterior view (Top) and the Johnson lateral view (Bottom). **D,** The MRI revealed the presence of 3 large bursae, which were excised at revision surgery. The removed mass was a viable fibrous sac filled with fibrin.

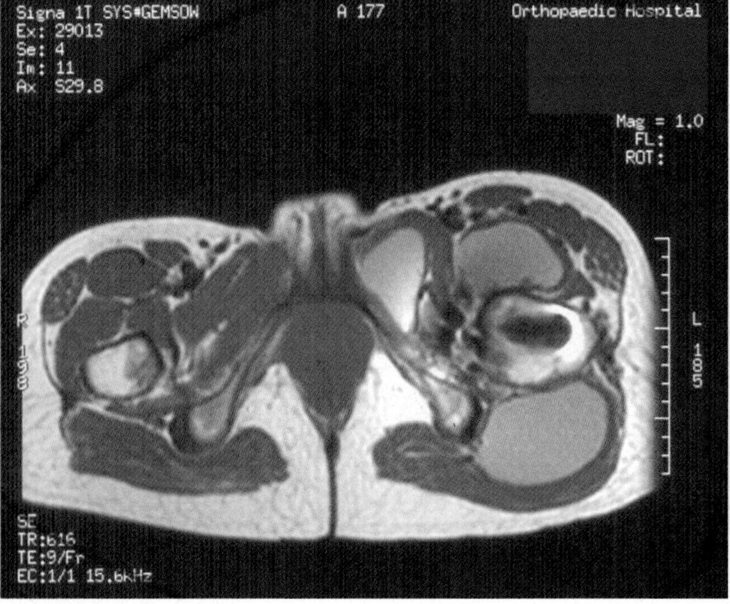

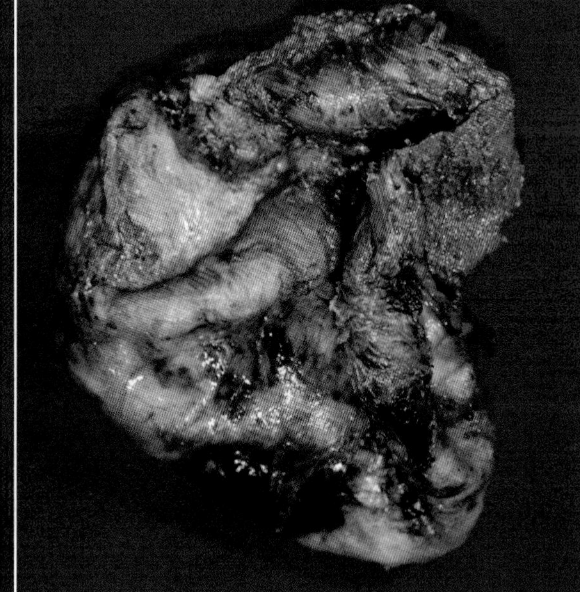

D

joint was excised (Fig. 18-1D) and she received a Profemur Z and Marathon liner with a 32-mm head. The patient subsequently developed a *Propionibacterium acnes* sepsis. A débridement was then performed and an antibiotic spacer inserted. Systemic vancomycin and rifampin IV antibiotics were administered for 6 weeks. Three months later, with normalization of ESR and CRP, we proceeded with the reimplantation of an anthropometric total hip (ATH) size 9 + 4 with a 60-mm polyethylene with a 40 ID cup. Cultures were negative, and 2 years postreimplantation, she has been able to resume all of her activities without pain and has a full range of motion.

The soft tissue mass was found to consist of fibrin lined by macrophages and giant cells, some of which contained visible metal. The mass was surrounded by a fibrous bursa–like sac, the walls of which contained occasional focal lymphocytic aggregates with some plasma cells, but these were not considered to be consistent with metal sensitivity. The measured wear of the removed femoral component was only 12 μ, or about 1 μ per year of use. The reason for the fluid production in this case remains a mystery.

Treatment of Patients with Unexplained Pain

In our series, three patients had pain scores of 6 and are characterized by having suggestion of an associated psychological condition. We recommend the use of a Minnesota Multiphasic Personality Test (MMPI), with the help of a psychologist, to assist in the evaluation when there are no findings to suggest a possible mechanical or biologic cause. If the patient has a low pain threshold or is in a life setting that is otherwise stressful, minor degrees of pain may be magnified and suggest surgical failure. Patients who are unhappy with their result should be carefully quizzed as to their degree of unhappiness about the care provided by the hospital or the surgeon. They should also be asked if there has been an intervening injury that, from their point of view, might have triggered or aggravated the pain.

We had several experiences in the early days of evaluating THR patients with unexplained pain in which we explored the hip in order to determine the possible cause of the pain. At surgery, there was no loosening and no other gross signs to explain the pain. Exchange of the prosthesis in these patients failed to relieve their symptoms. Sometimes no diagnosis was made other than the strong impression that emotional factors played a large part in the patient's disability. In our experience, exploration to determine the cause is rarely successful.

This is illustrated by one patient in our current hip resurfacing series, a 53-year-old man who came to our office with progressive pain in the hip for a duration of more than 1 year (Fig. 18-2). His UCLA scores were as follows: pain 3, walking 7, function 8, and activity level 4. His range of motion was only slightly restricted, and he had only moderate osteoarthritis at surgery. Eight months postoperatively, he still had persistent

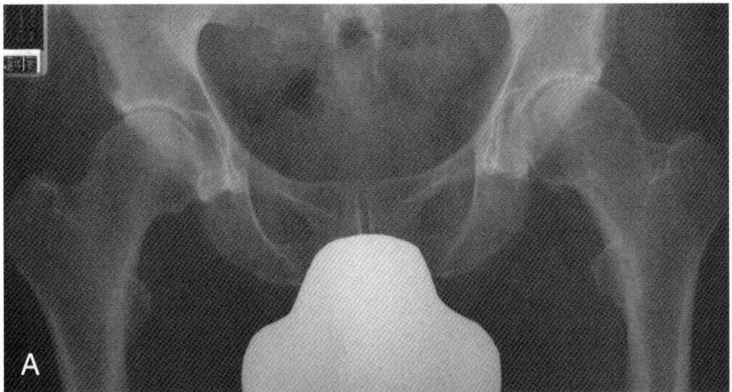

Figure 18-2 A, Anteroposterior radiograph of a 53-year-old man with primary osteoarthritis of the left hip. **B,** Anteroposterior and Johnson lateral views 4 years after surgery. The components are well positioned, with no sign of impingement. There is no heterotopic bone formation, yet the patient's University of California-Los Angeles scores are 7 for pain, 8 for walking and function, and 6 for activity.

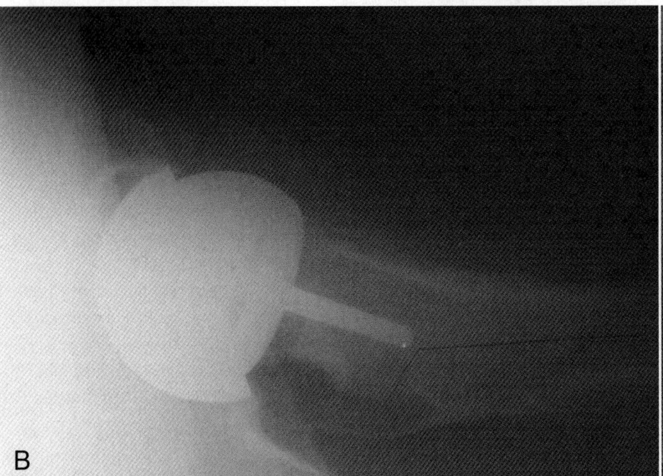

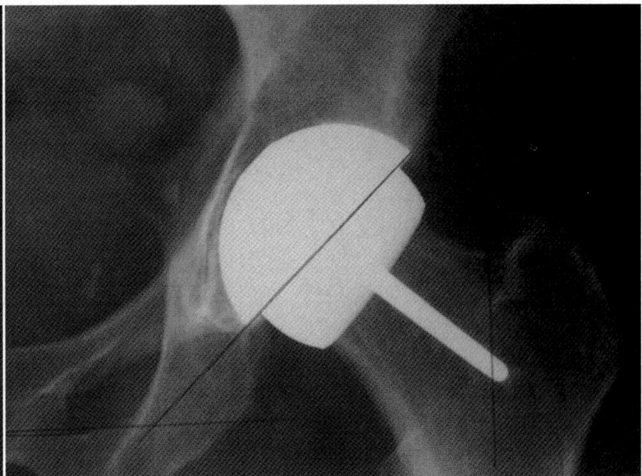

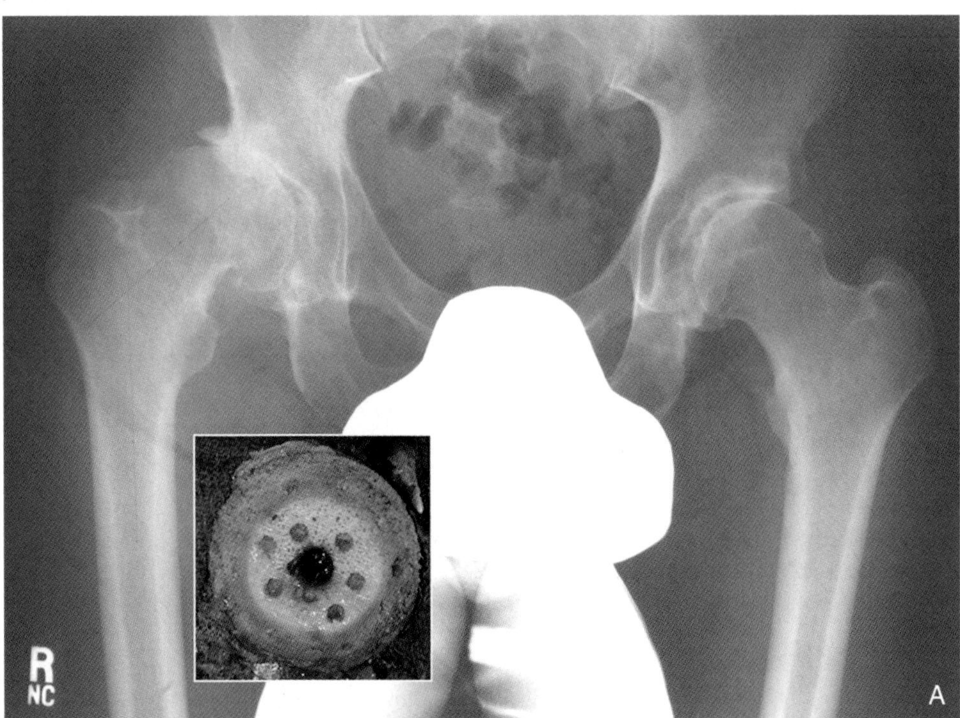

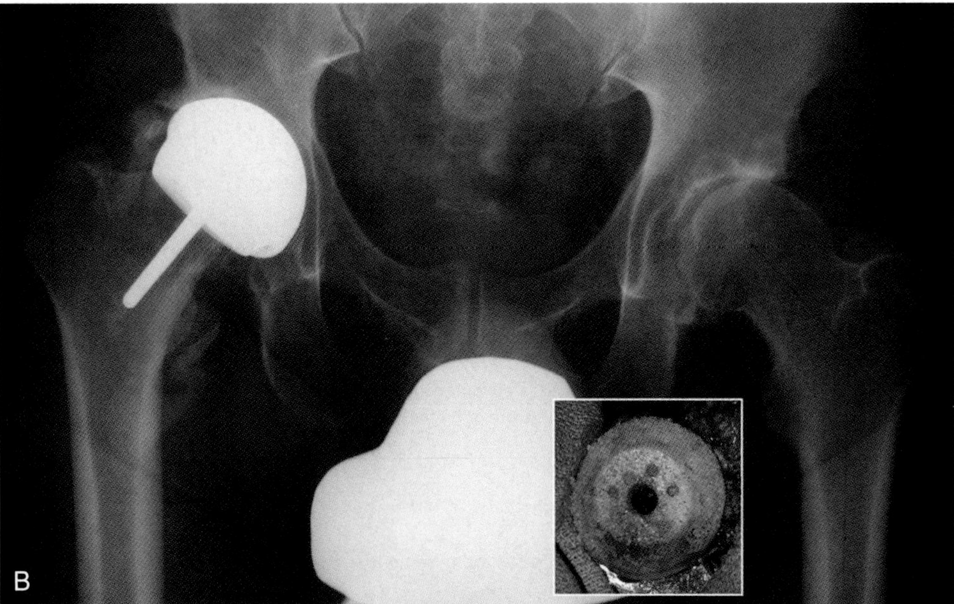

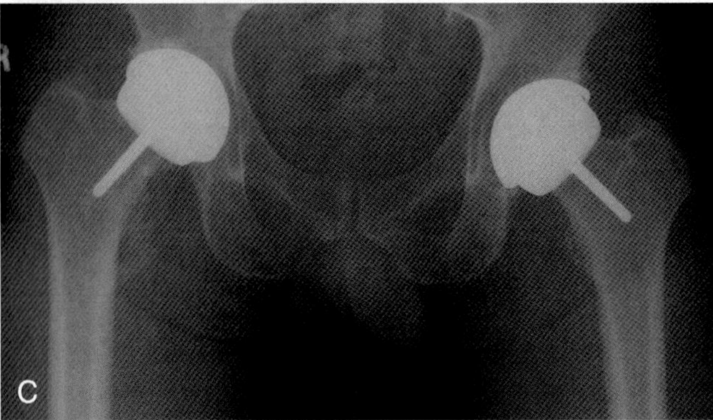

Figure 18-3 **A,** Anteroposterior radiograph of a 43-year-old man with bilateral primary osteoarthritis of the hips. The degenerative changes are much more pronounced on the right side, which was resurfaced first in a two-stage bilateral procedure. The insert shows the femoral head after reaming and good bone quality. **B,** Eight months after the first surgery, heterotopic ossification Brooker grade 3 has developed around the operated hip and the patient has become symptomatic on the left side with a marked thinning of the joint space. **C,** The resurfacing of the left hip was accompanied with a removal of heterotopic bone on the right side and radiation therapy in addition to the usual indomethacin (Indocin) prophylaxis. The patient has now been followed for 4.5 years after surgery on the right side and has resumed all his previous physical activities (including cycling and windsurfing) with University of California-Los Angeles hip scores of 10 for all categories on both sides.

though different and poorly localized pain, but was able to workout twice a week in the gym. He also had low back pain and underwent spine surgery 3 years postoperatively with apparently disc removal and nerve foraminotomy with some relief of radicular pain. However the hip pain continued, and he underwent exploratory surgery and removal of scar tissue at another hospital. The prosthesis was well fixed, with no definite cause for the patient's pain. The patient has now excellent painless full range of motion. His SF-12 scores worsened from a preoperative physical score of 41 and mental score of 49 to 4-year postoperative scores of 36 and 39, respectively, despite an absence of physical or radiologic explanation. At 7 years postoperatively, he has been only partially relieved by acupuncture and pain management with a variety of medications.

This case underscores the importance of first establishing a diagnosis to explain the source of the pain. Without a sound, accurate diagnosis, treatment, particularly surgical treatment, will frequently fail. An MMPI would have been useful.

The Treatment of Poorly Performing Hip Resurfacing

Trochanteric bursitis can generally be managed by anti-inflammatory agents supplemented with local injection of anesthetic and 1 or 2 mL of steroids. If hardware is present such as pins or wires used for prior trochanteric reattachment and the pain was relieved by injection only to return again, then removal of the hardware may be beneficial.

Iliopsoas bursitis has been reported with the BHR. The cause may be irritation locally due to the close proximity of the tendon to the acetabular component, which is more likely to occur if there is insufficient anteversion. Treatment consists of injection with local anesthesia and local steroids. Some have reportedly been relieved by iliopsoas tendon release. We have yet to make a definitive diagnosis of iliopsoas bursitis in our patients using the Conserve®Plus. Our surgical technique ensures that the low-profile socket is inserted well below the anterior wall of the pubis.

Heterotopic Bone

The incidence of significant heterotopic ossification (HO) restricting motion has been low and, due to technique changes, has not been a problem in the past 6 years. However, HO has been excised in three hips from the beginning of the series. A 44-year-old avid cyclist developed right osteoarthritis, and despite significant limitation of range of motion (90° flexion, 10° abduction-adduction arc, and 10° of rotation arc), he was still able to ride 4500 miles a year and snowboard, but this became impossible when the external rotation contracture increased (Fig. 18-3). The patient was resurfaced and indomethacin (Indocin) prophylaxis was given. Although pain was relieved and abduction-adduction improved to 40 degrees and rotation arc without contracture to 30 degrees, flexion was still limited to 90 degrees with a 25 degree flexion contracture due to grade III HO with a bridge anteriorly. Bike riding was more difficult, and his left hip became painful. He underwent contralateral hip resurfacing and excision of HO, and now has bilateral flexion of 135 degrees, 75 degrees of abduction-adduction arc, and 95 degrees of rotation arc. His pain, walking, function and, activity scores are all 10.

Summary

Assessment of the patient who has a failed or poorly functioning hip resurfacing is based on the history, physical examination, and pertinent radiographic and laboratory data. This may provide immediate answers, but often the cause for pain is unclear and further assessments may be required, including psychological tests. As shown by some of the case examples cited here, sometimes the true answer is elusive. Fortunately, in most cases, revision surgery provides relief, and can take advantage of newer, improved hip replacement technology.

CHAPTER 19

Treatment of Failed Hip Resurfacing

Harlan C. Amstutz

Scott T. Ball

Introduction

Currently, hip resurfacing is becoming popular in younger, active patients primarily due to perceived limitations of total hip replacement (THR). Historically, THRs have had a higher early failure rate in this population. Most practicing joint replacement surgeons have been faced with difficult total hip revisions for aseptic loosening. Although reconstruction of a failed THR can be successfully done with modern modular revision implants, it is nonetheless challenging surgery. For the patient, total hip revision surgery has increased morbidity and frequently diminished functional outcomes. Furthermore, bone loss can become extensive, and girdlestone resection arthroplasties are still occasionally necessary. Last, THRs are costly and have become a significant financial burden for the patient and the health care system.

The challenges of total hip revisions underscore the increasing interest in hip resurfacing for many orthopaedic surgeons and patients. Conversion of a failed hip resurfacing, particularly an isolated femoral side failure, is a very straightforward procedure. However, there are a few technical points that are specific to this procedure and are presented in the current chapter, along with our experience and the clinical outcomes to date of patients converted to a total hip for failed resurfacing.

Causes of Failure

Deep Infection

As with THR, infections may occur in a small percentage of patients. The type of treatment should be based on duration of infection (acute versus chronic), type of organism, and health of the host (patient). Patients with diabetes, obesity, malnutrition, or compromised immune status should be treated aggressively and most commonly will require resection of implants and delayed reimplantation of a total hip when the infection is cleared. Some organisms such as gram-negative bacteria are notoriously difficult to eradicate because they form a glycocalix (slime layer) on the implants, which even a scrub brush cannot entirely remove. This slime layer prevents antibiotic penetration and frequently results in recurrent infection. Consultation with an infectious disease expert is recommended.

Duration of infection is the last important determinant of treatment and can be broken down into acute postoperative (typically considered within 4 weeks of surgery), acute hematogenous (late infection that presents acutely) and subacute/chronic (more than 1 month after surgery or after onset of symptoms). With an acute infection (whether postoperative or acute hematogenous), débridement with retention of implants is recommended. For subacute and chronic infections, the components should be removed with interval placement of an antibiotic spacer and then delayed reimplantation when the infection is cleared.

In our series of more than 1150 total hip resurfacings, we have had six infections to date. One was an acute superficial postoperative infection, which was treated successfully with open débridement and systemic antibiotics. We have had three cases of acute-onset hematogenous deep sepsis, which were treated successfully with thorough débridement, retention of implants, and a prolonged course of organism specific intravenous antibiotics. These débridements were carried out 3, 5, and 30 days from onset of first symptoms.

A fifth patient presented with an insidious onset of symptoms approximately 6 months after surgery. He was afebrile but noticed mild swelling and noted that his hip was not performing as well as the other hip, which had also been resurfaced. It was presumed to be trochanteric bursitis, but a few months later, the symptoms had worsened and an aspiration demonstrated purulent material. Open débridement with retention of implants was attempted but failed. The patient was then definitively treated with resection of implants, a prolonged course of intravenous antibiotics and delayed reimplantation of a total hip. His cultures grew out Actinomyces, a spore-forming organism that is notoriously difficult to eradicate.

A sixth patient with rheumatoid arthritis presented 36 months after surgery with hematogenous sepsis from Streptococcus. The diagnosis and treatment was delayed by more than 1 month. At the time of surgery, a membrane was present under the femoral component, and therefore, retention of implants was not possible. She was treated with resection of implants, a thorough débridement, and direct exchange to a THR (see Fig. 16-3).

Isolated Femoral Side Failure

The most common mechanisms of failure of hip resurfacings are femoral neck fracture and femoral component aseptic loosening. In either case, these should be treated with a conversion to a total hip arthroplasty with a stemmed implant. Many patients ask if their failed resurfacing can be treated with a second resurfacing if the mode of failure is femoral loosening. Based on our prior experience, the unequivocal answer to this is no, because the quality of the remaining bone after a loosening failure is certainly going to be worse than at the time of resurfacing, and would therefore be likely predisposed to another failure.

With an isolated femoral side failure, retention of the acetabular component is the procedure of choice if the component is optimally positioned and rigidly fixed. Avoiding acetabular component removal will shorten the surgical time, bone and blood loss, and cost of treatment. However, retaining the acetabular component necessitates using a large femoral head made by the same manufacturer that matches the inner diameter of the existing shell. The previous operative report and implant record should be checked for implant sizing. Conversion options should be considered when a surgeon is selecting the initial resurfacing implant. The resurfacing surgeon should choose the preferred resurfacing device first based on their confidence in the given device, and second, based on whether or not the manufacturer has an optimal stemmed implant available with a large femoral head to match the monoblock resurfacing acetabular component in the event that the femoral side of the resurfacing fails.

At the time of conversion surgery, the hip should be approached through the surgeon's preferred approach. We prefer the posterior approach. As with any revision surgery, care should be taken with the electrocautery during the approach through scar tissue to avoid the sciatic nerve. In patients with a femoral neck fracture, the femoral head can be easily extracted. After the component is extracted, the remaining neck should be recut with an oscillating saw at a level determined by preoperative templating. In our experience, neck fractures have always been high enough that any primary total hip stem could be used (Fig. 19-1).

With femoral aseptic loosening or subsidence, the femoral component usually can be removed easily from the remaining bone. If not, the neck can be osteotomized with an oscillating saw at a level determined by preoperative planning and templating. The saw may encounter the metaphyseal stem of the component. The cut can be completed along the inferior/medial aspect of the neck with the saw. Then a half-inch osteotome or a narrow saw blade can be used to osteotomize around the metaphyseal stem and complete the neck cut on the lateral/superior side of the neck. The interval between the metaphyseal stem and the greater trochanter is relatively narrow, and care should be taken when osteotomizing this interval to protect against inadvertent damage to the greater trochanter.

After the femoral component has been removed and the neck cut has been made, the femur is prepared similar to a primary THR. The choice of implant is made according to the surgeon's preference (Fig. 19-2).

In all cases, the acetabular component should be inspected for damage. With metal-on-metal bearings, minor scratches can be accepted because these typically will polish out. If there is significant damage to the socket (which has not been seen in our experience), or if the component position exhibits more than 55 degrees of abduction angle, the socket should be removed.

Aseptic Loosening of the Acetabular Component

Just as with THRs, occasionally an acetabular component can loosen (typically a failure of initial ingrowth as opposed to late aseptic loosening). Patients frequently believe that a hip resurfacing offers a superior clinical result and may request that their femoral component be retained if they are undergoing revision for a loose shell. This is feasible but the revision is more challenging because the retained femoral head with the component in situ has a greater diameter than at the initial surgery and a larger pocket must be created to place it out of the way for acetabular preparation. The abductor muscles need to be stripped somewhat from the lateral wall of the pelvis much in the same way as when a primary resurfacing is performed. The surgeon's decision to attempt to retain the head during acetabular revision should be based on sound knowledge of pre-existing bone stock and bone preparation techniques. These patients should be counseled that revision to a THR with a stemmed femoral component may be desirable or necessary if a press-fit cup with an inner diameter matching the existing head cannot be stably implanted. If the femoral component is removed with a standard femoral neck osteotomy, exposure of the acetabulum is relatively easy and safe. If the femoral head is retained, its outside diameter must match the inside diameter of the new acetabular component.

In the event that both components are removed at the time of revision for a loose socket, a standard primary femoral stem is chosen according to the surgeon's preference, similar to a conversion of the femoral side only. A wider variety of options are available for the acetabular reconstruction and the implant can be chosen based on the size, shape and location of existing defects. In our series, three Conserve®Plus acetabular components required revision (despite being well fixed) because these conversions to THR occurred before the availability of the matching Big Femoral Head (BFH, Wright Medical Technology, Arlington, TN). There was not any significant acetabular bone loss in this process (average 3 mm) and a hemispherical component of slightly larger diameter was implanted. Should there be a loss of the anterior or pos-

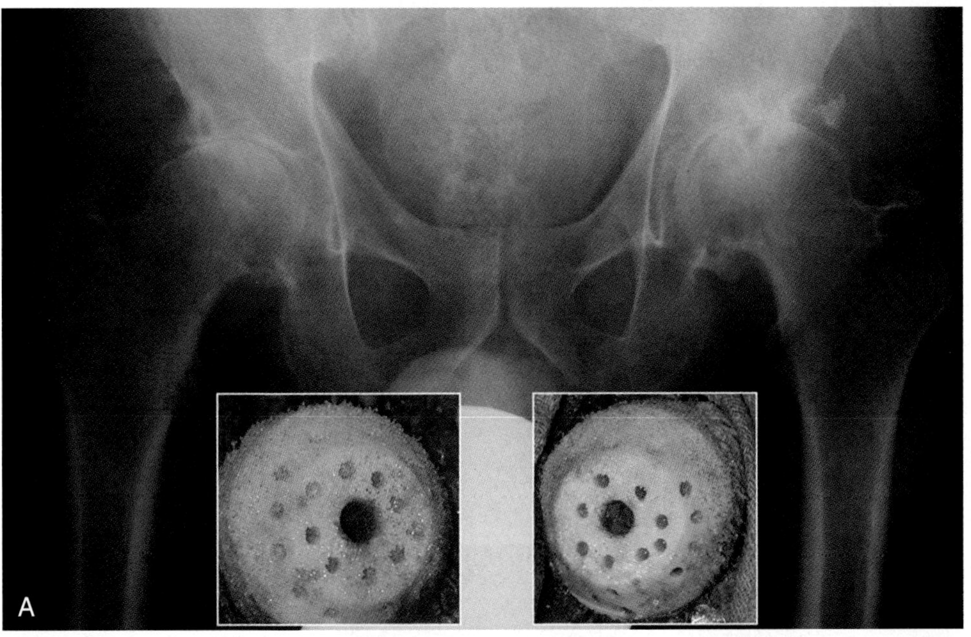

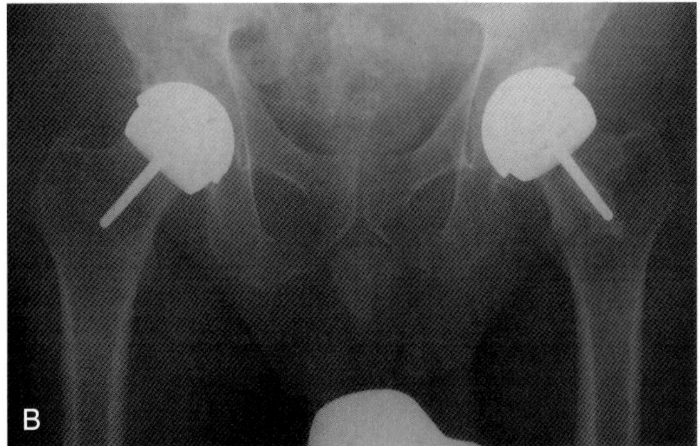

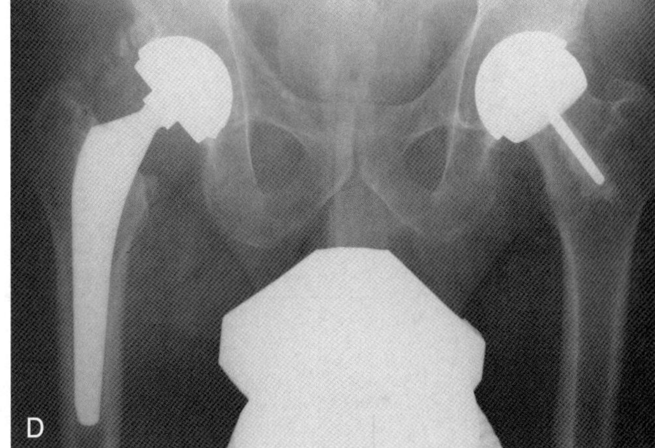

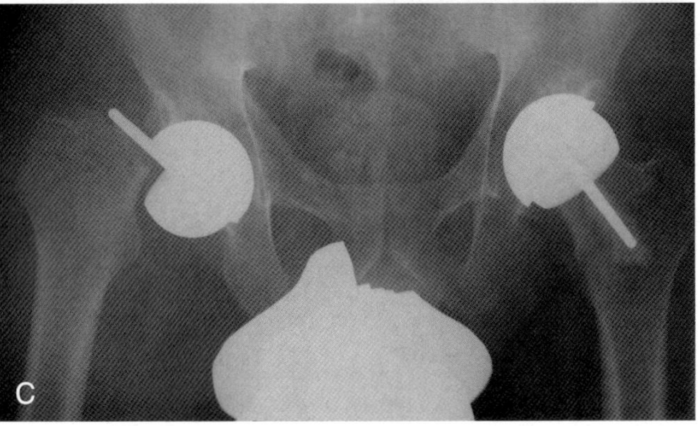

Figure 19-1 **A,** Anteroposterior pelvic radiograph of a 49-year-old man with bilateral primary osteoarthritis. The inserts show the excellent bone quality of the femoral heads after second-generation preparation. **B,** Anteroposterior pelvis radiograph taken 1 month after bilateral one-stage resurfacings: The right femoral head was reamed for a tight fit of the femoral component (<0.5-mm cement mantle performed to evaluate this type of bone preparation and cementing technique [see Chapters 7 and 9]). The left side had the metaphyseal stem cemented in whereas the stem was press-fit on the right side as part of our study to evaluate efficacy of stem cementation. **C,** Anteroposterior pelvis 2 months postoperatively; the right femoral neck fractured. **D,** The patient is shown 2 years after surgery; the right femoral component was converted to a standard grit-blasted anthropometric total hip (ATH) and a 50-mm Big Femoral Head articulating with the well-fixed acetabular component (56) that was retained at revision surgery. Clinical result is excellent, with comparable ROM, offset and equal leg lengths.

terior wall so that initial stability cannot be attained with the press-fit alone, then supplemental screw fixation should be used.

There are implants from some manufacturers that may address the problem. Wright Medical's Conserve®Plus hip line of implants (see Chapter 7) have several options to deal with the retained femoral component and isolated acetabular revision. The thick shell is 4 mm larger than the thin 3.5 mm shell, which allows upsizing of the acetabular component to obtain a new press-fit while retaining the same size femoral component. The Quadra-Fix socket has a superior phalange with the ability to add 1 to 3 machine screws to improve initial stability of fixation. The wall thickness is 4 mm. The Super-Fix socket is eccentric with 10 mm thickness superiorly and has a 14.5-

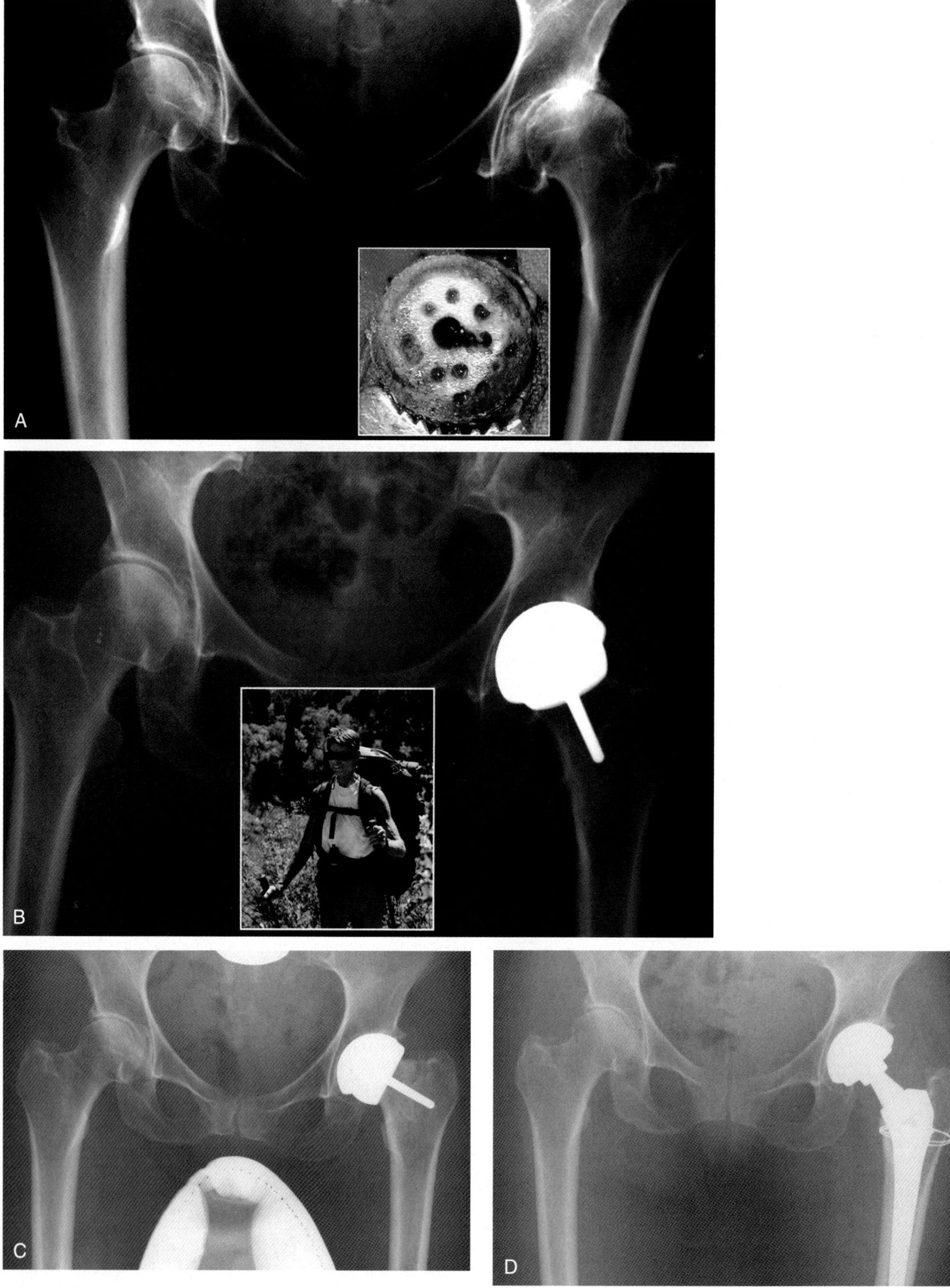

Figure 19-2 **A,** Anteroposterior pelvic radiograph of a 51-year-old fitness instructor with osteoarthritis of the left hip. There was possible mild dysplasia before the onset of large osteophytes in the floor of the acetabulum. Insert shows the femoral head before cementation of the femoral component (first-generation technique). **B,** Anteroposterior pelvis radiograph 1 year after resurfacing. The patient had returned to her occupation and extremely active lifestyle including spinning classes and mogul skiing. She is shown here backpacking in the Rocky Mountains (*insert*). **C,** Four years after surgery, the femoral component is loose and has tipped into varus. **D,** Revision surgery was performed. The well-fixed acetabular component was left in situ and matched with a 40-mm unipolar head and a profemur Z (Wright Medical Technology, Inc, Arlington, TN) femoral component. A short proximal fracture occurred on seating the component, which healed without incident after cerclage. Now 4 years post conversion to THR, her activity level is 8 on the University of California-Los Angeles scale.

mm difference between inner and outer diameter and is primarily used for more extensive bone loss and/or leg-length discrepancy. The eccentric superior portion of this socket allows placement of up to three cancellous screws for adjuvant fixation. We have not used the Super-Fix cup in treatment of failed resurfacings because other less invasive techniques were all that was necessary. However, they have been useful in three primary resurfacings with a combination of bone loss and leg-length discrepancy and in three primary THRs (BFH). The inferior fins on this cup provide excellent initial stability and supplemental screw fixation has not been necessary in any of these cases.

As with all revision surgery, preoperative planning is of paramount importance. The previous operative reports should be reviewed and the existing component size must be known. The manufacturers' representative should be notified well in advance so that all potential options can be available. Last, patients should be counseled that total revision may be necessary and a back-up system with a stemmed femoral component should be available in all cases.

Removal of an Ingrown Acetabular Component

Should an ingrown acetabular component need to be removed, curved sharp osteotomes should be used that match the outer radius of the socket to minimize bone removal. We recommend using available systems that use curved osteotomes of defined radius corresponding to the outer diameter of the shell (e.g., Explant by Zimmer, Universal Hip Cup Removal System by Innomed). These osteotomes are centered by placing a trial liner or impactor into the component. The device holds the center of this defined radius so that the osteotomes can be passed safely and precisely behind the socket, minimizing bone loss.

Results of Conversion to a Total Hip Replacement

The results of our conversions of a hip resurfacing to a total hip arthroplasty for femoral side failures was published in 2007.[1] The group of conversion patients were compared with an age-matched cohort of patients who underwent a stemmed primary total hip arthroplasty during the same period of time, to test the hypothesis that conversion of a failed hip resurfacing is similar to a primary total hip arthroplasty in terms of operative time, blood loss, complication rate, and clinical outcomes.

Twenty-one failed modern generation hip resurfacings (Conserve®Plus) in 20 patients with an average age of 50.2 years (23-72 years) were converted to a THR. In 18 hips, the acetabular component was retained and the femoral head diameter was maintained with a BFH. Three stable cups were removed because the conversion surgery predated the availability of the BFH. The control group consisted of 58 patients (64 hips) who underwent a primary THR, implanted during the same time period by the senior author. The average age of this control group was 50.8 years (range, 27-64 years).

There was no significant difference in operative time, blood loss, and complication rates between the conversions and the controls. The average follow-up was 46 months (range, 12-113 months) for the conversions and 57 months (24-105 months) for the controls. Clinical outcomes measures were comparable with average Harris Hip Scores of 92.2 and 90.3 for the hip resurfacing conversions and primary THRs, respectively. The UCLA activity scores were 6.8 and 6.4 in the conversion group and THR group, respectively. There have been no cases of aseptic loosening of the femoral or acetabular components in either group. The radiographic results were similar as well with no significant difference in the biomechanics of the reconstruction in terms of hip center, offset, stem position, and leg lengths. There have been no dislocations after conversion of a hip resurfacing. There was one minor femoral fracture, which occurred on stem insertion, was cerclaged, and healed without incident (Fig. 19-2D). Several other examples of failed hip resurfacings converted to a THR have been described throughout the various chapters of this book, such as Chapter 9 (Fig. 9-3), Chapter 12 (Figs. 12-6 and 12-7), Chapter 13 (Fig. 13-10), Chapter 14 (Fig. 14-9), Chapter 15 (Fig. 15-7), Chapter 16 (Fig. 16-3).

Of note, subsequent to publishing this study, one patient in the conversion group sustained a fracture of her femoral stem 40 months after conversion to the total hip and 70 months after her original hip resurfacing procedure performed at age 50. The patient played competitive singles tennis on a daily basis after both her resurfacing and conversion. The stem was the smallest size available but was a titanium alloy, double wedge–tapered stem which was grit-blasted. It was osseointegrated distally and fractured in the proximal one fourth. The stem was revised outside, but it is unlikely that the failed hip resurfacing was a factor because the proximal bone quality was excellent at conversion. It is possible that the rapid return to competitive tennis coupled with her small intramedullary canal and stem size were determining factors for the failure of the stem because no previous fractures have occurred with this stem design.

Discussion

The theoretical advantage of easy revisability of a resurfacing arthroplasty is strongly supported by the results we have seen in our patients. The surgery is similar to a primary THR in terms of operative time and blood loss. The reconstruction of the hip after conversion is similar to the primary THR in terms of position of the center of rotation, femoral offset, stem position and leg-length equality because primary femoral components can be used. Initial stability and fixation are reproducibly attainable because the intramedullary canal is virgin.

At an average follow-up of approximately 3.5 years in our study, all conversion patients reported good or excellent outcomes as measured by the Harris Hip score and Short Form-

12 (SF-12) scores. Furthermore, these patients have maintained a high level of activity with an average UCLA activity score of 6.8, and 10 of the 20 patients continuing to participate in sports regularly.

Historically, the most common complication of other types of conversion hip surgery and of revision total hip arthroplasty has been dislocation. Following conversion of a standard hemiarthroplasty to a total hip, dislocation has been reported in approximately 10% of patients,[2] and it has been reported in 2% of patients undergoing total hip arthroplasty after previous peri-acetabular osteotomy.[3] In a recent large series, the dislocation rate following revision THR was 7% to 11%.[4] In contrast, in our series of conversions of failed femoral components from resurfacing arthroplasty, there have been no dislocations and no infections. In our conversion hip patients, the absence of postoperative instability is likely related to the large femoral head size (average 43.5 mm). The increased stability of large femoral heads in the revision setting has been clearly established by a number of previous studies.[5-8]

Following resurfacing arthroplasty, normal stresses and bone density are maintained in the proximal femur.[9] For this reason, conversion to a total hip is similar to doing a primary total hip and femoral osseointegration generally occurs with a stemmed prosthesis. In contrast, femoral-side revision of failed conventional THA can be technically demanding and the results are less predictable with increased rates of dislocation, and septic and aseptic loosening.[10-13]

With the current generation of resurfacing implants, the metal acetabular shell is thin and therefore, minimal acetabular bone is removed at the time of the index procedure, similar to a traditional THA. The fixation of this porous-coated acetabular component has performed as well as similar porous coated components used for decades in THA.[14] Furthermore, osteolysis is rare with metal-on-metal bearings and has not been an issue in our patients. To maintain the conservative paradigm of the index procedure, it is preferable to retain the acetabular shell at the time of conversion of a failed femoral component, if possible.

Summary

In conclusion, resurfacing arthroplasty of the hip has been considered a conservative alternative to THR because it preserves femoral bone, which facilitates a safe and relatively easy conversion to THR in the event of a failure. Our experience supports this premise. Conversion of an isolated femoral failure is similar to a primary total hip in terms of surgical effort, blood loss, complication rate, and postoperative clinical outcomes. Furthermore, a total revision should also be more straightforward, again because removal of the femoral side is simply performed through the same type of femoral neck osteotomy as a primary total hip. Removal of the acetabular component can be done efficiently and safely with today's curved osteotomes. Because of the absence of osteolysis, we have not seen major acetabular bone loss issues in any of our Conserve®Plus patients. However, bone loss associated with other types of prosthesis have been observed. The exceptions are possibly cases of metal hypersensitivity in which bone loss may be encountered on cases of metallosis associated with a high vertical angle of socket implantation. Even deep infections, which can be disastrous with total hips, seem to be more straightforward to handle since the femoral canal is not violated with a hip resurfacing.

References

1. Ball ST, Le Duff MJ, Amstutz HC: Early results of conversion of a failed femoral component in hip resurfacing arthroplasty. J Bone Joint Surg Am 2007;89:735-741.
2. Sierra RJ, Cabanela ME: Conversion of failed hip hemiarthroplasties after femoral neck fractures. Clin Orthop Relat Res 2002;399:129-139.
3. Parvizi J, Burmeister H, Ganz R: Previous Bernese periacetabular osteotomy does not compromise the results of total hip arthroplasty. Clin Orthop Relat Res 2004;423:118-122.
4. Alberton GM, High WA, Morrey BF: Dislocation after revision total hip arthroplasty: an analysis of risk factors and treatment options. J Bone Joint Surg Am 2002;84:1788-1797.
5. Smith TM, Berend KR, Lombardi AV Jr, Emerson RH Jr, Mallory TH: Metal-on-metal total hip arthroplasty with large heads may prevent early dislocation. Clin Orthop Relat Res 2005;441: 137-142.
6. Amstutz HC, Le Duff MJ, Beaulé PE: Prevention and treatment of dislocation after total hip replacement using large diameter balls. Clin Orthop Relat Res 2004;429:108-116.
7. Berry DJ, von Knoch M, Schleck CD, Harmsen WS: Effect of femoral head diameter and operative approach on risk of dislocation after primary total hip arthroplasty. J Bone Joint Surg Am 2005;87:2456-2463.
8. Cuckler J, Moore K, Lombardi AJ, McPherson E, Emerson R: Large versus small femoral heads in metal-on-metal total hip arthroplasty. J Arthroplasty 2004;19(suppl 3):41-44.
9. Harty J, Devitt B, Harty L, Molloy M, McGuinness A: Dual energy X-ray absorptiometry analysis of peri-prosthetic stress shielding in the Birmingham resurfacing hip replacement. Arch Orthop Trauma Surg 2005;125:693-695.
10. Engh CA Jr, Ellis TJ, Koralewicz LM, McAuley JP, Engh CA Sr: Extensively porous-coated femoral revision for severe femoral bone loss: minimum 10-year follow-up. J Arthroplasty 2002;17: 955-960.
11. Moreland JR, Moreno MA: Cementless femoral revision arthroplasty of the hip: minimum 5 years followup. Clin Orthop Relat Res 2001;393:194-201.
12. Weeden S, Paprosky WL: Minimal 11-year follow-up of extensively porous-coated stems in femoral revision total hip arthroplasty. J Arthroplasty 2002;17(suppl 1):134-137.
13. Lawrence JM, Engh CA, Macalino GE, Lauro GR: Outcome of revision hip arthroplasty done without cement. J Bone Joint Surg Am 1994;76:965-973.
14. Engh CA, Griffin WL, Marx CL: Cementless acetabular components. J Bone Joint Surg Br 1990;72:53-59.

CHAPTER 20

Rehabilitation and Activity Following Total Hip Resurfacing

Thomas P. Schmalzried

Michel J. Le Duff

Introduction

The fundamental goal of orthopaedic rehabilitation is to assist the patient in achieving his or her functional goals. Consequently, rehabilitation is influenced by the wide range of patient aspirations, which may differ from their actual capabilities. The components of rehabilitation following total hip resurfacing include preoperative evaluation and counseling; preoperative exercises, when possible; a relatively structured in-patient program; and a relatively flexible outpatient program. Many patients are capable of resuming all of their prearthritic activities and function without any restrictions, including participation in impact sports. It will require decades of follow-up and survivorship analysis of large cohorts of patients in order to assess the advisability of any post-operative activity level.

Preoperative Evaluation and Counseling

The patient is the greatest source of variability, so the postoperative rehabilitation program should be flexible. In the preoperative patient evaluation, it is common to assess the patient's current level of function and activity, as is documented to a variable degree by a number of outcome instruments.[1-3] The parameters generally include walking distance, limp, stair climbing, sitting comfort, any difficulty with shoes and socks, and may also assess occupational and recreational functions (Chapter 6 and Fig. 20-1). A distinction can be made between their function (the highest degree of capability) and their activity (what the patient actually does on a regular basis). It is helpful to know what physical activities the patient performed before becoming limited by hip arthritis as well as what activities the patient would like to pursue after successful recovery from hip arthroplasty. The general health of the patient can be stratified by American Society of Anesthesiologists (ASA) class[4]:

ASA 1: Normal healthy patient

ASA 2: Patient with mild systemic disease with no functional limitations

ASA 3: Patient with moderate systemic disease with functional limitations

ASA 4: Patient with severe systemic disease that is a constant threat to life

ASA 5: Moribund patient who is not expected to survive another 24 hours with or without surgery

The physical examination can give insight into the general health and level of conditioning, which can be used to set patient expectations and guide rehabilitation. The body mass index (BMI, weight in kilograms divided by the square of height in meters; kg/m^2) defines individuals that are overweight (BMI >25) or obese (BMI >30) according to the generally accepted guidelines from the American Obesity Association. Overweight and obese patients should be encouraged to lose weight preoperatively. Lower BMI is associated with a lower risk of venous thromboembolism, infection and wound complications.[5,6] Patients often rationalize that they have gained weight because of limited activity imposed by their hip arthritis. Our experience indicates that this is unlikely as most patients continue to gain weight following successful joint replacement surgery.[7]

A Trendelenburg gait or the presence of the Trendelenburg sign is an indicator of abductor weakness. In general, the greater the preoperative weakness, the longer it will take the patient to gain the desired strength following surgery. Similar to knee arthroplasty, preoperative hip range of motion (ROM) is correlated to postoperative ROM.[8] The outcomes of total hip resurfacing are better with relatively early intervention, because this limits the degree of secondary changes from joint degeneration such as stiffness and muscle atrophy.[9] Obviously, disability of other lower extremity joints can affect rehabilitation and rehabilitation potential and stratification by Charnley

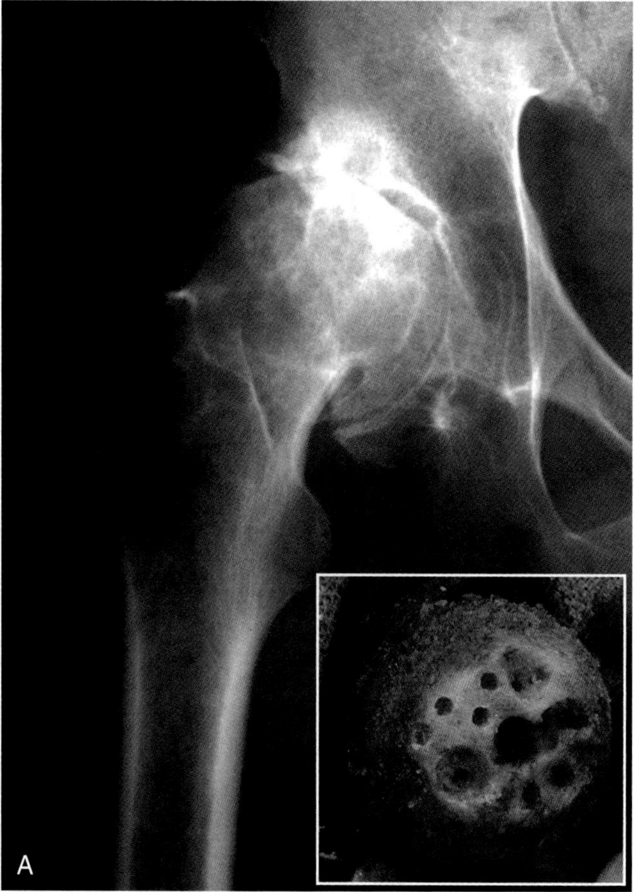

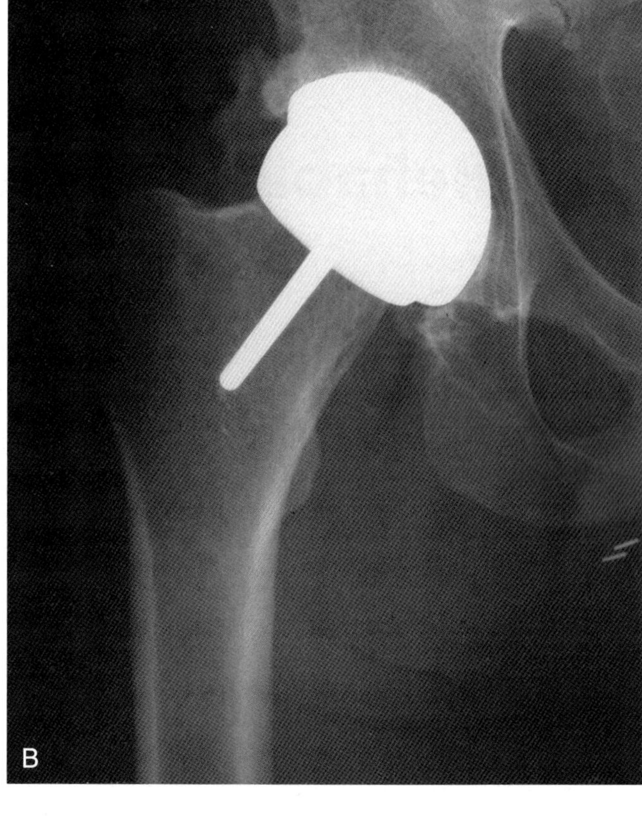

Figure 20-1 **A,** Pre-operative anteroposterior x-ray of a 44-year-old businessman with osteoarthritis of the right hip. The insert shows the femoral head with multiple defects before the application of cement. **B,** Eight years after surgery, the patient has been extremely active and resumed his usual physical activities with a frequency and intensity of participation unchanged from his prearthritic status. He developed a little heterotopic bone superiorly that does not affect his range of motion or hip scores in any way.

Class is useful (A = patients with involvement of only one hip; B = bilateral hip disability; C = disability of multiple joints or systemic illness).[10]

The information obtained in the preoperative assessment can be used to help set patient expectations and guide rehabilitation. Perhaps the strongest determinant of hospital length of stay (LOS) is the patient's expectation, and this can be set at the time of the initial evaluation. Healthy patients who are near their ideal body weight can generally be discharged the second day following total hip resurfacing (POD2). Other general guidelines include immediate encouragement of hip motion. Supervised outpatient physical therapy can begin the week following hospital discharge, given that the wound is healing satisfactorily. Progression to full-weight bearing occurs over the first month; however, a cane is preferred to a limp until recovery of strength, coordination and confidence allow a normal gait. Impact activities are uniformly discouraged during the first 3 postoperative months.

It is helpful to provide the patient with an overview of the hospitalization and the anticipated rehabilitation course for that patient, which may be more aggressive or more conservative depending on the general condition of the individual and their hip. A printed overview can help reinforce the message. The physician may comment on the patient's activity aspirations, especially if the physician believes those aspirations to be unreasonable or unattainable for that specific individual.

Preoperative preparation is limited by time and the painful hip joint. Weight loss, through judicious reduction in caloric mix and intake, should be pursued by overweight patients. Walking, cycling, swimming, and stretching of the hip and low back can be performed to tolerance. We do not generally prescribe supervised preoperative physical therapy for patients who have scheduled surgery. Once the decision to proceed with surgery has been made, the patient should consider the need for minor household modifications, such as a shower rail or chair. A tall, firm, chair with arms and an elevated toilet seat are helpful and these may be acquired pre-operatively.

Inpatient Rehabilitation

We have four general goals for rehabilitation following hip arthroplasty: (1) hip motion, (2) progressive weight bearing,

(3) usual activities of daily living, and (4) patient-specific activities including recreation and sports. The progress for the first three begins in the hospital as soon as practically possible. We favor regional anesthesia but the motor and sensory block may linger for the entire day of surgery. Because of this, the first physical therapy session is generally not scheduled until the morning after surgery. It is reasonable, however, for the inpatient physical therapist to visit the patient on the day of surgery, perform an assessment, and provide an educational overview of the in-patient program. We favor two supervised therapy sessions per day. Again, printed material can be helpful.

The patient can begin to actively flex the hip as soon as recovery from anesthesia allows. In this surgeon's experience, the risk of dislocation following total hip resurfacing is less than 1%, and none have occurred in the hospital. We do not use an abduction pillow or any other restraint on a regular basis. We encourage the patient to perform "heel slides" in bed as tolerated. Other bed exercises include gluteal and quad sets. Ankle dorsiflexion and plantar flexion can improve circulation and are encouraged on an hourly basis while the patient is awake. Healing occurs in two places: the patient's hip and in the patient's head. Encouraging early motion helps prevent stiffness and starts to build patient confidence in the new hip. We request that the therapist work with each patient to increase flexion to 120 degrees, abduction to 45 degrees, and external rotation to 45 degrees, as tolerated. This range of motion allows essentially all usual activities of daily living and hygiene, such as using the toilet, toenail and foot care. The author prefers a posterior approach with repair of the capsule and external rotation muscles. Because of this, we do not encourage adduction or internal rotation.

An important component of inpatient therapy is transfer training. This includes, lying to sitting, sitting to standing, and the reverse. Getting out of and into bed is initially a challenge for most patients. We request that the hospital bed be fitted with an overhead frame and a trapeze bar to assist with the early transfers. Such modifications are generally not available in the patient's home. For this reason, a discharge criterion is the ability to transfer into and out of bed with minimal assistance, which is generally limited to support of the operated leg.

We recommend that the patient sit in a chair as soon as medically possible. Lingering effects of anesthetics can cause orthostatic hypotension, which can limit sitting ability. We request that the patient sit in a relatively high chair as tolerated, starting with breakfast the first postoperative morning. The nursing staff should be trained in the bed-to-chair transfer, thus eliminating the need for a therapist for this activity. We recommend that patients be up in a chair for all meals. Flexion of the operated hip is allowed to 120 degrees (no need to limit further when seated). Reasonable hospital discharge criteria include a bed-to-chair transfer with minimal assistance and sitting tolerance of 1 hour.

The majority of femoral neck fractures occur within the first 6 weeks after surgery.[11,12] We favor partial weight bearing in the early postoperative phase to reduce the risk of femoral neck fracture. We recommend that weight bearing start at 50% and progress as tolerated to full over the following month. We are unaware of any randomized, prospective trial of immediate full weight bearing versus our progressive regimen. However, there is a physiologic "speed limit" for bone healing that is generally around 6 weeks and we prefer to be relatively conservative with regard to early weight bearing. Even if there is not violation of the cortex of the femoral neck (a so-called notch), the transition from reamed bone to unreamed bone is a stress riser. Healing is a process so graduated increases in hip loading are rational. The patient can transition to a single crutch or cane when they have sufficient strength and coordination to do so without limping. A reasonable hospital discharge criterion is the ability to ambulate with crutches for 100 feet. The patient also needs to be taught proper stair-climbing and descent technique and demonstrate sufficient proficiency to negotiate their home environment.

Outpatient Rehabilitation

All of the guidelines and exercises introduced in the hospital should continue as an outpatient with increases in exercise as tolerated. The primary goal of the sessions is education with the intent to discharge all patients to a home exercise program. At all times, the condition of the incision must be considered. If there is wound drainage of any character, it is recommended to limit physical activities until the drainage subsides. If the patient has access to a stationary bicycle, this can commence immediately. At this point in time, the goal is reciprocal motion, not strengthening: the resistance should be minimal and we recommend only about 5 to 10 minutes per day during the first 2 weeks. The incision must be completely healed before submersion of the wound in any way; bath tub, hot tub, whirlpool, swimming pool, etc. Subsequently, swimming and walking in chest-high water is a pleasant and effective adjunct to any rehabilitation program.

Supervised outpatient physical therapy 2 or 3 times per week helps direct recovery of motion, gait, coordination and strength during the first 6 weeks. In our experience, longer periods of supervised therapy are rarely needed. The therapist can guide and assist with range of motion exercises. In general, we do not limit the degree of flexion when combined with any abduction, nor do we limit abduction or external rotation. With a posterior approach and repair, we do not encourage internal rotation or abduction during the first 6 weeks. Range of motion can continue to improve for 12 months. The range of motion that is ultimately achieved is related to the preoperative range of motion. Hips that are stiff preoperatively will gain more motion than the hip that is flexible, but the flexible hips will still have more motion in the end.[8]

The therapist can directly assess the patient's gait and advise modifications as indicated, including additional loading of the operated hip and progression to a single crutch or cane. Most patients are capable of independent gait within the first postoperative month. Active and active-assisted exercises to strengthen hip flexion and abduction can be increased to tolerance. Again, preoperative strength and coordination will influence the return of active motion. Proprioceptive training exercises can commence immediately so long as the short-term load bearing limitations are respected.

Patients commonly inquire when they are allowed to drive a car. It should be recognized that the physician can assess only medical safety and not road safety. The patient must not be taking narcotic or sedative medication when driving. With left hip surgery, it is medically safe for most patients to drive a car with an automatic transmission as soon as they can get into and out of their vehicle, which is generally within 2 weeks of surgery. With right hip surgery, the patient must have sufficient strength and coordination to appropriately use the accelerator pedal and the brake pedal. It is medically safe for most patients to perform these functions within 4 weeks of surgery. We are unaware of scientific data to support any recommendation for the time to resume driving after hip arthroplasty. The patients drive at their own risk, regardless of the time frame.

Activity Following Total Hip Resurfacing

The last phase of rehabilitation is the return to or the pursuit of patient-specific activities including recreation and sports. The time frame for this phase of recovery is variable and essentially lifelong. We do not have any general activity restrictions for hip resurfacing patients but we do advise a "marathon mentality": for any new activity, start slow and progress as tolerated. A distinction should be made between capability and advisability of activity following hip arthroplasty. Experience of more than 10 years indicates that the current generation of hip arthroplasty technology is capable of running and other high-cycle-high-impact activities. However, it will require decades of follow-up and survivorship analysis of large cohorts of patients in order to assess the advisability of any postoperative activity level.

In a consecutive series (nonselected; all diagnoses) of 400 hips with metal-on-metal resurfacings, Amstutz et al[13] reported an average University of California-Los Angeles (UCLA) activity score of 7.7. Fifty-four percent of the patients had an activity score of 8, 9, or 10. In a series of patients with osteoarthritis, Daniel et al[14] reported UCLA scores of 8, 9 or 10 in 81% of the patients. In a comparison of concurrent total hip resurfacing and total hip replacement patients and outcomes, the average UCLA activity rating of the resurfacing patients was 8.2 whereas that of the total hips was 5.9. This difference in activity level is, at least in part, due to differences in the demographics of the two groups.[15] The activity level of a subset of total hip replacement patients with a large-diameter metal-on-metal bearing and demographics similar to that of the resurfacing group was 7.7.

The high average activity of the resurfacing patients is not due to any demonstrated increase in the functional capability of resurfacing compared to modern total hip arthroplasty. The difference is due to the aspirations and attitude of the resurfacing patient who chooses resurfacing with the intention of pursuing higher level activities and the knowledge that (in the event of failure) a total hip can be performed later (see Fig. 20-1). Again, it will require decades of follow-up and survivorship analysis of large cohorts of patients in order to assess the advisability of any postoperative activity level (for both resurfacing and total hip replacement).

What Types of Sporting Activities Do Our Patients Engage in?

Total hip arthroplasty (THA) was originally used with the primary goal to relieve pain and restore basic mobility for the patient. Encouraged by the success of the procedure, surgeons started implanting younger patients and the initial goals of hip arthroplasty shifted toward a more global restoration of the patient's original lifestyle. Wright et al[16] showed that, immediately after pain relief and walking function, returning to recreational activities was now the most important reason why patients undergo THA. These recreational activities, although diverse, often translate into sporting activities, especially for young patients for who sports constitute an important part of the overall physical activity.[17] The question of the effects of physical activity and sports in particular on the outcome of THA was raised in the early 1980s, and several studies have attempted to correlate a measurement of sporting activity with implant survivorship. Dubs et al[18] studied a cohort of 110 patients with average follow-up of 5.8 years (range, 1 to 14 years) and found that those with total hip replacements who did not participate in sports had a higher loosening rate than those who did. Ritter and Meding[19] found that participation in sports decreased after THA and did not affect significantly the outcome of THA. Kilgus et al[20] reviewed 1016 cases and separated active from nonactive patients based on their UCLA activity scores. They found that active patients were at greater risk of implant loosening than the less active ones, especially patients engaging in high impact (loosening risk times 2.3) versus low impact (loosening risk times 1.9) types of activities.

Such conflicting results suggest that variables other than the ones selected in these studies must be acting factors in the outcome of THA for active patients, and controlling for extraneous variables such as implant design, age of the patients or etiology seems necessary to establish valid comparisons or relationships. However what emerges as a possible explanation for the inconsistent results of the three previously mentioned studies is the methodology to assess patient participation in sports. Intuitively, it seems logical that the outcome of THA be affected by more than just what patients do after surgery but also by how much and how. To this date, the main failure mechanism for THA has been aseptic loosening due to polyethylene debris–induced periprosthetic osteolysis.[21-28] The relationship between a quantitative measure of patient activity and polyethylene wear has been established using devices able to record the number of hip cycles for a given amount of time.[29,30] This method of direct measurement of activity, although very accurate, is difficult to implement on a routine basis, in a clinical setting. In addition, when it comes to sporting activities, all hip cycles should not be considered having the same effect on the prosthesis: depending on the main mode of displacement associated with each activity, the magnitudes of the peak joint reaction forces can vary in great proportions.[31-33]

Thus, the study of hip resurfacing outcome in relationship to participation in sports would greatly benefit from a questionnaire integrating nature or type of activities engaged in by the patient, frequency of participation, duration of the sessions, and intensity of participation. Until longer survival data are gathered, the information collected can be used to describe the patterns of return to sporting activities of the resurfacing patient population.

Instrument

Data collection was performed using a survey available online as an encrypted document. The patients were given the possibility to report up to three sporting activities that they were participating in on a regular basis. For each sport mentioned (chosen out of an extensive list), the patient selected the frequency of participation and the duration of typical sessions (see Fig. 6-4). The intensity level was also recorded as patients were asked to indicate if they were participating competitively or for recreational purposes only. The patients also reported if they were beginners, intermediate, advanced, or expert for each activity selected. The survey was filled out at each clinical follow-up with a minimum of 1 year after surgery.

Subjects

The first 436 patients (500 hips) who received metal-on-metal surface arthoplasties (Conserve®Plus, Wright Medical Technology, Arlington, TN), were asked to fill out the sports activity survey at least 1 year after surgery and then yearly. The average age for the whole group was 48.6 years (range, 15 to 78 years), and men accounted for 74%. The average weight was 83.2 kg (range, 42 to 164 kg) and BMI 27.0 (range, 17.5 to 46.4). Initial etiologies included osteoarthritis (65%), developmental dysplasia of the hip (12%), osteonecrosis (8%), trauma (8%), and others (Legg-Calve-Perthes disease, slipped capital femoral epiphysis [SCFE], ankylosing spondylitis, rheumatoid disease, and melorheostosis, 7%). Overall, 7.2% of the cases had undergone previous surgeries. Sixty-four patients had bilateral metal-on-metal resurfacing arthroplasty (MMRA), and 16 patients had various types of hip arthroplasties on the contralateral hip.

Results

Three hundred and ninety-three patients filled out the survey, which represents 90% of the whole group. Popular activities patients engaged in were: walking/hiking (24% of the activities), cycling (14%), weight lifting (14%), swimming (9%), golf (10%), skiing (4%), tennis and yoga (each 3%). Other activities (19%) were numerous, each representing less than 3%.

Fifty-five percent of the patients listed three activities for regular participation. Patients engaged in activities more than twice a week 45% of the time and, in 40% of the activities, for more than 1 hour each time. Participation was mentioned as recreational 93% of the time versus 7% labeled competitive. Finally, the patients considered themselves experts 6% of the time, advanced 23%, intermediate 60%, and beginners 11% of the time.

Case Histories

The following case histories of very active patients treated with metal-on-metal resurfacing are illustrated with video footage available on the DVD provided with the present volume.

Patient # 1. Male; Date of Surgery: 6/1/99

Vice President of a technology company, he was 43 with very severe degenerative arthritis when he had his surgery. He had a bit of difficulty even with walking. He is a vigorous athlete who regularly engages in snowboarding, skiing, mountain biking, and tennis. Eight years after surgery, he is beginning to have symptoms from osteoarthritis on his contralateral hip, slightly limiting the frequency of his sporting activities. The patient's radiographic features are presented in Figure 20-1. His current pain, walking, function, and activity scores are 10, 9, 8 and 9, respectively.

Patient # 2. Male; Date of Surgery: 6/9/98

This patient is a 43-year-old ballet dancer and artistic director of a ballet company who developed osteoarthritis in both hips. He underwent bilateral metal-on-metal hip resurfacing in 1998. He returned to performing ballet within 10 months after a vigorous rehabilitation program and continued performing for more than 3 years. He now confines his activities to instructing and directing his ballet company, along with several hours of workouts daily. The patient's radiographic features are presented in Figure 12-5. His current pain, walking, function, and activity scores are 10, 10, 10, and 10, respectively.

Patient # 3. Female; Date of Surgery: 4/27/00

This patient is a 39-year-old martial arts instructor with a specialty in Tae Kwon-Do. She developed osteoarthritis possibly secondary to an injury incurred in an automobile accident. She was disabled for 2 years until she underwent hip resurfacing. She has resumed a very high level of activity including resuming her profession as a martial arts instructor. Her current pain, walking, function, and activity scores are 8, 10, 10, and 9, respectively.

Patient # 4. Male; Date of Surgery: 5/20/99

This patient is a 49-year-old machine shop owner who had progressive osteoarthritis for more than 7 years on both hips. The patient is a power lifter who had previously bench-pressed 500 pounds. The patient underwent simultaneous procedures on both hips 5 years ago. He has been doing extremely well and has returned to power lifting and can squat over 500 pounds again. He also plays golf regularly, jogs, and rides horses. His current pain, walking, function, and activity scores are 10, 10, 10 and 8, respectively.

Discussion

The overall results for the patient population studied show a very important participation in sports as postoperative mode of recreation. Only 5.8% of the patients who filled out the survey declared not engaging in any of the sporting activities suggested or other. If we consider that the patients who did not respond to the survey did not do any sports (which is most likely too conservative an assumption), there is still at least 84% of the patients who participate in sporting activities 1 year or more after surgery. This result correlates with those of Naal et al. in their descriptive report of patient sporting activity after hip resurfacing.[34]

Patients considered themselves beginners only 11% of the time, which indicates that they generally return after surgery to physical activities they already participated in instead of taking on new activities based on their new status. The predominance of activities like hiking and cycling suggests that patients elect primarily activities that provide cardiovascular benefits in the most controlled environment possible to avoid accidental trauma. These results are consistent with those of previous reports describing the nature of the sporting activities chosen by hip patients[19,35] after surgery but also the activities that are generally suggested or recommended by orthopaedic surgeons.[36,37]

References

1. Amstutz H, Thomas B, Jinnah R, Kim W, Grogan T, Yale C: Treatment of primary osteoarthritis of the hip. A comparison of total joint and surface replacement arthroplasty. J Bone Joint Surg 1984;66A:228-241.
2. Harris W: Traumatic arthritis of the hip after dislocation and acetabular fractures: treatment by mold arthroplasty. An end-result study using a new method of result evaluation. J Bone Joint Surg 1969;51A:737-755.
3. Ware J, Kosinski M, Keller S: A 12-Item Short-Form Health Survey: construction of scales and preliminary tests of reliability and validity. Med Care 1996;34:220-233.
4. Keats A: The ASA classification of physical status—a recapitulation. Anesthesiology 1978;49:233-236.
5. Mantilla C, Horlocker T, Schroeder D, Berry D, Brown D: Risk factors for clinically relevant pulmonary embolism and deep venous thrombosis in patients undergoing primary hip or knee arthroplasty. Anesthesiology 2003;99:552-560.
6. Guss D, Bhattacharyya T: Perioperative management of the obese orthopaedic patient. J Am Acad Orthop Surg 2006;14: 425-432.
7. Heisel C, Silva M, dela Rosa M, Schmalzried T: The effects of lower-extremity total joint replacement for arthritis on obesity. Orthopedics 2005;28:157-159.
8. dela Rosa M, Silva M, Heisel C, Reich M, Schmalzried T: Range of motion after total hip resurfacing. Orthopedics 2007;30: 352-357.
9. Schmalzried T, Silva M, de la Rosa M, Choi E, Fowble V: Optimizing patient selection and outcomes with total hip resurfacing. Clin Orthop Relat Res 2005;441:200-204.
10. Charnley J: Low Friction Arthroplasty of the Hip. New York: Springer-Verlag, 1979:
11. Cutts S, Datta A, Ayoub K, Rahman H, Lawrence T: Early failure modalities in hip resurfacing. Hip International 2005;15: 155-158.
12. Shimmin A, Back D: Femoral neck fractures following Birmingham hip resurfacing. J Bone Joint Surg Br 2005;87:463-464.
13. Amstutz H, Beaulé P, Dorey F, Le Duff M, Campbell P, Gruen T: Metal-on-metal hybrid surface arthroplasty: two to six year follow-up. J Bone Joint Surg 2004;86A:28-39.
14. Daniel J, Pynsent PB, McMinn D: Metal-on-metal resurfacing of the hip in patients under the age of 55 years with osteoarthritis. J Bone Joint Surg 2004;86B:177-188.
15. Schmalzried T, Fowble V, dela Rosa M: A comparison of total hip resurfacing and total hip replacement patients and outcomes. Clin Orthop Relat Res (in press).
16. Wright JG, Rudicel S, Feinstein AR: Ask patients what they want. Evaluation of individual complaints before total hip replacement. J Bone Joint Surg Br 1994;76:229-234.
17. Sequeira M, Rickenbach M, Wietlishbach V, Tullen B, Schutz Y: Physical activity assessment using a pedometer and its comparison with a questionnaire in a large population survey. Am J Epidemiol 1995;142:989-999.
18. Dubs L, Gschwend N, Munzinger U: Sport after total hip arthroplasty. Arch Orthop Trauma Surg 1983;101:161-169.
19. Ritter MA, Meding JB: Total hip arthroplasty. Can the patient play sports again? Orthopedics 1987;10:1447-1452.
20. Kilgus DJ, Dorey FJ, Finerman GA, Amstutz HC: Patient activity, sports participation, and impact loading on the durability of cemented total hip replacements. Clin Orthop Rel Res 1991;269:25-31.
21. Bauer TW, Schils J: The pathology of total joint arthroplasty.II. Mechanisms of implant failure. Skeletal Radiol 1999;28:483-497.
22. Cooper RA, McAllister CM, Borden LS, Bauer TW: Polyethylene debris-induced osteolysis and loosening in uncemented total hip arthroplasty. A cause of late failure. J Arthroplasty 1992;7:285-290.
23. Joshi AB, Markovic L, Ilchmann T: Polyethylene wear and calcar osteolysis. Am J Orthop 1999;28:45-48.
24. Manley MT, Serekian P: Wear debris. An environmental issue in total joint replacement. Clin Orthop Rel Res 1994;298:137-146.
25. Wroblewski BM: Osteolysis due to particle wear debris following total hip arthroplasty: the role of high-density polyethylene. Instr Course Lect 1994;43:289-294.
26. Willert HG, Bertram H, Buchhorn GH: Osteolysis in alloarthroplasty of the hip. The role of ultra-high molecular weight polyethylene wear particles. Clin Orthop Rel Res 1990;258:95-107.

27. Jacobs JJ, Shanbhag A, Glant TT, Black J, Galante JO: Wear debris in total joint replacements. J Am Acad Orthop Surg 1994;2: 212-220.
28. Sochart DH: Relationship of acetabular wear to osteolysis and loosening in total hip arthroplasty. Clin Orthop Rel Res 1999;135-150.
29. Feller J, Kay P, Hodgkinson J, Wroblewski B: Activity and socket wear in the Charnley low-friction arthroplasty. J Arthroplasty 1994;9:341-345.
30. Schmalzried TP, Shepherd EF, Dorey FJ, Jackson WO, dela Rosa M, Fa'vae F, McKellop HA, McClung CD, Martell J, Moreland JR, Amstutz HC: The John Charnley Award. Wear is a function of use, not time. Clin Orthop Rel Res 2000;381:36-46.
31. Van Den Bogert A, Read L, Nigg B: An analysis of hip joint loading during walking, running, and skiing. Med Sci Sports Exerc 1999;31:131-142.
32. Bergmann G, Graichen F, Rohlmann A: Hip joint loading during walking and running, measured in two patients. J Biomech 1993;26:969-990.
33. Bergmann G, Graichen F, Rohlmann A: Is staircase walking a risk for the fixation of hip implants? J Biomech 1995;28:535-553.
34. Naal F, Maffiuletti N, Munzinger U, Hersche O: Sports after hip resurfacing arthroplasty. Am J Sports Med 2007;[Epub ahead of print].
35. Margheritini F, Zeri A, Belli P, Giuliante A: Sport after total hip replacement. Hip International 1997;7:169-173.
36. McGrory BJ, Stuart MJ, Sim FH: Participation in sports after hip and knee arthroplasty: review of literature and survey of surgeon preferences. Mayo Clin Proc 1995;70:342-348.
37. Kuster M: Exercise recommendations after total joint replacement: a review of the current literature and proposal of scientifically based guidelines. Sports Med 2002;32:433-445.

CHAPTER 21

The Future of Hip Resurfacing

Harlan C. Amstutz

Where We Are Now?

One of the hottest topics today in orthopaedics is hip resurfacing. It is being performed all around the world, and in some centers, it has become the gold standard for the arthritic hip for the patient younger than 50 years of age. Results from the surgeon innovators and from controlled clinical trials are very good in patients with good bone quality. Patients are attracted to the minimally bone invasive concept of preserving the head and neck and avoiding an intramedullary stem. The procedure will be driven by patient demand, and the Internet will play an important role.

The versatility and durability of metal-on-metal, hybrid hip resurfacing devices far surpass the metal-on-polyethylene hip resurfacings of the 1970s and 1980s. Observing this marked improvement with my experience ranging from the THARIES to the Conserve®Plus over the years has been very gratifying. In particular, the durability of the Conserve®Plus socket has been excellent with no cases of loss of fixation or loosening. This porous bead technology for fixation has been very successful for 24 years with other socket systems.

On the femoral (other) side, however, I have found that the procedure is very technique dependent. The incidence of femoral loosening in patients with primary osteoarthritis and good bone quality has been rare, even from the beginning of implantation in 1996, and I have been surprised by the good results from hips with severe cystic defects (thanks to improved bone preparation and cementing techniques). The results of resurfacing in patients with high risk factors will need to be confirmed by others.

Because the surface area for femoral fixation is small compared with conventional stem-type devices, I have learned that meticulous attention to the preparation of the bone surfaces is critical and that optimizing fixation can likely mean years of increased durability. Efforts to improve fixation have continued each operating day, and as a result, patients with risk factors, such as cystic degeneration, can be successfully resurfaced. These techniques include a thorough cleaning of cysts, pulsatile lavage, and drying the bone with a Carbojet; and cementing the stem in select patients, as emphasized in Chapter 7. However, I continue to recommend that surgeons begin their surgical experience with patients with good bone quality and to refer patients with risk factors to more experienced resurfacing surgeons.

Although high-impact activities have not been associated with failure when the bone quality was ideal, very high activity levels have been found to reduce durability when there were deficiencies in bone stock with the early technique. Fortunately, with the newly devised techniques to improve femoral fixation, the durability of resurfacings in patients who have continued with high impact activities has been excellent, despite the presence of risk factors when they were operated upon. Results in those patients have been as good as less active patients, but further follow-up is needed to determine long-term efficacy. The progress in improved durability and the elimination of short-term failures may justify carefully applying the surface technology to older patients even though total hip arthroplasty, when using a big femoral head to obviate dislocation, is a very dependable alternative.

The results from the innovators of other resurfacing devices implanted in patients with good bone quality have also been very promising, although further detailed follow-up with complete radiographic analysis needs to be done. Carefully evaluated long-term results are critical, as with any procedure. The surgeons who perform large numbers of resurfacings find it challenging to do the necessary critical analysis simply because of the magnitude of the effort to do adequate follow-ups. In my experience, a minimum of one full-time person per 300 cases is needed to contact and remind the patients to come in for follow-up examinations, scan in the radiographs and enter the data for analysis. This effort, along with continued failure analysis, is essential in determining efficacy in order to refine designs and techniques. The reported results from surgeons and institutions with smaller case numbers and less experience are also important, particularly those with higher short-term failure rates.

Where Do We Go From Here?

With every major implant company and numerous smaller companies offering metal-on-metal hip resurfacing implants (at last count, 19 designs were available in Europe), the hip surgeon performing, or considering hip resurfacing faces a vast array of choices. Data to help sort between these devices are currently limited or unavailable. Evaluation of the various component designs (size, shape, and the length of the stem; socket profile and fixation surface), materials (as-cast, heat treated, forged and differential hardness), and techniques of implantation (with or without a cement mantle, various surgical approaches) all need the advantage of time to provide the information needed to sort out the optimal factors.

The materials now being employed to manufacture the prostheses are currently limited to cobalt chromium alloys, albeit with variations in metallurgy and tribologic factors: These variations should be evaluated as to both wear clinical performance with the advantage of additional decades. New, low-wear materials (for example, ceramics and ceramic coatings, diamond, and so on) will likely be tested. Are there other materials to be investigated? Will we use metal-backed improved cross-linked polyethylene versus metal or is the trade off of returning to thicker components just not appealing?

Long-term analysis of wear products and studies into the potential risks they pose will continue and will address the current concerns of the many critics of metal-on-metal prostheses. What are the consequences, or are they negligible compared with the advantages they bring? What is the significance of outliers? Will routine ion monitoring be important for this issue?

How can we prevent or at least understand hypersensitivity? Will preoperative laboratory testing become available? Clearly funded studies are required to answer such questions.

Technique and training are always evolving, and special attention should focus on improving the pin centering, perhaps even by the use of navigation. However, in my view, there will always be an art to resurfacing, which involves the surgeon preparing the femoral head to take the best advantage of the remaining bone. How thick should the cement mantle be . . . nil or .5 or 1 mm? What will be the role of cementless femoral components? Evaluation of the different surgical approaches needs to occur.

One other possible area of evolution of metal-on-metal resurfacing is the mode of fixation of the femoral component. This is a logical evolution based on the excellent durability of cementless total hip conventional stems and our previous experience with porous ingrowth femoral resurfacing components, despite the current success of using a cement grout which seems more favorable to resurfacing than to stem-type devices (because these generate much more severe stresses due to cantilever loading conditions). Currently, most major hip resurfacing manufacturers are developing a cementless, internally porous coated femoral shell.

One manufacturer (Corin Medical, Cirencester, UK – US distributed by Stryker, Inc.) already has some early experience with the cementless Cormet 2000 device but it is still too soon to evaluate the clinical performance of this prosthesis in comparison with the hybrid designs. A reported high rate of femoral neck narrowing with this device suggests that the success of this mode of fixation will rely on component design even more so than cemented components. The type of porous coating, the choice of surfaces to be porous coated, the length, shape and diameter of the metaphyseal stem will undoubtedly affect both initial fixation and bone-loading parameters. In addition, a very precise instrumentation should allow the surgeon to achieve a tight fit with full component seating and the preservation of blood supply to the femoral head might be a greater concern with this type of device to ensure osseointegration of the component. However, the main issue with this type of device will remain patient selection because patients with large femoral head defects may be at risk to start with a compromised initial fixation. Femoral bone grafting may be a suitable solution for these patients but will probably encounter some limitations with patients bound to resume high impact activities and who would benefit from the added interface area of a cemented metaphyseal stem.

Finally, educational tools and venues to teach and improve the surgeons' skills are paramount. Ultimately the success of the procedure will depend on eliminating short-term failures. Education focusing on indications and technique is therefore essential. Instruction should include workshops with plastic bones, cadavers, and observation of hip resurfacing done by experienced surgeons. Improved results also require eager and willing surgeons who will commit to a serious education program and who will not submit to external pressures to perform surgery before they are ready. Their first cases should be critiqued by an experienced surgeon. Continued follow-up and failure analysis will help us further understand the limitations of hip resurfacing and its applicability to all patients with hip arthritis.

I do believe the future of hip resurfacing is bright not only because of the recent successes but because there are now many bright young surgeons who have espoused the technique and will contribute new ideas and ways to improve the art and answer the questions raised. This interest is in stark contrast to the 1980s, when there was little interest or effort to improve resurfacing. The rebirth of the modern era of hip resurfacing has been particularly satisfying, building upon lessons learned and applying new technologies to achieve the goal of bone preservation.

Index

Note: Page numbers followed by f refer to figures; those followed by t refer to tables.

Q

R

S

T

U

V

W